# INFUSION CHEMOTHERAPY–IRRADIATION INTERACTIONS

## Principles and Applications to Organ Salvage and Prevention of Second Primary Neoplasms

# INFUSION CHEMOTHERAPY–IRRADIATION INTERACTIONS

## Principles and Applications to Organ Salvage and Prevention of Second Primary Neoplasms

*Editors:*

C. JULIAN ROSENTHAL, M.D., F.A.C.P.
Director of Research, Othmer Cancer Center,
Long Island College Hospital, Professor of Medicine and Oncology,
State University of New York, Health Science Center at Brooklyn,
339 Hicks Street, Brooklyn, New York 11201, USA

and

MARVIN ROTMAN, M.D.
Professor and Chairman, Radiation Oncology Department,
State University of New York, Health Science Center at Brooklyn,
Long Island College Hospital, Brookdale University Medical Center,
450 Clarkson Avenue, Brooklyn, New York 11203, USA

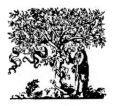

1998
ELSEVIER
Amsterdam – Lausanne – New York – Oxford – Shannon – Singapore – Tokyo

ELSEVIER SCIENCE B.V.
Sara Burgerhartstraat 25
P.O. Box 211, 1000 AE Amsterdam, The Netherlands

ISBN 0-444-82608-4

Printed in The Netherlands

**For their understanding, patience and love**
this book is dedicated

TO: *Sanda, Larry and Irene*
C. Julian Rosenthal


TO: *Marsha, David, Sonny, Dolly and Sydney*
Marvin Rotman

# Foreword

The need for combined modality therapy arises from the inability of surgery and radiation therapy to consistently cure intermediate stage solid tumors. This is due to the persistence of radiation resistant cells within the irradiated field or the early microscopic systemic spread of the disease. Sequential combined modality therapy has been investigated with some success. In particular, adjuvant chemotherapy has been shown to prolong survival rates in patients with colorectal cancer and breast cancer. Induction chemotherapy has been less consistently successful. Nevertheless, in stage IIIB non-small-cell lung cancer, increased time to progression and long-term survival rates have been reported utilizing this modality. Similarly in head and neck cancer, larynx preservation has been achieved.

*Concomitant chemoradiotherapy* is conceptually more intriguing than sequential approaches. In the ideal setting it still results in administration of systemically active chemotherapy (as do the sequential treatment approaches) while also allowing for a radiation sensitizing effect within the irradiated field. However, increased toxicities are almost unavoidable and are routinely observed. Furthermore, concomitant chemoradiotherapy is the logistically most complex and demanding form of combined modality therapy since physicians representing multiple specialties need to communicate and deliver protocol based therapy to a patient in a well coordinated fashion. For these reasons concomitant chemoradiotherapy has been less readily investigated and accepted. Neveretheless, when reviewing the literature, it is clear that patients with locoregionally advanced solid tumors can frequently benefit from the administration of concomitant chemoradiotherapy. Increased disease-free and/or overall survival rates have frequently been reported in a variety of solid tumors including esophageal cancer, rectal cancer, anal cancer, head and neck cancer, and non-small-cell and small-cell lung cancer. While in all of these settings acute toxicity is usually increased, a significant proportion of patients do appear to benefit from this more aggressive approach in the long run.

Drs. Rosenthal and Rotman have contributed to the literature of concomitant chemoradiotherapy through their own investigations. More importantly, they have repeatedly brought together investigators representing multiple specialties and interests from various parts of the world to discuss the basic and clinical principles and most recent trial results of concomitant chemoradiotherapy. This publication represents another major effort in this respect. Standard and recent investigational treatment approaches for all major tumor sites are reviewed. The basic integration of the more recent drugs with significant single agent activity in selected tumors, including the taxanes, are reviewed both with regard to their preclinical as well as clinical interactions with radiation. These drugs have already begun to impact on the standard therapies in patients with metastatic disease in several solid tumor types. It is hoped that their integration into the management of patients with locoregionally advanced disease will be more successful at increasing cure rates for these types of tumors.

Finally, biological principles of recent interests are explained and reviewed. As our understanding of these principles expands it can be hoped that further opportunities for novel and more successful therapies and prevention strategies will become available in the future.

*Everett E. Vokes*, M.D.
Professor of Medicine and Radiation Oncology
University of Chicago Medical Center
Chicago, Illinois

Scientific advances of the past quarter century have vastly expanded our knowledge and understanding of the biologic, etiologic and molecular mechanisms responsible for neoplasia. Concomitant with this unprecedented 'information explosion,' significant progress has been made in designing specific therapy for certain tumors, with improved outcomes no doubt attributable to the modeling of therapeutic interventions based, in many instances, upon these aforementioned scientific insights.

In this volume, Drs. Rosenthal and Rotman have assembled a series of chapters authored by well recognized experts, with a unifying theme of exploring the scientific basis of, and highlighting the clinically significant synergistic therapeutic interactions between chemotherapy and irradiation therapy. The reader is provided with a concise and readily understandable overview of the theoretical and experimental basis for radiation–chemotherapy interactions in the first chapter, co-authored by the editors. Subsequent chapters carefully address the pharmacokinetics of radiosensitizing agents, and explore the optimization of schedules for infusional therapy with concomitant radiation. Highlights of this volume include several chapters which provide useful overviews of the newest and most promising molecular approaches to cancer treatment: apoptosis as a target of therapeutic development; use of antiangiogenesis agents in cancer treatment; gene therapy and its applications to chemo–radiation therapy of cancer; and tumor suppression gene inactivation by SV40 mediated transformation.

Generalist physicians and specialists will find this text to be a useful resource that can provide answers to questions asked by patients, and that can help direct the clinician to appropriate sources for further inquiry in this most important and rapidly changing field.

*Stephan L. Kamholz*, M.D.
Professor & Chairman
Department of Medicine
State University of New York
Health Science Center at Brooklyn

# Preface

*"Truth in science can be defiined as the working hypothesis best suited to open the way to the next better one"*

Konrad Lorenz

The concomitant administration of chemotherapy and radiation therapy, that entered clinical practice for the last two decades, has aimed at reducing the local and regional recurrence rates of malignant tumors. It has a sound theoretical basis and is supported by many pre-clinical and clinical studies. It has been difficult, however, to extrapolate from the preclini-cal data guidelines for clinical applications. For this reason the design and execution of well conceived clinical trials have been crucial in this new field of clinical practice. An initial presentation of the experimental and clinical investigations in this field was made in a monograph we edited in 1991. Since then significant progress was made in the understand-ing of some of the mechanisms of chemotherapy–irradiation interaction while new agents like mitomycin C, paclitaxel, carboplatin have proven to be effective radiation sensitizers. Most importantly, several large phase III comparative trials have been completed during the last 6 years and have substantiated the fact that the protracted administration of specific chemotherapeutic agents with concomitant irradiation can lead to the permanent eradication of malignant tumors at certain sites, sparing the organ anatomy as well as its function. This has become a reality for all patients with squamous cell cancer of the anal canal and for a significant number of patients with rectal cancer, esophageal cancer, cancer of the vulva and uterus and bladder carcinoma as well as for some cases of cancer of the nasopharynx, oro-pharynx and larynx and selected cases of advanced loco-regional soft tissue sarcomas. For these reasons, we felt that a detailed review of the progress made during the last 6 years in the field of continuous infusion chemotherapy–irradiation interactions is warranted at this time. This publication provides this review in parallel with a description of the principles of the continuous infusion chemotherapy with concomitant radiation therapy.

During the last few years we have witnessed the translation to clinical practice of some of the significant advances molecular biologists have made in identifying the molecular events leading to carcinogenesis. For this reason we included in this publication four areas in which recent developments permit therapeutic applications that could be incorporated or could replace the current chemoradiation regimens. These areas are: apoptosis enhancement, sup-pressor gene repair, antiangiogenic therapy and gene therapy directed at specific DNA mu-tations or rearrangements .

With the rapid pace of progress made during the last 6 years, the concomitant chemo-therapy–irradiation regimens would soon become standard treatment for many neoplasms, permitting organ sparing. This could also lead to potential long term complications of these two modalities of treatment. For this reason we also included in this volume a section on chemo–radiation induced carcinogenesis followed by a section on the recent clinical advances in cancer chemoprevention that will, hopefully, decrease the risk of developing second primary neoplasms due to the administration of chemo–radiation therapy.

We attempted to organize the material in a rational sequence starting with an overview of the current status of the concomitant administration of irradiation and protracted infusion of chemotherapeutic agents and ending with a review of some theoretical and practical aspects of the use of computers in future research and clinical practice to optimize the benefits derived from the administration of the chemo–radiation regimens.

This publication would not have been possible without the effort of many individuals. I would like to thank first the contributors to various chapters for providing updated data of their work and of the field of their review as well as Dr. Marvin Rotman, the co-editor of this publication for his invaluable help in selecting and organizing the material included in this volume. I would also like to acknowledge the expert editorial review we received at Elsevier Science from Dr. Peter Harrison, the initial useful advice from Ms. Amanda Spiteri, the senior publishing editor, and Ms Lorna O'Brien. I also thank, for their expert secretarial assistance, Mrs Sandra Amrani, Ms Abiola Scotland and Ms Mary Ann Volare.

I hope that the data presented in various chapters and their discussion will give the readers useful information to apply to their clinical or experimental work and will, hopefully, generate in their minds new questions and new thoughts and ideas that may lead to further progress in cancer therapy.

*C. Julian Rosenthal*, M.D.

# List of contributors

H. ALI
Providence Cancer Center
Southfield, MI 48075, USA
Tel.: +1-800-341-0801
Fax: +1-810-424-2919

A. ALIMONTI
Laboratorio di Tossicologia Applicata
Istituto Superiore di Sanità
Viale Regina Elena 299, 00161 Roma, Italy

M. AL-SARRAF
Providence Cancer Center
Southfield, MI 48075, USA
Tel.: +1-800-341-0801, +1-810-424-3341
Fax: +1 810-424-2919

E.P. AMBINDER
Department of Medicine
Mount Sinai School of Medicine
1 Gustave Levy Place
New York, NY 10029, USA
Tel.: +1 212-289-2828
Fax: +1 212-860-9134

G. ASTARA
Department of Medical Oncology
Institute of Internal Medicine
University of Cagliari
09124 Cagliari, Italy
Tel.: +39-70-60-28-253
Fax: +39-70-66-36-51

H. AZIZ
Department of Radiation Oncology
Long Island College Hospital
339 Hicks Street
Brooklyn
NY 11201, USA
Tel.: +1 718-780-1801

F. BADELLINO
Division of Surgical Oncology
National Institute for Cancer Research
Genova, Italy

M. BAMBERG
Department of Radiotherapy
Section of Radiobiology and Molecular Environmental Research
Ebethard Karls University Tubingen
Rontgenweg 11
72076 Tubingen
Germany
Tel.: +49-7071-29-5962
Fax: +49-7071-29-7462

A.V. BEDINI
Istituto Nazionale di Tumori
Via Venezian 1
20133 Milano
Italy
Tel.: +39-2-2390601/384
Fax: +39-2-2360486

D. BELINA
Othmer Cancer Center and Departments of Medicine and Radiation Oncology
Long Island College Hospital
339 Hicks Street
Brooklyn
NY 11201, USA
Tel.: +1-718-270-2181

G. BERNARDO
National Institute for Cancer Research
Largo Rosanna Benzi 10
16132 Genova
Italy
Tel.: +39-10-5600670
Fax: +39-10-355562/5737505

J. BETKA
Department of Oncology
Charles University
U nemocnice 2
128 08 Prague 2
Czech Republic
Tel.: +420-2-294304
Fax: +420-2-298490

A. BIANCHI
Department of Medical Oncology
Institute of Internal Medicine
University of Cagliari
Via S. Giorgio 12
09124 Cagliari
Italy
Tel.: +39-70-60-28-253
Fax: +39-70-66-36-51, +39-70-60-28-253

A.W. BLACKSTOCK
Department of Radiation Oncology
Bowman Gray School of Medicine
Winston Salem
NC 27157, USA

G. BONCIARELLI
Dipartimento di Terapie Oncologiche Integrate
ULSS 21
37045 Legnago (VR), Italy
Tel.: +39-442-632275/632403/632364
Fax: +39-442-632469

E. BOVEN
Department of Medical Oncology
University Hospital Vrije Universiteit
De Boelelaan 1117
1081 HV Amsterdam
The Netherlands
Tel.: +31-20-4444300
Fax: +31-20-4444355

T. BRADLEY
Department of Medical Oncology
State University of New York
Health Science Center at Brooklyn
450 Clarkson Avenue
Brooklyn
NY 11203, USA
Tel.: +1-718-245-2785

A. BRAVERMAN
Department of Medical Oncology
State University of New York
Health Science Center at Brooklyn
450 Clarkson Avenue
Brooklyn
NY 11203, USA
Tel.: +1-718-270-2559

D.E. BRENNER
Division of Hematology-Oncology
Department of Internal Medicine
University of Michigan Medical School and
    Veterans Affairs Medical Center
Ann Arbor
MI 48109-0724, USA
Tel.: +1-313-647-1417

G. CANAVESE
Division of Surgical Oncology
National Institute for Cancer Research
Largo Rosanna Benzi 10
16132 Genova, Italy
Tel.: +39-10-5600670
Fax: +39-10-355562/5737505

C. CANEVALI
Dipartimento di Chimica Inorganica Metallor-
    ganica e Analitica
Centro CNR
Via Venezian 21
20133 Milano, Italy
Tel.: +39-2-26680688
Fax: +39-2-2362748

S. CAROLI
Laboratorio di Tossicologia Applicata
Istituto Superiore di Sanità
Viale Regina Elena 299
00161 Roma, Italy

P. CECH
Department of Oncology
Charles University
U nemocnice CZ128 08
Prague 2
Czech Republic
Tel.: +420-2-294304
Fax: +420-2-298490

P. CHANDRA
Department of Medical Oncology
State University of New York
Health Science Center at Brooklyn
450 Clarkson Avenue
Brooklyn
NY 11203, USA
Tel.: +1-718-270-1744

K. CHOI
State University of New York
Health Science Center at Brooklyn
450 Clarkson Avenue
Brooklyn
NY 11203, USA
Tel.: +1-718-270-2182

H. CHOY
Center for Radiation Oncology
Vanderbilt Medical Center
1301 22nd Avenue SB-902TVC
Nashville
TN 37232-5671, USA
Tel.: +1-615-343-9239

J. CIRRONE
Department of Radiation Oncology
State University of New York
Health Science Center at Brooklyn
450 Clarkson Avenue
Brooklyn
NY 11203, USA
Tel.: +1-718-270-1603

F. COSSU
Department of Radiation Therapy
University of Cagliari
09124 Cagliari
Italy
Tel.: +39-70-60-28-253
Fax: +39-70-66-36-51, +39-70-60-28-253

R.W. CRAIG
Department of Pharmacology and
    Toxicology
Dartmouth Medical School
Hanover
NH 03755-3835, USA
Tel.: +1-603-650-1657
Fax: +1-603-650-1631 (lab)

R.J. CRISTIANO
Section of Thoracic Molecular Oncology
Department of Thoracic and Cardiovascular
    Surgery, University of Texas
M.D. Anderson Cancer Center
1515 Holcombe Blvd.
Houston, TX 77030, USA
Tel.: +1-713-792-6932/6115 (lab)
Fax: +1-713-794-4901

B.J. CUMMINGS
Department of Radiation Oncology
Princess Margaret Hospital
610 University Avenue
Toronto, ON M5G 2M9, Canada
Tel.: +1-416-949-2129/924-0671
Fax: +1-416-946-2038

L. CURRELI
Department of Medical Oncology
Institute of Internal Medicine
University of Cagliari
Via S. Giorgi 12
09124 Cagliari, Italy
Tel.: +39-70-60-28-253
Fax: +39-70-66-36-51, +39-70-60-28-253

G. DASTOLI
National Institure for Cancer Research
Largo Rosanna Benzi 10
16132 Genova, Italy
Tel.: +39-10-5600670
Fax: +39-10-355562/5737505

J.A. DECAPRIO
Assistant Professor of Medicine
Dana-Farber Cancer Institute
Harvard Medical School
44 Binney Street, Boston
MA 02115, USA
Tel.: +1 617-632-3825
Fax: +1 617-632-4381

D. DESSÌ
Department of Medical Oncology
Institute of Internal Medicine
University of Cagliari
09124 Cagliari, Italy
Tel.: +39-70-60-28-253
Fax: +39-70-66-36-51, +39-70-60-28-253

G. DI COSTANZO
Service of Medical Oncology
S. Croce Hospital
v. Coppino 26
12100 Cuneo
Italy
Tel.: +39-171-441-309527/309531
Fax: +39-171-6995

A. EASTMAN
Department of Pharmacology and Toxicology
Dartmouth Medical School
Hanover
NH 03755-3835, USA
Tel.: +1-603-650-1657
Fax: +1-603-650-1631 (lab)

M.B. FENNERTY
Oregon Health Science University
OR, USA

V.D. FERRARI
Dipartimento di Terapie Oncologiche Integrate
ULSS 21, Via Gianelli 1
37045 Legnago (VR), Italy
Tel.: +39-442-632275/632403/632364
Fax: +39-442-632469

C. FILLINI
Division of Radiotherapy
S. Croce Hospital
v. Coppino 26
12100 Cuneo, Italy
Tel.: +39-171-441-309527/309531
Fax: +39-171-6995

V. GEBBIA
Chair and Service of Chemotherapy
University of Palermo
90127 Palermo
Italy

M. GHIANI
Department of Medical Oncology
Institute of Internal Medicine
University of Cagliari
Via S. Giorgi 12
09124 Cagliari, Italy
Tel.: +39-70-60-28-253
Fax: +39-70-66-36-51, +39-70-60-28-253

G. GIUDICE
Istituto Nazionale di Tumori
Via Venezian 1
20133 Milano, Italy

B.S. GLISSON
Department of Thoracic/Head and Neck Medical Oncology
The University of Texas
M.D. Anderson Cancer Center
1515 Holcombe Blvd., Box 80
Houston, TX 77030, USA
Tel.: +1-713-792-6363
Fax: +1-713-796-8655

A. GRAMAGLIA
Radiotherapy Department
Istituto Nazionale di Tumori
Via G. Venezian 1
20133 Milano, Italy
Tel.: +39-2-2390601/384
Fax: +39-2-2360486

G. GRECCHI
Service of Medical Oncology
S. Croce Hospital
v. Coppino 26
12100 Cuneo
Italy
Tel.: +39-171-441-309527/309531
Fax: +39-171-6995

R.S. HERBST
Dana-Farber Cancer Institute
44 Binney Street
Boston
MA 02115, USA
Tel.: +1-617-632-3122
Fax: +1-617-632-2411

W. HOFFMANN
Department of Radiotherapy
Section of Radiobiology and Molecular Environmental Research
Ebethard Karls University Tubingen
Rontgenweg 11
72076 Tubingen
Germany
Tel.: +49-7071-29-5962
Fax: +49-7071-29-7462

W.K. HONG
Department of Thoracic/Head and Neck Medical Oncology
The University of Texas
M. D. Anderson Cancer Center
1515 Holcombe Blvd., Box 80
Houston, TX 77030, USA
Tel.: +1-713-792-2121
Fax: +1-713-796-4901

H. HONOVÁ
Department of Oncology
Charles University
U nemocnice 2
128 08 Prague 2
Czech Republic
Tel.: +420-2-294304
Fax: +420-2-298490

L. ISNARDI
National Institute for Cancer Research
Largo Rosanna Benzi 10
16132 Genova, Italy
Tel.: +39-10-5600670
Fax: +39-10-355562/5737505

A. JIRILLO
Dipartimento di Terapie Oncologiche Integrate
ULSS 21
37045 Legnago (VR), Italy
Tel.: +39-442-632275/632403/632364
Fax: +39-442-632469

M.J. JOHN
Radiation Oncology
University of California San Francisco-Fresno
The Cancer Center at St Agnes
7130 North Millbrook Avenue Ste 112
Fresno, CA 93720, USA
Tel.: +1-209-449-5500
Fax: +1-209-449-5551

V.C. JORDAN
Department of Surgery and the Robert H. Lurie Cancer Center
Northwestern University Medical School
Olson Pavilion 8258
303 East Chicago Avenue
Chicago, IL 60611-3008, USA
Tel.: +1 312-908-4148
Fax: +1 312-908-1372

L. JUDAS
Department of Oncology
Charles University
U nemocnice 2
128 08 Prague 2, Czech Republic
Tel.: +420-2-294304
Fax: +420-2-298490

P. KASÍK
Department of Oncology
Charles University
U nemocnice 2
128 08 Prague 2, Czech Republic
Tel.: +420-2-294304
Fax: +420-2-298490

F.R. KHURI
Department of Thoracic/Head and Neck Medical Oncology
The University of Texas
M. D. Anderson Cancer Center
1515 Holcombe Blvd., Box 80
Houston, TX 77030, USA
Tel.: +1-713-792-6363
Fax: +1-713-794-4901

J. KLOZAR
Department of Oncology
Charles University
U nemocnice 2
128 08 Prague 2, Czech Republic
Tel.: +420-2-294304
Fax: +420-2-298490

K. KRISHNAN
Division of Hematology-Oncology
Department of Internal Medicine
James H. Quillen College of Medicine and Veterans Affairs Medical Centre
East Tennessee State University
Johnson City, TN, USA

J.M. KURIE
Department of Thoracic/Head and Neck Medical Oncology
The University of Texas
M. D. Anderson Cancer Center
1515 Holcombe Blvd., Box 80
Houston, TX 77030, USA
Tel.: +1-713-792-6363
Fax: +1-713-794-4901

P. LA CIURA
Service of Medical Oncology
S. Croce Hospital
v. Coppino 26, 12100 Cuneo, Italy
Tel.: +39-171-441-309527/309531
Fax: +39-171-6995

B. LAMPIS
Department of Medical Oncology
Institute of Internal Medicine
University of Cagliari
09124 Cagliari, Italy
Tel.: +39-70-60-28-253
Fax: +39-70-66-36-51, +39-70-60-28-253

S.M. LIPPMAN
Department of Thoracic/Head and Neck Medi-
  cal Oncology, University of Texas
M. D. Anderson Cancer Center
1515 Holcombe Blvd., Box 80
Houston, TX 77030, USA
Tel.: +1-713-792-0625

J. LOKICH
Department of Neoplastic Disease
The Cancer Center of Boston
Boston, MA 02120, USA
Tel.: +1-617-739-6605
Fax: +1-617-739-4819

F. LONARDI
Dipartimento di Terapie Oncologiche Integrate
ULSS 21
37045 Legnago (VR), Italy
Tel.: +39-442-632275/632403
Fax: +39-442-632469

M.R. MADIANO
Department of Haematology and Oncology
University of Arizona
Tucson, AZ, USA
Tel.: +1-520-324-2409
Fax: +1-520-624-7445

G. MANTOVANI
Department of Medical Oncology
Institute of Internal Medicine
University of Cagliari
09124 Cagliari, Italy
Tel.: +39-70-60-28-253
Fax: +39-70-66-36-51, +39-70-60-28-253

G. MARCHETTI
Division of Radiotherapy
S. Croce Hospital
v. Coppino 26
12100 Cuneo
Italy
Tel.: +39-171-441-309527/309531
Fax: +39-171-6995

E. MASONI
Dipartimento di Chimica Inorganica Metallor-
  ganica e Analitica
Centro CNR
Via Venezian 21
20133 Milano
Italy
Tel.: +39-2-26680688
Fax: +39-2-2362748

E. MASSA
Department of Medical Oncology
Institute of Internal Medicine
University of Cagliari
09124 Cagliari
Italy
Tel.: +39-70-60-28-253
Fax: +39-70-66-36-51, +39-70-60-28-253

A. MELANO
Division of Radiotherapy
S. Croce Hospital
v. Coppino 26
12100 Cuneo, Italy
Tel.: +39-171-441-309527/309531
Fax: +39-171-6995

M. MERLANO
Medical Oncology Department
S. Croce Hospital
12100 Cuneo, Italy
Tel.: +39-171-441-309527/309531
Fax: +39-171-6995

F. MILANI
Radiotherapy Department
Istituto Nazionale di Tumori
Via G. Venezian 1
20133 Milano
Italy
Tel.: +39-2-26680688
Fax: +39-2-2362748

F. MORAZZONI
Dipartimento di Chimica Inorganica Metallor-
  ganica e Analitica
Centro CNR, Via Venezian 21
20133 Milano
Italy
Tel.: +39-2-26680688/26680673
Fax: +39-2-2362748

M. MORROW
Department of Surgery and the Robert H. Lurie
  Cancer Center
Northwestern University Medical School
Chicago
IL 60611, USA
Tel.: +1 312-908-8060

D. NGUYEN
Section of Thoracic Molecular Oncology
Department of Thoracic and Cardiovascular
  Surgery, University of Texas
M.D. Anderson Cancer Center
1515 Holcombe Blvd.
Houston
TX 77030, USA
Tel.: +1-713-792-6932/6115
Fax: +1-713-794-4901

G. NICOLÒ
National Instirure for Cancer Research
Largo Rosanna Benzi 10
16132 Genova
Italy
Tel.: +39-10-5600670
Fax: +39-10-355562/5737505

G. NUMICO
National Instirure for Cancer Research
Largo Rosanna Benzi 10
16132 Genova, Italy
Tel.: +39-10-5600668
Fax: +39-10-355562

M. PALAZZI
Radiotherapy Department
Istituto Nazionale di Tumori
Via G. Venezian 1
20133 Milano
Italy
Tel.: +39-2-2390601/384
Fax: +39-2-2360486

R. PALUMBO
National Institute for Cancer Research
Largo Rosanna Benzi 10
16132 Genova, Italy
Tel.: +39-10-5600670
Fax: +39-10-355562/5737505

G. PAVANATO
Dipartimento di Terapie Oncologiche Integrate
ULSS 21
37045 Legnago (VR), Italy
Tel.: +39-442-632275/632403/632364
Fax: +39-442-632469

A. PELISSERO
Division of Radiotherapy
S. Croce Hospital
v. Coppino 26
12100 Cuneo, Italy
Tel.: +39-171-441-309527/309531
Fax: +39-171-6995

D. PERRONI
Service of Medical Oncology
S. Croce Hospital
v. Coppino 26
12100 Cuneo, Italy
Tel.: +39-171-441-309527/309531
Fax: +39-171-6995

F. PETRUCCI
Laboratorio di Tossicologia Applicata
Istituto Superiore di Sanità
Viale Regina Elena 299
00161 Roma, Italy

L. PETRUŽELKA
Department of Oncology
Charles University
U nemocnice 2
128 08 Prague 2, Czech Republic
Tel.: +420-2-294304
Fax: +420-2-298490

O. PŘIBYLOVÁ
Department of Oncology
Charles University
U nemocnice 2
128 08 Prague 2, Czech Republic
Tel.: +420-2-294304
Fax: +420-2-298490

E. PROTO
Department of Surgery
Otolaryngology Branch
University of Cagliari
Via S. Giorgio 12
09124 Cagliari, Italy


P. RAFFO
National Institute for Cancer Research
Largo Rosanna Benzi 10
16132 Genova, Italy
Tel.: +39-10-5600670
Fax: +39-10-355562/5737505


H. RAMBHIA
Othmer Cancer Center and Department of
    Medicine
Long Island College Hospital
339 Hicks Street, Brooklyn, NY 11201, USA


G. RAVASI
Thoracic Surgery Department
Istituto Nazionale di Tumori
Via G. Venezian 1
20133 Milano, Italy
Tel.: +39-2-26680688
Fax: +39-2-2362748


M. REGAZZI-BONORA
National Institute for Cancer Research
Largo Rosanna Benzi 10
16132 Genova, Italy
Tel.: +39-10-5600670
Fax: +39-10-355562/5737505


T.A. RICH
Department of Radiation Oncology
Box 383
University of Virginia
Health Sciences Center
Charlottesville, VA 22903, USA
Tel.: +1-804-924-5191
Fax: +1-803-982-3262


S. ROCKWELL
Department of Therapeutic Radiology
Yale University School of Medicine
P.O. Box 208040
New Haven, CT 06520-8040, USA
Tel.: +1-203-785-2963
Fax: +1-203-785-4622


H.P. RODEMANN
Department of Radiotherapy
Section of Radiobiology and Molecular Envi-
    ronmental Research
Ebethard Karls University Tubingen
Rontgenweg 11
72076 Tubingen, Germany
Tel.: +49-7071-29-5962
Fax: +49-7071-29-7462


B.S. ROSENSTEIN
Department of Radiation Oncology
Mount Sinai School of Medicine of the City
    University of New York
New York
NY 10029, USA
Tel.: +1-212-241-6158
Fax: +1-212-410-7194


C.J. ROSENTHAL
Othmer Cancer Center and Department of
    Medicine
Long Island College Hospital
339 Hicks Street
Brooklyn, NY 11201, USA
Tel.: +1 718-780-1480/1481
Fax: +1 718-780-2401


J.A. ROTH
Section of Thoracic Molecular Oncology
Department of Thoracic and Cardiovascular
    Surgery
University of Texas M.D. Anderson Cancer
    Center
1515 Holcombe Blvd.
Houston, TX 77030, USA
Tel.: +1-713-792-6932
Fax: +1-713-792-2121


M. ROTMAN
State University of New York
Health Science Center at Brooklyn
450 Clarkson Avenue
Brooklyn, NY 11203, USA
Tel.: +1 718-270-2181


M.T. RUFFIN IV
Department of Family Practice
University of Michigan Medical School and
    Veterans Affairs Medical Center
Ann Arbor, MI 48109-0724, USA

E. RUSSI
Division of Radiotherapy
S. Croce Hospital, v. Coppino 26
12100 Cuneo, Italy
Tel.: +39-171-441-309527/309531
Fax: +39-171-6995

M.C. SANTONA
Department of Medical Oncology
Institute of Internal Medicine
University of Cagliari
09124 Cagliari, Italy
Tel.: +39-70-60-28-253
Fax: +39-70-66-36-51, +39-70-60-28-253

A. SCHULSINGER
Department of Radiation Oncology
State University of New York
Health Science Center at Brooklyn
450 Clarkson Avenue
Brooklyn
NY 11203, USA
Tel.: +1-718-270-1593

D. SCHWARTZ
Department of Radiation Oncology
State University of New York
Health Science Center at Brooklyn
450 Clarkson Avenue
Brooklyn
NY 11203, USA
Tel.: +1-718-270-1593

B. SHANK
Radiation Oncology Department
Box 1236
Mount Sinai Medical Center
One Gustave L. Levy Place
New York
NY 10029-6574, USA
Tel.: +1-212-241-6158
Fax: +1-212-410-7194

C. SOHN
Department of Radiation Oncology
State University of New York
Health Science Center at Brooklyn
450 Clarkson Avenue
Brooklyn
NY 11203, USA
Tel.: +1-718-270-2181

F. SPITZ
Department of Surgical Oncology
University of Texas M.D. Anderson Cancer
  Center
1515 Holcombe Blvd.
Houston, TX 77030, USA
Tel.: +1-713-792-6932
Fax: +1-713-794-4901

G.N. STEMMERMAN
University of Cincinnati
Cincinnati
OH, USA

L. TAVECCHIO
Thoracic Surgery Department
Istituto Nazionale di Tumori
Via G. Venezian 1
20133 Milano, Italy
Tel.: +39-2-2390601/384
Fax: +39-2-2360486

S.G. TAYLOR
Rush University and the Cancer Center
Illinois Masonic Medical Center
901 West Wellington
Chicago, IL 60657, USA
Tel.: +1-312-296-7089/7731
Fax: +1-312-297-7731

B.A. TEICHER
Dana-Farber Cancer Institute
44 Binney Street
Boston, MA 02115, USA
Tel.: +1-617-632-3122
Fax: +1-617-632-2411

J.E. TEPPER
Department of Radiation Oncology
University of North Carolina at Chapel Hill
School of Medicine
Chapel Hill, NC 27599-7512, USA
Tel.: +1-919-966-7700
Fax: +1-919-966-7681

S. TOMA
National Institute for Cancer Research
Largo Rosanna Benzi 10
16132 Genova, Italy
Tel.: +39-10-5600670
Fax: +39-10-355562/5737505

M. TUBIANA
The Centre Antoine Béclère
45 rue des Saints-Pères
75006 Paris
France
Tel.: +33-1-42-86-22-95
Fax: +33-1-47-03-93-85

C.B. VAUGHN
Southfield Oncology Institute
27211 Lahser Road
Southfield
MI 48034, USA
Tel.: +1-810-356-2828

C. VECCHIO
National Institute for Cancer Research
Largo Rosanna Benzi 10
16132 Genova
Italy
Tel.: +39-10-5600670
Fax: +39-10-355562/5737505

S. VILLA
Radiotherapy Department
Istituto Nazionale di Tumori
Via G. Venezian 1
20133 Milano
Italy

W.H. WILSON
The Medicine Branch
Division of Clinical Sciences
National Cancer Institute
Building 10, Room 12-N-226
9000 Rockville Pike
Bethesda, MD 20892-1904, USA

L.-T. WU
Department of Medicine
Long Island College Hospital
339 Hicks Street
Brooklyn, NY 11201, USA
Tel.: +1-718-780-1480/1481

P. ZATLOUKAL
Department of Oncology
Charles University
U nemocnice 2
128 08 Prague 2, Czech Republic
Tel.: +420-2-294304
Fax: +420-2-298490

M. ZUCCHETTI
Istituto di Ricerche Farmacologiche "Mario
   Negri"
Via Eritrea 62
20157 Milano
Italy

# Contents

**Section III  Future Directions: Molecular Biology Advances – Potential Clinical Applications to Chemo–Radiation**

## Section IV  Chemo–Radiation Induced Carcinogenesis

## Section V    Advances in Cancer Chemo-Prevention

## Section VI  Computer Technology in Research and Clinical Practice

# SECTION I

# MODULATION OF RADIOTHERAPY BY BIOLOGICAL AND CHEMOTHERAPEUTIC AGENTS

*"It is in the realm of uncertainties that progress must lie."*
                                                      Edward Searles

C.J. Rosenthal and M. Rotman (Eds.), *Infusion Chemotherapy–Irradiation Interactions*
© 1998 Elsevier Science B.V. All rights reserved

# CHAPTER 1

# Infusion chemotherapy-irradiation interactions: an overview

## C. JULIAN ROSENTHAL[1,2] and MARVIN ROTMAN[1,2]

[1]*Othmer Cancer Center and Departments of Medicine, and Radiation Oncology, Long Island College Hospital, 339 Hicks Street, Brooklyn, NY 11201, USA, and* [2]*State University of New York, Health Science Center at Brooklyn, 450 Clarkson Avenue, Brooklyn, NY 11203, USA*

## 1. Introduction

Despite significant progress in understanding the molecular basis of carcinogenesis and in developing new therapeutic agents effective against malignant tumors, the last decades have brought only a small decrease in cancer mortality rate.

Overall, less than 15% of the patients with advanced cancer can be cured. Curability is attainable more frequently when therapy of malignant tumors is instituted at a time they are still localized at their site of origin. It varies between 30% and 90% in function of tumor size, its location and histology. Radiation therapy constitutes an effective treatment of many localized solid tumors. However, its curative potential is limited either by acquired or intrinsic radiation resistance or by the systemic dissemination of some malignant tumors before the primary tumor could be eradicated by surgery or irradiation. Chemotherapy on the other hand is active systemically but very few single agents or combinations can eradicate malignant tumors even when limited just at a small primary site.

To overcome the innate (intrinsic) or acquired radiation resistance of malignant cells an idea was developed 40 years ago of using chemotherapy to enhance the effectiveness of radiation and was first experimentally tested by Heidelberger et al. [1].

The successful clinical use of this approach had to await a better understanding of the factors that could permit the timing synchronization of the two modalities and the development of the technology for the administration of many chemotherapy agents by continuous protracted infusions at a constant rate throughout most of the radiation treatment, which is likely to secure for most chemotherapy agents the best synchronization with irradiation.

## 2. Experimental basis for radiation-protracted chemotherapy interaction

Prolonging the time over which tumor cells are exposed to drugs was tried early in the development of chemotherapy in the hope of enhancing the effectiveness of the drugs and, at the same time, of reducing their side effects because of the need for lower concentrations.

Shimoyama [2], in the course of in vitro studies on Yoshida ascites sarcoma cells, delineated two different groups among the antineoplastic agents whose performance was enhanced by prolonged contact with malignant cells and a third group that included the nitro-

soureas and most of the alkylating agents with the exception of cisplatin and cyclophosphamide whose prolonged contact with the sarcoma ascitic cells did not lead to improved
toxicity profile. Drugs in the first group (doxorubicin, bleomycin, mitomycin C, dactinomy-
cin, etc.) are cytotoxic to malignant cells when kept in contact for 24–96 h, at concentrations
100–500 times lower than when kept in contact with the same cells for just 30 min. Lower
concentrations of the drugs decrease their cytotoxic effect on normal cells. These in vitro
findings were confirmed by clinical studies of continuous infusion doxorubicin and bleomycin. There were significant reductions in myocardial toxicity from continuously infused
doxorubicin and in lung toxicity from protracted infusion of bleomycin.

For the second group of antineoplastic agents (5-fluorouracil (5-FU), cytosine arabino-
side, methotrexate, L-asparaginase, vinblastine, vincristine, cisplatin, etc.), protracted contact with malignant cells for more than 2 days increases their cytotoxic activity by 2–3 logs
as compared with only 30 min of contact. This is of particular importance since these drugs
rapidly reach a plateau level beyond which an increase in concentration is no longer reflected by an increase in cytotoxicity [2]. Clinical evidence, again, confirmed the benefits of
prolonged infusion for all these drugs with the exception of methotrexate. These experimental data were published 1 year after the first publication of a successful treatment of a
concomitant administration of radiation therapy with a chemotherapy agent, 5 fluorouracil
administered by Nigro et al. [3] by continuous intravenous infusion to patients with anal
carcinoma who refused surgery. The above mentioned experimental data together with a
growing number of other preclinical data have led to an increasing understanding of the
rationale behind this approach. This, in turn, has led to a growing amount of clinical investigation in the last decade into the multimodal use of a variety of other neoplastic agents, including cisplatin, doxorubicin, dacarbazine, bleomycin and more recently mitomycin C and
paclitaxel.

The exact mechanism by which these chemotherapeutic agents potentiate the radiation
therapy effect is, in most cases, poorly understood. Following the schematic classification of
chemical modifiers of cancer treatment recently reviewed by Coleman et al. [4] some of
these drugs (i.e., mitomycin C, anthracyclines, bleomycin, dacarbazine) could be considered
to be acting as hypoxic cell sensitizers primarily through their interference with the repair of
the DNA injury inflicted on neoplastic cells by radiation therapy. 5-FU belongs to another
class of radiosensitizers, the thymidine analogs, that are incorporated into the DNA of cy-
cling cells and make them more sensitive to irradiation. None of the chemotherapeutic
agents appear to belong to a third major class of radiosensitizers that enhance the radiation
effect through glutathione depletion of neoplastic cells like that induced by L-buthiomine
sulfoxide or diethylimaleate.


## 3. Cisplatin as radiation potentiator

cis-Diamminedichloroplatinum II (cis-DDP or cisplatin), the first of the group of platinum
coordination complexes used effectively against some human malignancies was found in
1974 by Wolinsky et al. [5] to potentiate irradiation effects on a rat experimental tumor. In
the late 1970s, studies by Douple and Richmond [6] on Escherichia coli bacteria, V-79 Chinese hamster cells, and mouse mammary carcinoma showed that cisplatin sensitizes hypoxic
cells to radiation by increasing DNA susceptibility to radiation damage. The effect can be
seen in the abrogation of the shoulder and the steepening of the exponential portion of the

single cell survival curve. At the same time, cisplatin inhibits the repair of potentially lethal radiation-induced damage to the DNA [6–9]. In order to produce these two major effects, however, it was found that cisplatin must be present at the time of irradiation as well as shortly after irradiation at a concentration of at least 10 M [8]. It was these findings that led to a number of experimental studies by Fu et al. [10] and by Douple et al. [11] into the kinetics and the efficacy of cisplatin and paraplatin (a second generation platinum compound) in potentiating radiation effects. A convincing experimental demonstration of the radiosensitizing effect of cisplatin was performed by Kyriazis et al. [12] on human bladder carcinoma implanted in nude mice. The mice receiving both modalities of therapy had a statistically significant improvement in response and survival over those receiving radiation alone. Other experimental data suggested that the cisplatin-radiation interaction is enhanced when radiation is administered by multiple fractions [13].

All the early clinical studies on the cisplatin–radiation interactions used only bolus intravenous administration of the drug [14,15]. While indicating a favorable trend, the results have been inconclusive in proving a cisplatin radiosensitizing effect. Better results were reported in studies using higher intermittent doses of cisplatin. A phase II trial [16] by the Radiation Therapy Oncology Group (RTOG) administered 100 mg/m$^2$ cisplatin every 3 weeks with appropriate hydration and antiemetics, to patients with stage III and IV head and neck neoplasms. Results from this study showed an improvement when compared with those from studies using fractionated smaller doses of 15–20 mg/m$^2$. Survival at 1 year of 66% and median survival of just over 2 years [16] were encouraging. In a recently reported pilot study [17] of patients with squamous cell carcinoma of the lung and head and neck who received high dose cisplatin (40 mg/m$^2$ per day for 5 consecutive days) for three cycles during radiation therapy a complete response rate of 100% was achieved. This suggests that dose may be important for cisplatin synergy with radiation. However, the toxicity of this regimen was significant and no information is available from this study concerning survival or duration of response.

Other recent therapeutic trials with carcinoma of the bladder have used cisplatin bolus injection every 3 weeks with concomitant irradiation to the bladder given to a total dose of 60 Gy in a split course [18] or non-split course [19,20]. Results indicate an improvement of approximately 20% in the complete response (CR) rate for patients with macroscopic residual tumor when compared with historical control studies in which cisplatin was administered sequentially after radiation therapy.

However, it was not until the phase I–II study by Rosenthal et al. [21] that the maximum tolerated dose and the overall toxicity of cisplatin as a potential radiosensitizer were assessed. Trials were set up in patients with squamous cell carcinoma of the lung, head and neck and esophagus [21], transitional cell carcinoma of the bladder [22] and advanced paranasal sinus and esophageal squamous cell carcinoma [23,24]. The phase I study on protracted continuous infusion [21] indicated that a daily dose of 5 mg/m$^2$ per day was well tolerated for a mean of 18 consecutive days. Increasing the daily dose led within a few days to intolerable gastrointestinal toxicity while prolonging the duration of the cisplatin infusion beyond 18 days led to unacceptable thrombocytopenia ($85 \pm 12 \times 10^3/\mu l$). However, this same study, as well as Sauer's study [22] found that cisplatin can be administered by continuous infusion over a shorter period of only 5 days up to a dose of 25 mg/m$^2$ per day with only moderate gastrointestinal toxicity.

Ongoing clinical trials are attempting to define further the role of continuous infusion cisplatin as a radiosensitizer in the treatment of other primary tumors.

## 4. 5-Fluorouracil as radiation potentiator

5-Fluorouracil is a pyrimidine analog that inhibits de novo synthesis of DNA by binding thymidylate synthetase. It also leads to synthesis of defective DNA due to its combination with an RNA precursor nucleotide. Its effects as a radiopotentiator could be due to its inhibition of the repair of sublethal damage produced by radiation [25].

The use of 5-FU in continuous infusion with concomitant irradiation began fortuitously in 1974 with Nigro's [3] application to the therapy of anal carcinoma of Seifert's observation [26] on the benefits of administration of 5-FU by continuous infusion. This initial favorable experience was followed by systematic preclinical studies carried out by Byfield et al. [27] which established the scheduling requisites for the effective use of infused 5-FU as a radiosensitizer of human tumors.

In 1980, Byfield et al. [28] expanded the use of concomitant irradiation with 5-FU infusion at a dose of 20 mg/kg per day for 5 consecutive days every 2 weeks to the treatment of unresectable squamous cell carcinoma of the esophagus. A complete clinical response was achieved in five out of six cases.

It was, however, only in 1982 that two reports of somewhat larger series of patients with anorectal carcinoma [29,30] clearly documented the curative effect of this concomitant combined modality therapy. Radiosensitization was achieved by the use of 5-FU at a dose of 1000 mg/m$^2$ per day administered by continuous infusion for 96–120 h every 2 weeks with one dose of mitomycin C (10 mg/m$^2$) on the 1st day of therapy only. All patients in these two series (a total of 32 patients) achieved complete remissions which were maintained at the time of reporting (2–36 months). Based on these results, combined concomitant modality therapy had replaced surgical resection in the treatment of squamous cell carcinoma of the anus; this represents, to date, the most successful application of concomitant modality therapy in the treatment of malignant tumors. It is a clear indication of the effectiveness of 5-FU infusion in enhancing the effects of radiation, which was found to be capable of inducing, by itself, complete lasting remissions but with a much higher rate (up to 25%) of local failures in patients with T$_3$ and T$_4$ lesions [31].

During the following years similar combined modality therapy was administered with varying degrees of success to squamous cell carcinomas at other sites. Coia et al. [32] reported in 1984 a 17-month median survival in patients with stage I and II squamous cell carcinoma of the esophagus. The regimen used was two cycles of 5-day infusion 5-FU with concomitant radiation therapy to a total dose of 60 Gy over a 6-week period. Recurrences in previously irradiated areas were reported in only 10% of cases.

Keane et al. [33] reported on a similar combined modality treatment administered to 35 patients with locally advanced esophageal squamous cell carcinoma (lesions larger than 5 cm in diameter), circumferential or extending outside the esophagus: 15 patients received just one cycle of 5-FU infusion while 20 received two cycles. The results of this pilot study were compared with matched controls from a previous series of patients with esophageal squamous cell carcinoma who received irradiation alone. In 18 out of 35 patients receiving the combined concomitant therapy, the tumor remained locally controlled. The 2-year actuarial rate of 30% and the local relapse-free rate of 47% compared favorably with the rates of 15% and 20%, respectively, noted in the patients receiving irradiation alone. Continuous course therapy resulted in better survival at 2 years (48% versus 13%) and in better local relapse-free rates (73% versus 29%) than the split-course irradiation. However, the slope of the survival curve was not changed for responding patients, indicating that the noted improvement may represent just a delay in death for those patients with advanced unresectable tumors. This was not the case for patients treated in the early stages by Coia et al. [34] who added mitomycin C to the 5 FU infusion radiation therapy regimen.


## 5.  Mitomycin C as radiation potentiator

Mitomycin C is an antitumor antibiotic which functions as an alkylating agent by opening its quinone ring after reductive activation which makes it more cytotoxic to hypoxic tumor cells than to the surrounding aerobic normal tissue cells. The potential contribution of mitomycin C as a radiosensitizer was suspected since the 1970s based on experimental animals data generated at Yale University [35].

The supradditive effects of mitomycin C given as a single i.v. bolus concomitantly with radiation therapy and 5-FU by continuous intravenous infusion was demonstrated by three randomized phase III studies in patients with head and neck tumors [36] with epidermoid anal cancer [37,38] and in the advanced cervical cancer [39]. In all three studies patients receiving mitomycin C with 5 FU and irradiation had a higher partial and complete response rate and a longer duration of their response than those receiving only 5-FU infusion and concomitant radiation therapy.

Experimental data [40] have shown, however, that the interaction between mitomycin C and radiation therapy is dependent on the timing of mitomycin C administration. In order to eliminate the need for difficult timing synchronization of the two modalities of treatment in clinical practice a phase I study of the administration of mitomycin C by continuous i.v. infusion with concomitant radiation therapy was carried out at our institution [41] in patients with colon carcinoma metastatic to the liver and is fully reviewed elsewhere in this volume.

This study established the MTD of mitomycin C by continuous intravenous infusion with concomitant radiation therapy at 1 mg/m$^2$ per day for 21 days while standard radiation (180 cGy/session) was delivered to the measurable metastatic lesions in the phase I study [41] and to the liver invaded by metastases from colon carcinoma in the phase II study. The response rate to this combined modality treatment was superior to the best results reported with 5-FU radiopotentiation as previously described or with intra hepatic artery or infusional chemotherapy. However, due to the small number of patients enrolled in this study, no definitive conclusions could be reached other than to continue testing this regimen in other tumors known to have brief responses to mitomycin C alone.


## 6.  Radiation potentiation by 5-FU and mitomycin C combination infusional chemotherapy

In parallel with the phase I and II studies probing mitomycin C by continuous intravenous infusion as radiation potentiator, during the last 5 years mitomycin was found to be effective when administered as a single dose by i.v. bolus in combination with 5-FU by continuous infusion for 4–5 days during the first and fourth week of delivery of radiation therapy (FUMIR). However, none of these studies showed a clear superiority of FUMIR to each of the two drugs administered alone with concomitant radiation therapy. FUMIR was administered by Leichman et al. [42] to 25 patients with squamous cell carcinoma of the esophagus in a shorter variant for only 3 weeks to a total radiation dose of 30 Gy. The complete remission rate of 25% was inferior to the result obtained by Coia et al. [32] with 5-FU infusion-RT. On the other side patients receiving only radiation therapy alone to the esophageal lesions to a total dose of 30 Gy achieved complete remission just in only 3% of cases [42].

Similar response rates of 22% were achieved in a group of squamous cell carcinoma patients receiving 60 Gy to the primary lesion and another group of patients receiving 5-FU, cisplatin and 30 Gy radiation [43]. The risk of distant metastases, the failure to improve cure rates when residual tumor was still present after preoperative 5-FU-mitomycin C [42] and the relatively high mortality rates following resection of residual esophageal cancer [43] suggest that patients in whom symptomatic residual tumor remains after treatment with FUMIR would do better with a palliative bypass rather than a radical esophageal resection. However, in early-stage patients achieving a complete response, survival is clearly improved. It remains to be determined whether or not surgical resection of the esophageal segment is necessary after complete remission is obtained through the administration of 5-FU with or without mitomycin C.

The FUMIR combined concomitant modality therapy was also used in the therapy of locally advanced squamous cell carcinoma of the cervix with disease expanding to both pelvic side walls or to the rectum and bladder. In these cases, irradiation alone is followed by a 75% risk of pelvic failure [39]. Twenty-seven patients were treated by Thomas et al. [39] at the Princess Margaret Cancer Institute with split-course radiation therapy with hyperfractionation. Two daily doses of 1.5 Gy were administered for 4 days together with 5-FU infusion and one dose of 6 mg/m$^2$ mitomycin C followed by single doses of 1.8 Gy radiation for another 6 days. This course was repeated once after a 24-day interval and was complemented by an intracavitary cesium 137 line source delivering a dose of 40 Gy at 2 cm from the applicator. Seventy-four percent of patients achieved complete remission (CR); in 65% of cases the CR was maintained at 3 years, but long-term follow-up results are not yet available.

The FUMIR combination was also used successfully in the therapy of locally advanced transitional cell carcinoma and squamous cell carcinoma of the bladder, initially by Rotman et al. [44,45] and by Russell et al. [46]. Of the 20 evaluable patients in the Rotman et al. [45,47] study 86% achieved CR after receiving 40–45 Gy in daily fractions for 5 days a week and an additional 20–25 Gy as a pelvic boost or a 30 Gy interstitial implant with concomitant 5-FU infusion at 25 mg/kg per 24 h for 5 days and one dose of mitomycin C at 10 mg/m$^2$ as i.v. bolus. These results compare favorably with CR rates of 31–49% reported by various investigators after the preoperative administration of 40–50 Gy alone [48,49]. The adjusted overall 5-year survival rate was projected at 53% with better rates for stages $A_2$ and $B_1$ (80%) than for $B_2$, C, and D (40%).

Finally the FUMIR combined concomitant modality therapy was also tested in a few studies in patients with adenocarcinoma at various sites, particularly the rectum and stomach. There were encouraging results from the rectal adenocarcinoma study [50]. Among 64 patients with locally advanced disease (ulcerated, fixed lesions at least 4 cm in diameter) complete response was attained in 12.5% of cases; operations were performed after a total tumor dose of 40 Gy was given over a period of 4 weeks with two cycles of 96 h infusion of 5-FU at a dose of 1000 mg/m$^2$ per day and one bolus injection of mitomycin C (10 mg/m$^2$). No nodal involvement was seen in 73.5% of cases while in historical control studies less than 50% of the patients are free of nodal involvement. The projected survival at 5 years of 64% was slightly better than in historical control studies. The data of FUMIR effectiveness in patients with adenocarcinoma are less convincing than those in patients with squamous cell carcinoma at various sites and transitional cell carcinoma of the bladder. The contribution of mitomcyin C to the radiosensitizing effect of 5-FU was recently demonstrated in an RTOG-ECOG study in which patients with squamous cell carcinoma of the anus received radiation therapy and concomitant infusional 5-FU alone or in combination with mitomycin C [38]. Residual disease and local recurrences were lower (8% and 16% respectively in the FUMIR arm than in the 5-FU-RT arm (15% and 34%). Disease free survival was statistically significantly better in the FUMIR arm (73% versus 51%; $P = 0.0002$) while the overall survival was 76% in the FUMIR arm versus 67% in the 5FU-RT arm ($P = 0.18$) [38].

Recent data have suggested that the radiosensitizing effect of infusion 5-FU could be also enhanced by its combination with cisplatin.

## 7.  Radiation potentiation by cisplatin–5-FU combination infusional chemotherapy

Four studies in patients with advanced head and neck squamous cell carcinoma using infusional 5-FU and cisplatin with concomitant radiation therapy have reported excellent results. Taylor et al. [51] administered cisplatin 60 mg/m$^2$ on day 1, 5-FU 800 mg/m$^2$ per day on days 1–5, and split-course radiation therapy also on days 1–5 with the cycle repeated every 2 weeks. This regimen led to a 98% overall response rate and a CR rate of 55% with a median survival of 37 months. A different regimen in which cisplatin was given at 75 mg/m$^2$ on days 1 and 43 with 5-FU administered by continuous infusion during a non-split course of radiation therapy for 3 weeks led to an overall response rate of 100% with 94% CR and 64% survival at 21 months [52]. Similarly Wendt et al. [53] administered a non-split course of radiation therapy following a hyperfractionation schema (twice daily 0.18 Gy per 8 day therapy) and a lower dose of 5-FU (350 mg/m$^2$ per day by continuous infusion on days 2–5). Finally, Al-Sarraf et al. [16] study showed that the cisplatin–5-FU infusion achieved twice the complete response rate of any previously reported regimen in advanced head and neck squamous cell carcinomas. It is notable that in respect to advanced head and neck squamous cell carcinoma, survival is not significantly better in patients achieving complete clinical remission than in good partial responders [51]. This indicates the difficulties encountered in determining complete responses by clinical evaluation or random endoscopic biopsies.

Recently two randomized phase III studies [54,55] in patients with advanced squamous cell carcinoma of the head and neck were reported and convincingly demonstrated the benefit of cisplatin–5-FU regimen addition to radiation therapy. Merlano et al. [54] reported in 1991 the results of a cooperative study of the Italian National Cancer Institute comparing radiotherapy alone with chemotherapy and radiation therapy. Four cycles of cisplatin 20 mg/m$^2$ per day i.v. and 5 FU 200 mg/m$^2$ per day ×5 days were alternated with three courses of radiotherapy 20 Gy each. Among 101 evaluated patients there was a 46% complete response in patients receiving combined modality therapy and only 28% in patients receiving radiation therapy alone; there was also a statistically significant difference in survival ($P < 0.05$) and event free survival (EFS) ($P < 0.003$).

Al Sarraf et al. [55] in behalf of the inter cooperative study groups reported on the significant better results seen in a group of 71 patients with nasopharyngeal cancer that received cisplatin 100 mg/m$^2$ on days 1, 22 and 43 of a radiation therapy regimen followed by 4 cycles of cisplatin and infusional 5 FU 1000 mg/m$^2$ ×4 days every 4 weeks; they had a

1 year survival of 80% and median progression free survival of 52 months versus 55% 1 year survival and 13 months PFS in the group that received radiation therapy alone.

A similar experience concerning potentiation of radiation therapy by concomitant chemotherapy was reported by John et al. [56,57] in patients with esophageal carcinoma. Infusional 5-FU was administered in combination with cisplatin or mitomycin C or high dose methotrexate with calcium leucovorin rescue. These sequential studies indicated that an increase in the total dose of radiation delivered to the primary lesion together with an increase in the number of drugs administered in combination with 5-FU led to a parallel increase in the complete response rate from 57 to 72% and finally to 100% and a decrease in the local failure rate from 50 to 15%. The superiority of chemotherapy with cisplatin on day 1 and infusional 5 FU on days 1–4 given at 3 weeks interval to 61 patients with squamous cell carcinoma of the esophagus was demonstrated by an intergroup phase III study [58] in which another 59 patients received radiation therapy alone. There was a 42% survival at 24 months for the combined modality arm versus only 10% survival in the radiation therapy alone arm. As in head and neck carcinomas, achieving complete clinical and histological response documented by a random endoscopic biopsy does not preclude local recurrences nor does it have a significant impact on 5-year survival rates as projected by the analysis of the two early studies by John et al. It is of note that in the studies concerning locally advanced esophageal carcinoma approximately 25% of all cases were adenocarcinomas and that in these cases and those with squamous cell carcinoma histology results were similar.

The improved response rates of adenocarcinoma of the esophagus to a combination of infusional 5-FU with cisplatin and concomitant radiation was confirmed by a study of 21 patients with adenocarcinoma of the gastro-esophageal junction. These patients received three cycles of 5-FU (1000 mg/m$^2$ per day) and cisplatin (20 mg/m$^2$ per day) infusion for 96 h, concomitantly with 5 Gy radiation therapy [59]. In 16 cases the treatment was followed by radical surgery which revealed complete histological responses in five cases, microscopic tumors in six and gross tumors in five. This is better than the response found in historical controls but inferior to that reported for cases of squamous cell carcinoma of the esophagus. In the same study, while patients' median survival was improved vis-à-vis that of historical controls, no improvement in long-term survival was noted.

Finally, the infusional 5-FU cisplatin combination was successfully used in patients with squamous cell carcinoma of the cervix [60]. This led to a decrease in the rate of recurrence at 3 years from 60% in historical controls in whom radiation therapy was administered with concomitant 5-FU alone to 35% in the relatively small series of patients who received cisplatin as well as 5-FU infusion with concomitant irradiation.

Despite significant progress in the rate and duration of response, these studies of combined cisplatin–5-FU infusional therapy with concomitant radiation therapy indicate that in squamous cell carcinoma of the head and neck, esophagus and cervix, as well as in the few adenocarcinomas tested cure is not yet achievable at a statistically significant rate.

## 8. Radiation potentiation by cisplatin–5-FU combination infusional chemotherapy and oral hydroxyurea

Hydroxyurea is a potent inhibitor of the enzyme ribonucleotide reductase which leads to inhibition of DNA synthesis only in cells that are actively synthesizing DNA during the period of drug exposure. As an inhibitor of DNA repair hydroxyurea may potentially interact with alkylating agents or irradiation to enhance cytotoxicity. It may simply have additive effects with radiation as an S phase specific agent [61] and also inhibits the excision repair of thymine dimers and single strand DNA breaks induced by irradiation [62]. Hydroxyurea also is able to synchronize cells by preventing their entry from the radiosensitive $G_1$ phase to the relatively radioresistant S phase of the cell cycle [63].

Early clinical trials of radiation therapy with concomitant hydroxyurea showed mixed results in patients with head and neck cancer with benefits reported by Richards and Chambers [64] and no advantage found by Stefani et al. [65]. The results were, however, clearly favorable in patients with carcinoma of the cervix [66].

For this reason Vokes and associates tested in several trials [67–69] the effect of the addition of hydroxyurea to 5-FU by continuous intravenous infusion (800 mg/m$^2$ per day ×5 days) in an attempt to increase the radiation enhancing effect.

Among 15 evaluable patients that had received prior radiation there were 6 complete responders and 8 partial responders [68].

Among 17 evaluable patients who received the above regimen as first line therapy there were 12 complete responders while the other 5 patients had partial responses. The median survival of patients in group I was of 8 months while those in group II had a median survival of 14 months [68].

These data are among the best ever reported reasons why hydroxyurea continues to be tested in other combinations [69] and at different dose levels.


## 9.  Radiation potentiation by doxorubicin

Doxorubicin (adriamycin) is an antitumor antibiotic from the anthracyclines family which has the broadest clinical applications in the treatment of malignant neoplasms. It is toxic to the cells through its ability to intercalate in the DNA and RNA structure as well as through three distinct chemical interactions; two reactions in the cells result from transferring one electron which ultimately generate free toxic intracellular superoxide anion radicals. The third reaction consists of carbonyl reduction of the chromophore side chain and produces the alcohol metabolite of doxorubicin, doxorubicinol, which also has potent antiproliferative and antineoplastic actions.

The in vitro interaction between doxorubicin and irradiation in mammalian tumor cells has been studied since 1977 [70]. The combination was found to be synergistic at lower doses and additive when the doxorubicin dose was increased to more than 0.15 mg/kg body weight. Despite this finding, and despite early clinical trials showing that single pulses of doxorubicin in conventional doses (40–60 mg/m$^2$ per day every 3 weeks) were well tolerated [71] the predominant view for many years was that doxorubicin administered concomitantly with radiation therapy led to increased toxicity represented by enteritis, esophagitis, cardiomyopathy [72] and a skin recall phenomenon [73].

The radiopotentiating effects on certain neoplasms (sarcomas and some hepatocellular carcinomas) of doxorubicin administered by continuous infusion concomitantly with irradiation and the clinical feasibility of this approach were first reported by Rosenthal et al. [74]. The use of this regimen was based on prior reports [75] showing a significant reduction in doxorubicin cardiotoxicity when administered over periods of 96 h as compared with a bolus intravenous administration of an equal dose. The kinetics of the doxorubicin infusion [74] indicate an initial delay of approximately 16 h in reaching maximum serum level probably due to doxorubicin's initial diffusion to various tissues from where it is subsequently released. A steady level is reached after 30 h of the 120 h infusion.

In the preliminary pilot study [75] 4 out of 9 patients with locally advanced or metastatic soft tissue sarcomas achieved complete response at the level of all lesions that received radiation therapy concomitantly with the 5-day cycle of continuous infusion doxorubicin at a concentration of 12 mg/m$^2$ per day. The cycles were repeated every 3–4 weeks (split-course therapy). Two out of the original 3 patients with advanced loco-regional recurrent disease without distant metastases who achieved complete remission have maintained their remission longer than 5 years and are probably cured. The same regimen was administered to another 11 cases with similarly beneficial results [76]. There were 4 partial and 4 complete responses with a mean duration of the response of $152 \pm 12$ weeks for patients in complete remission and of $32 \pm 7$ weeks for patients achieving partial remissions. Of interest is the fact that complete remission as well as maximum tumor size reduction in patients with only partial remissions were all achieved at a significantly lower total dose of radiation therapy (mean 38 Gy) than the amount needed in historical controls to achieve equal results using conventional non-split course radiation therapy (mean 65 Gy). Similar results were also reported by Toma et al. [77] and Palumbo et al. [78] and are discussed elsewhere in this volume. By giving to their patients G-CSF after the completion of doxorubicin infusion these investigators could administer the cycles of therapy at 3 weeks instead of 4-week intervals. They noted 3 complete responses and 17 partial remissions among 35 patients with soft tissue sarcomas with an overall response rate of 57%. The overall median survival of these patients was of 12 months for the whole group and of 22.2 months for the responders. However, 13 of the responders underwent radical surgery after 2–3 cycles of combined therapy; their median survival was of 38 months.

The results of the same regimen of doxorubicin by continuous infusion and concomitant split course radiation therapy administered to 12 patients with hepatocellular carcinoma [79] also indicated some antineoplastic activity for this combination only when three cycles of doxorubicin (60 mg/m$^2$ per 5 day cycle) and at least 24 Gy radiation therapy were delivered. There were 4 partial remissions among 7 patients that completed the treatment. The other 5 patients received just one or two cycles due to disease progression [79].

Thus it appears that doxorubicin has an enhancing effect on the radiation treatment of soft tissue sarcomas and to a lesser extent of hepatomas. Its use as a possible radiation potentiator agent is still under investigation; this effect could be further enhanced by the incorporation of doxorubicin in liposome as in doxil, an agent that has recently significantly improved the results of the therapy of Kaposi's sarcoma.

## 10. Bleomycin as radiation potentiator

Bleomycin is a unique antitumor antibiotic isolated from a soil *Streptomyces*. It acts as a nuclease causing DNA strand scissions and release of thymidine from the DNA strand. Because of this, bleomycin interferes with DNA cellular repair that follows cell irradiation and such it could have a radiosensitizing effect.

For a relatively brief period bleomycin was frequently used in studies testing the potential radiation enhancing effect of chemotherapeutic agents especially in patients with head and neck squamous cell carcinoma.

While Cachin et al. [80] reported only borderline advantage for bleomycin administered weekly during the radiation treatment of 86 patients with advanced head and neck cancer, Shanta and Krishmanvitta [81] and Fu et al. [82] reported statistically significant differences in overall responses in favor of radiation therapy administered with concurrent bleomycin 15–30 mg. i.v. or i.m. two to three times weekly during the duration of irradiation as compared with results in patients that received radiation therapy alone (80% versus 20% in Shanta's study; 67% versus 45% in the Fu et al. study). In the latter study patients also received maintenance therapy with methotrexate and bleomycin.

However, due to high incidence of pulmonary interstitial fibrosis following protracted use of bleomycin, its clinical study as potential radiation sensitizer was abandoned. It was replaced during the last 4 years by the excitement created by early favorable results of paclitaxel as radiation sensitizer.

## 11. Paclitaxel as radiation potentiator

As member of the taxanes class of antineoplastic compounds paclitaxel main activity is to bind to microtubules during the $G_2/M$ phases and to make them resistant to depolymerization. This results in irreversible damage due to the cell arrest in the $G_2/M$ phases of the cell cycle; this could, at its turn result in increased cell sensitivity to irradiation due to increase synchronization of malignant cells [83]. In preclinical studies the radiation sensitizing enhancement effect of paclitaxel was demonstrated in human derived cell lines from an astrocytoma [84], from an ovarian carcinoma [85] and a head and neck squamous cell carcinoma [86].

It was soon realized that the radiosensitizing effect of paclitaxel was also due to its activity as an inducer of cell apoptosis [87] as well as to its role as potentiator of cell reoxygenation [88]. These data led Choy et al. [89] to conduct an initial phase I clinical study of paclitaxel administered with concomitant radiation therapy as a weekly 3 h infusion whose MTD was established at 60 mg/m². It was soon realized that paclitaxel cytotoxic effect increases up to a certain concentration (5–10 nmol/l) above which it becomes highly dependent on exposure time [90]. This led Wilson et al. to perform a phase I study [91] of paclitaxel administered by 96 h continuous intravenous infusion whose MTD was established at 140 mg/m² per 96 h. A similar schedule of paclitaxel was administered by Rambhia et al. [93] in a phase I study in conjunction with daily standard doses of radiation therapy. Its MTD was established at 130 mg/m² per 96 h.

Following these initial observations several phase II studies of paclitaxel with concomitant radiation therapy were performed and many other are in course of completion. Chamberlain et al. [93] and Glantz et al. [94] conducted phase I/II studies of weekly paclitaxel administered over 3 h infusion and daily radiation therapy to recurrent or residual brain tumors; an improved median survival to 9.2 months versus the expected 3.5 months was reported for this group of previously treated patients. Glantz and Choy et al. have recently updated the results of their phase I/II studies in patients with brain tumors and non-small cell carcinoma of the lung [95]. Among the patients with recurrent glioblastoma multiforme in 12 patients who underwent reoperation for recurrent lesions at the original tumor site accelerated radiation necrosis was noted after a median of 49 days following completion of treatment.

Among 29 evaluable patients with NSCLC who received weekly paclitaxel and concomitant radiation therapy 2 had a complete response and 23 a partial response for an 86% overall response rate. At 12 months followup the survival rate among these patients was 61% while their median survival was not yet reached [95]. In a parallel phase I/II study in stage IIIB non-small cell carcinoma of the lung [96] Wolf et al. reported a 75% response rate among 24 evaluable patients.

Several teams of investigators [97,98] have recently reported on the concomitant administration of thoracic radiotherapy and paclitaxel in combination with carboplatin in patients with locally advanced non-small cell carcinoma of the lung. An 82% overall response was reported among 23 patients who received weekly paclitaxel 50 mg/m$^2$ and carboplatin at AUC of 2 with concomitant radiation over 6–7 weeks followed by 2 cycles of paclitaxel/carboplatin at 3 weeks interval [97]. Bonomi et al. [99] have administered also etoposide together with paclitaxel and carboplatin in 9 patients that underwent successful pulmonary resection. Two of these cases presented histologic complete remission at the time of surgery.

Paclitaxel as radiosensitizer have been recently tested in combination with other radiation potentiators in the therapy of head and neck cancer. Haraf et al. [100] reported a 95% response rate with 59% complete remissions among 22 evaluable patients with locally advanced cancer who received paclitaxel low dose continuous infusion (15–25 mg/m$^2$ per day) in combination with 5-FU infusion and oral hydroxyurea. A combination of paclitaxel (200 mg/m$^2$ as 3 h infusion) and carboplatin dosed to an area under the curve of 7 (mg-min/ml) given every 4 weeks during radiation treatment led to an overall response rate of 20% among 28 patients with advanced nasopharyngeal cancer [100]. Better results were reported after the administration of weekly paclitaxel at an MTD of 40 mg/m$^2$ per week and carboplatin at 100 mg/m$^2$ per week during the duration of radiation therapy to 18 patients with unresectable squamous cell carcinoma of the head and neck. There were two complete and 6 partial responses among 11 evaluable patients [102]. Limiting toxicities in all these studies were represented by neutropenia with its accompanying complication and mucositis that can be severe.

Paclitaxel as radiosensitizer is currently tested in many centers for its potential capability to improve results of the therapy of locally advanced tumors of the esophagus, pancreas, stomach. It is tested in combination with cisplatin and 40 Gy concurrent radiation in esophageal cancers [103]. In pancreatic cancer a weekly 3 h infusion of 50 mg/m$^2$ paclitaxel concomitant with irradiation to the pancreas for 5–6 weeks led to a 27% partial response rate among 11 patients with measurable disease [104].

Paclitaxel possible admixture with some of the other radiation potentiator agents is also under investigation.

## 12. Admixture of radiation enhancing chemotherapeutic agents

The admixture of some of the radiation enhancing drugs previously described in the same solution for combined concomitant administration with radiation therapy represents an area of investigative interest for two reasons: its potential superior results as compared with the radiation enhancing effect of each of the components of the admixture and its significant ease of administration at lower cost as compared with the need for separate central venous ports or separate peripheral intravenous access for each of the admixture components.

So far there are no systematic studies of such radiation sensitizer admixtures; likely because it was first necessary to establish the radiation enhancing effect of each of the chemotherapeutic agents before attempting to admix them. Once the best radiation enhancing agents are identified their possible use as an admixture could be explored. This is currently done in several centers.

The major practical issue in any admixture of different drugs in the same solution is related to the stability of the pharmacological effects of the individual drugs in this new environment. A comprehensive review of the current information concerning the stability of various chemotherapeutic agents in various solutions was published by Williams and Lokich [105]. It offers the basis for developing new studies of the potential benefits of the admixtures of some of the proven radiation potentiator agents previously reviewed.

From the data presented by Williams and Lokich only a few radiation potentiators appear stable in normal saline solutions for up to 7 days:

– cisplatin (up to 0.2 mg/ml) and etoposide (up to 0.4 mg/m$^2$)
– cisplatin (up to 1 mg/ml) and floxuridine (up to 10 mg/m$^2$); the latter is a more stable metabolite of 5-FU
– carboplatin (up to 1 mg/ml) and etoposide (up to 0.2 mg/ml).

The majority of the other radiation potentiators were not studied in admixtures.

## 13.  Future directions

From this relatively brief and by no means exhaustive review of the progress made in the study of radiation interaction with chemotherapeutic agents that could enhance its antineoplastic effect it becomes apparent that this field is still in its early development.

Future progress is expected from different directions of investigation:

– New drugs are tested for their potential radiation enhancing effect. Among them gemcitabine and the topotecans appear to have significant radiosensitizing effect in preclinical studies.
– Phase III clinical studies are carried out to prove that the addition of a chemotherapy agent to radiation results in a synergistic antineoplastic effect of these two therapeutic modalities.
– The study of the admixture in the same solution of the best radiosensitizing chemotherapeutic agents should also lead to possible therapeutic benefits.
– Finally, significant progress could be expected from the new advances in understanding the molecular event conducive to carcinogenesis which would lead to the development of treatments especially targeted at these events (some of them are presented in the 5th section of this volume). These new therapies could replace or be incorporated in the current chemo-radiation regimens which is expected to increase their curability rate while decreasing their toxicities and side effects.

## References

1.  Heidelberger C, Greisbach C, Montag BJ, et al. Studies in fluorinated pyrimidine. II Effects of transplanted tumor: Cancer Res 18: 305–317, 1958.
2.  Shimoyama M. The cytocidal action of alkylating agents and anticancer antibodies against in vitro cultured Yoshida ascites sarcoma cells. Jpn Soc Cancer Ther 10: 63–72, 1975.

3.    Nigro ND, Vaitkevicius VK, Considine Jr B. Combined therapy for cancer of the anal canal: a preliminary report. Dis Colon Rectum 17: 354–336, 1974

4.    Coleman NA, Bump EA, Kramer RA. Chemical modifiers of cancer treatment. J Clin Oncol 6: 709–733, 1988.

5.    Wolinsky I, Swiniorsky J, Kensler CI, Venditi JM. Combination radiotherapy and chemotherapy for P388 lymphocytic leukemia in vitro. Cancer Treatment Rep 4: 73–76, 1974.

6.    Douple EB, Richmond RC, Logan ME. Preclinical studies with platinum compounds. J Clin Hematol Oncol 7: 585–603, 1977.

7.    Douple EB. Keynote address: platinum-radiation interactions. NCI Monogr 6: 315–319, 1988.

8.    Douple EB, Tollen MD, Spencer F. Platinum levels in murine tumor following intraperitoneal administration of cisplatin or paraplatin. NCI Monogr 6: 129–132, 1988.

9.    DeWitt L. Combined treatment of radiation and cisdiammine dichloroplatinum(II). A review of experimental and clinical data. Int J Radiat Oncol Biol Phys 13: 403–426, 1987.

10.   Fu KK, Rayner PA, Lam KN. Modification of continuous low dose rate irradiation by concurrent chemotherapy infusion. Int J Radiat Oncol Biol Phys 10: 1473–1478, 1984.

11.   Douple EB, Willis ML, Jones EL. Radiopotentiation in a murine tumor (MTG-B) by continuous infusion platinum. In: Rotman M, Rosenthal CJ (Eds), Concomitant Continuous Infusion Chemotherapy and Radiotherapy. Berlin: Springer, pp. 191–196, 1991.

12.   Kyriazis AP, Yagoda A, Kereiasker JG, et al. Experimental studies on the radiation modifying effect of Cis-diamminedichloroplatinum II (DDP) in human bladder transitional cell carcinomas grown in nude mice. Cancer 52: 452–457, 1983.

13.   Dritschilo A, Piro AJ, Kelman AD. The effect of cisplatin on the repair of radiation damage in plateau phase Chinese hamster (V-79) cells. Int J Radiat Oncol Biol Phys 5: 1345–1349, 1979.

14.   Reimer RR, Gahbauer R and Bukowski RM. Simultaneous treatment with cisplatin and radiation therapy for advanced solid tumors: a pilot study. Cancer Treat Rep 6: 19–222, 1981.

15.   Soloway MS, Kard M, Scheinberry M, et al. Concurrent radiation and cisplatin in the treatment of advanced bladder cancer: a preliminary report. J Urol 128: 1031–1033, 1982.

16.   Al-Sarraf M, Pajak TF, Marciol VA, et al. Concurrent radiotherapy and chemotherapy with cisplatin in inoperable squamous cell carcinoma of the head and neck. Cancer 59: 259, 265, 1987.

17.   Wheeler P, Salter M, Stephans S, et al. Simultaneous therapy with high dose cisplatin and radiation for unresectable squamous cell cancer of the head and neck: a phase I-II study. NCI Monogr 6: 339–341, 1988.

18.   Jakse G, Raushmeier H, Fritsch E, et al. Die Intergrier at radiotherapic and chemotherapic des lokal fortyeschrittenen harnblesenkarcinomas. Akt Urol 17: 68–73, 1986.

19.   Coppin C and Brown E. Concurrent cisplatin with radiation for locally advanced bladder cancer: a pilot study suggesting improved survival. Proc Am Soc Clin Oncol 5: 99, 1986.

20.   Shipley WU, Prant GR, Einstein AB, et al. Treatment of invasive bladder cancer by cisplatin and radiation in patients unsuited for surgery. J Am Med Assoc 258: 931–935, 1987.

21.   Rosenthal CJ, Rotman M, Choi K, Sand J. Cisplatin by continuous infusion with concurrent radiation in malignant tumors (a phase I-II study). In: Rosenthal CJ, Rotman M. (Eds), Clinical Applications of Continuous Infusion Chemotherapy and Concomitant Radiation Therapy. New York: Plenum Press, pp. 177–180, 1986.

22.   Sauer R, Schrott KM, Dunst J, et al. Preliminary results in the treatment of invasive bladder carcinoma with radiotherapy and cisplatinum. Int J Radiat Oncol Biol Phys 15: 871–875, 1988.

23.   Rotman M, Choi K, Isaacson S, et al. Treatment of recurrent carcinoma of the paranasal sinuses using concomitant infusion cis-platinum and radiation therapy. In: Rosenthal CJ, Rotman M. (Eds), Clinical Applications of Continuous Infusion Chemotherapy and Concomitant Radiation Therapy. New York: Plenum Press, pp. 189–194, 1986.

24.   Choi K, Rotman M, Aziz H, Stark RS, Rosenthal CJU, Marti J. Locally advanced paranasal sinus and nasopharyngeal cancers. Effects of hyperfractionated radiation and concomitant continuous infusion cisplatin. In: Rotman M, Rosenthal CJ (Eds), Concomitant Continuous Infusion Chemotherapy and Radiotherapy. Berlin: Springer, pp. 197–204, 1991.

25.   Vietti J, Eggerding F, Valeriote E. Combined effect of radiation and 5-FU on survival on transplanted leukemia cells. J Natl Cancer Inst 47: 865–870, 1971.

26.   Seifert P, Baker LH, Reed ML, Vaitkevicius KV. Comparison of continuously infused 5-fluorouracil with bolus injection in patients with colorectal adenocarcinoma. Cancer 36: 123–128, 1975.

27. Byfield JE, Chan PYM, Seargran SL. Radiosensitization of 5 FU: molecular origins and clinical scheduling implications. Proc Am Assoc Cancer Res 18: 74(abstr), 1977.
28. Byfield JE, Barone R, Mendelsohn J, et al. Infusional 5-fluorouracil and x-ray therapy for nonresectable esophageal cancer. Cancer 45: 703–708, 1980.
29. Sishy B, Remington JH, Hinson J, et al. Definitive treatment of anal-canal carcinoma by means of radiation therapy and chemotherapy. Dis Colon Rectum 25: 686–688, 1982.
30. Cummings BJ, Rider WD, Harwood AR. Combined radical radiation therapy and chemotherapy for esophageal carcinoma. Am J Clin Oncol 7: 653, 1982.
31. Papillon J. Radiation therapy in the management of the epidermoid carcinoma of the anal region. Dis Colon 17: 181–187, 1974.
32. Coia LR, Eugstrom PF, Paul A, et al. A pilot study of combined radiotherapy and chemotherapy for esophageal carcinoma. Am J Clin Oncol 7: 653, 1984.
33. Keane TJ, Harwood AR, Elhakim T, et al. Radical radiation therapy with 5-fluorouracil infusion and mitomycin C for esophageal squamous cell carcinoma. Radiother Oncol 4: 205–210, 1985.
34. Coia LR, Stafford P, Engstrom PF, et al. The use of infusional 5 fluorouracil, mitomycin C and radiation as the primary management of esophageal cancer. In: Rotman M, Rosenthal CJ (Eds), Concomitant Continuous Infusion Chemotherapy and Radiotherapy. Berlin: Springer, pp. 143–148, 1991.
35. Routh AM, Barton B, Lee CPY. Effect of caffeine in L-cells exposed to Mitomycin C. Cancer Res 30: 2724–2729, 1970.
36. Weissberg JB, Sou YH, Papac RJ, et al. Randomized clinical trial of mitomycin C as an adjunct to radiotherapy in head and neck cancer. Int J Radiat Oncol Biol Phys 17: 3–9, 1989.
37. Cummings BJ, Keane TG, O'Sullivan B. Epidermoid anal cancer. Treatment by radiation and 5 fluorouracil with or without mitomycin C. Int J Radiat Oncol Biol Phys 21: 1115–1125, 1991.
38. Flam M, John M, Pajak TF, et al. Role of mitomycin in combination with fluorouracil and radiotherapy and of salvage chemoradiation in the definitive non-surgical treatment of the epidermoid carcinoma of the anal canal: results of a Phase III randomized Intergroup study. J Clin Oncol 14: 2527–2539, 1996.
39. Thomas G, Dembo A, Fyles A, et al. Concurrent chemoradiation in advanced cervical cancer. Gynecol Oncol 328: 446–451, 1990.
40. Grau C, Overgaard J. Radiosensitizing and cytotoxic properties of mitomycin C in C3H mouse mammary carcinoma in vivo. Int J Radiat Oncol Biol Phys 20: 265–269, 1991.
41. Rosenthal CJ, Rotman M, Choi KN, et al. Rapid tumor lysis induced by mitomycin C (MC) administered by continuous infusion (CI) with concomitant radiation therapy (RT). A phase I study (Abstr). Proc Am. Assoc Cancer Res 32: 391, 1991.
42. Leichman L, Steiger Z, Seydel HG, Vaitkevicius VK. Combined preoperative chemotherapy and radiation therapy for cancer of the esophagus: the Wayne State University, Southwest Oncology Group and Radiation Therapy Oncology Group experience. Semin Oncol 11: 178–185, 1984.
43. Cummings BJ, Keane TJ, Harwood AR, Thomas GM. Combined modality therapy with 5-fluorouracil, mitomycin C and radiation therapy for squamous cell cancers. In: Rosenthal CJ, Rotman M (Eds), Clinical Applications of Continuous Infusion Chemotherapy and Concomitant Radiation Therapy. New York: Plenum Press, 1986, pp. 133–147.
44. Rotman M, Macchia R, Silverstein M, et al. Treatment of bladder carcinoma with concomitant infusion chemotherapy and irradiation. In: Rosenthal CJ, Rotman M (Eds), Clinical Applications of Continuous Infusion Chemotherapy and Concomitant Radiation Therapy. New York: Plenum Press, pp. 149–153, 1986.
45. Rotman M, Macchia R, Silverstein M, et al. Treatment of advanced bladder carcinoma with irradiation and concomitant 5-fluorouracil infusion. Cancer 59: 710–714, 1987.
46. Russell KJ, Boileou MA, Tretori RC, et al. Transitional cell carcinoma of the urinary bladder: histologic clearance with combined 5-FU chemotherapy and radiation therapy. Preliminary results of bladder preservation study. Radiology 167: 848, 1988.
47. Rotman M, Aziz H, Parruzzo M, et al. Treatment of advanced transitional cell Ca. of the bladder with irradiation and concomitant 5-fluorouracil infusion. Int J Radiat Oncol Biol Phys 19: 1131–1137, 1990.
48. Bloom HJD, Henry W, Wallace D, Skeet R. Treatment of T3 bladder cancer. A controlled trial of preoperative radiotherapy and radical mastectomy versus radical radiotherapy. Br J Urol 54: 136–151, 1982.
49. van der Werf-Messing G, Friedall GH, Menon RS, et al. Carcinoma of the urinary bladder T2 Nx Mo treated by preoperative irradiation followed by cystectomy. Int J Radiat Oncol Biol Phys 8: 1849–1855, 1982.

50. Haghbin M, Sishy B, Hinson EJ. Combined modality preoperative therapy in poor prognostic rectal adenocarcinoma. Radiat Oncol 13: 75–81, 1988.

51. Taylor SG IV, Murthy AK, Caldarelli DD, et al. Improved control in advanced head and neck cancer with simultaneous radiation and cisplatin/5-FU chemotherapy. Cancer Treat Rep 69: 938–939, 1985.

52. Adelstein D. Sharan V, Earle A, et al. Simultaneous radiotherapy and chemotherapy with 5 fluorouracil and cisplatin for locally confined squamous cell head and neck cancer. NCI Monogr 6: 347–351, 1988.

53. Wendt TC, Wustrow TPU, Hortenstein RC, et al. Accelerated split course radiotherapy and simultaneous cis-dichloro diammine platinum and 5-fluorouracil chemotherapy with folinic acid enhancement for unresectable carcinoma of the head and neck. Radiat Oncol 10: 277–284, 1987.

54. Merlano N, Corvo R, Margarino G, et al. Combined chemotherapy and radiation therapy in advanced inoperable squamous cell carcinoma of the head and neck. The final report of a randomized trial Cancer 67: 915–921, 1991.

55. Al Sarraf M, LeBlanc M, Giri PGS, et al. Superiority of chemo-radiotherapy (CT-RT) versus radiotherapy (RT) in patients (pts.) with locally advanced nasopharengeal cancer. Preliminary results of intergroup (0099) randomized study. Proc Am Soc Clin Oncol 15: 882(Abstr), 1996.

56. John M, Flam M, Wittlinger P, Mowry PA. Inoperable esophageal carcinoma: results of aggressive synchronous radiotherapy and chemotherapy, a pilot study. Am J Clin Oncol 10: 310–316, 1987.

57. John MJ, Flam M, Mowry PA, et al. Radiotherapy alone and chemoradiation for nonmetastatic esophageal carcinoma. A critical review of chemoradiation. Cancer 63: 2397–2403, 1989.

58. Herskovic A, Mortz K, Al Sarraf M, et al. Intergroup esophageal study: comparison of radiotherapy (RT) to radio chemotherapy combination: A phase III trial (Abstract). Proc Am Soc Clin Oncol 10: 407, 1991.

59. Burton GV, Wolfe WG, Crocker I, et al. Adenocarcinoma of the gastroesophageal function: preoperative cisplatin and concomitant continuous infusion 5-fluorouracil and radiation therapy. In: Rotman M, Rosenthal CJ (Eds), Concomitant Continuous Infusion Chemotherapy and Radiotherapy. Berlin: Springer, pp. 255–258, 1991.

60. John M, Cooke K, Flam M, et al. Preliminary results of concomitant radiotherapy and chemotherapy in advanced cervical carcinoma. Gynecol Oncol 28: 101–110, 1987.

61. Donehower RC. Hydroxyurea. In: Chabner BA, Collins JM (Eds), Cancer Chemotherapy: Principles and Practice. Philadelphia, PA: Lippincott, pp. 424–448, 1990.

62. From RJ, Kute DW: Effect of 1-beta-D-arabinofuranosylcytosine and hydroyurea on the repair of x-ray-induced DNA single-strand breaks in human leukemia blasts. Biochem Pharmacol 34: 2557–2560, 1985.

63. Sinclair WK: The combined effect of hydroxyurea and x-rays on Chinese hamster cells in vitro. Cancer Res 28: 198–206, 1968.

64. Richards GJ, Chambers RG. Hydroxyurea: a radiosensitizer in the treatment of neoplasms of the head and neck. Am J Roentgen Radium Nucl Med 55: 555–565, 1969.

65. Stefano S, Ells RW, Abata J. Hydroxyurea and radiotherapy in head and neck cancer. Radiology 101: 391, 1971.

66. Piter MS, Barlo JJ, Vongtame V, et al. Hydroxyurea: a radiation potentiator in carcinoma of the uterine cervix. Am J Obstet Gynecol 147: 803–808, 1983.

67. Vokes EE, Panje WR, Shilsky RI, et al. Hydroxyurea, fluorouracil and concomitant radiotherapy in poor prognosis head and neck cancer. A phase I-II study. J Clin Oncol 7: 761–768, 1989.

68. Vokes EE, Choi KE, Schilsky RL, et al: Cisplatin, fluorouracil and high dose leucovorin for recurrent or metastatic head and neck cancer. J Clin Oncol 6: 618–626, 1988.

69. Vokes EE, Moormeier JA, Ratain MJ, et al. 5-fluorouracil leucovorin, hydroxyurea and escalating doses of continuous infusion cisplatin with concomitant radiotherapy. A clinical and pharmacologic study. Cancer Chemother Pharmacol 29: 178–184, 1992.

70. Byfield JE, Lynch M, Kulhaman I, Chan PYM. Cellular effects of combined adriamycin and x-ray irradiation in human tumor cells. Cancer 19: 194–204, 1977.

71. Byfield JE, Watring WG, Kemkin SR, et al. Adriamycin: a useful adjuvant drug for combination radiation therapy. Proc Am Assoc Cancer Res - Am Soc Clin Oncol 16: 253(Abstr), 1977.

72. Rosen G, Tefft M, Martinez A, et al. Combination chemotherapy and radiation therapy in the treatment of metastatic osteogenic sarcoma. Cancer 35: 622–630, 1975.

73. Cassidy JR. Radiation-Adriamycin interaction; preliminary clinical observations. Cancer 36: 946–948, 1975.

74. Rosenthal CJ, Rotman M, Bhutiani M. Concomitant radiation therapy and doxorubicin by continuous infusion in advanced malignancies: a phase I-II study: evidence of synergistic effects in soft tissue sarco-

mas and hepatomas. In: Rosenthal CJ, Rotman M (Eds), Clinical Applications of Continuous Infusion Chemotherapy and Concomitant Radiation Therapy. New York: Plenum Press, pp. 159–176, 1986.

75.   Rosenthal CJ, Rotman M. Pilot study of interaction of radiation therapy with doxorubicin by continuous infusion. NCI Monogr 6: 285–290, 1988.

76.   Rosenthal CJ, Rotman M. Concomitant continuous infusion adriamycin and radiation. Evidence of synergistic effects in soft tissue sarcomas. In: Rotman M, Rosenthal CJ (Eds), Concomitant Continuous Infusion Chemotherapy and Radiotherapy. Berlin: Springer, pp. 271–279, 1991.

77.   Toma S, Palumbo R, Grimaldi A, et al. Concomitant radiation-doxorubicin administration in locally advanced or metastatic soft tissue sarcomas. In: Banzet P, Holland JF, Khagot D, Weil M (Eds), Cancer Treatment, An update. Berlin: Springer, pp. 581–583, 1994.

78.   Palumbo R, Grimaldi A, Canovese G, et al. Concomitant radiotherapy at low doses in locally advanced and/or metastatic soft tissue sarcomas (STS): long term follow up. Ann Oncol 7: 117(Abstr), 562P, 1996.

79.   Stark RS, Rosenthal CJ, Rotman M. Infusion Adriamycin and radiation in hepatomas. In: Rotman M, Rosenthal CJ (Eds), Concomitant Continuous Infusion Chemotherapy and Radiotherapy. Berlin: Springer, pp. 281–284, 1991.

80.   Cachin Y, Jortag A, Sanchott, et al. Preliminary results of a randomized EORTC study comparing radiotherapy and concomitant bleomycin to radiotherapy alone in epidermoid carcinoma of the oropharynx. Eur J Cancer 13: 1389, 1977.

81.   Shanta V, Krishmanvitta S. Combined bleomycin and radiotherapy in oral cancer. Clin Radiol 31: 617, 1980.

82.   Fu KK, Philipp T, Salveerberg T, et al. Combined radiotherapy and chemotherapy with bleomycin and methotrexate for advanced, inoperable head and neck cancer. J Clin Oncol 5: 1410, 1987.

83.   Schiff PB, Horwitz SB. Taxol stabilizes microtubules in mouse fibroblast cells. Proc Natl Acad Sci USA 77: 1561–1565, 1980.

84.   Tischler RB, Geard CR, Hall EJ, et al. Taxol sensitizes human astrocytoma cell lines to radiation. Cancer Res 52: 3459–3497, 1992.

85.   Stern A, Sevin BU, Perras J. Taxol sensitizes human ovarian cancer cells to radiation. Cancer Res 48: 252–258, 1993.

86.   Hoffman W, Rodeman HP, Balka C, et al. Paclitaxel in simultaneous radiochemotherapy of head and neck cancer: preclinical and clinical studies. Semin Oncol 24(Suppl 2): 72–77, 1997.

87.   Milos L, Hunter N, Kurdoglu B, et al. Apoptotic death of mitotically arrested cells in murine tumors treated with taxol. Proc Am Assoc Cancer Res 35: 314, 1994.

88.   Milos L., Hunter N, Kurdoglu B, et al. Enhancement of tumor radioresponse of a murine mammary carcinoma by paclitaxel. Cancer Res 54: 3506–3510, 1994.

89.   Choy H, Akerley W, Safron H, et al. Phase I Trial of outpatient weekly paclitaxel and concurrent radiation therapy for advanced non small cell carcinoma of the lung. J Clin Oncol 12: 2682–2686, 1994.

90.   Lopes NM, Adams EG, Pitts TW, et al. Cell kill kinetics and cell cycle effects of taxol on human and hamster ovarian cell lines. Cancer Chemother Pharmacol 32: 234–242, 1993.

91.   Wilson HH, Berg SI, Bryant G, et al. Paclitaxel in doxorubicin refractory or mitoxantrone refractory breast cancer. A phase I/II trial of 96 h infusion. J Clin Oncol 12: 1621–1629, 1994.

92.   Rambhia H, Aziz H, Rotman M, et al. Paclitaxel 96 h i.v. infusion with concomitant radiation therapy. Phase I study. Proc Am Soc Clin Oncol 14: 473, 1563, 1995.

93.   Chamberlain MC, Kormanik P. Salvage chemotherapy with paclitaxel for recurrent primary brain tumors. J Clin Oncol 13: 2066–2071, 1995.

94.   Glantz M, Choy H, Kearns M, et al. Phase I study of weekly outpatient paclitaxel and concurrent cranial irradiation in adults with astrocytoma. J Clin Oncol 14: 600–609, 1996.

95.   Glantz M, Choy H, Akerley W, et al. Weekly paclitaxel with and without concurrent radiation therapy: toxicity, pharmacokinetics and response. Semin Oncol 23(Suppl 16): 128–135, 1996.

96.   Wolf M, Faora C, Goery C, et al. Paclitaxel and simultaneous radiation in stage III A/B non small cell carcinoma of the lung. Semin Oncol 23(Suppl 16): 108–112, 1996.

97.   Choy H, Akerly W, Safran H. Paclitaxel plus carboplatin and concurrent radiation therapy for patients with locally advanced non small cell lung cancer. Semin Oncol 23(Suppl 16): 117–119, 1996.

98.   Belani CP, Aisner J, Bahri S, et al. Chemoradiotherapy in non small cell cancer: paclitaxel/carboplatin/ radiotherapy in regionally advanced disease. Semin Oncol 23(Suppl 16): 113–116, 1996.

99.   Bonomi P, Siddiqui S, Lincoln S, et al. Escalating palitaxel doses and thoracic radiotherapy as preoperative or definitive treatment for stage III non small cell lung cancer. Semin Oncol 23(Suppl 16): 102–107, 1996.

100.  Haraf DJ, Stenson K, List M, et al. Continuous infusion paclitaxel, 5-fluorouracil and hydroxyurea with concomitant radiotherapy in patients with advanced or recurrent head and neck cancer. Semin Oncol 24(Suppl 2): 68–71, 1997.
101.  Fountziakis G, Athanassiadis A, Samantas E, et al. Paclitaxel and carboplatin in recurrent or metastatic head and neck cancer: a phase II study. Semin Oncol 24(Suppl 2): 58–64, 1992.
102.  Conley B, Jacobs M, Suntyharolingan, et al. A pilot trial of paclitaxel, carboplain and concurrent radiotherapy for unresectable squamous cell carcinoma of the head and neck. Semin Oncol 24(Suppl 2): 78–81, 1997.
103.  Safran H, King T, Hesketh P, et al. A phase II study of neo adjuvant paclitaxel, cisplatin and radiation therapy followed by esophagectomy. Proc Am Soc Clin Oncol 15: 218(Abstr), 1996.
104.  Safran H, Choy H, Sikov W, et al. Phase I study of paclitaxel and concurrent radiation for locally advanced gastric, pancreatic cancer. J Clin Oncol 15: 901–907, 1996.
105.  Williams DA, Lokich J. A review of the stability and compatibility of antineoplastic drugs for multiple drug infusions. Cancer Chemother Pharmacol 31: 171–181, 1992.

C.J. Rosenthal and M. Rotman (Eds.), *Infusion Chemotherapy–Irradiation Interactions*

# CHAPTER 2

# Optimal scheduling of chemo–radiotherapy regimens

## JACOB LOKICH

*Department of Neoplastic Disease, The Cancer Center of Boston, Boston, MA 02120, USA*

## 1. Introduction

Combined modality therapy for regional cancers utilizing infusional chemotherapy in conjunction with standard fractionation or hyperfractionation radiation has become common practice for a number of tumor categories. Clinical questions remain regarding the optimal chemotherapy regimen as well as method of administration and the optimal sequence of interdigitation of the two modalities. The purpose of this review is to focus on these two questions in developing the use of infusional chemotherapy administered concomitantly with radiation for the following tumors: head and neck cancer, esophageal cancer, lung cancer and rectal cancer.

## 2. Infusional (fractionated) chemotherapy

Infusional as opposed to bolus delivery of chemotherapy is becoming increasingly commonplace in oncologic practice based upon our understanding of the pharmacokinetics of drugs and the dynamics of tumor cell growth. In fact, the vast majority of chemotherapeutic agents are schedule dependent with an increased level of activity when the exposure time is extended [1]. As detailed in Table 1, the cell kill concentration for infusion relative to bolus administration in in vitro experimental systems predicts a schedule dependency for each of the class of drugs indicated and is most prominent for the anti-metabolite class.

The major radiation sensitizing agents are listed in Table 2. Of the six agents, the major sensitizing agent being employed is 5-fluorouracil (5-FU). All six of the agents have the capacity of being administered on an infusion schedule or in a schedule dependent fashion with hydroxyurea administered as an oral agent concomitant with radiation. There are limited data to date on the use of paclitaxel as a radiation sensitizing agent and on an infusion schedule but preliminary reports suggest that it will be a radiation sensitizing agent.

## 3. Tactical radiation schemas

In the context of concomitant administration of chemotherapy with radiation, three common treatment plans are: (1) simultaneous administration throughout the period of radiation for 4–6 weeks, (2) intermittent infusion for 4 days at the beginning of a standard fractionation radiation and at the end, and (3) intermittent delivery of both radiation and chemotherapy.

Table 1

Schedule of dependency of antineoplastic drugs

| Agent | Cell kill concentration | | Schedule dependency ratio |
|---|---|---|---|
| | bolus | infusion | |
| 5-Fluorouracil | 220 | 0.23 | 957 |
| Methotrexate | 97 | 0.32 | 303 |
| Bleomycin | 3.5 | 0.012 | 292 |
| Etoposide | 3.3 | 0.032 | 103 |
| Cisplatin | 19 | 0.030 | 63 |
| Melphalan | 1.3 | 0.13 | 10 |
| Doxorubicin | 0.13 | 0.022 | 5.9 |

Each of these schematics has their proponents. Continuous infusion chemotherapy through-out radiation may be viewed as "fractionated" chemotherapy and for optimal radiation sen-sitization, the simultaneous delivery of the chemotherapy is desirable. Each of the tactical sequences described in Fig. 1 has been applied for one or more of the tumor categories to be discussed.

## 4.   Head and neck cancer

Head and neck cancer represents one of the areas in which chemotherapy has been extraor-dinarily successful in inducing tumor regression. Modern combination chemotherapy trials utilize 5-FU and cisplatin with infusional schedules to achieve response rates upwards of 90% and two-thirds of the patients achieve complete clinical responses [2]. Present strate-gies to improve even this response rate include modulating the 5-FU with hydroxyurea, leu-covorin and/or interferon and the combined application of these multi-drug agents adminis-tered on an infusional schedule in conjunction with radiation [3].

Taylor has comprehensively reviewed the use of single agent chemotherapy in conjunc-tion with radiation therapy for head and neck cancer [4]. Table 3 describes the composite trials reviewed by Taylor involving five different chemotherapeutic agents. For 5-FU, 13 individual trials have been carried out although only three were randomized trials utilizing a control group. However, in two of the three randomized trials with 5-fluouracil and radia-tion, there was a demonstrated survival advantage. None of these trials involved infusional delivery although subsequent phase I and phase II trials of fluorouracil have indicated ac-tivity for combined infusional 5-FU and radiation. In the initial phase I trial, 5-FU was ad-

Table 2

Radiation sensitizing antineoplastic agents

5-Fluorouracil
Hydroxyurea
Cisplatin
Etoposide
Taxol    = paclitaxel
Doxorubicin

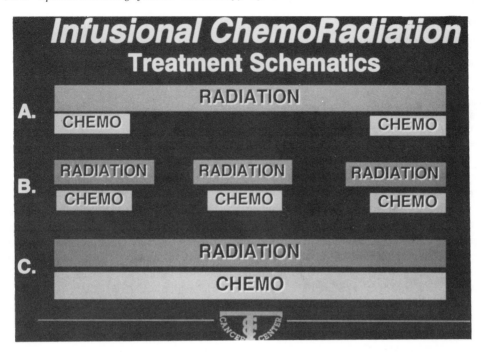

Fig. 1. The three tactical schedules for combining chemotherapy with concomitant radiation.

ministered at a dose of 250 mg/m$^2$ per day utilizing standard fractionation radiation and 9 of 14 patients achieved a complete response [5]. An expanded phase II trial was reported in 1993 involving 35 patients. The complete response rate was 22 of 35 and although there was increased local toxicity, the 2-year survival in this group of patients was 62% compared to 23% in historical controls [6].

For the other agents listed in Table 3, none utilized an infusional schedule. One trial using low dose daily bleomycin suggested a synergistic effect but there were no randomized trials. For hydroxyurea, there were two randomized trials comparing radiation alone to radiation plus hydroxyurea but an optimal schedule for hydroxyurea was not established. Finally, for methotrexate and for the platinum analogues, although there were three random-

Table 3

Single agent chemoradiotherapy trials

| Agent no. | Trials | No. of patients/ trial | Conclusion |
| --- | --- | --- | --- |
| Bleomycin | 10 | 7–82 | Low dose daily BLM, probably synergistic |
| 5-Fluorouracil | 13[a] | 18–151 | Survival advantage in 2/3 randomized trials |
| Hydroxyurea | 8[b] | 15–423 | No advantage |
| Methotrexate | 6 | 21–156 | Increased toxicity |
| Platinum analogues | 13[c] | 16–124 | No advantage |

[a]3/13 randomized trials.
[b]3/8 randomized trials.
[c]1/13 randomized trials.

Table 4

Infusional chemoradiotherapy trials: split course 5-FU + cisplatin

| Reference | No. of patients | CR % | Survival |
|---|---|---|---|
| Taylor et al. [7] | 53 | 55 | Median 37 months |
| Wendt et al. [8] | 62 | 79 | 53% at 2 years |
| Vokes et al. [9] | 31 | 81 | NA |
| ECOG [10] | 52 | 77 | Median 37 months |

ized trials, there was only one randomized trial utilizing platinum. There was no advantage demonstrated.

The use of multi-drug regimens combining 5-FU with cisplatin and concomitant simultaneous radiation has been explored in four trials (Table 4). These four studies accrued patients with advanced stage III head and neck cancer; were inoperable for cure and were previously untreated. The treatment involved concomitant infusional 5-FU and cisplatin with radiation. The most recent trial by the Eastern Cooperative Group was a phase II trial in 52 patients. This trial was compared to a predecessor trial which was a phase III trial comparing radiation alone to radiation plus weekly cisplatin. In the latter study, the control arm had a 45% CR rate and a 24% 4-year survival. With concomitant chemotherapy in the subsequent trial, the CR rate was 77% and the 4-year survival was 49%. Both of these are statistically significant as indicated by the *P* values although it must be emphasized that these are consecutive trials and do not represent direct randomized comparisons of chemotherapy with radiation versus radiation alone.

In summary for head and neck cancer, the simultaneous administration of infusional chemotherapy with radiation therapy for locally advanced disease achieves complete response rates in more than two-thirds of patients. There is as yet no defined survival advantage over radiation alone in the context of optimal phase III trials. Nonetheless, ongoing trials comparing chemoradiation and radiation may be fruitful. It is surprising that with such high response rate that survival to date has yet gone unaffected.

## 5. Esophageal cancer

The combined modality approach to esophageal cancer utilizing infusional chemotherapy with radiation represents an extension of the experience of infusional chemotherapy and radiation for anal cancer developed initially at Wayne State University. The initial strategy employed short term infusion of 5-FU with mitomycin C and low dose radiation as preoperative therapy and in the initial series 5 of 20 patients were rendered pathologically free of disease [11]. This experience has been extended to other institutions and combined modality therapy without surgery has been advocated by some [12].

In the modern era two large studies have addressed the preoperative use of combined infusional chemotherapy and radiation therapy. Poplin et al. reported on 113 patients receiving low dose radiation to 3000 rad in conjunction with short term infusional 5-FU and cisplatin. Sixty-two percent of the patients were resected and 25% had a pathologic complete response but the median survival was only 12 months for the whole group [13].

Protracted infusion fluorouracil delivering chemotherapy throughout the period of higher doses of radiation was developed as a pilot feasibility study by Rich et al. [14]. They demonstrated that low dose infusional 5-FU could be administered in conjunction with standard fractionation radiation to doses as high as 6000 rad and in a small population of patients with esophageal cancer, Lokich et al. demonstrated an 80% response rate in patients not coming to surgery [15]. Utilizing a similar 5-FU regimen in conjunction with radiation with standard fractionation or hyperfractionation and with the addition of cisplatin and vinblastine, Forestiere et al. treated 43 patients preoperatively [16]. Eighty-four percent were resected with 24% pathologic CR rate. In this group of patients, the median survival was extended to 23–32 months. The authors concluded also that this therapy was equally effective in epidermoid as well as adenocarcinomas.

Two studies have addressed definitive treatment utilizing infusional chemotherapy and radiation without the addition of surgery. In a phase III comparative trial, Herskovic et al. randomized patients to receive either radiation alone or radiation in conjunction with 5-FU infusion and cisplatin [17]. In this trial, chemotherapy added substantially and significantly to radiation with a 43% 2-year survival in the combined modality arm. In a report by Coia et al., 57 patients treated with infusional 5-FU and mitomycin C along with radiation to 6000 rad, the median survival was 18 months [13].

In summary, one can state that combined modality therapy utilizing infusional chemotherapy with radiation is effective in esophageal cancer and that combined chemotherapy and radiation is superior to radiation alone. Ongoing trials are addressing the role of comparing either chemotherapy alone or combined chemotherapy, radiation and surgery to surgery only. Such phase III trials are being carried out by the Radiation Therapy Oncology Group and the EORTC. Following completion of these studies, a reasonable question to be raised is whether or not organ sparing surgery can be employed for tumors of the esophagus. In this context, a comparative trial of combined modality chemotherapy radiation without operation versus operation only will be a necessary next step.

## 6.  Lung cancer

Lung cancer, both small cell and non-small cell variants, commonly are treated with combined chemotherapy and radiation. For small cell carcinoma, induction chemotherapy is generally followed in sequence with radiation therapy particularly for limited stage disease but also for complete responders in advanced or extensive stage disease. A major issue in controversy for the combined modality approach to small cell lung cancer is the timing of radiation in conjunction with chemotherapy and more recent trials have emphasized the need for concomitant or very early introduction of radiation. Infusional chemotherapy schedules have not been employed in conjunction with radiation therapy for this histologic subtype of lung cancer.

For non-small cell lung cancer, both squamous cell and adenocarcinoma types, combined modality therapy is commonly employed in the 1/3 or so patients within this histologic subtype that present with stage IIIA or IIIB disease. A number of clinical trials of concomitant and sequential combined chemotherapy and radiation with and without surgery have substantiated the contribution of chemotherapy to radiation [18].

Early single agent bolus chemotherapy with concomitant radiation trials involved 5-FU, hydroxyurea or bleomycin [19]. In these phase III trials carried out in the 1970s, the contribution of the chemotherapy to radiation was substantiated although the trials accrued few patients and statistical validation was not possible. In the trial employing 5-FU with radiation, this agent was administered as a bolus, and there was a survival difference in adenocarcinomas only [20]. In the trial utilizing hydroxyurea, only 53 patients were entered and there was no statistically significant difference [21]. The radiation was administered as split course. Finally, with single agent bleomycin in a very small study involving only 33 patients with bleomycin administered twice a week, there was a 13-month median survival compared to 6 months for radiation alone [22].

Single agent combined infusion with radiation for stage III disease has been carried in more modern clinical trials using either 5-FU or cisplatin. In the first study reported by Lokich et al., protracted 5-FU infusion was administered in conjunction with standard fractionation radiation simultaneously [23]. In the initial series of 30 patients with stage IIIB disease, there was a 10% cure rate and this experience has been continued with an expanded accrual of approximately 50 patients. Protracted delivery of cisplatin either using a daily bolus schedule or a continuous infusion schedule has also been evaluated. In the study by Schaake-Koning, standard fractionation radiation to a dose of 5500 rad was administered in conjunction with daily bolus cisplatin or weekly cisplatin or no cisplatin [24]. In this randomized trial, reported in 1992, the 1-year local disease free survival was 59% for the arm receiving daily bolus cisplatin compared to 42% for the radiation only arm. Furthermore, Bedini et al. reported on the use of infusional cisplatin in conjunction with a split course standard fractionation radiation schema and achieved an 86% response rate [25].

More recent trials of infusional chemotherapy with radiation have employed infusional fluorouracil with bolus platinum with or without additional agents in predominantly phase II trials utilizing either continuous standard fractionation radiation or split course standard fraction radiation. In the initial report by Taylor et al., continuous infusion fluorouracil with cisplatin administered once a month and radiation administered for 5 consecutive days using a split course treatment every other week was followed by surgery. In 64 patients entered, there was a 66% resectability rate and a 2-year survival of 40%. Within this group too, approximately 25% of patients resected demonstrated no evidence of tumor pathologically [26]. Weiden et al. utilized a similar regimen with continuous radiation in 76 patients and demonstrated 42% resectability rate [27]. Rowland et al. added etoposide to the two drug regimen concomitant with radiation and in 57 patients, 79% were found to be resectable with a 40% 2-year survival [28]. Strauss et al. added vinblastine to the 5-FU continuous infusion with cisplatin and utilized standard continuous fractionation radiation and of 32 patients a 67% resectability rate was established [29]. Finally, in 1993, Wozniak et al. reported on the combination of etoposide plus cisplatin administered as a continuous infusion low doses throughout standard fractionation radiation. In 59 patients, there was a 69% resectability rate with 40% 2-year survival [30].

Within these five trials, there appears to be no advantage for one regimen over the other. Although resectability varied within the 60–70% range, the 2-year survival was similar for all regimens. Therefore, an optimal drug combination or method of administration with radiation has not been established. Extrapolating from the 2-year survival of 40% with combined infusional chemotherapy and radiation compared to the 10% cure rate for radiation alone, it seems reasonable to conclude that combined modality therapy is superior to radiation alone. The specific contribution of surgery needs to be established since approximately 25% of patients who are deemed to be resectable have no pathologic evidence of tumor.

## 7. Rectal cancer

The role of radiation therapy in reducing local recurrence for rectal cancer has been studied by the Gastrointestinal Tumor Study Group which established the contribution of chemotherapy to radiation in a prospective randomized trial initiated in 1975 [31]. This study was a four arm study comparing bolus chemotherapy with radiation to radiation alone, chemotherapy alone and surgery alone. This study reported both a disease free survival advantage as well as an overall survival advantage at 7 years for combined modality therapy, 67% compared to 32% for no adjuvant therapy. This study was expanded by the North Central Oncology Group which compared radiation alone to radiation preceded by and followed by chemotherapy and demonstrated a decrease in local occurrence and distant metastasis and an improved survival with the addition of chemotherapy to radiation [32].

The superiority of infusional 5-FU over bolus 5-FU in patients with advanced colon cancer [33] as well as the feasibility of administration of infusional 5-FU in conjunction with radiation prompted an Intergroup clinical trial using a phase III trial designed to compare infusional 5-FU to bolus 5-FU in adjuvant treatment of rectal cancer with both groups receiving radiation therapy following resection. In this study, with more than 600 patients entered on the two arms, the group receiving infusional 5-FU with radiation is superior to the group receiving bolus 5-FU with radiation in terms of relapse free survival and overall survival (76 versus 68%) and there was a reduction in both local recurrence and distant metastasis [34].

This trial sets the standard for adjuvant therapy for rectal cancer which should be considered to be infusional 5-FU with radiation. The approach has also been applied in recurrent rectal tumors with pathologic complete remissions [35]. The clinical alert and recommendation by the National Cancer Institute however, mandates the use of bolus 5-FU at 500 mg/m$^2$ per day for 5 days in conjunction with radiation. The risk of this dose and schedule for 5-FU in terms of both morbidity and mortality however is not justified particularly in the context of the Intergroup trial demonstrating the superiority in terms of survival of infusional delivery.

## 8. Organ sparing and infusional chemoradiation

In addition to the four selected tumors in which infusional chemotherapy and radiation therapy are being employed for regional disease a number of other tumor categories have combined chemotherapy and radiation to achieve local tumor control with organ sparing. The specific advantage of this approach is to reduce the morbidity of radical surgery. These tumors include anal cancer, bladder cancer and carcinoma of the larynx.

Anal cancer, up to 1975, was routinely managed surgically using abdominal resection and permanent colostomy. However, with the use of infusional 5-FU and mitomycin C in conjunction with radiation, the curability of most of these lesions without surgery has resulted in reserving the radical surgical procedure only to a salvage role and is necessary in less than 10% of patients [36]. The contribution of mitomycin C to this regimen is debatable and the essential components appear to be infusional fluorouracil and radiation.

Bladder cancer remains commonly treated with radical cystectomy for locally advanced disease. However, a number of clinical trials employing fluorouracil infusion with radiation [37] or cisplatin combined with radiation [38] have achieved substantial response and local control without surgery. Combined modality treatment employing a regimen of cisplatin, methotrexate and vinblastine with radiation utilizing a bolus regimen has also been employed to achieve bladder sparing [39]. One could reasonably suggest that the interdigitation of fluorouracil with cisplatin administered as an infusion may have intrinsic advantages over the latter regimen.

For advanced cancer of the larynx, traditional therapy has been surgical involving a total laryngectomy with its consequent morbidity. The combined use of induction chemotherapy with infusional fluorouracil and cisplatin added to radiation therapy with laryngeal sparing has been compared in a phase III trial to surgical therapy with radiation [40]. There are no survival differences in the two groups and although the local recurrence rate is higher in the group treated without surgery, 65% of the patients in the non surgical group survived without having to endure a laryngectomy thus contributing substantially to their quality of life.

## Summary

Combined chemotherapy and radiation therapy is increasingly being applied for definitive therapy of regional cancers. Although a variety of integration schemas for the two modalities are presently employed, it seems likely that the simultaneous delivery of both modalities should be optimal and that 'fractionated' chemotherapy and 'infusional' radiation therapy should be administered coincident with each other in order to obtain maximal synergy. A novel tactical approach for chemo-sensitive tumors is to apply induction chemotherapy initially as neo-adjuvant to minimize the tumor burden and thereby maximize the effect of combined chemo-radiotherapy.

The use of chemotherapy administered as an infusion has applicability to a broad spectrum of tumors and for the common agents being explored for radiation sensitization, including fluorouracil, platinum analogues, hydroxyurea, etc., the infusional schedule is rationale and optimal.

In terms of the radiation, a variety of schedules have been employed including continuous or split course and even hyperfractionation. The optimal schedule of radiation administration has not been established but may be variable related to the type of tumor and the type of chemotherapeutic agent to be applied.

Infusional chemotherapy in conjunction with standard fractionation radiation therapy has become the standard of care for esophageal cancer, rectal cancer and anal cancer. It is being applied increasingly for head and neck cancer and is likely to achieve an impact on survival in this disease although to date, studies are not definitive. For non-small cell lung cancer, combined modality therapy has become common practice but the specific role of infusional chemotherapy has not been addressed in prospective comparative trials. For other tumors, phase II trials and less commonly phase III trials utilizing infusional chemotherapy with radiation have provided a basis for organ sparing treatment resulting in improved quality of life for patients with bladder cancer, laryngeal cancer and possibly other gastrointestinal cancers.

## Acknowledgements

Supported by The Cancer Center Research Foundation.

## References

1.   Mitchell RB, Ratain MJ, Vogelzang NJ. Experimental rationale for continuous infusion chemotherapy. In: Lokich J (Ed), Cancer Chemotherapy by Infusion, 2nd edn. Chicago, IL: Precept Press, 1990.

2.   Dreyfuss AL, Clark JR, Wright JE, et al. Continuous infusion high-dose leucovorin with 5-fluorouracil and cisplatin for untreated stage IV carcinoma of the head and neck. Ann Intern Med 112: 167–172, 1990.

3.   Vokes E, Weichselbaum RR, Mick R, et al. Favorable long-term survival following induction chemotherapy with cisplatin, fluorouracil, and leucovorin and concomitant chemoradiotherapy for locally advanced head and neck cancer. J Natl Cancer Inst 84: 877–882, 1992.

4.   Taylor S. Head and neck cancer. In: Lokich J, Byfield J (Eds), Combined Modality Cancer Therapy: Radiation and Infusional Chemotherapy. Chicago, IL: Precept Press, 1991, pp. 75–98.

5.   Weppelmann B, Wheeler RH, Peters GE, et al. A phase I study of prolonged infusion 5-fluorouracil and concomitant radiation therapy in patients with squamous cell cancer of the head and neck. J Radiat Oncol 20: 357–360, 1991.

6.   Olver IN, Hughes PG, Smith JG, et al. Concurrent radiotherapy and continuous ambulatory infusion 5-fluorouracil in advanced head and neck cancer. Proc Am Soc Clin Oncol 890: 1993.

7.   Taylor SG IV, Murrthy AK, Caldarelli DD, et al. Combined simultaneous cisplatin/fluorouracil chemotherapy and split course radiation in head and neck cancer. J Clin Oncol 7: 846–856, 1989.

8.   Wendt TG, Hartestein RC, Wustrow TPU, Lisner J. Cisplatin, fluorouracil with leucovorin calcium enhancement, and synchronous accelerated radiotherapy in the management of locally advanced head and neck cancer: a phase II study. J Clin Oncol 7: 471–476, 1989.

9.   Vokes EE, Panje WR, Schilsky RL, et al. Hydroxyurea, fluorouracil and concomitant radiotherapy in poor-prognosis head and neck cancer: a phase I-II study. J Clin Oncol 7: 761–766, 1989.

10.  Adelstein DJ, Kalish LA, Adams GL, et al. Concurrent radiation therapy and chemotherapy for locally unresectable squamous cell head and neck cancer: an Eastern Cooperative Oncology Group pilot study. J Clin Oncol 11: 2136–2142, 1993.

11.  Leichman L, Steiger Z, Seydel HG, et al. Preoperative chemotherapy plus radiation therapy for patients with cancer of the esophagus: potentially curative approach. J Clin Oncol 2: 75–79, 1984.

12.  Coia LR, Engstrom PF, Paul AR, et al. Long-term results of infusional 5-FU, mitomycin-C and radiation as primary management of esophageal carcinoma. Int J Radiat Oncol Biol Phys 20: 29–36, 1991.

13.  Poplin E, Fleming T, Leichman L, et al. combined therapies for squamous cell carcinoma of the esophagus, a Southwest Oncology Group Study (SWOG 8037). J Clin Oncol 5: 622–628, 1987.

14.  Rich TA, Lokich JJ, Chaffey JT. a pilot study of protracted venous infusion of 5-fluorouracil and concomitant radiation therapy. J Clin Oncol 3: 402–406, 1985.

15.  Lokich JJ, Shea M, Chaffey J. Sequential infusional 5-fluorouracil followed by concomitant radiation therapy for tumors of the esophagus and gastroesophageal junction. Cancer 60: 275–279, 1987.

16.  Forastiere AA, Orringer MB, Perez-Tamayo C, et al. Preoperative chemoradiation followed by transhiatal esophagectomy for carcinoma of the esophagus: final report. J Clin Oncol 11: 1118–1123, 1993.

17.  Herskovic A, Martz K, Al-Sarraf M. Combined chemotherapy and radiotherapy compared with radiotherapy alone in patients with cancer of the esophagus. N Engl J Med 326: 1593–1598, 1992.

18.  Belani CP. Multimodality management of regionally advanced non-small-cell lung cancer. Semin Oncol 20: 302–314, 1993.

19.  Bonomi P, Reddy S, Faber LP. Lung cancer. In: Lokich J, Byfield J (Eds), Combined Modality Cancer Therapy: Radiation and Infusional Chemotherapy. Chicago, IL: Precept Press, 1991, pp. 63–74.

20.  Carr DT, Childs DS, Lee RE. Radiotherapy plus 5-FU compared to radiotherapy alone for inoperable and unresectable bronchogenic carcinoma. Cancer 29: 375–380, 1972.

21.  Landgren RC, Hussey DH, Barkley HT, et al. Split course irradiation compared to split course irradiation plus hydroxyurea in inoperable bronchogenic carcinoma – a randomized study of 53 patients. Cancer 34: 1598–1601, 1974.

22.  Chan PYM, Byfield JE, Kagan AR, et al. Unresectable squamous cell carcinoma of the lung and its management by combined bleomycin and radiotherapy. Cancer 37: 2671–2676, 1976.

23.  Lokich JJ, Chaffey J, Neptune W. Concomitant 5-fluorouracil infusion and high-dose radiation for stage III non small cell lung cancer. Cancer 64: 1021–1025, 1989.

24.  Schaake-Koning C, Vanden Bogart W, Dalesio O. Effects of concomitant cisplatin and radiotherapy on inoperable non-small-cell lung cancer. N Engl J Med 326: 324–530, 1992.

25.   Bedini AV, Tavecchio L, Milani F, et al. Prolonged venous infusion of cisplatin and concurrent radiation therapy for lung carcinoma. Cancer 67: 357–362, 1991.

26.   Taylor SG IV, Trybula M, Bonomi P, et al. Simultaneous cisplatin-fluorouracil infusion and radiation followed by surgical resection in regionally localized stage III non-small cell lung cancer. Ann Thorac Surg 43: 87–91, 1987.

27.   Weiden P, Pinatodosi S. Preoperative chemotherapy in stage III non-small cell lung cancer. A phaseIi study of the lung cancer study group (LCSG). Proc Am Soc Clin Oncol 7: 197, 1988.

28.   Rowland K, Bonomi P, Taylor IV SG, et al. Phase II trial of etoposide, cisplatin, 5-FU and concurrent split course radiation in stage IIIa, and IIIb non-small cell lung cancer. Proc Am Soc Clin Oncol 7: 203, 1988.

29.   Straus G, Sherman L, Matthiesen O, et al. Concurrent chemotherapy and radiotherrapy followed by surgery in marginally resectable stage IIIa non-small cell lung cancer. A Cancer and Acute Leukemia Group B study. Proc Am Soc Clin Oncol 3: 215, 1988.

30.   Wozniak A, Kraut M, Herskovic A, et al. Phase II trial of etoposide, cisplatin, 5-FU and concurrent split course radiation in stage IIIa and IIIb non small cell lung cancer. Proc Am Soc Clin Oncol 12: 333(Abstr 1109), 1993.

31.   Douglass Jr HO, Moertel CG, Mayer BJ, et al. Survival after postoperative combination treatment of rectal cancer. N Engl J Med 315: 1294–1295, 1986.

32.   Krook JE, Moertel CG, Gunderson LL, et al. Effective surgical adjuvant therapy for high-risk rectal carcinoma. N Engl J Med 324:709–715, 1991.

33.   Lokich JJ, Ahlgren J, Gullo J, et al. A prospective randomized comparison of continuous infusional 5-fluorouracil with a conventional bolus schedule in metastatic colorectal carcinoma: A Mid-Atlantic Oncology Program Study. J Clin Oncol 7: 425–432, 1989.

34.   O'Connell M, Martenson J, Rich T, et al. Protracted venous infusion (PVI) 5-fluorouracil (5-FU) as a component of effective combined modality post-operative surgical adjuvant therapy for high-risk rectal cancer (abstract). Proc Am Soc Clin Oncol 12: 193, 1993.

35.   DePaoli A, Boz G, Innocente R, et al. Concurrent 5-FU ling term continuous infusion (CI) and radiation therapy (RT) for unresectable rectal cancer (RC). Proc Am Soc Clin Oncol 12: 634, 1993.

36.   Sischy B, Doggett HLS, Krall JM, et al. Definitive irradiation and chemotherapy for radiosensitization in management of anal carcinoma: interim report on radiation therapy oncology group study no. 8314. J Natl Cancer Inst 81: 850–856, 1989.

37.   Rotman M, Aziz H. Bladder cancer. In: Lokich J, Byfield J (Eds), Combined Modality Cancer Therapy: Radiation and Infusional Chemotherapy. Chicago, IL: Precept Press, 1991, pp. 199–208.

38.   Chauvet B, Brewer Y, Felix-Faure C, et al. Combined radiation therapy and cisplatin for locally advanced carcinoma of the urinary bladder. Cancer 72: 2213–2218, 1993.

39.   Kaufman DS, Shipley WU, Griffin PP, et al. Selective bladder preservation by combination treatment of invasive bladder cancer. N Engl J Med 329: 1377–1382, 1993.

40.   Veterans Affairs Laryngeal Cancer Study Group. Induction, chemotherapy plus radiation compared with surgery plus radiation in patients with advanced laryngeal cancer. N Engl J Med 324: 1685–1690, 1991.

C.J. Rosenthal and M. Rotman (Eds.), *Infusion Chemotherapy–Irradiation Interactions*

# CHAPTER 3

# Retinoids and cytokines in combination with ionizing radiation in squamous cell carcinomas – preclinical and clinical results

W. HOFFMANN, M. BAMBERG and H. PETER RODEMANN

*Department of Radiotherapy, Section of Radiobiology and Molecular Environmental Research,
Ebethard Karls University Tubingen, Rontgenweg 11, 72076 Tubingen, Germany*

## 1. Introduction

While the interest in retinoic acid (RA) and interferon-$\alpha$ (IFN-$\alpha$) in cancer therapy as separate treatment modalities had gained in the past, a strong rationale to combine these agents has emerged out of various preclinical studies demonstrating their different mechanisms of action and enhanced in vitro activity in a variety of human hematologic and solid tumor cell lines [1–5]. By using a combination of isotretinoin and recombinant IFN-$\alpha$, excellent therapeutic effects have been reported in the treatment of squamous cell carcinoma of the skin and the cervix [6–13]. Phase I and II trials for other tumor entities are currently performed [14–19].

Recently, it has been demonstrated that irradiation of normal and transformed human skin fibroblasts results predominantly in an induction of terminal differentiation of theses cells [20,21]. Furthermore, pretreatment with all-*trans*-RA significantly enhances the radiosensitivity of both normal and transformed human fibroblasts as well as mouse melanoma cells. This radiomodulating effect of RA may be due to an induction of differentiation divisions as indicated by the expression of certain proliferation and differentiation markers, e.g., melanin synthesis [22].

IFN-$\alpha$ acting as an antiproliferative and differentiation modulating cytokine has also been described to affect the radiosensitivity of tumor cells in vitro. The mechanism of this phenomenon has not yet been totally revealed, but it has been suggested that IFN-$\alpha$ may potentate radiotoxicity through an inference with cellular DNA repair processes resulting in an accumulation of sublethal radiation damage [23].

## 2. Preclinical results

By the use of several established human squamous cell carcinoma cell lines of the head and neck and of cervical cancer, the effects of single agent treatment with all-*trans* RA, IFN-$\alpha$ in combination with single dose irradiation (IR, 2 Gy) as well as of the combined treatment modality employing RA, IFN-$\alpha$ and IR on colony formation and cell survival (surviving fraction at 2 Gy, SF2) were analyzed.

## 2.1.  Materials and methods

### 2.1.1.  Cells
Three head and neck cancer cell lines (HTB 43, SCC-9 and SCC4) and two cervical cancer cell lines (C4-I and HTB 35) purchased from the American Tissue Culture Collection (USA) were used in this study. All cell lines were cultured in minimal essential medium (MEM; Gibco) supplemented with 10% fetal calf serum and standard amounts of antibiotics (penicillin 557 IU/ml; streptomycin 740 IU/ml). Cells were routinely subcultured once per week using 0.05% trypsin. Medium was renewed twice weekly. Using this protocol the doubling time of the cell lines could be calculated to range between 23 and 48 h. After receiving and propagating the cells for five passages, sufficient amounts of cells were frozen and stored in liquid nitrogen. All experiments were performed with cells four passages after thawing. At this passage level the cell attachment and plating efficiency of the five cell lines was reproducible throughout all experiments.

### 2.1.2.  Colony formation assay
Cells were seeded at a density of 50 cells per $cm^2$ in 6-well tissue culture plates (Falcon, Becton Dickinson) and incubated for 12 days under various treatment protocols. For determination of plating efficiency, cells were seeded as above and incubated for 12 days to allow colony formation from single plated cells. Cell cultures were fixed with 3.7% paraformaldehyde in PBS and 70% ethanol (10 min each) and stained using a two-step staining procedure with Coomassie and Giemsa. The fraction of surviving cells was determined by counting the number of colonies bigger than 50 cells formed under the various conditions. The numbers were blotted as the surviving fraction versus control (100%).

### 2.1.3.  Treatment procedures
Twenty-four hours after plating cells were treated for the subsequent incubation period (12 days) with all-*trans*-RA (Hoffmann-La Roche) and/or interferon-$\alpha$ (Roferon-A3, Hoffmann-La Roche) in various concentrations (RA 1.0 or 10 $\mu$M; IFN 0.5, 5.0, 50 and 500 IU/ml). Control cultures received medium plus solvent solutions. During the subsequent incubation procedures, no further addition of the compounds was performed.

### 2.1.4.  Irradiation procedure
Treated or untreated cells were irradiated 24 h after adding the compounds or solvents to the culture medium with a single dose of 2 Gy of ionizing radiation generated by a linear accelerator (4 MV photons MEVATRON 60/Siemens, dose rate 2 Gy/min).

## 2.2.  Results

### 2.2.1.  Effects of RA and IFN-$\alpha$ on the colony formation of squamous cell carcinomas
Treatment of squamous cell carcinoma cell lines of the cervix resulted with all-*trans* retinoic acid (10 $\mu$M) in a decrease of colony formation by about 90% in HTB 35 and about 95% in C4-I. When the cell lines were treated with a combination of both compounds inhibition of colony formation was almost complete. In the two cell lines, HTB 35 and C4-I, a concentration of 50 IU/ml interferon-$\alpha$ reduced colony formation by approximately 80-85% as compared to the untreated controls.

For the head and neck cancer cell lines treatment with all-*trans* retinoic acid (10 $\mu$M) decreased colony formation by about 45% (HTB 43), 26% (SCC4) and 66% (SCC9). Incubation with IFN-$\alpha$ (50 IU/ml) led to an inhibition of colony formation of 35% (HTB 43), 36% (SCC 4) and 37% (SCC 9). For all three cell lines the combined treatment with both compounds resulted in a more pronounced decrease of colony formation as compared to the effects of the single agent treatment.

### 2.2.2.   Colony formation of the squamous cell lines as a function of RA and IFN-$\alpha$ pretreatment in combination with irradiation

The radiosensitivity of the cell lines was determined and the surviving fraction at 2 Gy, $SF_2$, could be demonstrated to range between 0.4 and 0.95 (C4-I, $SF_2$ 0.4; HTB 35, $SF_2$ 0.6; HTB 43, $SF_2$ 0.6; SCC 4, $SF_2$ 0.95; SCC 9, $SF_2$ 0.4). If treatment with either RA or IFN-$\alpha$ alone was followed by an irradiation with a single dose of 2 Gy, colony formation was reduced in the cervical cancer cell lines HTB 35 and C4-I by about 95 and 80%, respectively, as compared to unirradiated controls. Combination of RA and IFN-$\alpha$ followed by irradiation abolished colony formation almost completely in both cell lines.

In comparison to the cervical cancer cell lines cells from head and neck tumors (HTB 43, pharyngeal cancer; SCC 4, SCC 9 tongue cancer) were less sensitive towards single agent pretreatment followed by irradiation. Combined pretreatment of RA and IFN-$\alpha$ and subsequent single dose irradiation with 2 Gy, however, led to a pronounced inhibitory effect on the clonogenicity of these cell lines by about 80 and 95% as compared to unirradiated controls.

## 3.   Clinical results

Clinically, the combination of 13-*cis* retinoic acid (13cRA) and interferon-$\alpha$ (IFN-$\alpha$) has been studied in a variety of tumor types and was identified to have, among others, substantial activity in advanced squamous cell carcinomas (SCCs) of the skin and the cervix [7,8, 10–13]. Since radiotherapy (XRT) is a substantial part of the treatment of SCC, the question arises as to whether the therapeutic results obtainable with radiation alone can be further improved by using the additive effect of a systemic treatment with 13cRA and IFN-$\alpha$. The rationale for this approach is based on experimental data since both IFN-$\alpha$ and retinoids have been demonstrated to synergistically potentate the radiation toxicity of human SCC cells [4,5,24]. In addition, it has been shown that vitamin A and its derivates potentate the response of experimental animal tumors to radiation [25,26].

We evaluated prospectively the feasibility and toxicity of such a combination using 13cRA and IFN together with simultaneous radiation in SCCs of different origin, and compared our results with a group of patients treated systemically with 13cRA and IFN-$\alpha$ alone [9].

### 3.1.   Treatment and drug administration

*Group A.* Twenty-seven patients underwent external beam irradiation using linear accelerators. Doses given ranged between 50 and 70 Gy in 1.8–2.0 daily fractions over 5–8 weeks (ICRU report 50) depending on tumor type, stage and treatment intention (for patients' characteristics, see Table 1). Patients received 13cRA, 0.5 mg/kg body weight, orally once a day and IFN-$\alpha$, $3 \times 10^6$ IU s.c., 3 times a week.

*Group B.* Thirty patients receiving systemic treatment alone were treated with 1.0 mg/kg body weight 13cRA orally and IFN-$\alpha$, $3 \times 10^6$ IU s.c., once a day.

## 3.2.  Results

### 3.2.1.  Hematological toxicity
In both treatment groups A and B, myelotoxicity was moderate and did not exceed WHO grade II in most cases. None of the patients required blood transfusion or antibiotic treatment. In 3 patients out of group B, who are irradiated for cervical ($n = 2$) and head and neck ($n = 1$) cancer, WHO grade III leucopenia ($1.0–1.9 \mu l$) led to interruption of trial medication for 7 days. In group A, only 2 patients developed grade III toxicity, with leucopenia in a head and neck cancer patient and in one patient with esophageal cancer with anemia combined with thrombocytopenia, causing treatment interruption for 7 and 10 days, respectively.

### 3.2.2.  Non-hematological toxicity
Fatigue and "flu-like symptoms" occurred in 35% of all cases. Fever on the days of IFN medication could easily be managed using paracetamol $3 \times 500$ mg p.o. and was always transient. Three out of 5 patients with head and neck cancer in group A developed grade III mucositis in the course of radiotherapy. Combined treatment (RA/IFN + Radiatio) induced slightly pronounced toxicity scores of mucositis and skin toxicity compared with patients treated systemically only (mean severity of side effects, Table 2).

### 3.2.3.  Response
*Group A.* four partial responses were observed outside the irradiation field ($2\times$ cervical cancer, $1\times$ head and neck cancer, $1\times$ NSCLC). Median duration of response was 152 days and 50 days for the patients with cervical cancer.

*Group B.* Treatment with RA/IFN-$\alpha$ alone led to three partial responses in patients with cervical cancer. All together, 7 patients out of a total of 36 evaluable for response responded to the systemic treatment with a partial remission.

The overall response rate of all 16 cervical cancer patients evaluable for response was 5

Table 1

Patients' characteristics

|  | Group A (13cRA/IFN-$\alpha$/XRT) | Group B (13cRA/IFN-$\alpha$) |
|---|---|---|
| *Eligible (total n = 57)* | 27 | 30 |
|    Male | 12 | 18 |
|    Female | 15 | 12 |
| Performance status (ECOG) | 0–1 | 0–2 |
| Age (range, years) | 27–71 | 38–70 |
| | | |
| *Tumor type* | | |
|    Cervix | 13 | 12 |
|    Head and neck | 5 | 10 |
|    NSLC | 8 | 5 |
|    Esophagus | 1 | 3 |

Table 2

Mean severity of side effects

| Side effects | Tumor type | | | | | |
| --- | --- | --- | --- | --- | --- | --- |
| | Cervix | | Head and neck | | Lung | |
| | Group A | Group B | Group A | Group B | Group A | Group B |
| Anemia | 0.46 | 0.92 | 0.60 | 0.50 | 0.38 | 0.40 |
| Leucopenia | 0.92 | 0.75 | 1.40[a] | 1.00[a] | 0.50 | 0.00 |
| Thrombocytopenia | 0.15 | 0.00 | 0.00 | 0.00 | 0.00 | 0.00 |
| SGOT/SGPT | 0.15 | 0.50 | 0.00 | 0.20 | 0.00 | 0.20 |
| Mucositis | 0.85 | 0.33 | 1.80[a] | 0.80 | 0.63 | 0.20 |
| Nausea | 1.31[a] | 0.66 | 0.40 | 0.70 | 1.00[a] | 0.80 |
| Diarrhea | 0.62 | 0.25 | 0.20 | 0.00 | 0.13 | 0.00 |
| Pulmonary toxicity | 0.38 | 0.08 | 1.40[a] | 1.20[a] | 1.25[a] | 1.40[a] |
| Fever | 0.38 | 0.70 | 1.20[a] | 0.40 | 1.00[a] | 0.40 |
| Skin/cheilitis | 1.38[a] | 0.75 | 1.60[a] | 1.20[a] | 1.25[a] | 1.20[a] |

Mean severity (MS) of side effects (WHO toxicity score). Values represent calculated mean of side effects.
$MS = (n_1 \times 1) + (n_2 \times 2) + (n_3 \times 3) + (n_4 \times 4) / n_0 + n_1 + n_2 + n_3 + n_4$
where $n_1$, number of cases with Grade 1 toxicity; $n_2$, number of cases with Grade 2 toxicity; $n_3$, number of cases with Grade 3 toxicity; $n_4$, number of cases with Grade 4 toxicity.
[a]WHO values > 1.

out of 16 (31%; 95% CI 11–59%). Mean duration of response was 106 days in patients with cervical cancer (Table 3).

## 4. Conclusions

In patients with solid tumors, toxicity of systemic treatment with RA/IFN-$\alpha$ alone has been previously described to be mild and to consist mainly of fatigue and skin changes [10,11]. We have integrated the regimen of 13cRA and IFN-$\alpha$ into standard comprehensive radio-

Table 3

Responses

| Tumor type | Evaluable | CR | PR | SD | PD |
| --- | --- | --- | --- | --- | --- |
| *Group A (13cRA/IFN-$\alpha$/XRT)* | | | | | |
| Cervix | 4 | 0 | 2 | 1 | 1 |
| Head and neck | 1 | 0 | 1 | 0 | 0 |
| NSCLC | 1 | 0 | 1 | 0 | 0 |
| Esophagus | 1 | 0 | 0 | 1 | 0 |
| *Group B (13cRA/IFN-$\alpha$)* | | | | | |
| Cervix | 12 | 0 | 3 | 6 | 3 |
| Head and neck | 9 | 0 | 0 | 8 | 1 |
| NSCLC | 5 | 0 | 0 | 3 | 2 |
| Esophagus | 3 | 0 | 0 | 3 | 0 |

CR, complete response; PR, partial response; SD, stable disease; PD, progressive disease.

therapy of SCCs of different sites. In combination with radiotherapy acute toxicity is revealed to be moderate and generally does not exceed the toxicity seen with radiation only. With the regimen used, the comparison between toxicity of combination treatment with a group of patients treated with systemic treatment alone revealed a very mild increase of acute toxicity only. Hematological toxicity was mild and transient in both treatment groups, necessitating treatment interruption in a few cases only. Among non-hematological manifestations of toxicity in patients with cervical cancer, diarrhea was more pronounced with systemic treatment plus radiation. Systemic treatment in combination with irradiation led to remissions in group A, with 4 partial responses outside the irradiation field (2× cervical cancer, 1× NSCLC and 1× head and neck cancer). Together with the two partial responses in cervical cancer observed in group B, out of all 16 patients with cervical cancer evaluable for responses, the partial response rate was about 30%. This confirms other observations describing only casuistic responses in patients with head and neck tumors, NSCLC or esophageal cancer, suggesting that biological differences among different tumors, including different etiologies, account for the responsiveness of skin and cervical cancers and the relative failure of other SCCs [9]. Another possible explanation is under investigation – namely, whether the coincidence of cervical cancers with human papilloma viruses (HPV) infection could explain the susceptibility of these tumors to this kind of treatment since both IFN-$\alpha$ and retinoids are known to exert anti-viral effects [13].

Since the combination of RA and IFN-$\alpha$ has been shown to be effective in advanced SCC and since the addition of ionizing radiation tests on both a preclinical and clinical rationale, we conclude that this treatment is indeed feasible. We suggest that further evaluation of the 13cRA/IFN combination in phase I/II trials as an adjunct to radiotherapy might define the ultimate role of the combination.

## Acknowledgements

This work was supported by a grant from the Deutsche Krebshilfe, Dr. Mildred Scheel Stiftung (W59/94/Ho2).

## References

1. Angioli R, Sevin BU, Perras JP, et al. In vitro potentiation of radiation cytotoxicity by recombinant interferons in cervical cancer cell lines. Cancer 71: 3717–3725, 1993.
2. Bollag W, Peck R, Frey J. Inhibition of proliferation by retinoids, cytokines and their combination in four human transformed epithelial cell lines. Cancer Lett 62: 167–172, 1992.
3. Frey JR, Peck R, Bollag W. Antiproliferative activity of retinoids, interferon-$\alpha$ and their combination in five human transformed cell lines. Cancer Lett 57: 223–227, 1991.
4. Hoffmann W, Bamberg M, Rodemann HP. Antiproliferative effects of ionizing radiation, all-trans-retinoic acid and interferon-$\alpha$ on cultured human squamous cell carcinomas. Radiat Oncol Invest 2: 12–19, 1994.
5. Hoffmann W, Kley J, Schiller U, et al. Retinoids and interferon-alpha enhance the anti proliferative effect of radiation in cultured human squamous cell carcinoma cell lines. Proc Am Soc Clin Oncol 14: 1683, 1995.
6. Alberts DS, Modiano MR, Shamdas GJ. Phase II trial of 13-cis-retinoic acid plus interferon-$\alpha$ for advanced, heavily treated squamous cell carcinoma of the cervix. Proc Am Soc Clin Oncol 29: 852, 1993.
7. Bollag W, Holdener E. Retinoids in cancer prevention and therapy. Ann Oncol 3: 513–526, 1992.

8.   Conley B, Wu R, Finley M. Relationship of toxicity to pharmocokinetics of all-trans-retinoic acid in a phase I trial in solid tumor patients. Proc Am Soc Clin Oncol 29: 342, 1993.

9.   Hoffmann W, Schiebe M, Hirnle P, et al. 13-cis retinoic acid and inter feron-alpha ± irradiation in the treatment of squamous cell carcinomas. Int J Cancer 70: 475–477, 1997.

10.  Lippman SM, Kavanagh JJ, Espinoza PM, et al. 13-cis-retinoic acid plus interferon-$\alpha$. Highly active systemic therapy for squamous cell carcinoma of the cervix. J Natl Cancer Inst 4: 241–245, 1992.

11.  Lippman, SM, Parkinson DR, Itri M, et al. 13-cis-retinoic acid and interferon-$\alpha$-2a. effective combination therapy for advanced squamous cell carcinoma of the skin. J Natl Cancer Inst 84: 235–240, 1992b.

12.  Lippman SM, Kavanagh JJ, Paredes M. 13-cis-retinoic acid, interferon-$\alpha$ 2a and radiotherapy for locally advanced cancer of the cervix. Proc Am Soc Clin Oncol 29: 816, 1993.

13.  Lippman SM, Kavanagh JJ, Paredes M. 13cRA, IFN-alpha and radiotherapy for locally advanced cancer of the cervix. Proc Am Soc Clin Oncol 12: 259, 1993.

14.  Dmitrovsky, D, Bosi GJ. Active cancer therapy combining 13-cis-retinoic acid with interferon-alpha. J Natl Cancer Inst 84: 241–245, 1992.

15.  Gross G, Logan DM, Maroun JA. Small cell lung carcinoma and colonic carcinoma cell proliferation is partially inhibited by 13-cis-retinoic acid, all-trans-retinoic acid or $\alpha$-interferon in vitro. Proc Am Soc Clin Oncol 29: 309, 1993.

16.  Rinaldi DA, Lippman SM, Burris HA. Phase II study of 13-cis-retinoic acid and $\alpha$-2$\alpha$-interferon in patients with advanced squamous cell lung cancer. Proc Am Soc Clin Oncol 29: 1191, 1993.

17.  Roth AD, Abele R, Alberto P. 13-cis-retinoic acid plus interferon-$\alpha$. A phase II clinical study in squamous cell carcinoma of the lung and the head and neck. Oncology 51: 84–86, 1994.

18.  Toma S, Palumbo R, Vincenti M. Efficacy of recombinant interferon-$\alpha$ and 13-cis-retinoic acid in the treatment of squamous cell carcinomas. Ann Oncol 5: 463–465, 1994.

19.  Yung WKA, Simaga M, Levin VA. 13-cis-retinoic acid. A new and potentially effective agent for recurrent malignant astrocytomas. Proc Am Soc Clin Oncol 29: 497, 1993.

20.  Rodemann HP, Bayreuther K, Franz PI, et al. Selective enrichment and biochemical characterization of seven human skin fibroblast cell types in vitro. Exp Cell Res 180: 84–93, 1989.

21.  Rodemann HP, Peterson HP, Schwenke K, von Wangenheim KH. Terminal differentiation of human fibro blasts is induced by radiation. Scanning Microsc Int 5: 1135–1143, 1991.

22.  Schiller U, Ulrich W, Bamberg M, Rodemann HP. Retinoic acid modulates the radiosensitivity of tumor cells by inducing differentiation divisions. Eur J Cell Biol 63(Suppl 40): 195, 1994.

23.  Bonnen E, von Wussow P. Interferone und andere Therapiemodalitäten. In: Niederle N, von Wussow P (Eds), Interferone. Berlin: Springer, pp. 420–436, 1990.

24.  Hoffmann W, Schlak I, Schiller U, et al. Growth modulating effects of all-trans retinoic acid, inferferon-$\alpha$ and ionizing radiation in human head and neck and cervical cancer cell lines. Ann Oncol 5: 7–10, 1994.

25.  Seifter E, Rettura G, Padava J. Regression of C3HBA mouse tumor due to x-ray therapy combined with supplemental $\beta$-carotene or vitamin A. J Natl Cancer Inst 71: 409–417, 1983.

26.  Tannock IF, Sutt HD, Marshal N. Vitamin A and the radiation response of experimental tumors. J Natl Cancer Inst 48: 731–741, 1972.

C.J. Rosenthal and M. Rotman (Eds.), *Infusion Chemotherapy–Irradiation Interactions*
© 1998 Elsevier Science B.V. All rights reserved

CHAPTER 4

# Mechanisms of interaction between 5-fluorouracil and radiation: implications for continuous infusion chemotherapy

JOEL E. TEPPER[1] and A. WILLIAM BLACKSTOCK[2]

*[1]Department of Radiation Oncology, University of North Carolina at Chapel Hill, School of Medicine, Chapel Hill, NC 27599-7512, USA and [2]Department of Radiation Oncology, Bowman Gray School of Medicine, Winston Salem, NC 27157, USA*

Both radiation therapy and chemotherapy have been used for many years in the treatment of malignant disease. 5-Fluorouracil (5-FU) is one of the older chemotherapeutic agents, and was discovered by Heidelberger [1] based on the proposed mechanism of action. The concept of using both modalities together was put forth in the 1960s [2–4] and combined modality therapy with these two agents has been employed in a variety of malignancies since that time.

The initial studies demonstrating a beneficial combined modality effect in the clinical trial setting were performed at the Mayo Clinic [3] and demonstrated, for a variety of gastrointestinal malignancies, that there was an improved therapeutic outcome when bolus 5-FU was used with radiation therapy in contrast to the use of radiation therapy alone. These studies relied on a 3-day bolus regimen of chemotherapy at a dose which would not be expected to have any significant effect when used alone. Since that time, a number of clinical studies have been done to evaluate the use of combined modality therapy in a variety of anatomical sites. Interestingly, although many new chemotherapeutic drugs have been developed since that time, 5-FU has remained the drug most commonly used in combined radiation therapy/chemotherapy studies. This combination has been used in tumors of the esophagus [6], stomach [5], pancreas [7,8], rectum [9,10], anus [11,12], head and neck [13], and to a lesser extent in colon, lung and uterine cervix cancers and is now standard therapy in at least some of these sites.

5-FU is thought to have as its primary mode of action inhibition of the enzyme thymidylate synthase leading to the depletion of thymidine triphosphate and thus decreased formation of DNA. However, it can have a number of other effects including incorporation of fluorouracil triphosphate into RNA or the incorporation of the deoxy fluorinated triphosphate into DNA. Each of these can have adverse effects which could lead to cell death.

Despite the extensive use of concurrent radiation therapy and 5-FU based chemotherapy, there is surprisingly little definitive information on the mode of action of the combination. This is not for lack of trying. A large number of laboratory studies have been done to determine the mode of interaction between the agents. Obtaining this information is critical if we are to optimize the combination therapy. Knowing the mode of action will affect the timing and dosing of the two agents and may allow us to develop improvements of therapy based on a knowledge of the basic biology. Possibilities that have been suggested for the interaction have included: (1) drug induced alterations of nucleotide pools making effective DNA repair less efficient [14–16]; (2) 5-FU modulating cell cycle distribution and putting cells into a radiosensitive phase of the cell cycle [17]; (3) incorporation of 5-FU into DNA or into RNA; and (4) the possibility that radiation is in fact enhancing the cell killing of 5-FU rather than 5-FU producing radiation sensitization [18–20]. Determining the mechanism of the interaction is critical if we are to be able to modulate the effect, maximize the cell killing produced by the combination and determine in which situations the combination is likely to be of benefit.

Some of the original studies on the interaction were performed by Byfield [18,19]. His data suggest that the interaction is affected by both the concentration of the drug and the duration of exposure of cells to 5-FU. Interestingly, his data also show that sensitization is seen almost entirely when the cell lines were sensitive to cell killing from 5-FU alone. Based on these pieces of information, he suggested that the combination regimen produces a benefit based on chemosensitization by radiation therapy. His data also provide information on the optimal method of delivering 5-FU when sensitization is desired. The sensitizing effect is most pronounced when 5-FU is delivered after the radiation therapy rather than before. This timing effect supports the notion of chemosensitization. It also suggests that the method in which the two agents were combined in many clinics (radiation therapy after the 5-FU) may not be ideal. In fact, in most clinical trials of the combination, the timing of the radiation therapy with respect to 5-FU administration was not defined. It is possible that the relatively small benefit seen in those clinical trials would have been much larger if optimal timing had been employed.

Another implication of the data of Byfield is that a long term continuous infusion of 5-FU, by increasing the duration of the exposure of tumor cells to the drug, would be more effective. Although at the time that his in vitro studies were done there were not good techniques to deliver long term infusions in vivo, with the advent of portable infusion pumps and indwelling catheters, this mode of delivery has become quite feasible. An intermediate strategy of delivering 5-FU with a continuous infusion over 4–5 days is also feasible and has also became popular in specific clinical situations. The total amount of drug delivered is highest with the long term infusion, somewhat less with the short term (4 day) infusion, and lowest with the standard bolus approach.

Although the data of Byfield is of interest, there is certainly no agreement as to the mode of action of the combination. Lawrence et al. [15–17] have done extensive studies on the interaction, primarily using floxuridine (5-fluoro-2'-deoxyuridine, FduUrd or FUdR) to simplify the assessment (lack of RNA effects with FUdR). His data do not support the concept of radiation therapy producing chemosensitization, do not demonstrate a necessity for having the cell line sensitive to 5-FU in order to produce sensitization and do not support the concept of maximal cell kill when the radiation therapy is delivered prior to chemotherapy. Rather, his studies show that floxuridine exposure prior to radiation is more effective than after radiation, that sensitization enhances thymidylate synthase (TS) inhibition and is associated with a decrease in the number of DNA double strand breaks and sublethal damage repair.

Given the discrepancies in the experimental results described above, we decided to utilize an entirely different methodology to determine the mechanism of the 5-FU–radiation interaction. Data exist suggesting that tumors that retain 5-FU (as measured by F-19 nuclear magnetic resonance spectroscopy (NMRS)) have a better response to 5-FU based chemo-

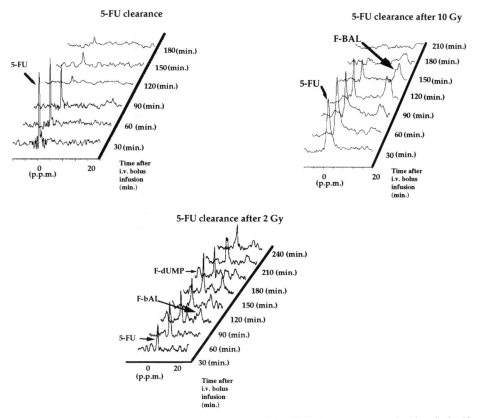

Fig. 1. F-19 NMR spectroscopy in animals after injection of either 5-FU alone or pre-treated with radiation therapy at doses of 2 Gy and 10 Gy. After the radiation therapy pre-treatment there is prolonged retention of both
5-FU and the metabolite 5-fluoro-$\beta$-alanine. The retention is greater at the higher radiation dose.

therapy [21]. Given some of the earlier data, we thought that it was possible that radiation
therapy was producing an improved chemotherapy response by increasing the tumor retention of the fluorinated pyrimidine. Thus, we embarked on a series of experiments utilizing
F-19 NMR spectroscopy to determine if this hypothesis is true.

With F-19 NMR spectroscopy one can obtain spectra at various times after injection of
the fluorine compound. One can detect the presence of the parent compound and, depending
on the strength of the NMR system, specific metabolites. Higher magnetic strengths improve the resolution of the system and can allow one to detect specific metabolites in shorter
periods of time.

Experiments were performed utilizing nude mice injected subcutaneously with $10^6$ human colon adenocarcinoma (HT-29) cells and these results have been previously reported
[20]. Animals were treated when the tumors were 1.0 cm in diameter which occurred approximately 3 weeks after the injection. All animals received an intravenous injection of
100 mg/kg of 5-FU. Animals in the first group received 5-FU alone, while animals in a second group received a single dose of 10 Gy of irradiation prior to the 5-FU. Animals then
were evaluated with NMR spectroscopy, using a 2 Tesla NMR spectroscopy system, at
varying times after the drug injection.

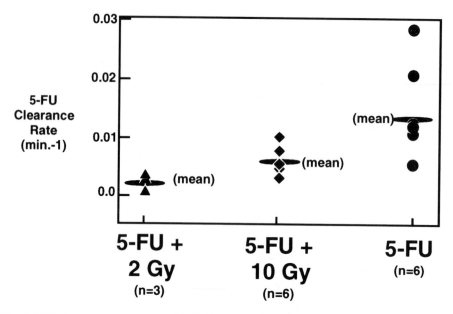

Fig. 2. 5-FU clearance rates as measured by F-19 NMR spectroscopy after injection of 5-FU alone or with pre-treatment with 2 Gy or 10 Gy of radiation therapy. The clearance rates are markedly decreased with the addition of radiation therapy, and there is a suggestion that this is a dose dependent phenomenon.

Typical spectra for animals treated with 5-FU, but with or without radiation therapy, are shown in Fig. 1. As can be seen, in animals which were pretreated with radiation, the 5-FU peak is maintained for substantially longer periods of time than for animals treated with 5-FU alone. There is a suggestion that the amount of 5-FU retention is dependent on the radiation dose. In addition, a peak representing the inactive metabolite, fluoro-$\beta$-alanine is much more pronounced in the animals that had been preirradiated. One can take this information and calculate the 5-FU clearance rates both with and without preirradiation. This calculation shows a three-fold difference in the clearance rates, from 0.00178/min without radiation to 0.00055/min with irradiation (Fig. 2). This large difference could result in tumor cells being exposed to the chemotherapeutic agent for substantially longer periods of time when pre-irradiated, thus producing a better therapeutic result.

A second set of experiments have also been performed to determine if this effect is resulting from retention of 5-FU in the tumor interstitium or whether there is a true intracellular effect (Blackstock et al., unpublished data). Similar experiments to those described above were performed except that after 5-FU exposure the cells were trypsinized and intracellular concentrations were determined by high performance liquid chromatography. After a dose of 2 Gy there was a 1.5-fold increase in the level of 5-FU and a 3-fold increase in the active metabolite 5-fluoro-2-deoxyuridine (FdUMP). A 5-fold increase in FdUMP was seen after pretreatment with 5 Gy of radiation, although no increase in 5-FU levels were seen. This could be secondary to the previously observed increase in levels of thymidine kinase after irradiation [22], which could lead to increased transformation of 5-FU to FdUMP.

These data are potentially quite relevant to the use of combined modality therapy in the clinic. If these differences hold up in patients, the use of radiation therapy could selectively cause increased retention of the chemotherapeutic agent in the tumor mass without any increase in systemic toxicity. Since the timing of the radiation is critical in this interaction, the exact timing of administration could have enormous impact on the therapeutic efficacy. It is indeed possible (and perhaps likely) that radiation therapy and 5-FU interact in a number of different ways. There may be a direct effect of 5-FU on the radiation therapy by modulation of DNA injury, with this effect being maximized when radiation therapy is delivered after the 5-FU. A second effect is that of increased drug retention when the drug is delivered after the radiation therapy. Since these two modes of action have very different implications for timing of drug delivery, it is important to distinguish between them.

Another possible method of dealing with the problem is to give 5-FU by a long term continuous infusion. This will, of course, result in chemotherapy being delivered before, during and after the radiation therapy, thereby taking advantage of both modes of drug–radiation interaction. A potential problem with this approach is that the amount of drug being delivered at any point in time is less with continuous infusion therapy. If this results in a low concentration of drug at the time that the radiation therapy is delivered, there would be less of an opportunity for sensitization. However, since drug serum concentrations tend to be higher with continuous infusion therapy than would be predicted by a simple extrapolation of the known half-life of 5-FU, this might not be a major problem.

## Summary

The mode of interaction between 5-FU chemotherapy and radiation therapy has been studied for many years but is still unclear. There is evidence for a number of different mechanisms of action, and it is possible that there are a number of different ways in which these agents interact in any given clinical situation, although one mechanism or another may dominate at various times. Further information as to the mechanisms of interaction will be important if we are to optimize the use of these agents clinically.

## References

1.   Heidelberger C, Griesbach L, Montag B, et al. Studies on fluorinated pyrimidines: II. Effects on transplanted tumors. Cancer Res 18: 305–317, 1958.
2.   Bagshaw M. Possible role of potentiators in radiation therapy. Am J Roentgen 85: 822–833, 1961.
3.   Vermund H, Hodgett J, Ansfield F. Effect of combined roentgen irradiation and chemotherapy on transplanted tumors in mice. Am J Roentgen 85: 559–567, 1961.
4.   Vietti T, Eggerding F, Valeriote F. Combined effect of X radiation on 5-fluorouracil on survival of transplanted leukemic cells. J Natl Cancer Inst 47: 865–870, 1971.
5.   Moertel C, Childs D, Reitemeier R, et al. Combined 5-Fluorouracil and supervoltage radiation therapy of locally unresectable gastrointestinal cancer. Lancet 2: 865–867, 1969.
6.   Herskovic A, Leichman L, Lattin P, et al. Chemo/radiation with and without surgery in the thoracic esophagus: the Wayne State experiment. N Engl J Med 24: 1593–1598, 1992.
7.   Moertel CG, Frytak S, Hahn RG, et al. Therapy of locally unresectable pancreatic carcinoma: a randomized comparison of high dose (6000 rads) radiation alone, moderate dose radiation (4000 rads + 5-fluorouracil), and high dose radiation + 5-fluorouracil. Cancer 48: 1705–1710, 1981.
8.   Gastrointestinal Tumor Study Group. Therapy of locally unresected pancreatic carcinoma: a randomized comparison of high dose (6000 rads) radiation alone, moderate dose radiation (4000 rads + 5-fluorouracil), and high dose radiation + 5-fluorouracil. Cancer 48: 1705–1710, 1981.
9.   Lawrence T, Maybaum J, Ensmigner W. Infusional fluoropyrimidines as radiation sensitizers: clinical implications of laboratory findings. Infusion Chemother 1995, in press.

10.   Gastrointestinal Tumor Study Group. Radiation therapy and fluorouracil with or without semustine for the treatment of patients with surgical adjuvant adenocarcinoma of the rectum. J Clin Oncol 10: 549–557, 1992.

11.   Nigro N, Sydel H, Considine B, et al. Combined preoperative radiation and chemotherapy for squamous cell carcinoma of the anal canal. Cancer 51: 1826–1829, 1983.

12.   Flam M, John M, Pajak T, et al. Role of mitomycin in combination with fluorouracil and radiotherapy, and of salvage chemoradiation in the definitive nonsurgical treatment of epidermoid carcinoma of the anal canal: results of a phase III randomized intergroup study. J Clin Oncol 14: 2527–2539, 1996.

13.   Sailer S, Weissler M, Melin S, et al. Toxicity and preliminary results from a trial of hyperfractionated radiation with or without simultaneous 5-fluorouracil-cisplatin in advanced head and neck squamous cell carcinomas. Semin Radiat Oncol 2: 38–40, 1992.

14.   McGinn C, Shewach D, Lawrence T. Radiosensitizing nucleosides. J Natl Cancer Inst 88: 1193–1203, 1996.

15.   Canman C, Tang H, Normolle D, et al. Variations in patterns of DNA damage induced in human colorectal tumor cells by 5-fluorodeoxyuridine: implications for mechanisms of resistance and cytotoxicity. Proc Natl Acad Sci USA 89: 10474–10478, 1992.

16.   Lawrence T, Davis M, Maybaum J. Dependence of 5-fluorouracil-mediated radiosenitization on DNA-directed effects. Int J Radiat Oncol Biol Phys 29: 519–523, 1994.

17.   Miller E, Kinsella T. Radiosensitization by fluorodeoxyuridine: effects on thymidylates synthase inhibition and cell synchronization. Cancer Res 52: 1687–1694, 1992.

18.   Byfield J, Calabro-Jones P, Klisak I, Kulhanian F. Pharmacologic requirements for obtaining sensitization of human tumor cells in vitro to combined 5-fluorouracil of ftorafur and x-rays. Int J Radiat Oncol Biol Phys 8: 1923–1933, 1982.

19.   Calabro-Jones P, Byfield J, Ward J, et al. Time-dose relationships for 5-fluorouracil cytotoxicity against human epithelial cancer cells in vitro. Cancer Res 42: 4413–4420, 1982.

20.   Blackstock AW, Kwock L, Gill M, et al. Tumor retention of 5-fluorouracil following irradiation observed using fluorine-19 nuclear magnetic resonance spectroscopy. Int J Radiat Oncol Biol Phys 30: 160, 1994.

21.   Presant C, Wolf W, Albright M, et al. Human tumor fluorouracil trapping: clinical correlations of in vivo 19f nuclear magnetic resonance spectroscopy pharmacokinetics. J Clin Oncol 8: 1868–1873, 1990.

22.   Boothman D, Davis T, Sahihdak W. Enhanced expression of thymidine kinase in human cells following ionizing radiation. Int J Radiat Oncol Biol Phys 30: 391–398, 1994.

C.J. Rosenthal and M. Rotman (Eds.), *Infusion Chemotherapy–Irradiation Interactions*

45

# CHAPTER 5

# Early clinical trials using platinum compounds as radiosensitizers

EPIE BOVEN

*Department of Medical Oncology, University Hospital Vrije Universiteit, De Boelelaan 1117,
1081 HV Amsterdam, The Netherlands*

## 1. Introduction

Cis-diamminedichloroplatinum(II), or cisplatin, is the first platinum compound in clinical use and has shown activity against a wide variety of human solid tumors. At a relatively early stage, cisplatin was also found to have radiosensitizing properties. Research on the mechanisms of interaction has mainly taken place in cell culture systems and in animal tumor models. Results have varied from showing marked sensitization to none at all. Since then, four drug-radiation mechanisms have been described that might be exploited separately or together [1]:

–  hypoxic cell radiosensitization due to the electron affinity of platinum compounds,
–  DNA targeting due to their alkylating property,
–  inhibition of recovery from radiation damage,
–  thiol interaction.

It appears that for radiosensitization by conventional cytostatic agents a good response to the drug alone is necessary in order to see any enhancement of radiation response [2]. This also appears to be the case for cisplatin [3]. Patients with tumors responsive to the platinum compound would therefore seem a reasonable choice to include in studies on cisplatin–radiotherapy. Based on this hypothesis, clinical trials have been carried out in non-small cell lung cancer, head and neck cancer, cancer of the esophagus, cervix, vulva and the bladder.

Extrapolation from in vivo studies to the clinic seems to be difficult in the determination of the optimum dose and time relationships for combinations on radiation and platinum compounds [4]. In several animal tumor models it has been shown that the most significant enhancement occurred with daily cisplatin concurrently given with daily radiation. Carboplatin has also been investigated as a radiosensitizer. Whether it is superior to cisplatin in the combined modality approach is presently unknown [4].

Concomitant chemoradiotherapy in the clinic is usually being investigated in locally advanced primary tumors. The most important goal is to improve complete remission and survival rates. Decreased toxicity and a reduced incidence of severe long-term sequelae with improved quality of life have become important secondary endpoints [4]. These are exemplified by the possibilities of organ preservation for larynx, esophagus, anal canal and bladder.

## 2. Daily cisplatin as a radiosensitizer

In the early 1980s, our group conducted a feasibility study on the daily administration of cisplatin in combination with radiation [5]. Twenty-one patients, 16 with primary tumors and 5 with localized metastases, received radiotherapy using various techniques and time dose volume factors. Fifteen patients were treated with two fractions of 125 cGy/day delivered by a 4 MeV linear accelerator. Six patients received a single daily dose, mostly of 180 cGy. Most patients had adequate total doses (50–60 Gy). Cisplatin was administered within 15–30 min after each radiation session.

The first group of 14 patients received a daily dose of cisplatin of 8 mg/m$^2$ either as one single injection or divided in two doses in the case of two daily radiation fractions. In this group of patients, severe leukopenia (5 patients grade 4) and thrombocytopenia (2 patients grade 3–4) required postponement of the combined treatment modality in 4 patients for 18–35 days. The 7 patients in the second group received a reduced dose of cisplatin of 6 mg/m$^2$ per day and showed only moderate myelosuppression. This daily cisplatin treatment did not require i.v. hydration in order to maintain normal renal function. Oral fluid intake of at least 2 l daily was prescribed.

Our group has carried out a phase II trial of daily cisplatin and radiation in locally advanced non-small cell lung cancer patients [6,7]. The regimen consisted of radiation doses of 300 cGy for 4 days every week for 4 weeks with a 2-week split in between. Each radiation dose was followed by an i.v. injection of cisplatin 6 mg/m$^2$ within 30 min. Hydration consisted of oral fluid intake of 2 l daily, enabling the patient to receive the treatment on an outpatient basis. Of 40 patients entered into the study, 37 were evaluable for toxicity and 33 for response. The overall response rate was 65% and in 22% of patients the response was complete. Median duration of local control was 7 months and of overall survival was 10.5 months. Of importance, median duration of complete responders was 29.5 months. Side-effects were tolerable; late toxicities included transient asymptomatic pneumonitis, 5 patients developed bullous lesions within the fibrotic area, one patient developed radiation myelopathy and another suffered from a vertebral collapse without evidence of associated tumor.

## 3. Non-small cell lung cancer

Since our group reported on the results of cisplatin combined with radiation in locally advanced non-small cell lung cancer [6,7] several others have followed this approach (Table 1). Havemann et al. [8] have administered cisplatin weekly on the first radiation day. They observed a response rate of 66.6%. Reboul et al. [9] have designed a schedule where cisplatin was given continuously 20 mg/m$^2$ per day for 5 days in the second week of the two cycles of radiation. The complete response rate was 65.9% with an overall response of 81.7%. In the 11 patients that underwent resection, 3/11 did not have pathological evidence of tumor. Other phase II trials have been reported where cisplatin was combined with other cytostatic agents [10–13]. The group of Taylor [10] has treated stage III patients with radiation, cisplatin and 5-fluorouracil every other week to enable surgical resection. Of 64 patients there were 8% complete and 48% partial responses. In the 39 patients that underwent the planned operation, only 9 were histologically free of disease. Pisch et al. [11] have not found an increased resectability of stage IIIB tumors nor was any surgical specimen free of

Table 1

Phase II trials of cisplatin and radiation in stage III non-small cell lung cancer

| Patients | Radiation | Total dose (Gy) | Chemotherapy[a] | Median survival (months) | Survival 2-years (%) | Ref. |
|---|---|---|---|---|---|---|
| 33 | 3 Gy 4×/week 2(2)[b] 2 weeks | 48 | CDDP 6 mg/m$^2$/day (+30 min) | 10.5 | n.s.[c] | [6] |
| 30 | 2 Gy 5×/week 3(2)[b] 2 weeks | 50 | CDDP 20 mg/m$^2$/week | 14 | 20 | [8] |
| 85 | 2 Gy 5×/week 4(2)[b] 3 weeks | 70 | CDDP 20 mg/m$^2$/day days 1–5 (continuously) weeks 2,8 | 11.4 | 27.5 | [9] |
| 64 | 2 Gy 5×/week weeks 1,3,5,7 | 40 | CDDP 60 mg/m$^2$ day 1 5FU 800 mg/m$^2$/day days 1–5 weeks 1,3,5,7 | 16 | n.s. | [10] |
| 47 | 2 Gy × 2, 5×/week weeks 1,4,7 | 60 | CDDP 30 mg/m$^2$/day days 1–3 VP16 80 mg/m$^2$/day days 1–3 5FU 900 mg/m$^2$/day days 1–4 weeks 1,4,7 | 12.5 | 43 | [11] |
| 42 | 1.2 Gy × 2, 29 days; 6 weeks | 69.6 | CDDP 75 mg/m$^2$ days 1,29,50 VBL 5 mg/m$^2$/week x5 | 12.2 | 28 | [12] |
| 126 | 1.8 Gy 5×/week 5 weeks | 45 | CDDP 50 mg/m$^2$ days 1,8,29,36 VP16 50 mg/m$^2$/day days 1–5, 29–33 | IIIA 13 IIIB 17 | 37 39 | [13] |

[a]CDDP, cisplatin; VP16, etoposide; 5FU, 5-fluorouracil; VBL, vinblastine
[b]Two-week interval.
[c]n.s., not stated.

cancer. Albain et al. [13] have been able to remove 85% of IIIA and 80% of IIIB tumors after the combination of cisplatin and etoposide with radiation. They did not measure a survival difference between the groups. The strongest predictor of long-term survival after thoracotomy was absence of mediastinal lymph node metastases.

The past few years at least five reports have appeared on radiotherapy alone compared with chemoradiotherapy including a platinum compound in locally advanced non-small cell lung cancer (Table 2). As an extension of our phase II study in which we combined cisplatin 6 mg/m$^2$ per day with daily fractions of radiation, Schaake-Koning et al. [13] have carried out a phase III trial on radiotherapy alone versus radiotherapy plus weekly cisplatin 30 mg/m$^2$ versus radiotherapy plus daily cisplatin 6 mg/m$^2$. Survival was significantly improved in the radiotherapy–daily cisplatin group as compared with radiotherapy alone ($P = 0.009$) which was especially due to improved control of local disease ($P = 0.003$). Patients treated with cisplatin had substantial complaints of nausea and vomiting. Pulmonary side-effects were similar in the three treatment arms. Trovó et al. [14] have not reported a survival advantage of daily cisplatin 6 mg/m$^2$ and radiation, but the total dose of radiation was lower than that of Schaake-Koning et al. [13]. The group of Blanke [15] have measured a slightly higher response rate ($P = 0.076$) of radiation combined with 3-weekly cisplatin (50%) as compared with radiation alone (38%), but the median survival was not different between the treatment arms. Jeremic et al. [16,17] have studied carboplatin as a radiosensitizer and combined the drug with etoposide. In the first hyperfractionated radiation trial of three treatment arms, a survival benefit was noted for the patients where carboplatin and

Table 2

Phase III trials of platinum compounds and radiation in stage III non-small cell lung cancer

| Patients | Radiation | Total dose (Gy) | Chemotherapy[a] | Median survival (months) | Survival 2-years (%) | Ref. |
|---|---|---|---|---|---|---|
| 331 | 3 Gy × 10, 2.5 Gy ×10; 2(3–4)[b] 2 weeks | 55 | I none | n.s.[c] | 13 | [14] |
| | | | II CDDP 30 mg/m$^2$/week | n.s. | 19 | |
| | | | III CDDP 6 mg/m$^2$/day (–1 h) | n.s. | 26[d] | |
| 173 | 3 Gy 5×/week 3 weeks | 45 | I none | 10.3 | n.s. | [15] |
| | | | II CDDP 6 mg/m$^2$/day (–1 h) | 10.0 | n.s. | |
| 240 | 1.8–2.0 Gy 5×/week | 60–65 | I none | 46 weeks | 13 | [16] |
| | | | II CDDP 70 mg/m$^2$ q 3 weeks | 43 weeks | 18 | |
| 169 | 1.2 Gy × 2 5×/week | 64.8 | I none | 8 | 25 | [17] |
| | | | II carbo 100 mg days 1,2 VP16 100 mg days 1–3 weekly | 18 | 35[d] | |
| | | | III carbo 200 mg days 1,2 VP16 100 mg days 1–5 weeks 1,3,5 | 13 | 27 | |
| 131 | 1.2 Gy × 2 5×/week | 69.6 | I none | 14 | 26 | [18] |
| | | | II carbo 50 mg daily VP16 50 mg daily | 22 | 43d | |

[a]CDDP, cisplatin; carbo, carboplatin; VP16, etoposide.
[b]3–4-week interval.
[c]n.s., not stated.
[d]Significant versus radiation alone.

etoposide were given weekly as compared with radiation alone ($P = 0.0027$) [16]. Patients on chemotherapy suffered from a slightly higher incidence of acute and late grade 4 side-effects. In the second trial, radiation was again given twice-a-day together with daily doses of carboplatin and etoposide and compared with radiation alone [17]. A survival benefit was noted in the chemoradiotherapy arm ($P = 0.021$) as was a reduced incidence of local recurrences ($P = 0.015$). The two groups showed a similar rate of acute and late grade 4 side-effects.

## 4. Head and neck cancer

For patients with locally advanced head and neck cancer, several attempts have been made to improve local control from radiotherapy by the addition of cisplatin. Also studies have been carried out with the combination either as neoadjuvant therapy to facilitate surgery or larynx preservation or as adjuvant therapy to improve local control after surgery.

The effective chemotherapy regimen of cisplatin and continuous-infusion 5-fluorouracil in head and neck cancer has been combined with radiotherapy in a number of trials in stage III/IV disease (Table 3). Taylor et al. [19] have reported a complete response rate of 55% and a median overall survival of 37 months which were improved with respect to previous data on radiotherapy alone. Also in the studies of Wendt et al. [20] and Adelstein et al. [22]

Table 3

Phase II trials of cisplatin and radiation in stage III/IV head and neck cancer

| Patients | Radiation | Total dose (Gy) | Chemotherapy[a] | Median progression-free survival (months) | Median survival (months) | Ref. |
|---|---|---|---|---|---|---|
| 53 | 2 Gy 5×/week every other week | 70 | CDDP 60 mg/m$^2$ day 1 5FU 800 mg/m$^2$/day days 1–5 every other week | 51 | 37 | [19] |
| 62 | 1.8 Gy × 2, days 3–11, 22–44 | 70.2 | CDDP 60 mg/m$^2$ day 1 5FU 350 mg/m$^2$/day days 2–5 LV 100 mg/m$^2$/day days 2–5 weeks 1,3 | 60 ± 7% at 2 years | 52 ± 8% at 2 years | [20] |
| 46 | 125 cGy × 2 5×/week | 70 | CDDP 12 mg/m$^2$/day days 1–5 5FU 600 mg/m$^2$/day days 1–5 weeks 1,6 | 65% at 2 years | 73% at 2 years | [21] |
| 57 | 2 Gy 5×/week weeks 1–3, 9–11 | 60–68 | CDDP 75 mg/m$^2$/day 5FU 1000 mg/m$^2$/day days 1–4 weeks 1,5,9 | 26 | 37 | [22] |

[a]CDDP, cisplatin; 5FU, 5-fluorouracil; LV, leucovorin

complete responses were observed frequently and amounted to 81 and 77%, respectively. Brizel et al. [21] have reported complete responses in 92% of the primary tumors and in 71% of patients with neck disease at presentation. The major toxicities were weight loss of 10% or more [19,21] and severe mucositis. Some patients required enteral feeding tubes.

In a randomized trial in stage III/IV head and neck cancer, Bachaud et al. [23] have measured a better disease-free survival after surgery when radiotherapy was combined with weekly cisplatin 50 mg i.v. than after radiotherapy alone (respectively 65 and 41% at 2 years; $P < 0.01$). The total dose of radiation was 54–70 Gy depending on the extent of disease. The rate of locoregional failures was significantly higher in the radiotherapy alone group ($P < 0.05$). Side-effects, consisting of >10% body weight loss, mucositis, nausea and vomiting, as well as neutropenia, were more frequent in the chemoradiotherapy group, but were reversible in all instances. Another randomized trial carried out by Taylor et al. [24] has contained two groups of 107 patients each receiving either cisplatin 100 mg/m$^2$ on day 1 and 5-fluorouracil 1000 mg/m$^2$ per day continuously days 1–5 every 3 weeks for 3 cycles followed by 70 Gy of radiation or cisplatin 60 mg/m$^2$ on day 1 and 5-fluorouracil 800 mg/m$^2$ per day continuously on days 1–5 concurrently with radiation 2 Gy/day, on days 1–5 every other week for 7 cycles. The overall responses were 78 and 93%, respectively ($P = 0.006$). Initially all patients were considered to have inoperable disease; after chemoradiotherapy a total of 28 patients underwent surgery that included resection of the primary tumor. The progression-free survival was better in the concomitant treatment group ($P = 0.003$). No overall survival benefit was apparent for either regimen; sites of failure included the primary tumor site, regional neck disease and/or distant metastases. More supportive care was necessary in the concomitant arm due to radiation-induced mucositis.

## 5.  Cancer of the esophagus

A randomized trial in patients with squamous cell carcinoma or adenocarcinoma of the esophagus has been carried out by Herskovic et al. [25]. The group has compared cisplatin 75 mg/m$^2$ on day 1 and 5-fluorouracil 1000 mg/m$^2$ continuously for 4 days in weeks 1, 5, 8 and 11 plus radiotherapy in a dose of 50 Gy versus radiotherapy alone in a dose of 64 Gy in a total number of 121 patients. The survival in the combined modality group was 38% at 2 years, whereas this was 10% in the radiotherapy only group ($P < 0.001$). Severe side-effects, however, occurred in 44 and 25% of the patients, respectively. Reddy et al. [26] have treated 77 patients with squamous cell carcinoma either with radiotherapy alone (60–70 Gy) or combined with cisplatin 100 mg/m$^2$ on day 1 and 5-fluorouracil 1000 mg/m$^2$ per day continuously on days 2–5 every 4 weeks. Again, a survival benefit was noted for the concomitant arm: at 2 years 30% versus 7% ($P = 0.02$). Few patients suffered from treatment-related complications; dysphagia and the occurrence of fistulae developed in patients with persistent or progressive cancer. Forastiere et al. [27] have studied preoperative chemoradiotherapy in 43 patients with advanced squamous cell carcinoma or adenocarcinoma of the esophagus or cardia. Patients received cisplatin 20 mg/m$^2$ per day continuously on days 1–5 and 17–21, vinblastine 1 mg/m$^2$ per day bolus days 1–4 and 17–20 and 5-fluorouracil 300 mg/m$^2$ per day continuously on days 1–21 plus radiation 3750 cGy in 15 (250 cGy) or 45 Gy in 15 (150 cGy ×2) fractions. Of 41 patients, 36 had a potentially curative resection; 10/41 were tumor-free in the esophagus and adjacent lymph nodes. The median survival of all 43 patients was 29 months; 34% were alive at 5 years. The results of this regimen appeared to be improved over those reported with surgery alone. The majority of patients, however, experienced severe leukopenia and required nutritional support.

## 6.  Cervical cancer

A number of trials have been designed to improve the local control of advanced cancer of the cervix by adding cisplatin and other cytostatic agents to radiation (Table 4). In most instances cisplatin was given intermittently 50–60 mg/m$^2$ every 10–21 days except for the group of Morris et al. [31]. This group administered cisplatin plus floxuridine through bilateral intra-arterial catheters in the anterior division of the internal iliac arteries. Locoregional control of disease was high in all trials and amounted from 78 to 95%. The survival at 2 years was 61% in the study of Resbeut et al. [29] and this was 60% at 4 years in the study of Pearcey et al. [30]. In general, acute toxicity consisted of nausea, vomiting, myelosuppression and local gastrointestinal side-effects, such as diarrhea. Some late complications were renal insufficiency [29], chronic enteritis [29,30], rectovaginal or vesicovaginal fistulae [30].

## 7.  Cancer of the vulva

A small study has been reported in patients with advanced vulvar cancer who have been treated with radiation (40–50 Gy) concurrently given with cisplatin 4 mg/m$^2$ per day and 5-fluorouracil 250 mg/m$^2$ per day both continuously for 4 days every week for 4 weeks [32].

Table 4

Phase II trials of cisplatin and radiation in advanced cervical cancer

| Patients | Radiation | Chemotherapy[a] | Response (%) | Ref. |
|---|---|---|---|---|
| 19 | 50 Gy pelvis (28 fr)<br>60 Gy brachytherapy<br>40 Gy nodes | Cisplatin 50 mg/m$^2$ days 1,22,43<br>MMC 10 mg/m$^2$ days 1,43 | Local 95 | [28] |
| 40 | 45 Gy pelvis (33 days)<br>15 Gy brachytherapy<br>55–60 Gy nodes | Cisplatin 60 mg/m$^2$ days 1,21<br>5FU 600 mg/m$^2$/day days 1–4,<br>21–24 | Local 80 | [29] |
| 60 | 45 Gy pelvis (25 fr)<br>35–40 Gy brachytherapy<br>40–45 Gy nodes | Cisplatin 50 mg/m$^2$<br>days 1,11,21,31 | Local 78 | [30] |
| 16 | 40 Gy pelvis (20 fr)<br>brachytherapy<br>60–65 Gy nodes | FUDR i.a. 6.5–27 mg/m$^2$/day<br>days 1–5 weeks 1,2<br>Cisplatin i.a. 2–8 mg/m$^2$/day<br>days 1–5 weeks 3,4 | Local 88 | [31] |

[a]MMC, mitomycin C; 5FU, 5-fluorouracil; FDUR, floxuridine

Eleven of 12 patients had a partial clinical response. Four of 8 patients that underwent vulvar resection had no residual disease. Chemoradiotherapy was tolerated well.

## 8. Bladder cancer

An early study in clinical $T_2$ to $T_4$ bladder cancer on cisplatin 70 mg/m$^2$ given every 3 weeks for 8 courses concurrently with full dose radiation (63–68 Gy) in the first 7.5–10 weeks of treatment resulted in 13 complete responders of 17 evaluable patients [33]. Nausea and vomiting occurred in 74% of patients and in 3 patients significant side-effects developed: renal failure, systemic sepsis and transient small bowel obstruction. Chauvet et al. [34] have treated 69 patients with inoperable invasive bladder cancer with a regimen consisting of a radiation dose to the bladder of 55–60 Gy and the pelvic area of 40–45 Gy with concomitant continuous infusion cisplatin 20–25 mg/m$^2$ per day for 5 days in weeks 2 and 5 of radiation. In 18 patients, a macroscopically complete transurethral resection was carried out preceding chemoradiotherapy. Of 63 evaluable patients 48 achieved a complete response. The actuarial overall 3-year survival rate was 37.1% for all patients. In general, toxicity of this regimen was mild and acceptable.

In the study of Kaufman et al. [35] an attempt has been made to preserve the bladder in patients with $T_2$ to $T_4$ invasive bladder cancer. Patients underwent transurethral resection first, then received two cycles methotrexate–cisplatin–vinblastine and completed the treatment with radiation 45 Gy over a period of 5 weeks given concurrently with cisplatin 70 mg/m$^2$ on days 1 and 22. Consolidation chemoradiotherapy of 24.8 Gy and another cycle of cisplatin was given to patients that achieved a complete response or to incomplete responders unfit for surgery. Of the 53 patients entered into the trial, 46 patients completed the treatment; 8/10 incomplete responders underwent radical cystectomy and 34/36 patients with a complete response or unfit for surgery completed consolidation chemotherapy. At 2 years 45% of the patients were alive and free of disease. Of the 28 patients who achieved a complete response after initial treatment, 89% had functioning tumor-free bladders. The toxicity of this intensive treatment regimen was quite high. Eleven patients could not complete the chemoradiotherapy part because of renal dysfunction, intolerable incontinence, fatigue, cardiopulmonary failure or refused further treatment.

Mizoguchi et al. [36] have combined intraarterial cisplatin infusion with radiation in 23 patients with invasive bladder cancer. Cisplatin at a dose of 50 mg was infused into the internal iliac artery twice a week over 3 weeks concurrently with 30 Gy radiation in 15 fractions. In 2/6 patients who underwent total cystectomy, a complete response was noted. Preservation of bladder function by transurethral resection of the residual tumor was achieved in 17 patients. The overall response rate was 87%. Side-effects were tolerable and consisted of nausea, vomiting, myelosuppression and nephrotoxicity.

## 9. Conclusions

Early clinical trials using platinum compounds and more specifically cisplatin as radiosensitizer combined with radiotherapy have shown the feasibility of this approach. Side-effects are tolerable, but are increased in frequency as compared with radiotherapy alone. The frequency of late local toxicity appears to be slightly higher, and depends on the choice of the cytostatic agent as well as the presence of persistent tumor lesions. Randomized trials comparing cisplatin–radiotherapy versus radiotherapy alone have frequently reported improved local control. Cisplatin-sensitive tumor types appear to benefit most from the combination. Thus far, there is no control on the formation of distant metastases. This means that the combined modality approach does not consistently improve the overall survival. Of major interest is the role of chemoradiotherapy in organ preservation. Future studies should be restricted to well-controlled randomized trials and focus on the optimization of the dosing and the schedule when cisplatin is used as a radiation-enhancing compound.

## References

1. Nias AHW. Radiation and platinum drug interaction. Int J Radiat Biol 48: 297–314, 1985.
2. Steel GG. The search for therapeutic gain in the combination of radiotherapy and chemotherapy. Radiother Oncol 11: 31–53, 1988.
3. Begg AC. Cisplatin and radiation: interaction probabilities and therapeutic possibilities. Int J Radiat Oncol Biol Phys 19: 1183–1189, 1990.
4. Vokes EE. Interaction of chemotherapy and radiation. Semin Oncol 20: 70–79, 1993.
5. Keizer HJ, Karim ABMF, Njo KH, et al. Feasibility study on daily administration of cis-diamminedichloroplatinum (II) in combination with radiotherapy. Radiother Oncol 1: 227–234, 1984.
6. Van Harskamp G, Boven E, Vermorken JB, et al. Phase II trial of combined radiotherapy and daily low-dose cisplatin for inoperable, locally advanced non-small cell lung cancer. Int J Radiat Oncol Biol Phys 13: 1735–1738, 1987.
7. Boven E, Tierie AH, Stam J, Pinedo HM. Combined radiation therapy and daily low-dose cisplatin for inoperable, locally advanced non-small cell lung cancer: results of a phase II trial. Semin Oncol 15(Suppl 7): 18–19, 1988.
8. Havemann K, Wolf M, Görg C, et al. Preclinical and clinical experience with cisplatin and carboplatin and simultaneous radiation in non-small cell lung cancer. Ann Oncol 3(Suppl 3): S33-S37, 1992.
9. Reboul F, Vincent P, Chauvet B, et al. Radiation therapy with concomitant continuous infusion cisplatin for unresectable non-small cell lung carcinoma. Int J Radiat Oncol Biol Phys 28: 1251–1256, 1994.

10. Taylor SG, Trybula M, Bonomi PD, et al. Simultaneous cisplatin fluorouracil infusion and radiation followed by surgical resection in regionally localized stage III, non-small cell lung cancer. Ann Thorac Surg 43: 87–91, 1987.

11. Pisch J, Berson AM, Malamud S, et al. Chemoradiation in advanced non-small cell lung cancer. Int J Radiat Oncol Biol Phys 33: 185–188, 1995.

12. Byhardt RW, Scott CB, Ettinger DS, et al. Concurrent hyperfractionated irradiation and chemotherapy for unresectable non-small cell lung cancer. Cancer 75: 2337–2344, 1995.

13. Albain KS, Rusch VW, Crowley JJ, et al. Concurrent cisplatin/etoposide plus chest radiotherapy followed by surgery for stages IIIA (N2) and IIIB non-small cell lung cancer: mature results of Southwest Oncology Group phase II study 8805. J Clin Oncol 13: 1880–1892, 1995.

14. Schaake-Koning C, Van den Bogaert W, Dalesio O, et al. Effects of concomitant cisplatin and radiotherapy on inoperable non-small cell lung cancer. N Engl J Med 326: 524–530, 1992.

15. Trovó MG, Minatel E, Franchin G, et al. Radiotherapy versus radiotherapy enhanced by cisplatin in stage III non-small cell lung cancer. Int J Radiat Oncol Biol Phys 24: 11–15, 1992.

16. Blanke C, Ansari R, Mantravadi R, et al. Phase III trial of thoracic irradiation with or without cisplatin for locally advanced unresectable non-small cell lung cancer: a Hoosier Oncology Group protocol. J Clin Oncol 13: 1425–1429, 1995.

17. Jeremic B, Shibamoto Y, Acimovic L, Djuric L. Randomized trial of hyperfractionated radiation therapy with or without concurrent chemotherapy for stage III non-small cell lung cancer. J Clin Oncol 13: 452–458, 1995.

18. Jeremic B, Shibamoto Y, Acimovic L, Milisavljevic S. Hyperfractionated radiation therapy with or without concurrent low-dose daily carboplatin/etoposide for stage III non-small cell lung cancer: a randomized study. J Clin Oncol 14: 1065–1070, 1996.

19. Taylor SG, Murthy AK, Caldarelli DD, et al. Combined simultaneous cisplatin/ fluorouracil chemotherapy and split course radiation in head and neck cancer. J Clin Oncol 7: 846–856, 1989.

20. Wendt TG, Hartenstein RC, Wustrow TPU, Lissner J. Cisplatin, fluorouracil with leucovorin calcium enhancement, and synchronous accelerated radiotherapy in the management of locally advanced head and neck cancer: a phase II study. J Clin Oncol 7: 471–476, 1989.

21. Brizel DM, Leopold KA, Fisher SR, et al. A phase I/II trial of twice daily irradiation and concurrent chemotherapy for locally advanced squamous cell carcinoma of the head and neck. Int J Radiat Oncol Biol Phys 28: 213–220, 1993.

22. Adelstein DJ, Kalish LA, Adams GL, et al. Concurrent radiation therapy and chemotherapy for locally unresectable squamous cell head and neck cancer: an Eastern Cooperative Oncology Group pilot study. J Clin Oncol 11: 2136–2142, 1993

23. Bachaud JM, David JM, Boussin G, Daly N. Combined postoperative radiotherapy and weekly cisplatin infusion for locally advanced squamous cell carcinoma of the head and neck: preliminary report of a randomized trial. Int J Radiat Oncol Biol Phys 20: 243–246, 1991.

24. Taylor SG, Murthy AK, Vannetzel JM, et al. Randomized comparison of neoadjuvant cisplatin and fluorouracil infusion followed by radiation versus concomitant treatment in advanced head and neck cancer. J Clin Oncol 12: 385–395, 1994.

25. Herskovic A, Martz K, Al-Sarraf M, et al. Combined chemotherapy and radiotherapy compared with radiotherapy alone in patients with cancer of the esophagus. N Engl J Med 326: 1593–1598, 1992.

26. Reddy SP, Lad T, Mullane M, et al. Radiotherapy alone compared with radiotherapy and chemotherapy in patients with squamous cell carcinoma of the esophagus. Am J Clin Oncol 18: 376–381, 1995.

27. Forastiere AA, Orringer MB, Perez-Tamayo C, et al. Preoperative chemoradiation followed by transhiatal esophagectomy for carcinoma of the esophagus: final report. J Clin Oncol 11: 1118–1123, 1993.

28. Malviya VK, Deppe G, Kim Y, Gove N. Concurrent radiation therapy, cis-platinum, and mitomycin C in patients with poor prognosis cancer of the cervix: a pilot study. Am J Clin Oncol 12: 434–437, 1989.

29. Resbeut M, Cowen D, Viens P, et al. Concomitant chemoradiation prior to surgery in the treatment of advanced cervical carcinoma. Gynecol Oncol 54: 68–75, 1994.

30. Pearcey RG, Stuart GCE, MacLean GD, et al. Phase II study to evaluate the toxicity and efficacy of concurrent cisplatin and radiation therapy in the treatment of patients with locally advanced squamous cell carcinoma of the cervix. Gynecol Oncol 58: 34–41, 1995.

31. Morris M, Eifel PJ, Burke TW, et al. Treatment of locally advanced cervical cancer with concurrent radiation and intra-arterial chemotherapy. Gynecol Oncol 57: 72–78, 1995.

32.  Eifel PJ, Morris M, Burke TW, et al. Prolonged continuous infusion cisplatin and 5-fluorouracil with radiation for locally advanced carcinoma of the vulva. Gynecol Oncol 59: 51–56, 1995.
33.  Shipley WU, Coombs LJ, Einstein AB, et al. Cisplatin and full dose irradiation for patients with invasive bladder carcinoma: a preliminary report of tolerance and local response. J Urol 132: 899–903, 1984.
34.  Chauvet B, Brewer Y, Félix-Faure C, et al. Combined radiation therapy and cisplatin for locally advanced carcinoma of the urinary bladder. Cancer 72: 2213–2218, 1993.
35.  Kaufman DS, Shipley WU, Griffin PP, et al. Selective bladder preservation by combination treatment of invasive bladder cancer. N Engl J Med 329: 1377–1382, 1993.
36.  Mizoguchi H, Nomura Y, Terada K, et al. Combined intraarterial cisplatin infusion and radiation therapy for invasive bladder cancer. Int J Urol 2: 17–23, 1995.

C.J. Rosenthal and M. Rotman (Eds.), *Infusion Chemotherapy–Irradiation Interactions*

# *cis*-Dichlorodiammine platinum(II) given in low-dose continuous infusion with concurrent radiotherapy to patients affected by inoperable lung carcinoma: a pharmacokinetic approach

FRANCA MORAZZONI[1], CARMEN CANEVALI[1], MASSIMO ZUCCHETTI[2],
SERGIO CAROLI[3], ALESSANDRO ALIMONTI[3], FRANCESCO PETRUCCI[3],
GABRIELLA GIUDICE[4], ENRICO MASONI[1]
and AMEDEO VITTORIO BEDINI[4]

[1] *Dipartimento di Chimica Inorganica Metallorganica e Analitica, Centro CNR, Via Venezian 21, 20133 Milano, Italy* [2], *Istituto di Ricerche Farmacologiche " Mario Negri", Via Eritrea 62 , 20157 Milano, Italy,* [3] *Laboratorio di Tossicologia Applicata, Istituto Superiore di Sanità, Viale Regina Elena 299, 00161 Roma, Italy and* [4] *Istituto Nazionale Tumori, Via Venezian 1, 20133 Milano, Italy*

## *1. Introduction*

The standard treatment for patients with locally advanced inoperable non-small cell lung carcinoma (NSCLC) is radiotherapy (RT), but the related chance of cure is indeed dismal, the long-term survival rate being 0–5%. Locoregional failure is the principal cause of death and accounts for 70% of all deaths [1].

Many investigational programs on radiopotentiation have been performed with the aim of improving survival through the achievement of a better response rate and better locoregional control. A combination therapy, radiation treatment and concurrent *cis*-dichloro diammine platinum (CDDP) infusion, is one of the most developed techniques employed after preclinical and clinical investigations.

Several clinical experiences have been reported on low-dose CDDP and RT in NSCLC [2–9]. However, the effort to ameliorate the therapeutic index of the schedules was based on a cocktail of empirically mixed ingredients since no major information is available on the pharmacokinetics of CDDP delivery at low dose and/or by repeated continuous intravenous infusion (RCVI). To fill this gap and with the aim of further optimizing future treatment plans we projected the study reported in the present paper.

Analytical problems due to extremely low levels of drug or drug metabolites in blood were solved in the investigation on a first group of 22 patients. However, the results of this study were deduced from too small a number of samples to provide a pharmacologic rationale regarding the efficiency of our therapeutic schedule. In the investigation of a second group of 16 patients the results were definitely rectified by taking the following steps:

– analytical levels of Pt were reconsidered by collecting a larger number of samples from patients followed throughout the therapy;
– decay trends of the infused drug were determined and the related pharmacokinetic parameters calculated.

## 2. Patients and methods

### 2.1. Administration procedure and selection of patients

At the time of the pharmacokinetic evaluation of the present study, the regimen under investigation at the National Cancer Institute of Milan was of a weekly dose of 10 Gy given in 5 fractions from Monday to Friday, and a concurrent 100-h infusion of CDDP, delivered at a daily dose of 4 mg/m$^2$ by means of a central venous catheter and a portable pump; the treatment was repeated for 5 (first group of patients) or 6 (second group of patients) consecutive weeks (Fig. 1). CDDP infusion was started just before the first weekly administration of radiotherapy (RT), and suspended on Friday, after the last. The weekly schedule delivered a total RT dose of 60 Gy and a CDDP total dose of roughly 96 mg/m$^2$. This regimen was evaluated in one feasibility and one phase II study.

Histologically proven NSCLC, informed consent, physical examination, chest X-rays, bronchoscopy, and computed studies of brain, chest, and upper abdomen were entry criteria. Exclusion criteria were: pleural effusion, inability to be ambulatory, age >75 years, previous treatment, impaired cardiac or renal function, abnormal blood cell counts.

Further entry criteria of 5 patients enrolled in the phase II study were stage IIIa-N2, functional operability and absence of superior vena cava syndrome.

Toxicity and response criteria followed the Eastern Cooperative Oncology Group (ECOG) [10] and World Health Organization (WHO) [11] rules, respectively. The patients' clinical response was assessed by means of computed studies of brain, chest, and upper abdomen about 45 days after the end of treatment.

### 2.2. Sampling procedure

Patients were sampled before the start (on Monday) and at the end (on Friday) of the continuous weekly infusion. The disappearance of platinum from plasma and ultrafiltrate plasma was observed in patients who were sampled at the end of the first and fifth weeks of treatment at the following times after the end of infusion: 0.5, 1, 4, 7, 10 and 24 h.

Blood samples (10 ml) were collected in heparinized tubes and centrifuged at 2500 rev./min for 15 min at 4°C to obtain plasma. This plasma (about 5 ml) was separated and subdivided in two portions: A and B. Portion B (about 2.5 ml) was stored in cryotubes (NUNC,

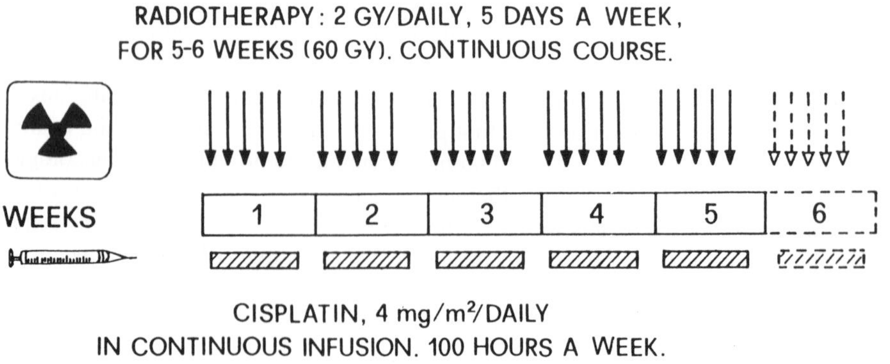

RADIOTHERAPY: 2 GY/DAILY, 5 DAYS A WEEK, FOR 5-6 WEEKS (60 GY). CONTINUOUS COURSE.

CISPLATIN, 4 mg/m$^2$/DAILY IN CONTINUOUS INFUSION. 100 HOURS A WEEK.

Fig. 1. Scheme of the treatment.

Denmark) at −20°C until the analysis of total Pt. Portion A (about 2.5 ml) was centrifuged at 5000 rev./min for 90 min at 4°C using Centriflo ultrafiltration membrane cones having a cutoff value of 50 000 kDa (Amicon Corp., USA). Further centrifugation was performed at 5000 rev./min for 60 min at 4°C on Centricon-10 microconcentrators (Amicon Corp., USA) having a cutoff value of 10 000 kDa. However, no residual fraction was obtained. The ultrafiltrate was stored at −20°C in cryotubes (NUNC, Denmark) until the analysis of platinum.

## 2.3.   Analytical procedure

Samples were thawed in a warm bath immediately before analysis. Determinations of platinum in plasma were accomplished by inductively coupled plasma-atomic emission spectrometry (ICP-AES) by diluting samples 1:3 (vol/vol) with Milli-Q (Millipore) water. No detectable level of the element was measured in water used for dilution. Calibration was performed using Pt(II) standard solutions in Milli-Q water. Matrix effects due to plasmatic components proved to be irrelevant within the concentration range under investigation. Basic information on the apparatus and experimental conditions is given in Table 1. Determination of platinum in ultrafiltrate plasma was carried out by inductively coupled plasma-mass spectrometry (ICP.MS) after 1:4 (v/v) dilution of samples with Milli-Q water. Calibration was performed by using standard addition method. The instrumental specifications and analytical conditions are reported in Table 2. ICP-MS spectrometer, employing an ultrasonic U 5000 AT nebulizer (Cetac, Omaha, NB) allowed an overall measurement precision of 0.015 $\mu$g/l.

## 2.4.   Pharmacokinetic and statistical analysis

Fittings curves of the experimental Pt concentrations versus time during the weeks of infusion were calculated using the routine FORTRAN VA04A program on the appropriate function [12].

Pt decay curves at the end of first and fifth weeks of infusion were determined in plasma and in ultrafiltrate plasma by fitting the data on a general non-linear fitting program [13], in accordance with the biexponential function:

Table 1

ICP-AES apparatus specifications and analytical conditions for the determination of Pt

| | |
| --- | --- |
| Spectrometer | Instruments SA, Jobin-Yvon 24 Sequential (France) |
| Monochromator | Czerny-Turner mounting |
| Nebulizer | Meinhard pneumatic |
| RF Power | 1.0 kW |
| Auxiliary gas flow | 14 l/min |
| Sheath gas flow | 0.2 l/min |
| Aerosol gas flow | 0.35 l/min |
| Sample feed | 0.50 ml/min |
| Analyte line [Pt(II)] | 214.42 nm |
| Reference line [C] | 193.09 nm |
| Integration period | 300 ms |

$$[Pt] = A \exp(-\alpha t) + B \exp(-\beta t) \tag{1}$$

The 24 h post-infusion area under the curves of [Pt] concentration versus time (AUC), distribution ($t_{1/2}\, \alpha$) and terminal ($t_{1/2}\, \beta$) half life were obtained from the fitting of the decay curves.

The variability of pharmacokinetic results was compared by analysis of variance. A probability $P = 0.05$ or less was considered significant (Duncan test).

## 3.  Results

### 3.1.  Clinical results

All the patients were evaluable for their locoregional response, the objective response rate having been 75%. The minimum follow-up period was 12 months. Complete clinical data were available in all the cases. The first site of progression was found within the irradiated area in 12.5% of cases.

Figure 2 shows the Pt concentration levels in plasma, $[Pt]^{tot}$, and in ultrafiltrate plasma, $[Pt]^{uf}$, of the first group of 22 patients. The values of platinum levels determined on Mondays and Fridays during the 5 weeks of infusion, reported in Table 3, were appropriately fitted by the curve of continuous infusions $[Pt] = K(1 - \exp(-kt))$; $[Pt] = [Pt]_{Friday}$ on days 4, 11, 18, 25, 32; $[Pt] = [Pt]_{Monday}$ on days 7,14,21,28,35; $t = $ time in days. The percentage of Pt in ultrafiltrate plasma versus that in plasma, calculated from the fitting curves, was about 3% and did not vary with the therapy duration.

Figure 3 shows the values of platinum in plasma, $[Pt]^{tot}$, and in ultrafiltrate plasma,$[Pt]^{uf}$, determined in the second group of patients during the 6 weeks of therapy and also on days 1, 2 and 3 of the first infusion week. $[Pt]^{tot}$ increased rapidly during the first week of therapy, then more slowly in the following weeks. The levels on Monday,$[Pt]^{tot}_{Monday}$, (i.e., the first day of the infusion) were roughly 2 times lower than those on Friday, $[Pt]^{tot}_{Friday}$, (i.e., the last day of the infusion); however, although drug administration was interrupted weekly on Friday, $[Pt]^{tot}_{Friday}$ at the end of each week became comparable or slightly higher than at

Table 2

ICP-MS apparatus specifications and analytical conditions for the determination of Pt

| | |
|---|---|
| Spectrometer | Elan 5000 ICP-MS (Perkin-Elmer, USA) |
| Nebulizer | Cross flow, Scott chamber |
| RF Power | 1.0 kW |
| Plasma gas flow | 16 ml/min |
| Auxiliary gas flow | 1 ml/min |
| Aerosol gas flow | 1 ml/min |
| Sample feed | 1 ml/min |
| Element/Mass | Pt/195 |
| Optimization | on signal: $^{103}$Rh, $^{24}$Mg, $^{208}$Pb |
| Replicate time | 15000 ms |
| Dwell time | 300 ms |
| Sweeps for readings | 5 |
| Readings/ licate | 3 |
| Sc...g mode | Peak hop transient |

Table 3

Platinum levels on Mondays and Fridays during the 5 weeks of infusion

| Weeks | Total Pt ($\mu$g/l)[a] | | Free Pt ($\mu$g/l)* | | Percentage of free Pt versus total Pt | |
|-------|------------------------|--------|---------------------|--------|---------|--------|
|       | Friday | Monday | Friday | Monday | Friday | Monday |
| 1st | 238 (195–294) | 148 (158–209) | 8.6 (4.2–11.5) | 5.0 (2.0–6.2) | 3.59 | 3.37 |
| 2nd | 341 (218–478) | 237 (101–299) | 11.0 (5.6–18.1) | 7.4 (4.6–16.3) | 3.23 | 3.12 |
| 3rd | 356 (260–528) | 290 (199–412) | 11.2 (6.0–19.2) | 8.6 (3.3–15.4) | 3.15 | 2.96 |
| 4th | 358 (265–438) | 322 (203–376) | 11.2 (6.5–18.5) | 9.2 (2.9–13.0) | 3.13 | 2.86 |
| 5th | 358 (265–572) | 341 (364–444) | 11.2 (7.7–13.8) | 9.4 (10.8–12.8) | 3.12 | 2.75 |

[a]Calculated values (the minimum and the maximum of the experimental values are shown within parentheses).

the end of the previous week. Also in this case the $[Pt]^{tot}_{Friday}$ values throughout the therapy appropriately fitted the curve characteristic of continuous infusions $[Pt] = K(1 - \exp(-kt))$ (Table 4 and Fig. 3).

From the end of the first administration week and during the 6 weeks of therapy, $[Pt]^{uf}_{Friday}$ showed values that increased less compared with those of the corresponding $[Pt]^{tot}_{Friday}$ (Table 4 and Fig. 3). In the case of $[Pt]^{uf}_{Friday}$ the standard deviation of data was much higher (Fig. 3) than for all the other Pt concentration values. $[Pt]^{uf}_{Friday}$ ranged from 16 to 22% of $[Pt]^{tot}_{Friday}$. The values of $[Pt]^{uf}_{Monday}$ were 20–40 times lower than $[Pt]^{uf}_{Friday}$,

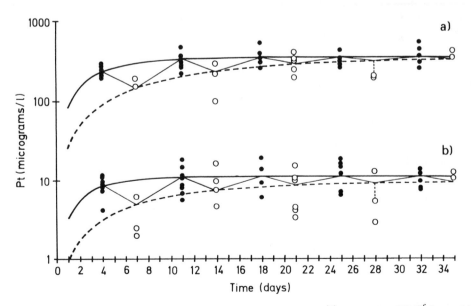

Fig. 2. Plasma concentration levels and best fitting curves generated for $[Pt]^{tot}$ (curves a) and $[Pt]^{uf}$ (curves b) on Fridays and on Mondays, reported versus sampling day. Each point represents the Pt concentration for an individual patient. Solid circles stand for the concentrations measured on Friday, open circles for those on Monday.

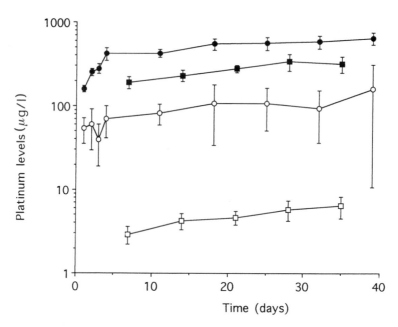

Fig. 3. Mean values ± the standard deviation value of plasma concentration levels ($\mu$g/l) for $[Pt]^{tot}$ (solid symbols) and $[Pt]^{uf}$ (open symbols) on Fridays (○) and on Mondays (□) reported versus sampling day.

representing 1.5–2 % of $[Pt]^{tot}_{Monday}$. The percentages of Pt in ultrafiltrate plasma on Monday were always statistically lower ($P < 0.01$) than those on Friday.

Figure 4 shows the disappearance of $[Pt]^{tot}$ and $[Pt]^{uf}$ at the end of the first and fifth infusion weeks. In most patients a biexponential decay of both Pt species was observed. $[Pt]^{tot}$ levels appeared higher after the fifth than after the first infusion week, while the corresponding $[Pt]^{uf}$ levels showed less marked differences. These results confirmed the trend of both $[Pt]^{tot}_{Friday}$ and $[Pt]^{uf}_{Friday}$ during the 6 weeks of drug administration: $[Pt]^{tot}_{Friday}$ values increased during therapy, while $[Pt]^{uf}_{Friday}$ values were more or less unvaried.

Tables 5 and 6 show the pharmacokinetic parameters determined in patients for Pt in plasma and in ultrafiltrate plasma, respectively.

In the case of platinum in plasma, the mean values of $C_{max}$ (the maximum value of the Pt concentration) and of AUC (the value of the area under the decay curve in the time range 0–24 h) obtained the fifth week were about 2-fold those of the first week. Also the mean $\beta$ half-life of total Pt approximately doubled, but the difference was not statistically significant.

Table 4

Mean (±SD) platinum levels determined at the end of weekly infusion of 4 mg/m$^2$ per day of CDDP

|  | First week | Sixth week | $P^a$ |
|---|---|---|---|
| $[Pt]^{tot}_{Friday}$ ($\mu$g/l) | 356 ± 62 | 649 ± 116 | <0.01 |
| $[Pt]^{uf}_{Friday}$ ($\mu$g/l) | 78 ± 31 | 114 ± 87 |  |

[a]Statistic difference assessed by Duncan test.

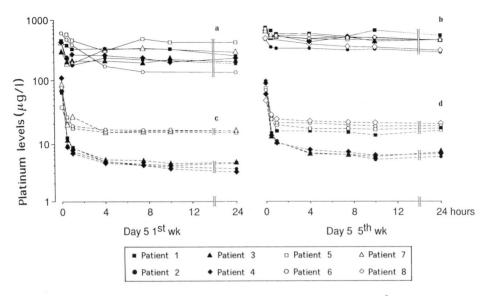

Fig. 4. Pt decay curves at the end of the first (lines a and b referred to [Pt]$^{tot}$ and [Pt]$^{uf}$ respectively ) and of the fifth infusion week (lines c and d referred to [Pt]$^{tot}$ and [Pt]$^{uf}$ respectively). Each curve was associated with single patient as in the legend.

Instead, as shown in Table 6, the pharmacokinetic parameters of platinum in ultrafiltrate plasma were found to be similar for the first and fifth weeks of treatment.

From the data in Fig. 4, it can be assumed that the percentage of platinum in ultrafiltrate versus platinum in plasma, about 20% immediately after the end of the weekly infusion, decreases to about 3% after 30 min. Thus we realized that during the pharmacokinetic evaluations on the group of 22 patients, the time between the drawing and the plasma ultrafiltration was too long with respect to the time employed by platinum to bind plasma proteins.

## 4. Discussion and conclusions

Radiotherapy and concurrent low-dose CDDP given in both bolus administration and continuous infusion for radioenhancement purposes has been object of several investigations on non-small cell lung cancer [2–9].

One recent large three-arm phase III study [14] focused on the radioenhancement effects of bolus CDDP and the impact of its dose fractionation. The study revealed a significantly improved outcome for the patients given the integrated treatment, over those who underwent only RT. Moreover, five bolus administrations a week of daily 6 mg/m$^2$ of CDDP had a favorable impact on short- and mid-term survival compared with a single shot delivery of the cumulative weekly dose of 30 mg/m$^2$. This improved result was due to better locoregional control, however toxicity was quite high.

We have been investigating the effects of the hyperfractionation of CDDP dose up to its extreme application, as is the continuous infusion, in the clinical setting since 1988. Our first phase II trial [3] consisted of a weekly CDDP dose of 30 mg/m$^2$, given as a 120-h infu-

Table 5

Pharmacokinetic parameters of platinum plasma determined in patients

| Patient no. | $C_{max}$ $(\mu g/l)$ | $t_{1/2}\alpha$ (h) | $t_{1/2}\beta$ (h) | AUC 24 h $(\mu g/l/h)$ |
|---|---|---|---|---|
| (a) *After 1 week of continuous infusion* | | | | |
| 1 | 444 | 0.17 | 51 | 7691 |
| 2 | n.d. | n.d. | 120 | 5271 |
| 3 | 304 | n.d. | n.d. | 5210 |
| 4 | 441 | 0.03 | 135 | 5594 |
| 5 | 589 | n.d. | 143 | 10396- |
| 6 | 622 | 1.5 | 84 | 6873 |
| 7 | 450 | n.d. | 132 | 2224 |
| Mean | 475 | 0.57 | 111 | 6180 |
| ±SD (N) | 115 (6) | 0.81 (3) | 36 (6) | 2526 (7) |
| CV (%) | 24 | 142 | 32 | 41 |
| (b) *After 5 weeks of continuous infusion* | | | | |
| 1 | 755 | 0.40 | 647 | 13847 |
| 2 | 480 | 0.14 | 100 | 7776 |
| 3 | 655 | 0.030 | 164 | 11594 |
| 4 | 674 | 0.030 | 152 | 11920 |
| 5 | 649 | 0.29 | 323 | 11629 |
| 6 | 709 | 0.090 | 93 | 11987 |
| 8 | 494 | n.d. | 60 | 8808 |
| Mean | 631 | 0.16 | 220 | 11080 |
| ±SD (N) | 105 (7) | 0.15 (6) | 207 (7) | 2074 (7) |
| CV (%) | 17 | 94 | 94 | 19 |

sion together with, each week, a 50-Gy split radiation course, similar in design to that of the above-mentioned randomized study [14]. A very high rate (80%) of clinical objective responses was observed. A pathological complete response was assessed in only one of 38 cases and toxicity was mild to moderate. In our second phase II study [2], a lower dose of CDDP, 4 mg/m², was administered daily. Five 100-h weekly infusions over 5 consecutive weeks were administered since a 50-Gy 5-week continuous course of RT was adopted. Again toxicity was mild to moderate, and the clinical response rate superimposable. However a greater than 20% pathological complete response rate was surgically proven.

Despite the promising clinical results any further development of an integration schedule needed a previous evaluation of the pharmacokinetics of CDDP administration by continuous infusion at low dose. Thus the present study is the first to report pharmacokinetic information on platinum in plasma and in ultrafiltrate plasma of lung carcinoma patients receiving prolonged infusions of CDDP concurrent with radiotherapy.

In vitro experiments [6] have shown that platinum concentration is required to potentiate the cytotoxic effect of radiation against NSCLC cell line EPLC in the range 1–2.5 $\mu M$ (190–400 $\mu g/l$ of Pt). Skov et al. [15] showed that CDDP 0.1 $\mu M$ (19 $\mu g/l$) for 2 h potentiated the cytotoxic effect of radiation on hypoxic V79 Chinese hamster cells.

A large variability of CDDP concentrations for an identical dose of delivered drug was seen in our patients, as has already been pointed out by Reece et al. [16]. However it appeared that the steady state level of platinum in ultrafiltrate plasma achieved with our infusion, namely 110 $\mu g/l$, was in the same order of magnitude as those found to be active in vitro as radiopotentiators. Furthermore the repeated continuous infusions allowed a very

Table 6

Pharmacokinetic parameters of platinum in ultrafiltrate plasma determined in patients

| Patient no. | $C_{max}$ ($\mu$g/l) | $t_{1/2}\alpha$ (h) | $t_{1/2}\beta$ (h) | AUC 24 h ($\mu$g/l/h) |
|---|---|---|---|---|
| *(a) After 1 week of continuous infusion* | | | | |
| 1 | 66 | 0.15 | 38 | 127 |
| 2 | n.d. | n.d. | 17 | 220 |
| 3 | 74 | 0.13 | 35 | 135 |
| 4 | 112 | 0.090 | 19 | 121 |
| 5 | 37 | 0.23 | 279 | 358 |
| 6 | 79 | 0.19 | 172 | 398 |
| 7 | 89 | 0.11 | 93 | 401 |
| 8 | 55 | 0.21 | n.d. | 450 |
| Mean | 73 | 0.16 | 93 | 276 |
| ±SD ($N$) | 24 (7) | 0.053 (7) | 99 (7) | 140 (8) |
| CV (%) | 33 | 33 | 106 | 51 |
| *(b) After 5 weeks of continuous infusion* | | | | |
| 1 | 97 | 0.16 | 54 | 376 |
| 2 | 91 | 0.14 | 33 | 168 |
| 3 | 98 | 0.12 | 63 | 179 |
| 4 | 61 | 0.14 | 45 | 172 |
| 5 | 76 | 0.19 | 275 | 413 |
| 6 | 71 | 0.13 | 121 | 461 |
| 8 | 48 | 0.25 | 211 | 517 |
| Mean | 77 | 0.16 | 115 | 327 |
| ±SD ($N$) | 19 (7) | 0.045 (7) | 94 (7) | 150 (7) |
| CV (%) | 25 | 28 | 82 | 46 |

prolonged exposure to ultrafiltrable platinum species, greater than that achieved after a bolus administration; in fact the binding of CDDP to plasma proteins is of considerable importance in the pharmacokinetics of drug and <10% of platinum is protein unbound, or the pharmacologically active species, half an hour from the end of the administration [17].

Total platinum tended to accumulate in the body after our repeated infusions, in agreement with some previous studies [18]. Platinum in ultrafiltrate plasma remained at a constant level avoiding peaks of concentration that play a role in the degree of toxicity [16]. In fact, compared with the daily bolus administration reported in the already mentioned three-arm phase III study [14], the same dose given in continuous infusion was of very low toxicity in our experience [3,4].

In our study, platinum in ultrafiltrate plasma showed a half-life of several hours. This was unexpected, considering that free CDDP is known to disappear from plasma very quickly [1]. Moreover the $[Pt]^{uf}_{Friday}$ values reported in the present study have relevant standard deviations with respect to the $[Pt]^{uf}_{Monday}$ values, suggesting that different Pt species (CDDP metabolytes) are present in the ultrafiltrate plasma for different decay times. Although the chemical composition of ultrafiltrable platinum is unknown, it is likely that a major fraction is represented by small peptides bonding platinum, that are ultrafiltrable by filters with a size of 10 000 kDa. Platinum bound to low molecular weight proteins showed less variance and was still detectable three days from the end of the infusion, i.e., on Monday. This may be relevant, as it cannot be excluded that the mechanism proposed by several authors for radiopotentiating the action of CDDP [19] could be operative also in the case of

Pt bound to low molecular weight proteins. In this case the long life of the platinum species in ultrafiltrate plasma could enhance the radiopotentiating action. Given present-day knowledge, this idea is totally hypothetical and studies to chemically identify any platinum containing species and to investigate their pharmacological properties are warranted.

The unhomogeneity of the patients sampled in this work, especially because of the disease's advanced stage, precludes any meaningful evaluation on the treatment impact on survival. However, we can conclude that the locoregional progression was very low, occurring in only two patients, and toxicity was negligible. These results agree with those reported in our previous phase II studies [2–4]. At the same time, the pharmacokinetic results suggest that, throughout therapy, prolonged continuous CDDP venous infusions at the reported doses are the key to ensuring constant very high percentage of platinum in ultrafiltrate plasma (roughly 20%) and a platinum level sufficient for radioenhancement ($110 \, \mu/l$), without any concentration peaks of platinum-free proteins.

## Summary

The pharmacokinetics of *cis*-dichlorodiammine platinum(II) (CDDP), given as a continuous infusion with concurrent radiotherapy to patients with locally advanced inoperable non-small cell lung carcinoma (NSCLC), was investigated in two groups of patients of 22 and 16 patients, respectively. For the first group the regimen, repeated for 5 consecutive weeks, consisted of weekly 10 Gy radiotherapy (RT) given in 5 fractions from Monday to Friday, and concurrent 100-h infusion of CDDP delivered at a daily dose of 4 mg/m$^2$ by a central venous catheter and a portable pump. For the other group, the same regimen was repeated for 6 consecutive weeks. Throughout the weeks of therapy, the platinum levels were determined in plasma and in ultrafiltrate plasma by inductively coupled plasma atomic emission spectrometry (ICP-AES) and inductively coupled plasma mass spectrometry (ICP-MS), respectively. Mean levels of platinum in plasma [Pt]$^{tot}$ increased from the first to the last week of infusion, while mean levels of platinum in ultrafiltrate plasma, [Pt]$^{uf}$, showed no marked variation throughout the therapy. [Pt]$^{uf}$ was in the first group of patients around 3% of [Pt]$^{tot}$ and in the second group it ranged from 16% to 22% of [Pt]$^{tot}$. Pt decay levels, measured in the group of 16 patients for 24 h at the end of the first and fifth weeks of infusion, demonstrated that in the group of 22 patients the separation of the plasma fraction containing high molecular weight proteins was not fast enough to minimize the interaction of such proteins with CDDP. Thus the group of 16 patients was taken as representative of the pharmacokinetics. Pt decay curves allowed the calculation of the Pt half-life and the area under the decay curves. The mean value of the area under the decay curve (AUC), [Pt]$^{tot}$ versus time in the time range 0–24 h from the end of the fifth infusion week, was about twice that from the end of the first week; instead the mean AUC values did not vary for the [Pt]$^{uf}$ versus time curves. The mean values of the $\alpha$ half-life of Pt in the ultrafiltrate plasma were in accordance with the literature; however an unexpected very long $\beta$ half-life was found (more than 100 h). Thus it was suggested that Pt species, different from free CDDP, would be present in the ultrafiltrate plasma; such species probably involve metal bound to low-molecular weight proteins. Throughout the therapy, the toxic effects in all patients were negligible, and 75% of them had an objective locoregional reduction of disease. In only two cases was an intra- RT- field progression of disease observed. Based on these data, it can be concluded that cisplatin present at the level of $110 \, \mu g/l$ in the ultrafiltrate plasma, in the reported scheme of continuous intravenous infusion, has an enhancing effect on radiation and avoids concentration peaks of protein unbound platinum. The constant and very high percentage of platinum in ultrafiltrate plasma and the absence of peaks of concentration are very probably the key for the high efficiency and the low toxicity of our scheme.

## Acknowledgements

Supported by a grant from Consiglio Nazionale delle Ricerche.

## References

1.   Saunders MI, Bennet MH, Dische S, Anderson PJ. Primary tumor control after radiotherapy for carcinoma of the bronchus. Int J Radiat Oncol Biol Phys 10: 499–501, 1984.
2.   Bedini AV, Ravasi G. T4 and/or non resectable N2 lung carcinoma: cisplatin, radiotherapy and systematic adjuvant surgery Preliminary data of a phase II study. J Chemother 8(Suppl 3): 41, 1996, in press.
3.   Bedini AV, Tavecchio L, Milani F, et al. Prolonged venous infusion of cisplatin and concurrent radiation therapy for lung carcinoma. Cancer 67: 357–362, 1991.
4.   Bedini AV, Tavecchio L, Milani F, et al. Non resectable stage iiia-b lung carcinoma: a phase ii study on continuous infusion of cisplatin and concurrent radiotherapy (plus adjuvant surgery). Lung Cancer 10: 73–84, 1993.
5.   Ellerbroek NA, Fossella FV, Rich TA, et al. Low dose continuous infusio cisplatin combined with external beam irradiation for advanced colorectal adenocarcinoma and unresectable non-small cell lung carcinoma. Int J Radiat Oncol Biol Phys 20: 351–355, 1991.
6.   Havemann K, Wolf M, Gorg C, et al. Preclinical and clinical experience with cisplatin and carboplatin and simultaneous radiation in non-small cell lung cancer. Ann Oncol 3(Suppl 3): S33–S37, 1992.
7.   Soresi E, Clerici M, Grilli R, et al. A randomized clinical trial comparing radiation therapy and radiation therapy plus cis-dicholoammine platinum(II) in the treatment of locally advanced non-small cell lung cancer. Semin Oncol 15: 20–25, 1988.
8.   Trovò MG, Minatel E, Franchin G, et al. Radiotherapy versus radiotherapy enhanced by cisplatin in stage III non-small cell lung cancer. Int J Radiat Oncol Biol Phys 24: 11–15, 1992.
9.   Van Harskamp G, Boven E, Vermoken JB, et al. Phase II trial combined radiotherapy and daily low-dose cisplatin for inoperable locally advanced non-small cell lung cancer (NSCLC). Int J Radiat Oncol Biol Phys 13: 1735–1738, 1987.
10.  Oken MM, Davis TE, Creech RH, et al. Toxicity and response criteria of the Eastern Cooperative Oncology Group. Am J Clin Oncol 5: 649–655, 1982.
11.  Miller AB, Hoogstraten B, Staquet M, Winkler RA. Reporting results of cancer treatment. Cancer 47: 207–214, 1981.
12.  Powell MJD. An efficient method for finding the minimum of a function of several variable without calculating derivatives. Comput J 7: 155–162, 1964.
13.  Sacchi Landriani G, Guardabasso V, Rocchetti M. NL-FIT: a microcomputer program for non linear fitting. Comput Programs Biomed 16: 35, 1983.
14.  Schaake-Koning C, Van den Bogaert W, Dalesio O, et al. Effects of concomitant cisplatin and radiotherapy on inoperable non-small-cell lung cancer. N Engl J Med 236: 524–530, 1992.
15.  Skov K, Mac Phail S. Interaction of platinum drugs with clinically relevant X-ray doses in mammalian cells: a comparison of cisplatin, carboplatin, iproplatin, and tetraplatin. Int J Radiat Oncol Biol Phys 20: 221–225, 1991.
16.  Reece P, Stafford I, Russel J, et al. Creatinine clearance as predictor of ultrafilterable platinum plasma levels and nephrotoxicity. J Clin Oncol 5: 304–309, 1987.
17.  Vokes EE, Ackland SP, Vogelzang NJ. Cisplatin, carboplatin, and gallium nitrate. In: Lokich JJ (Ed), Cancer Chemotherapy by Infusion, 2nd edn. Chicago, IL: Precept Press, pp. 176–196, 1990.

18.    Groen HJM, van der Leest AHD, de Vries EGE, et al. Continuous carboplatin infusion during 6 weeks radiotherapy in locally inoperable non small-cell lung cancer: a phase I and pharmacokinetic study. Br J Cancer 72: 992–997, 1995.

19.    Dewit L. Combined treatment of radiation and cis-diamminedichloroplatinum(II): a review of experimental and clinical data. Int J Radiat Oncol Biol Phys 13: 403–426, 1987.

C.J. Rosenthal and M. Rotman (Eds.), *Infusion Chemotherapy–Irradiation Interactions*

# CHAPTER 7

# Infusional schedules of platinum compounds and 5-fluorouracil in the chemoradiotherapy of solid tumors

GIANLUIGI GRECCHI[1], PIETRO LA CIURA[1], ANTONIO PELISSERO[2], ELVIO RUSSI[2], CLAUDIA FILLINI[2], ANTONELLA MELANO[2], GIANNA DI COSTANZO[1], DAVIDE PERRONI[1] and GIUSEPPE MARCHETTI[2]

[1]*Service of Medical Oncology,* [2]*Division of Radiotherapy, S. Croce Hospital, v. Coppino 26, 12100, Cuneo, Italy*

## 1. Introduction

Many patients with regionally advanced solid tumors suffer from progressive disease either for local and distant relapses, or both; the improvement of local and systemic tumor control remains an important goal of clinical research. In those diseases in which there is a prolonged phase of regional growth, before systemic progression, the integration of chemotherapy and radiotherapy seems to offer the better chance of controlling the tumor, when inoperable. These modalities are used today mainly with sequential or alternating schedules; nevertheless, the concomitant administration of both modalities, seems preferable on a preclinical basis. However, this modality carries some problems, due to the enhancement of the toxicity of both treatments, when given at clinically active doses and schedules. A number of different schedules of concurrent multimodality therapy have been applied up to now, in view of the theoretical advantage of radiosensitization with improved local control, and reduction in total treatment time. The main issue is clearly the administration of chemotherapy in active doses and schedules, without altering the radiotherapy course, and hopefully without unfavorable effects to normal tissues. Up to now only in a few series have we seen a clear advantage with a good therapeutic index for some patients; therefore the optimal drug combination and schedule are yet to be found [1].

Both platinum compounds and fluorouracil have radiosensitizing effects through different mechanisms, but these are greatly dependent on the administration modality (by pulse or by continuous infusion, especially for fluorouracil). Their toxicities are also different, with prevalent hematological toxicity for the platinum analogue carboplatin, mucosal toxicity for fluorouracil, when given with concurrent radiotherapy, and renal toxicity for cisplatin [2,3]. The fluoropyrimidines have radiosensitizing properties, when given by continuous infusion, due to their ability to inhibit DNA lethal and sublethal damage repair, by altering the nucleotide metabolism, and to their synchronizing effects on the cellular cycle [4,6]. Encouraging preliminary data in the 1980s suggested the feasibility of prolonged infusion of fluoropyrimidines in conjunction with the radiotherapy, in gastrointestinal and urinary cancers, as well as in those of the respiratory tract [9–14]. The first reports used short term continuous infusions for 96–120 h during the first and the last week of the radiotherapy program, with some degree of mucosal and hematological toxicity due to the drug infusion. The experience of other groups, with fluorouracil given daily at the dose of 200–300 mg/m$^2$ per day, during the entire radiotherapy program, showed feasibility and excellent activity at the expense of a slightly higher degree of mucositis in 35–45% of patients, and the appearance of hand–foot syndrome in 15–20% of patients [10,12].

For platinum compounds, the mechanisms by which they enhance radiation effects are both chemical and biochemical. The former works through the formation of reactive free radicals or altered binding of Pt complexes to DNA, and appears to be more potent in hypoxic cells. It needs, however, a higher free platinum concentration in tissues, usually not easily achievable during clinical use. The latter works by interfering with biochemical processes that normally limit radiation damage, and needs less free platinum in tissues [2,5]. Among platinum compounds, cisplatin should be administered with adequate hydration and enhanced diuresis, even in prolonged schedule [5,7,8]. On the other hand, the analogue carboplatin is easily given without hydration, has a low aquation rate, and accumulates as free platinum progressively in cells when administered by continuous infusion. Its toxicity is mainly hematological, and is related to the individual glomerular filtration rate [3]. Preliminary trials showed the feasibility of prolonged administration of carboplatin at 30 $mg/m^2$ per day, for as many as 21 consecutive days [15]. For these reasons, we first evaluated the feasibility of a schedule of concomitant radiotherapy and prolonged infusion of carboplatin at 25 $mg/m^2$ per day, in order to evaluate its tolerability, and secondly the feasibility and activity of a schedule of carboplatin, at the same dosage, for 7 days, given on alternate weeks with fluorouracil, administered at 300 $mg/m^2$ per day, for 7 consecutive days. On a third series of patients, we substituted carboplatin with cisplatin, given at 5 $mg/m^2$ per day, as shown in older phase 1 studies [7,8], due to the greater activity of this compound on squamous cancer of the gastrointestinal and respiratory tract. Our aim was to verify the activity and tolerance of this infusional combination of two drugs with different radiosensitizing properties and probably not overlapping toxicities, combining them with a conventional radiotherapy treatment on an outpatient basis.

## 2. Materials and methods

Concomitant chemotherapy with carboplatin at 25 $mg/m^2$ per day was initially offered to patients with advanced esophageal cancers, proposed for palliative radiotherapy. The drug was given by a portable device, usually a peristaltic pump (CADD, Pharmacia Deltec Inc., St Paul, MN), or an elastomeric device (Infusor , Baxter Corp., Deerfield, IL), after implantation of a central venous access. Patients had a careful evaluation and staging with esophagogram, CT scan of the thorax and upper abdomen, bronchoscopy, complete blood chemistries, ORL evaluation, after the endoscopy with pathologic confirmation of diagnosis. Eligible patients had to have no contraindications to central venous access, and a good performance status (ECOG score of 2 or less). The drug was infused without interruption for the entire duration of the administration of radiation unless the patient demonstrated progressive disease or an adverse effect from the chemotherapy. For the patients developing drug related toxicity, the drug was interrupted for a minimum of 7 days, and restarted at the recovery from the adverse event. Radiation therapy was delivered at the rate of 1.8–2 Gy/day, 5 days/week, usually with a three field technique, in an ambulatory setting. Some patients were initially treated with radiotherapy in a split schedule, to improve tolerability, but later on this seemed unnecessary. Patients were monitored weekly, with complete physical examinations and blood counts. Supportive nutritional care was insured by means of a thorough dietary evaluation and the use of an endoscopic-percutaneus enterostomy, or eventually a pharingostomy feeding tube. Within 1 month after completion of radiation therapy, an assessment of therapeutic intervention was undertaken, utilizing the same algorithm used at the beginning. For patients with measurable/evaluable lesions, a complete response (CR) was defined as 100% regression of all visible/evaluable tumor by all parameters. Partial response (PR) was defined as 50% or greater reduction of the product of the measurable diameters of the tumor, and quantified upon the esophagogram/ esophagoscopy with biopsy/ CT scan evidence, together with the clinical evaluation and the restoration of food transit. Supportive care included esophageal dilatation, when needed. Response duration was measured from the initiation of therapy, as was survival. Toxicity was evaluated according to World Health Organization criteria [20]. Appropriate reductions for chemotherapy were instituted for mild cytopenia (white blood cell (WBC) count grade 1, <4000/mm$^3$, grade 2, <3000, and platelets (Plt) grade 1, <100 000 and grade 2, <75 000). Chemotherapy was delayed for 1 week or more for grade 2 or superior toxicity, or grade 1 persistent toxicity. Informed consent was obtained. In the following series, a similar strategy was used also for patients with tumors of the respiratory tract, with the exception of the schedule of chemotherapy, which consisted firstly of carboplatin, given at 25 mg/m$^2$ per day for 1 week, and fluorouracil, given at 300 mg/m$^2$ per day for the following week, alternated during the entire radiation program. In the third and last group of patients, cisplatin was administered in place of carboplatin, at 5 mg/m$^2$ per day, without hydration. Chemotherapy for induction or consolidation was allowed in sensitive tumors, but the evaluation of the response was in any case based on the evidence obtained at the beginning of radiation. The first group consisted of 6 patients with advanced squamous esophageal cancers (stage III), median age 60 years, and were treated from 1992 to 1993; the second group comprised 9 patients with far advanced stage III esophageal cancers, 8 squamous, 1 with adenocarcinoma, with median age 64 years, treated from 1993 to 1994. Three patients were treated in this group with preoperative intent, 2 underwent surgery, 1 had curative surgery. The third group consisted of 18 patients with various tumors, treated from 1995; all patients had a tumor that could be encompassed by a single radiotherapy field. The accrual is going on. Up to now, 5 esophageal cancers, 3 tumors of the cardias, 2 gastric cancers, 3 lung cancers, 1 mediastinal MUO, 4 oropharyngeal tumors have been treated. Four received split course radiation. The characteristics of this population are described in Table 1; all presented far advanced cancers, deemed inoperable at diagnosis or at surgical exploration.

## 3. Results

A total of 33 patients were evaluated in this series. Group 1 included 6 patients, treated from the beginning of 1992, with advanced esophageal tumors of squamous histology. There were no complete responders, 1 partial response, 2 patients presented progressive disease. Clinical improvement was observed in 3 out of 6 patients, with partial restoration of food transit. Hematological toxicity was common; there were 5 episodes of WHO grade 1 WBC toxicity, 2 of grade 2 WBC toxicity, 1 episode of grade 1 and 2 episodes of grade 2 Plt toxicity. One patient experienced a grade 2 peripheral neurotoxicity, and 2 patients had severe esophagitis, on a herpetic and micotic basis. In all the patients the hematological toxicity appeared on the 4th or 5th week of treatment, and chemotherapy had to be interrupted for a

Table 1

RT plus cisplatin and fluorouracil on alternate weeks: patient characteristics

| No. | Patient | Age | Sex | Tumor | Stage | RT (Gy) | Other treatments |
|-----|---------|-----|-----|-------|-------|---------|------------------|
| 1 | R.M. | 74 | M | Cardias, ca. | T3N1M0 | 55.8 | Surgery |
| 2 | B.L. | 66 | F | Cardias, ca. | T4N2M0 | 50; split | CT: c.i.FU/DDP and b.MMC |
| 3 | B.V. | 71 | M | Cardias, ca. | T4N2M0 | 55; split | CT: c.i.FU/DDP and b.Mtx/FUfa |
| 4 | B.T. | 72 | F | Cardias, ca. | T4N2M0 | 50; split | CT: c.i.FU/DDP and b.MMC |
| 5 | B.F. | 70 | M | Cardias, ca. | T3N1M0 | 54 | CT: c.i.FU/DDP |
| 6 | P.A. | 64 | M | Cer.esoph., sq. | T4N1M0 | 62 | – |
| 7 | L.F. | 55 | M | Th.esoph., sq. | T4N1M0 | 63 | CT: b.DDP /c.i.FU |
| 8 | R.R. | 69 | M | Di.esoph., sq. | T3N1M0 | 65.2 | CT: b.DDP/c.i.FU |
| 9 | C.G. | 67 | M | Th.esoph., sq. | T3N1M0 | 65.6 | CT: b.DDP/c.i.FU |
| 10 | C.M. | 57 | M | Di.esoph., sq. | T3N1M0 | 61 | – |
| 11 | G.A. | 58 | F | Lung, ca. | T2N3M0 | 52, split | CT: b.DDP, b.NRB |
| 12 | B.G. | 71 | F | Lung, sq. | T2N1M0 | 62.4 | CT: b.DDP, b.NRB |
| 13 | O.G. | 50 | M | Mediast.MUO, ca. | TxN3M0 | 65.4 | – |
| 14 | A.P. | 67 | M | Lung, sq. | T3N3M0 | 65 | CT: b.DDP, b.NRB |
| 15 | A.R. | 51 | M | Ba.tongue, sq. | T4N1M0 | 69 | Surgery |
| 16 | A.V. | 51 | M | Ba.tongue, sq. | T4N1M0 | 69 | CT: b.DDP,c.i.Fu |
| 17 | B.E. | 65 | F | Re.mol.gingiva, sq. | T4N1M0 | 69 | – |
| 18 | B.G. | 56 | M | Tonsil, sq. | T4N0M0 | 66.9 | – |
| 19 | S.M. | 59 | M | Ba.tongue, sq. | T4N1M0 | 69 | – |

Abbreviations: CT, chemotherapy; RT, radiotherapy; c.i., continuous infusion; b., bolus; M, male; F, female; ca., adeno-carcinoma; sq., squamous carcinoma; mediast., mediastinal; MUO, metastases unknown origin; cer., cervical; th., thoracic; di., distal; esoph., esophagus; ba., basis; re.mol., retromolar.

week or more in all cases. Radiation therapy doses ranged from 45 to 61 Gy. Median survival was 6 months, ranging from 2 to 12 months.

Owing to these figures, the subsequent patients were treated with the alternate week schedule of infusional carboplatin and fluorouracil. This group comprised 9 esophageal cancers, all in advanced stage III. Six patients underwent radiation therapy at 59–67 Gy (median 62 Gy), while three patients had 40–46 Gy for preoperative intent. Two of these had surgical exploration, one was resected. Toxicity in the group (in 52 cumulative weeks of chemoradiotherapy) was: WBC grade 1, 5 episodes; WBC grade 2, 1 episode; WBC grade 3, 1 episode; Plt grade 1, 3 episodes; Plt grade 1, 3 episodes; Plt grade 2, 1 episode; anemia grade 1, 4 episodes; requiring transfusions, 1 patient; mucositis grade 1, 2 episodes; other toxicities, not registered, except actinic grade 1 mucositis in 6 patients, and painful ulcer in one (micotic esophagitis). Responses were: 1 pathological CR; 5 PR (2 > 75%); 1 stable disease (SD); 2 progressions (PD). The median survival was 9 months (range 7–21). Clinical improvement: 4 out of 9, with normal food transit restored in 2 patients. Preliminary results of these series have already been published [16,18,19].

In the third group of 19 patients (Table 1), treated with infusional cisplatin and fluorouracil on alternate weeks, all the patients were evaluable for toxicity, and 18 for response. At a median followup of 11 months (range 2–24 months), 3 patients died, and the others are alive, 6 with persistent or relapsing disease. Responses are shown in Table 2, and toxicities in Table 3.

Table 2

RT plus cisplatin and fluorouracil on alternate weeks: patient response–survival

| Pt | Tumor | OR:CT scan | OR: EGDS-FBS | OR: tu.hyst. | Clinical benefit | Transit | TTP | Survival from RT | Survival from hist. diagnosis |
|----|-------|-----------|------------|------------|-----------------|---------|-----|-----------------|---------------------------|
| 1 | Cardias, ca. | PR | CR | Surgery: neg. | +++ | +++ | NED | 23+ | 24+ |
| 2 | Cardias, ca. | SD | CR | Neg. | +++ | +++ | 6 | 13 | 16 |
| 3 | Cardias, ca. | SD | SD | Pos. | +++ | ++ | 12 | 18+ | 21+ |
| 4 | Cardias, ca. | SD | CR | Neg. | ++ | +++ | 10 | 17+ | 19+ |
| 5 | Cardias, ca. | PR | PR | n.e. | +++ | +++ | – | 9+ | 10+ |
| 6 | Cer.esoph.,sq. | CR | CR | Neg. | +++ | +++ | NED | 16+ | 19+ |
| 7 | Th.esoph., sq. | PR | CR | Neg | +++ | +++ | – | 12+ | 15+ |
| 8 | Di.esoph., sq. | PR | CR | Neg | +++ | +++ | – | 7+ | 11+ |
| 9 | Th.esoph., sq. | PR | PR | Neg | ++ | + | 2nd eso.tu | 6+ | 9+ |
| 10 | Di.esoph., sq. | n.e | n.e. | n.e. | ++ | +++ | n.e. | 3+ | 5+ |
| 11 | Lung, ca. | CR | CR | Neg. | +++ | – | n.e./hem | 18 | 25 |
| 12 | Lung, sq. | CR | n.e. | n.e. | +++ | – | NED | 6+ | 10+ |
| 13 | Med. MUO,ca | SD | n.e. | n.e. | + | – | n.e./hem | 7 | 11 |
| 14 | Lung, sq. | PR | n.e. | n.e. | ++ | n.e. | – | 4+ | 9+ |
| 15 | Ba.tongue, sq. | PR | PR | T2N0 (surg) | ++ | – | 11 | 13.5 | 14.5 |
| 16 | Ba.tongue, sq. | CR | CR | Neg | +++ | – | NED | 11+ | 12+ |
| 17 | Re.mol.gingiva,sq. | PR | CR | Neg | +++ | – | 4 | 7 | 9 |
| 18 | Tonsil, sq. | PR | n.e. | n.e. | +++ | – | – | 9+ | 12+ |
| 19 | Ba.tongue, sq. | PR | PR | n.e. | ++ | – | – | 4+ | 5+ |

Abbreviations, Pt, patient; RT, radiotherapy; CT, computerized tomography; ca., adeno-carcinoma; sq., squamous carcinoma; med., mediastinal; MUO, metastases unknown origin; cer., cervical; th., thoracic; di., distal; esoph., eso., esophagus; ba., basis; re.mol., retromolar; OR, observed response; PR, partial response; SD, stable, or minimal response; NED, non evidence of disease; EGDS, esophagogastroscopy; FBS, fibrobroncoscopy; his., histology; neg., negative; n.e., not evaluable/evaluated; 2nd tu.,second tumor; hem., massive hemoftosis. Survival is expressed in months, either from RT beginning or from histologic diagnosis.

Hematological and non-hematological toxicities were mainly mild, with absolutely no episodes of grade III–IV toxicity, apart from stomatitis in oropharyngeal tumors.

At the present time, the situation for this group of patients is depicted in Table 2. It is not possible to give any data about the survival of this population, due to the small number of events; clearly a longer period is needed. The tolerance of this schedule is fairly good, with 37 weeks with hematological grade I–II toxicity among a total of 128 weeks of combined treatment. Considering the controversial issue of evaluating responses and staging of these patients, among 18 evaluable patients, the responses were: 9 complete, at endoscopy or at clinical evaluation, with 1 additional lung patient presenting a complete CT scan response, not evaluable by endoscopy. Two patients presented stable disease, and 6 partial responses. Eleven biopsies were obtained: 10 showed a negative histology, 1 positive. The clinical counterparts are, on the other hand, the recovery of normal food transit in all the esophageal or esophago-gastric patients, and the prolonged time without symptoms enjoyed by a consistent subgroup of them, as well for the few patients with lung cancers.

Table 3

RT plus cisplatin and fluorouracil on alternate weeks: toxicities and dose modifications

|          | Grade I | Grade II | Grade III | CT 75% red. | CT 50% red. | CT stopped |
|----------|---------|----------|-----------|-------------|-------------|------------|
| WBC      | 30      | 7        | 0         |             |             |            |
| Plt      | 4       | 2        | 0         |             |             |            |
| Hb       | 5       | 2        | 0         |             |             |            |
| Mucositis| 3       | 2        | 6         | 32          | 2           | 6          |
| Nausea   | 11      | 7        | –         |             |             |            |
| Vomit    | 7       | 6        | 2         |             |             |            |
| PPDE     | 1       | –        | –         |             |             |            |

Weeks of toxicity and dose reductions among 128 weeks of concurrent chemoradiotherapy. Abbreviations: red., reduction.; WBC, granulocytes total number; Plt, platelets; Hb, hemoglobin; PPDE, palmoplantar erytrodysestesia.

## 4. Discussion

We report a heterogeneous series of patients with advanced tumors of the proximal gastro-enteric and respiratory tract, treated with infusional platinum compounds with and without fluorouracil and concomitant radiation. We observed initially a good tolerance for the double drug schedule on alternate weeks therapy. The results reported by us, in this very preliminary experience of long term infusional carboplatin and radiotherapy [16], are consistent with the published literature. Other authors [17] subsequently reported some problem with the administration of the drug for the entire radiation course; we aimed nevertheless for this issue in the setting up of this experience.

The initial selection of a group of patients with esophageal disease was made according to the model of this disease. Its natural history is in fact characterized by a long phase of local growth, with very limited survival after locoregional treatments, like surgery and radiotherapy alone or in combination. The drug resistance occurs relatively late in the course of this disease, whereas other squamous tumors of the head and neck have a longer history even in advanced stages. Afterwards we experienced this schedule for some oropharyngeal tumors, and for lung tumors with a chemoradiotherapy consolidation strategy.

In the reported series, the schedule with prolonged infusion of cisplatin and fluorouracil, seems to have the most encouraging activity. Among the group of esophageal and esophago-gastric junction tumors, the clinical response was complete in 6 out of 9 evaluable patients, with two partial responses and one stable disease (one additional patient is too early for evaluation). The clinical palliation result was excellent in many patients, with 8 experiencing a complete and 2 of 10 a near total restoration of food transit. This response translated into a high percentage (>50%) of patients surviving for more than 1 year with normal food transit; 8 of 10 removed the gastro-jejunostomy. Due to the short follow up, we cannot draw conclusive data. At a median followup of about 10 months, 1 patient with far advanced cancer at laparotomy died at 13 months; the one who underwent surgery is a long survivor, free of disease at 23 months. In the group of advanced lung tumors, treated with induction chemotherapy and consolidation chemoradiotherapy, 1 patient experienced a survival of 25 months from the diagnosis. The others are under observation at 6 and 8 months, while the patient with mediastinal MUO had no response, and died at 7 months of massive hemoftosis. The group with oropharyngeal cancers seems to present activity figures super-imposable on other combined treatments, but the number of patients is too small to draw conclusions. Nevertheless, the toxicity observed during the treatment was very favorable: with the exception of the oropharyngeal tumors, who presented the highest percentage of stomatitis, a severe (grade III or IV) toxicity was never observed. Furthermore, the radiation therapy plan was never altered. All the patients received a form of therapy during those days in which radiation was not given. This combination may be a proposal for solving the problem of the elapsed treatment days, which is a critical item for radiotherapy quality control, and moreover offers the possibility of overcoming the resistance acquired in induction treatments, as stressed elsewhere [21,22]. Finally, we like to emphasize that this schedule carries the administration of a form of systemic treatment. The mean cumulative dose of cisplatin delivered during the whole radiation treatment is in fact in the order of 100 mg/m$^2$, and that of fluorouracil is 10.600 mg/m$^2$. This schedule, which appears very tolerable in a fully outpatient basis, allows double systemic therapy to be given, which may exert its effects both locally and systemically on those days in which radiotherapy is off.

## 5. Conclusions

Radiation therapy is an effective treatment for many tumors, when they have mainly loco-regional growth. The curative capability of this modality, however, is related to the intrinsic or acquired radiation resistance and to the systemic dissemination of many cancers. The cure rate remains low despite the use of combined surgery and radiation; efforts to increase the curative potential of radiotherapy include the administration of chemotherapy, either in a sequential or alternating manner, or a concurrent one. Many preclinical studies denote that the latter has a striking rationale, since many mechanisms of interaction may be operative. Some of these are constituted by the inhibition of lethal-sublethal damage repair, or cell cycle synchronization, as well as the elimination of cells with intrinsic resistance to one modality by the other. Moreover, concomitant administration of radiotherapy and chemotherapy carries a potential activity against different cell subpopulations, with different characteristics, or environmental and cell cycle conditions. Furthermore, concomitant administration of both modalities, allows local and systemic treatment to be given in a shorter time. Prolonged drug exposure seems to optimize the interaction between chemotherapy and irradiation; on the other hand, the continuous infusion administration of drugs has shown increased therapeutic index, by lowering at least the drug related toxicity. In this series we tested some of the potentially useful combinations in this setting, in patients with advanced disease and frequently poor performance status, and observed a favorable clinical tolerability, and possibly a beneficial palliation, sustained for a long time in some cases. This seems to confirm a role for this schedule, and in our opinion warrants further evaluation in disease oriented randomized trials.

## Summary

The main objectives of cancer treatment are to maximize the local control of the tumor, to prevent regional recurrence, and to promote long term survival or cure. Concomitant administration of chemotherapy and radiation therapy holds promise in improving tumor control by increased therapeutic activity. Combined modality therapy – chemotherapy and radiotherapy – is also used for palliation in many regionally advanced tumors, but the optimal drug combination and schedule are not firmly established. In order to reach an optimal synergism between the two modalities, and to avoid overlapping treatment related toxicities, we tried to combine drugs known as radiosensitizers, such as platinum compounds and fluorouracil, given in a prolonged infusion, with radiotherapy, given either by usual fractionation, or on a split course. Three consecutive series of patients with locally far advanced tumors of the upper gastrointestinal or respiratory tract, who were undergoing palliative radiotherapy, were evaluated. They were treated with three different schedules of drugs given by continuous infusion: carboplatin alone or carboplatin combined with fluorouracil on alternate weeks, or cisplatin combined with fluorouracil on alternate weeks, given by infusion throughout the radiotherapy course. The last schedule was the best tolerated and had the highest clinical activity, with patients experiencing unusual long term palliation.

## *References*

1.   Vokes EE, Weichselbaum RR. Concomitant chemoradiotherapy: rationale and clinical experiences in patients with solid tumors. J Clin Oncol 8: 911–934, 1990.
2.   Double EB, Richmond RC. Enhancement of the potentiation of radiotherapy by platinum drugs in a mouse tumor. Int J Radiat Oncol Biol Phys 8: 501–503, 1982
3.   Coughlin CT, Richmond RC. Biologic and clinical development of cisplatin compounds combined with radiation: concepts, utility, projections for new trials, and emergence of carboplatin. Semin Oncol 16 4(Suppl 6): 31–43, 1989.
4.   Byfield JE. Clinical basis for radiation and infusional chemotherapy. In: Lokich JJ, Byfield JE (Eds), Combined Modality Cancer Therapy. Radiation and Infusional Chemotherapy. Chicago, IL: Precept Press, pp. 15–47, 1991.
5.   Wheeler RH, Spencer S. Cisplatin plus radiation therapy. J Infus Chemother 5: 61–66, 1995.
6.   Lawrence TS, Maybaum J, Ensminger WD. Infusional fluoropyrimidines as radiation sensitizers: clinical implications of laboratory findings. J Infus Chemother 4: 1203, 1994.
7.   Rosenthal CJ, Rotman M, Choi K, Sand J: Cisplatin by continuous infusion with concurrent radiation in malignant tumors (a phase I–II study). In: Rosenthal CJ, Rotman M (Eds), Clinical Applications of Continuous Infusion Chemotherapy and Concomitant Radiation Therapy. New York: Plenum Press, pp. 177–180, 1986.
8.   Bedini AV, Tavecchio L, Milani F, et al. Prolonged venous infusion of cisplatin and concurrent radiation therapy for lung carcinoma. Cancer 67: 357–362, 1991.
9.   Taylor SG IV, Trybula M, Bonomi P, et al. Simultaneous cisplatin-fluorouracil infusion and radiation followed by surgical resection in regionally localized stage III non small cell lung cancer. Ann Thor Surg 43: 87–91, 1987.
10.  Lokich JJ, Chafey J, Neptune W. Concomitant 5-fluorouracil infusion and high dose radiation for stage III non small cell lung cancer. Cancer 64: 1021–1025, 1989.
11.  Rich TA, Lokich JJ, Chaffey JT. A pilot study of protracted venous infusion of 5 fluorouracil and concomitant radiation therapy. J Clin Oncol 3: 402–406, 1985.
12.  Lokich JJ, Shea M, Chaffey J. Sequential infusion 5 fluorouracil followed by concomitant radiation therapy for tumours of the esophagus and gastroesophageal junction. Cancer 60: 275–279, 1987.
13.  Coia LR, Engstrom PF, Paul AR, et al. Long term results of infusional 5-FU, mitomycin-C and radiation as primary management of esophageal carcinoma. Int Radiat Oncol Biol Phys 20: 29–36, 1991.
14.  Weppelmann B, Wheleer RH, Peters GE, et al. A phase I study of prolonged infusion 5-fluorouracil and concomitant radiation therapy in patients with squamous cell cancer of the head and neck. J Radiat Oncol 20: 357–360, 1991.
15.  Smit EF, Willemse PH, Sleijfer DT, et al. Continuous infusion carboplatin on a 21-day schedule: a phase I and pharmacokinetic study. J Clin Oncol 9: 100–110, 1991.

16.  Grecchi GL, La Ciura P, Lauria G, et al. Continuous infusion carboplatin and radiotherapy: tolerance and feasibility through a portable device. Eur Cancer News 5: 9–10, 1992.

17.  Ausili Cefaro G, Marmiroli L, Nardone L, et al. Long term continuous infusion of carboplatin and concomitant radiotherapy in head and neck carcinoma: report on toxicity. Proc Am Soc Clin Oncol 12: 902, 1993.

18.  Grecchi GL, La Ciura P. Concomitant chemotherapy and radiation in oesophageal cancer: continuous alternating infusion of 5-fluorouracil and carboplatin. In: Einhorn J, Nord CE, Norrby SR (Eds), Recent Advances in Chemotherapy - Proc 18th Int Congr Chemotherapy, Stockholm, 1993. Washington, DC: American Society for Microbiology, pp. 841–842, 1994.

19.  Grecchi GL, La Ciura P, Di Costanzo G, et al. Radiation enhancement in combined treatment of solid tumors: evaluation of different schedules of infusional platinum compounds and 5-FU. Proc Am Soc Clin Oncol 15: 1671, 1996.

20.  Miller AB, Hoogstraten B, Staquet A, Winkler A. Reporting results of cancer treatment. Cancer 47: 207–214, 1981.

21.  Ensley JF, Ahmad K, Kish JA, et al. Improved response to radiation and concurrent cisplatinum in patients with advanced head and neck cancers that fail induction chemotherapy. Proc Am Soc Clin Oncol 8: 168, 1989.

22.  Pajak TF, Laramore GE, Marcial VA, et al. Elapsed treatment days - a critical item for radiotherapy quality control review in head and neck trials: RTOG report. Int J Radiat Oncol Biol Phys 20: 13–20, 1991.

C.J. Rosenthal and M. Rotman (Eds.), *Infusion Chemotherapy–Irradiation Interactions*
© 1998 Elsevier Science B.V. All rights reserved

# CHAPTER 8

# Hypoxia directed drugs: use with irradiation

## SARA ROCKWELL

*Department of Therapeutic Radiology, Yale University School of Medicine, P.O. Box 208040,
New Haven, CT 06520-8040, USA*

## 1. Introduction

The bioreductive alkylating agent mitomycin C was the first agent entered into clinical trials designed to test the hypothesis that a drug with selective toxicity to hypoxic cells could be used in combination with radiotherapy to improve the treatment of solid tumors. The initial randomized, prospective clinical trial of mitomycin C as an adjunct to radiotherapy in the treatment of carcinoma of the head and neck began at Yale in 1980 [1–3]. The success of this initial trial has led to a series of additional trials with mitomycin C in carcinoma of the head and neck and carcinoma of the cervix at Yale, through collaborations with colleagues in Venezuela, and through the International Atomic Energy Association [2–5]. Laboratory studies at Yale and elsewhere showing that a related bioreductive alkylating agent (porfiromycin) had greater selectivity in its toxicity to hypoxic cells [6,7] have resulted in the initiation of clinical trials testing porfiromycin as an adjunct to radiotherapy [4]. In addition, the concept of using hypoxia-selective drugs as adjuncts to radiotherapy is being investigated in a number of institutions, using a number of hypoxia-selective drugs, most notably tirapazamine and E09 [8,9]. There is therefore intense current interest, at many academic cancer centers, in the concept of using hypoxia-selective drugs as adjuncts to radiotherapy. This chapter reviews the considerations underlying the design of therapeutic regimens using hypoxia-selective agents and reviews laboratory data on the effects of mitomycin C and porfiromycin which are important to the design of such trials.

## 2. Targeting tumor subpopulations

The basic concept underlying the use of mitomycin C and porfiromycin as adjuncts to radiotherapy is that both of these drugs are more toxic to cells treated under hypoxia than to cells treated under aerobic conditions (Fig. 1), while radiation is more toxic to aerobic cells than to cells irradiated under hypoxia (Fig. 2). The selective toxicity of ionizing radiation to aerobic cells reflects the participation of molecular oxygen ($O_2$) in the radiation chemistry that leads to the production of cytotoxic damage. The radiation biology literature contains rich investigations of the mechanisms and implications of radiosensitization by oxygen [10,11] and the radiotherapy literature contains reports of many clinical trials based on approaches which might circumvent the radioprotective effects of hypoxia by oxygenating, sensitizing, or killing the hypoxic tumor cells (for reviews see [8,10,12,13]). The increased sensitivity of hypoxic cells to mitomycin C and porfiromycin reflects differences in the enzymatic activation and metabolism of these drugs by cells in different environments [14–16]. At normal physiologic pH under aerobic conditions, cells activate mitomycin C or porfiromycin to reactive intermediates which produce monofunctional alkylation of DNA, interstrand DNA crosslinks and intrastrand DNA crosslinks. Under hypoxia, the pattern of enzymatic activation changes, resulting in increased numbers of both monoadducts and crosslinks and in an increased proportion of crosslinks. The increased cytotoxicity of the drugs in hypoxia therefore reflects both an increased amount of damage and a change to a more toxic spectrum of lesions.

Cells do not need to be preincubated in hypoxia for long periods of time to acquire resistance to mitomycin C and porfiromycin [7,17,18]. Rather, resistance develops rapidly, apparently reflecting changes in the activities of existing enzymes. Cells made acutely hypoxic are sensitive to these drugs, while cells incubated in hypoxia, then reoxygenated, rapidly reacquire aerobic resistance. Radiosensitization by oxygen reflects chemical reactions involving $O_2$ [11]. For this reason, it is the presence of oxygen during irradiation which is critical in determining the radiosensitivity of cells. The induction of hypoxia after irradiation does not alter cellular radiosensitivity. Cells incubated in hypoxia, then oxygenated immediately before irradiation are fully radiosensitive. It is therefore the environment of the cells at the moment of treatment which determines their response to both radiation and bioreductive drugs. This fact is of great theoretical importance to the design of regimens combining radiotherapy with bioreductive drugs.

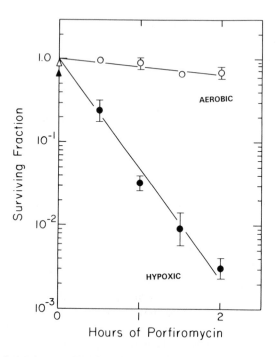

Fig. 1. Toxicity of porfiromycin to aerobic (○) and hypoxic (●) cells in vitro. Exponentially growing cell cultures were treated with 1 μm porfiromycin and cells were assayed for survival by colony formation. Points: means ± SEMs. Reprinted from [6].

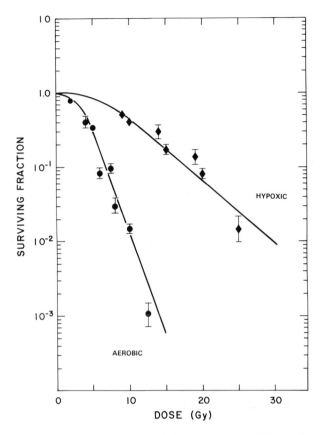

Fig. 2. Toxicity of radiation to aerobic (●) and hypoxic (◆) cells. Exponentially growing cell cultures were irradiated with 250 kV X-rays and cells were assayed for survival by colony formation. Points: means ± SEMs. Reprinted from [10].

## 3. Pharmacokinetic considerations

The theory underlying the use of bioreductive drugs with radiation differs fundamentally from that underlying the use of radiosensitizers. Radiosensitizers are used to modify the intrinsic radiosensitivity of the cells. Maximal radiosensitization is therefore obtained when maximal concentrations of the radiosensitizing moiety (free drug in the case of a chemical radiosensitizer such as misonidazole; maximal concentrations halogenated nucleotide incorporated into DNA in the case of IUdR) is present at the moment of irradiation. The planning of regimens for combining radiosensitizers with radiotherapy therefore must consider the detailed pharmacokinetics and mechanism of action of the specific drug being used. Moreover, both the sequence and the timing of the treatments will be critical in determining the outcome of therapy. In contrast, regimens combining radiotherapy with bioreductive drugs utilize the cytotoxicities of the two agents. The development of optimal treatment regimens using such combinations therefore depends on the nature of the selective cytotoxicities of the two agents, the interactions, if any, between the lesions produced by the drug and by radiation, and the nature in the changes in the microenvironments within tumors with time, both in treated and in untreated tumors. The development of optimal regimens for combining these drugs and radiation therefore requires considerable laboratory data and clinical information on the effects of the agents.


## 4.  Cell culture data

Cell culture systems were used to examine the effects of the sequence and of the time between treatments on the cytotoxicity of the regimens combining radiation with either mitomycin C or porfiromycin [6,7,18–20]. The results obtained with the two drugs were analogous. Initial experiments examined the effects of regimens in which mitomycin and radiation were given concomitantly or in close sequence. In these experiments, dose-response curves were performed for radiation alone, for drug alone, and for regimens combining drug plus radiation (e.g., Fig. 3). Isobologram analyses were performed as described by Steel and Peckham [21]. These analyses showed that the combined-modality regimens produced ad-

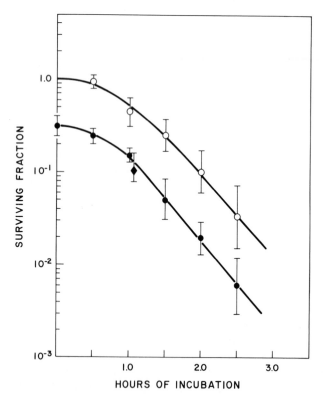

Fig. 3. One set of experiments examining the interactions of radiation and mitomycin C in vitro. Effect of irradiation on the survival of aerobic EMT6 cells treated in vitro with 1.5 $\mu$M mitomycin C for different periods of time. O, mitomycin C only; ●, mitomycin C + 5 Gy of X-rays delivered immediately before the beginning of drug treatment; ◆, mitomycin C + 5 Gy X-rays, with irradiation delivered during the final few minutes of drug treatment. Points: means ± SEMs. Reprinted from [19].

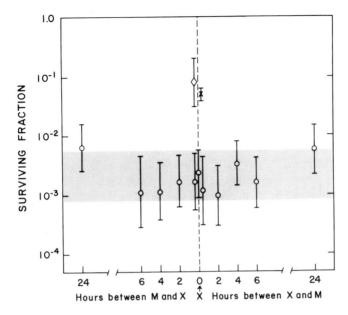

Fig. 4. Effect of the treatment sequence and of the interval between treatments on the survival of cells from exponentially growing, aerobic cultures of EMT6 cells exposed to mitomycin C and radiation. The axis shows the time
between irradiation and the drug treatment. Points: means ± SEMs. ×, X-rays only (7.5 Gy); ◇, 1.5 $\mu$M mitomycin C, 2 h; ○, both treatments; stippled area, area of additivity, calculated from single agent dose-response curves.
Reprinted from [19].

ditive cytotoxicities and suggested that the cytotoxicities of the two agents were independent. In other words, there appeared to be no significant interaction between the cytotoxicities of these two agents in these simple model systems. This was true both for cells treated
under aerobic conditions and for cells treated under acute hypoxia. The sensitivities of the
cells to the bioreductive drugs and to radiation were modulated by hypoxia, as described
above; however, the cytotoxicities of the drugs and radiation remained additive and independent either in air or in hypoxia.

Additional experiments were undertaken to examine the effect of the sequence of treatment with mitomycin C and radiation. In these experiments, exponentially growing cell
cultures were given both a 2 h treatment with 1.5 $\mu$M mitomycin C and 7.5 Gy of radiation;
mitomycin C was given at times ranging from 24 h before irradiation to 24 h after irradiation. As shown in Fig. 4, the sequence and the time between treatments had little effect on
the cytotoxicity of the combined-modality regimens. Treatment with mitomycin C and radiation separated by 24 h produced subadditive cytotoxicities, probably reflecting the proliferation of the surviving cells in the cultures (the cell cycle time in these cultures was
~12 h). However, all regimens with shorter intervals between drug and radiation resulted in
equivalent, additive, cytotoxicities. These data suggest that the efficacies of regimens combining mitomycin C with radiation are not influenced significantly by the details of the sequence or timing of the treatments in this simple model system where the environment of
the cells is uniform as a function of time.

The data shown in Fig. 4 provide no evidence of the temporal variations that would be
expected to occur if cell cycle effects influenced the sequence- and timing-dependence of

regimens combining mitomycin C and radiation. Although the cytotoxicity of radiation and mitomycin C both vary with the age of the cell [22,23], these variations are small relative to those seen with some cell cycle dependent anticancer drugs; MC and radiation are cytotoxic throughout the cell cycle. In addition, radiation and bioreductive drugs are toxic both to proliferating and to quiescent cells [24,25]. Both radiation and mitomycin C cause delayed cell death, which can occur several cell cycles after treatment. The proliferation patterns of both surviving and dying cells are perturbed after treatment, with cells delayed in passing critical checkpoints during the cell cycle [22,23]. Thus, although data from the experiments described above revealed no temporal variations that might reflect synchronization or cell cycle effects, it is possible that such effects would occur in other systems. However, because the cell cycle times of human tumor cells are longer and far more variable than those of the EMT6 cells used in these experiments, it is unlikely that such effects could be defined in human tumors and used as a guide to optimize such combined-modality therapy.

For solid tumors in vivo, the situation is more complex than with the cell culture systems described above, because of the microenvironmental heterogeneity in the solid malignancies [12,26]. It is now clear that these microenvironments are not static. Instead, fluctuations in blood flow through individual tumor blood vessels lead to temporal variations in the microenvironments of specific tumor regions, even in untreated tumors [27,28]. Treatment of the tumor with radiation or drug may result in additional alterations of the tumor microenvironment, as illustrated by the reoxygenation observed in experimental rodent tumors after irradiation [29]. The concept underlying the use of bioreductive alkylating agents with radiation is that radiation should be preferentially toxic to aerobic cells while the drug should be preferentially toxic to hypoxic cells, and that the concordant attack on these two cell populations should result in very efficacious treatment of the tumor. Because cells move from one population to another, optimal treatment with this combination should result from administering the agents concomitantly. That is, drug should be given during the course fractionated radiotherapy, rather than before the initiation of radiotherapy or after the completion of the radiotherapy course. Moreover, it would seem reasonable to administer the drug shortly before or shortly after irradiation, rather than separating the delivery by several hours or delivering drug on a separate day from irradiation.

## 5.  Administration of drugs: bolus versus fraction versus infusion

Another factor which must be considered in the design of clinical trials using bioreductive drugs and radiation is how to administer the drug. In chemotherapeutic regimens, mitomycin C and porfiromycin generally have been delivered as large bolus doses given once every 6 weeks [30–35]. Studies in cell culture [36–37] showed that the cytotoxicity of mitomycin C or porfiromycin to EMT6 cells or Chinese hamster cells was proportional to the concentration times the time ($C \times T$). Thus, treatment of EMT6 cells with mitomycin C at $2 \, \mu$M for 0.5 h, with $1 \, \mu$M for 1 h, with $0.5 \, \mu$M for 2 h, and with $0.1 \, \mu$M for 10 h all produced equivalent cytotoxicities. Cell culture studies [37] also revealed no significant repair of sublethal damage between mitomycin treatments and give no reason to predict that either the toxicities or the antineoplastic effects of the drug would be altered by protracting or fractionating the drug treatment over intervals short enough that proliferation did not occur during the treatment regimen.

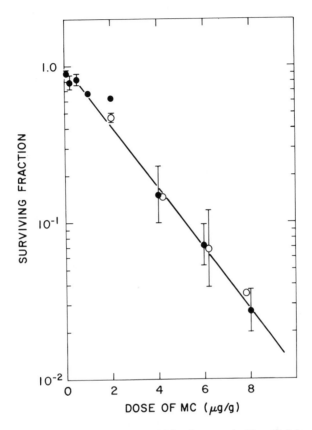

Fig. 5. Survival of cells in solid EMT6 tumors in BALB/c mice treated with graded doses of mitomycin C. ●, survival assayed 2 h after injection of mitomycin C; ○, survival assayed 24 hr after injection of mitomycin C. The similarity of the 2 and 24 h data suggests that there is no significant repair of potentially lethal mitomycin C damage by these tumor cells. Points: means ± SEMs. Reprinted from [35].

The survival curves for cells from EMT6 tumors treated with either mitomycin C or porfiromycin were exponential, with no evidence of a shoulder which might suggest the possibility of repair of sublethal damage with fractionated or protracted treatment (Fig. 5) [7,35]. Delaying explantation and assay for cell survival until 24 h after treatment revealed no repair of potentially lethal damage from these drugs (Fig. 5) [7,35]. In studies with EMT6 tumors in mice, we ask whether the antineoplastic effects of the drug were altered by moving from single doses to fractionated treatments with smaller doses or to infusion of drug over 2, 5 or 24 h [35]. When mitomycin C or porfiromycin was given as a single agent, the effect of a large rapid injection of drug appeared to be identical to that of two smaller doses adding up to the same total dose or to that of an infusion over periods of up to 24 h (Fig. 6, Table 1).

Studies examining the toxicity of mitomycin C to BALB/c mice had similar outcomes [35]. For mitomycin C and porfiromycin the survival curves for bone marrow stem cells (CFU-S, CFU-GM, and CFU-K) were exponential, with no evidence of a shoulder which might indicate the presence of repairable sublethal damage [7,35]. The toxic (lethal) effects of mitomycin C were indistinguishable whether mitomycin C was given as a acute injection

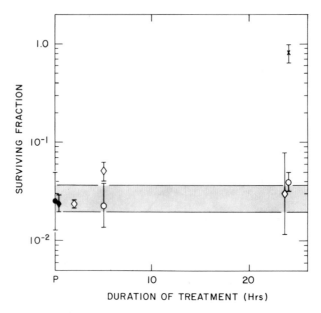

Fig. 6. Survival of cells in solid EMT6 tumors in BALB/c mice treated with a total dose of 8 μg/g mitomycin C. ○, drug given in two equal injections; ◇, drug infused continuously; ●, ◆, corresponding single-dose controls; stippled area, mean ± SEM from pooled controls. Points: means ± SEMs. None of the survivals for protracted or fractionated treatments differed significantly from the survivals measured after the single, rapid treatments. Reprinted from [35].

or as an infusion over 2, 5 or 24 h (Fig. 7, left panel) [35]. The toxicity of mitomycin C decreased when the drug was given as daily doses over 1, 2, or 3 weeks (Fig. 7, right panel), from 8.3 μg/g for a single fraction to 9.0 μg/g for 5 daily treatments, 12.4 μg/g for 10 daily treatments, and approximately 18 μg/g for 20 daily treatments over 4 weeks.

Table 1

Survival of cells in EMT6 tumor treated with 15 Gy of X-rays, 20 μg/g of porfiromycin, or various regimens combining these two treatments

| Treatment | Surviving fraction |
|---|---|
| POR (injection) | 0.0944 (0.0768–0.116) |
| POR (infused over 2 h) | 0.113 (0.0565–0.227) |
| X | 0.0524 (0.0441–0.0623) |
| POR + 1 h + X | 0.00185 (0.00133–0.00257) |
| POR (infused over 2 hr) + X | 0.00108 (0.000556–0.00208) |
| POR + 5 min + X | 0.00283 (0.00179–0.00445) |
| X + 5 min + POR | 0.00312 (0.00270–0.00360) |
| X + 4 h + POR | 0.00230 (0.00141–0.00375) |

Cell survival was assayed immediately after infusion of POR or 1 h after injection of POR. Surviving fractions are shown with SEMs.

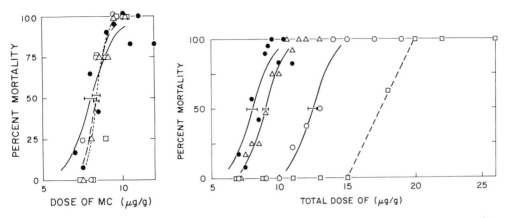

Fig. 7. Effect of continuous infusion (left panel) or fractionation (right panel) on the toxicity of mitomycin C to BALB/c mice. Left: single injection (●) versus infusion over 2 (○), 5 (△) or 24 (□) h. Right: single injection (●) versus 5 (△), 10 (○), or 20 (□) doses given as 1 treatment/day, 5 days/week. Bars: LD$_{50}$ ± SD, determined by probit analyses. Reprinted from [35].

The decreased toxicity seen with very protracted treatments was accompanied by a decrease in antineoplastic efficacy [35]. Tumor growth delay studies with EMT6 tumors showed similar growth delays for tumors treated with a single large dose of mitomycin C and for tumors treated with the same total dose in two equal fractions, separated by intervals of 5 or 24 h. Treatments with 5, 10, or 20 daily doses of mitomycin C yielded smaller growth delays. Moreover, 10 and 20 fraction regimens using doses shown to be equitoxic to the single dose yielded tumor growth delays that were equal to and smaller than the single treatment, respectively. Therefore, none of the fractionated regimens yielded a therapeutic ratio which was higher than that of mitomycin C used in a large single dose.

These data are in agreement with data from early clinical trials testing mitomycin C and porfiromycin as single chemotherapeutic agents, which suggested that both of these drugs had maximal therapeutic ratios when used in large, infrequent doses, as opposed to more highly fractionated treatment regimens [30–34]. It would be logical to assume that these drugs would be of maximal utility as adjuncts to radiotherapy when used in doses and with intervals that were similar to those which are most effective in single-agent and multi-agent chemotherapy; strong evidence from animal or modeling studies would be needed to justify consideration of combined-modality regimens using mitomycin C or porfiromycin treatment protocols which had proven less effective in single-agent chemotherapeutic regimens. As described below, our studies provide no reason to expect that protracted or fractionated drug treatments should be superior to large infrequent drug doses when mitomycin C and porfiromycin are used with radiotherapy.

## 6. Sequence and timing of drug and radiation treatments

The next question which arises in planning regimens combining radiotherapy with bioreductive drugs is that of the sequence and timing of the drug and radiation treatments. It seems intuitively obvious that drug and radiation should be given close together in time (on the same day), in order to maximize the effect of the preferential toxicities of the drug and radiation to different cell populations. Studies with cell cultures, described above, suggest that the toxicities of the drug and radiation are independent, and that the sequence and timing of the drug and radiation treatments are independent for exponentially growing cell cultures in a uniform environment. Studies with tumors in experimental animals were used to explore further the interactions of radiation with mitomycin C and with porfiromycin. One series of studies, reported in detail elsewhere [6,7], examined dose response curves for radiation alone, porfiromycin alone, and several regimens combining large doses porfiromycin with single doses of radiation given 1 h later. Analyses of these data, detailed elsewhere [7], showed that the regimens combining porfiromycin with radiation produced supra-additive cytotoxicity in the tumors, which appeared to reflect the preferential toxicity of the drug and radiation to different cell populations. Additional experiments, shown in Table 1, examined in more detail the relative effects of the sequence of porfiromycin and radiation and of the mode of administration of the drug (injection versus infusion). The details of the sequencing and timing of the drug and radiation had little effect on the cytotoxicity of the combined modality regimen. Similar data were obtained for mitomycin C and radiation combined in different sequences and with different intervals between treatments [5,20,38]. Taken together, these data suggest that the detailed sequencing and timing of the individual drug and radiation treatments probably are not critical in the design of regimens combining bioreductive drugs with radiation. This stands in marked contrast to the case with radiosensitizers or cell cycle-modulating drugs, where the sequence and timing of the individual treatments must be very carefully planned to obtain beneficial effects.

The final question remaining to be answered in the development of regimens combining bioreductive drugs and radiation is the question of when during fractionated radiotherapy the drug should be administered. In a simple modeling exercise, our dose-response curves for porfiromycin and for radiation as single agents were used to model the effect of various combined-modality regimens (Table 2). Three extreme regimens were considered: a regimen in which a large dose of drug was given with the first of 30 fractions of radiotherapy; a regimen in which a large single dose of drug was given with the last of 30 fractions of radiotherapy; and a regimen in which 30 small doses of drug were given daily, with each dose of radiation. We further assumed that changes in the oxygenation of the viable (surviving) tumor cells during the course of therapy were the critical factors modulating the cytotoxicity of the drug and radiation. Our data on the aerobic and hypoxic cytotoxicities of porfiromy-

Table 2

Results of modeling exercise predicting the effects of three different regimens of porfiromycin treatment as adjuncts to fractionated radiotherapy

| Assumed model of tumor oxygenation | Best drug regimen during therapy |
|---|---|
| No reoxygenation - oxygen status of cells constant during RT | 3 regimens equal |
| Reoxygenation to original hypoxic fraction between each fraction, oxic/hypoxic cells mix | 3 regimens equal |
| Hypoxic fraction falls during RT | Large single drug treatment at start of RT |
| Hypoxic fraction increases during RT | Large single drug treatment at end of RT |

These modeling results suggest no benefit to fractionating the drug treatment.

cin and radiation were used to model the overall cytotoxicity for each regimen, for each of four possible scenarios.

The first scenario assumed that there was no change in the oxygenation of the tumor cells during treatment; i.e., a cell that was aerobic at the beginning of the first radiotherapy treatment remained aerobic throughout the treatment, while a cell that was initially hypoxic remained hypoxic and viable through the full course of radiotherapy. In this scenario, a large dose of porfiromycin with the first radiation fraction, a large dose of porfiromycin with the last fraction, and small porfiromycin doses with every fraction all produced the same overall tumor cell survival at the end of therapy.

The second scenario assumed that reoxygenation to the initial hypoxic fraction occurred between each of the treatments, with complete mixing of the aerobic and hypoxic cell populations. This scenario might be expected to occur, for example, in tumors in which hypoxia was dominated by transient fluctuations in tumor blood flow. In this case, a large single dose of drug given with first radiation treatment, a large single dose of drug given with the last radiation treatment, and small doses of drug with each radiation treatment all produced equivalent overall cytotoxicities.

The third scenario considered was that of a tumor in which the hypoxic fraction fell during radiotherapy. This situation has been hypothesized to occur in some tumors as a result of rapid cell death and tumor shrinkage during treatment. In this case, the modeling showed that a large single drug treatment at the beginning of therapy was superior.

The last scenario considered was that in which the hypoxic fraction in the tumor increased during radiotherapy, as has been hypothesized in some tumors in which damage to the vasculature results in decreasing perfusion with progressive irradiation. Under this scenario, the model predicts that a single large drug treatment at the end of radiotherapy would be superior.

It is impossible at the present time to determine which of the four models of tumor oxygenation during therapy is most relevant to the treatment of human malignancies. Animal data can be found to support each of the four models. There is no way to know which (if any) of the animal tumor model systems is a valid model for a specific type of human tumor being treated in a clinical trial. Moreover, data on the oxygenation of human tumors during radiotherapy are still fragmentary. Those which do exist are based largely on gross measurements of tissue oxygenation or tissue metabolism. During the latter part of a 6-week course of successful therapy, such measurements of gross tissue oxygen tensions are most likely to reflect the status of the dying cells which comprise the vast bulk of the residual tumor mass. Because cells sterilized by radiation and bioreductive drugs cannot be distinguished from surviving cells, any histologic or tissue-level measurements of tumor physiology or tumor oxygenation made late in therapy will reflect the status of the dying cells, and may or may not reflect the oxygenation of the (relatively rare) surviving cells which determined the success or failure of treatment. There are essentially no data on the oxygenation of the clonogenic, surviving cells of human tumors during radiotherapy. It is important that none of these simple models provides an example of the situation in which treatment with many small fractions of drug would be superior to a large single treatment when the drug is used with conventionally fractionated radiotherapy. Because of considerations such as these, our clinical trials testing mitomycin C and porfiromycin as adjuncts to radiotherapy used two maximally tolerated doses of drug, one given during the first week of radiotherapy and one given 6 weeks later, at the end of radiotherapy.

There are, of course, many additional factors which could influence the efficacy and therapeutic ratio of different regimens combining radiotherapy with bioreductive drugs. These would include, for example, changes in cell proliferation during treatment, most notably the presence of accelerated repopulation, changes in perfusion during radiotherapy which resulted in improvement or worsening of drug delivery, or the development of drug resistance in the treated tumor cell population. However, consideration of such factors does not improve the predictability of the modeling.

Therefore, current data on the interactions of radiation and bioreductive drugs in vitro and in animal model systems can offer only general guidelines for the design of optimal regimens for combining these agents. The radiotherapy and chemotherapy courses should be concomitant. A maximal effect of the combination would be obtained by attacking the hypoxic and aerobic cell populations simultaneously. This means that drug and radiation treatments should be given close together (certainly on the same day); however, the detailed sequencing and timing of the individual treatments probably is not critical. The therapeutic ratio of the bioreductive drugs mitomycin C and porfiromycin, given as single agents, is largest when these drugs are given in large, infrequent bolus doses. Neither mathematical modeling of the outcome of combined modality regimens nor laboratory data obtained using cell culture and animal model systems provide evidence to suggest that other regimens, using more highly fractionated drug treatments or protracted infusions, should provide superior efficacy when these drugs are used as adjuncts to radiotherapy. In the absence of data to the contrary, it seemed appropriate to begin clinical evaluations of regimens combining bioreductive drugs and radiation by combining regimens that would be optimal for drug alone and radiotherapy alone; thus a regimen using a maximally tolerated dose of drug during the first week of a 6-week course of standard, daily fractionated radiotherapy and another near the end of radiotherapy was the logical starting point with which to evaluate clinical regimens combining bioreductive drugs and radiotherapy. The outcome of these trials, described elsewhere [1–5], suggests that these regimens are of value.

*Summary*

Mitomycin C and porfiromycin are being tested widely as adjuncts to radiotherapy in the treatment of carcinoma the head and neck and carcinoma of the cervix. These trials utilize the selective cytotoxicity of these bioreductive alkylating agents to hypoxic cells along with the selective toxicity of radiation to aerobic cell populations, in consort, to achieve a greater therapeutic ratio from the combined-modality regimens. The design of therapeutic regimens which combine hypoxia-selective drugs with radiotherapy differs in many ways from design of regimens using radiosensitizers or combining radiotherapy with conventional adjuvant chemotherapy. This chapter reviews the theoretical considerations, laboratory experiments, clinical data, and mathematical modeling which should be considered in the design of clinical regimens combining the bioreductive alkylating agents with radiotherapy. These considerations suggest that optimal use of hypoxia-selective drugs with radiotherapy must employ concomitant treatment regimens, in which drug is delivered during the course of fractionated radiotherapy. With the bioreductive alkylating agents mitomycin C and porfiromycin, this review suggests that one or two large doses of drug will be superior or equal to drug regimens incorporating more highly fractionated treatments or continuous infusions.

## Acknowledgments

Research reviewed in this paper was supported in part by Grant EDT62 from the American Cancer Society

## References

1.  Weissberg JB, Son YH, Papac RJ, et al. Randomized clinical trial of mitomycin C as an adjunct to radio-therapy in head and neck cancer. Int J Radiat Oncol Biol Phys 17: 3–9, 1989.
2.  Fischer JJ, Haffty BG, Son YH, et al. Bioreductive alkylating agents and radiation therapy in the treatment of squamous cell carcinoma of the head and neck region. In: Dobrosky W (Ed), Bioreductive Drugs, Sensi-tizers, Oxygen, and Radiotherapy. Austria: Facultas Universitatsverlag, pp. 167–179, 1993.
3.  Haffty BG, Son YH, Sasaki CT, et al. Mitomycin C as an adjunct to postoperative radiation therapy in squamous cell carcinoma of the head and neck: results from two randomized clinical trials. Int J Radiat Oncol Biol Phys 27: 241–250, 1993.
4.  Haffty BG, Son YH, Wilson LD, et al. The bioreductive alkylating agent porfiromycin in combination with radiation therapy in the management of squamous cell carcinoma of the head and neck. Radiat Oncol In-vest, in press.
5.  Haffty BG, Son YH, Papac RJ, et al. Chemotherapy as an adjunct to radiation in the treatment of squamous cell carcinoma of the head and neck. results of the Yale mitomycin C randomized trials. J Clin Oncol 15: 268–276, 1997.
6.  Keyes SR, Rockwell S, Sartorelli AC. Porfiromycin as a bioreductive alkylating agent with selective toxic-ity to hypoxic EMT6 tumor cells in vivo and in vitro. Cancer Res 45: 3642–3645, 1985.
7.  Rockwell S, Keyes SR, Sartorelli AC. Preclinical studies of porfiromycin as an adjunct to radiotherapy. Radiat Res 116: 100–113, 1988.
8.  Coleman CN. Conference summary: the ninth international conference on the chemical modifiers of cancer treatment. Br J Cancer 74: 5297–5302, 1996.
9.  Brown JM. SR4233 (tirapazamine): a new anticancer drug exploiting hypoxia in solid tumors. Br J Cancer 67: 1163–1170, 1993.
10. Rockwell S. Hypoxic cells as targets for cancer chemotherapy. In: Cheng Y-C, Goz B, Minkoff M (Eds), Development of Target Oriented Anticancer Drugs. New York: Raven Press, pp. 157–172, 1983.
11. Quintiliani M. The oxygen effect in radiation inactivation of DNA and enzymes. Int J Radiat Biol 50: 573–594, 1986.
12. Moulder JE, Rockwell S. Tumor hypoxia: its impact on cancer therapy. Cancer Metast Rev 5: 313–341, 1987.
13. Rockwell S. Use of hypoxia-directed drugs in the therapy of solid tumors. Semin Oncol 19: 29–40, 1992.
14. Tomasz M, Hughes CS, Chowdary D, et al. Isolation, identification, and assay of [$^3$H]-porfiromycin ad-ducts of EMT6 mouse mammary tumor cell DNA: effects of hypoxia and dicumarol on adduct patterns. Cancer Commun 3: 213–223, 1991.
15. Rockwell S, Sartorelli AC, Tomasz M, Kennedy KA. Cellular pharmacology of quinone bioreductive al-kylating agents. Cancer Metast Rev 12: 165–176, 1993.
16. Bizanek R, Chowdary D, Arai H, et al. Adducts of mitomycin C and DNA in EMT6 mouse mammary tumor cells. Effects of hypoxia and dicumarol on adduct patterns. Cancer Res 53: 5127–5134, 1993.
17. Rockwell S, Kennedy KA, Sartorelli AC. Mitomycin-C as a prototype bioreductive alkylating agent:  In vitro studies of metabolism and cytotoxicity. Int J Radiat Oncol Biol Phys 8: 753–755, 1982.
18. Rockwell S. Effect of some proliferative and environmental factors on the toxicity of mitomycin C to tu-mor cells in vitro. Int J Cancer 38: 229–235, 1986.
19. Rockwell S. Cytotoxicities of mitomycin C and x-rays to aerobic and hypoxic cells in vitro. Int J Radiat Oncol Biol Phys 8: 1035–1039, 1982.
20. Rockwell S, Sartorelli AC. Interactions between mitomycin C and radiation. In: Hill BT, Bellamy AS (Eds), Antitumor Drug-Radiation Interactions. Boca Raton, FL: CRC Press, pp. 125–139, 1990.
21. Steel GG, Peckham MJ. Exploitable mechanisms in combined radiotherapy-chemotherapy: the concept of additivity. Int J Radiat Oncol Biol Phys 5: 85–91, 1979.

22.   Sinclair WK. Cyclic x-ray responses in mammalian cells in vivo. Radiat Res 33: 620–643, 1968.

23.   Barlogie B, Drewinko B. Lethal and cytokinetic effects of mitomycin C on cultured human colon cancer cells. Cancer Res 40: 1973–1980, 1980.

24.   Rockwell S, Hughes CS. Effects of mitomycin C and porfiromycin on exponentially growing and plateau phase cultures. Cell Prolif 27: 153–163, 1994.

25.   Rockwell S. Influence of a 1400-gauss magnetic field on the radiosensitivity and recovery of EMT6 cells in vitro. Int J Radiat Biol 31: 153–160, 1977.

26.   Rockwell S, Knisely JPS. Hypoxia and angiogenesis in experimental tumor models: therapeutic implications. In: Goldberg ID, Rosen EM (Eds), Regulation of Angiogenesis. Basel: Birkhauser, pp. 335–356, 1996.

27.   Jain RK. Determinants of tumor blood flow: a review. Cancer Res 48: 2641–2658, 1988.

28.   Chaplin DJ, Olive PL, Durand RE. Intermittent blood flow in a murine tumor: radiobiological effects. Cancer Res 47: 597–601, 1982.

29.   Kallman RF. The phenomenon of reoxygenation and its implications for fractionated radiotherapy. Radiology 105: 135–142, 1972.

30.   Crooke ST, Bradner WT. Mitomycin C: a review. Cancer Treatment Rev 3: 121–139, 1976.

31.   Godfrey TE, Wilbur DW. Clinical experience with mitomycin C in large infrequent doses. Cancer 29: 1647–1652, 1972.

32.   Carter SK. Porfiromycin (NSC-56410) - clinical brochure. Cancer Chemother Rep 31: 87–97, 1968.

33.   Baker LH, Izbicki RM, Vaitevicius VK. Phase II study of porfiromycin vs mitomycin C utilizing acute intermittent schedules. Med Pediatr Oncol 2: 207–213, 1976.

34.   Doll DC, Weiss RB, Issel BF. Mitomycin: ten years after approval for marketing. J Clin Oncol 3: 276–286, 1985.

35.   Rockwell S, Nierenburg M, Irvin CG. Effects of the mode of administration of mitomycin on tumor and marrow response and on the therapeutic ratio. Cancer Treatment Rep 71: 927–934, 1987.

36.   Marshall RS, Rauth AM. Oxygen and exposure kinetics as factors influencing the cytotoxicity of porfiromycin, a mitomycin C analogue in Chinese hamster ovary cells. Cancer Res 48: 5655–5659, 1988.

37.   Hughes CS, Irvin CG, Rockwell S. Effect of deficiencies in DNA repair on the toxicity of mitomycin C and porfiromycin to CHO cells under aerobic and hypoxic conditions. Cancer Commun 3: 29–35, 1991.

38.   Rockwell S. Effects of mitomycin C alone and in combination with x-rays on EMT6 mouse mammary tumors in vivo. J Natl Cancer Inst 71: 765–771, 1983.

C.J. Rosenthal and M. Rotman (Eds.), *Infusion Chemotherapy–Irradiation Interactions*

91

CHAPTER 9

# Interaction of mitomycin C by continuous intravenous infusion and radiation in the treatment of colon carcinoma metastatic to the liver: evidence for a synergistic effect

C. JULIAN ROSENTHAL[1-4], HASSAN AZIZ[3,4], DANIEL BELINA[1-3],
KWAN CHOI[4] and MARVIN ROTMAN[2-4]

[1]*Othmer Cancer Center and Departments of* [2]*Medicine, and* [3]*Radiation Oncology, Long Island College Hospital, 339 Hicks Street, Brooklyn, NY 11201, USA, and* [4]*State University of New York, Health Science Center at Brooklyn, 450 Clarkson Avenue, Brooklyn, NY 11203, USA*

## 1. Introduction and background

### 1.1. Rationale for hypoxic cell radiosensitization

It has been known for more than 4 decades [1–3] that severely hypoxic cells are approximately three times more resistant to ionizing irradiation than the aerobic cells. This is due to the fact that molecular oxygen in very low concentrations (7 times lower than its venous blood tension) is a potent radiosensitizer through the release of free radicals that can react with DNA and proteins causing mutations or cell killing. Consequently, solid tumors that frequently contain areas of poor blood perfusion resulting in temporary or chronic hypoxia can become radioresistant.

### 1.2. Preclinical studies on agents promoting hypoxic cells radiosensitization

Experimental studies on transplanted mouse and rat tumors showed that 10–20% of the viable clonogenic cells were hypoxic [4–6]. Their percentage did not vary with serial transplantations nor with the degree of tumor differentiation, nor its origin except that leukemias and lymphomas generally appeared to be better oxygenated. Many hypoxic cells are viable and are capable of causing tumor recurrence after large single doses of radiotherapy and to influence the response of tumors to various fractionated radiotherapy regimens as well as to combined radiotherapy–chemotherapy regimens [7].

Animal studies have shown that the outcome of radiation therapy can be improved by using agents that circumvent the effects of hypoxia by oxygenating or killing the hypoxic tumor cells [7–11]. Because normal tissues contain few or no severely hypoxic cells, regimens incorporating such agents improve the responses of solid tumors without producing concomitant increase in radiation toxicity.

Hypoxia directed drugs were thought to be valuable not as single agents but rather in combination with radiotherapy or with drugs that selectively kill aerobic cells [12].

Hypoxic tumor cells theoretically could be targeted through a number of different mechanisms. Hypoxia could be indirectly induced by perturbations of the micro environment (i.e., by inducing low glucose levels, high lactate levels, low levels of nutrients or low intracellular pH). Hypoxic cells are less able than aerobic cells to maintain a relatively large transmembrane pH (up to 0.5 pH units) due to a drop in their intracellular pH. It was hypothesized that drugs that are chemically activated at low pH or by enzymes functioning only at low pH as well as those that have their influx modulated by alterations of the cell membrane at low pH could selectively target the hypoxic cells. The first generation of cytotoxic agents targeted at hypoxic cells proved to be either ineffective (i.e., 5-thio-D-glucose) or too toxic for normal tissues (i.e., misonidazole and derivatives that induced neurotoxicity). At Yale University in 1970, the mitomycins [13] were found in experimental animals to be more toxic against hypoxic tumor cells than to aerobic cells during their interactions with caffeine. The mitomycins are a family of antitumor antibiotics derived from *Streptomyces caespitosus*, related to porfiromycin that were found capable to suppress bacterial replication. Mitomycin C was found to function as an alkylating agent due to the fact that the quinone ring in its structure can be reduced by one electron transfer to form free radicals and to open its aziridine ring which then functions as an aklylator. However, it has only been since the late 1980s that Rockwell and Sartorelli have shown that, in order to produce cytotoxic damage, these bioreductive alkylating agents require reductive activation. In addition, mitomycin C was found to be more toxic at low pH than at physiologic pH. Tested on various experimental tumors, the regimens combining mitomycin C with irradiation consistently produced greater cytotoxicity, longer growth delay and better tumor control than the radiation therapy alone. The effect was shown to be supra-additive [14]. This was further increased when the N-methyl aziridyl analogue of mitomycin C, the porfiromycin, was used [15].

*1.3.   Early clinical trials on mitomycin C–radiation interaction*

These data led to an initial pilot randomized study [16] that showed that during the radiation treatment of loco-regional (Stage II–III) squamous cell carcinoma of the head and neck, mitomycin C administered as an i.v. bolus injection significantly increased loco-regional control when compared with irradiation alone without increasing normal tissue reactions [16]. These data were convincingly confirmed in the therapy of squamous cell carcinoma of the anus [17] and cervix [18] in which patients treated with mitomycin C and 5-fluorouracil (5-FU) adjunct to radiation therapy did better than those that receive only 5-FU with radiation therapy.

*1.4.   Rationale for the administration of mitomycin C by continuous intravenous infusion for radiation potentiation*

From experimental studies on a C3H mouse mammary carcinoma it was shown by Grau and Overgaard [19] that the interactions between mitomycin C (MMC) and radiation therapy are dependent on the timing of MMC administration. MMC has significantly enhanced the tumor growth delay induced by irradiation alone when administered 15 min before irradiation while no enhancement was seen when administered 4 h after irradiation [19]. Because these data cannot be confirmed in humans without very large clinical trials carried out over many years, it is logical to assume that in order to optimize the interaction between MMC and radiation therapy, it would be advantageous to have a steady level of MMC in the serum. This could be achieved only through its continuous i.v. administration during the whole period of radiation therapy delivery because MMC is rapidly cleared from the circulating plasma; its half-life in circulating blood is 12 h [20]. Preliminary studies by Lokich et al. [21] indicated that MMC by continuous intravenous infusion can be safely delivered up to 1.2 mg/m$^2$ per day for a maximum of 21 days. If the MMC administration continued beyond the 21st day, patients consistently developed thrombocytopenia (<50 000/$\mu$l) and granulocytopenia (<1000/$\mu$l).

We postulated that a similar continuous infusion administered during radiation therapy may enhance its cytotoxic effect on existing tumor cells (especially against those hypoxic centrally located) and could lead to their demise at a total dose lower than the one necessary for irradiation alone to be cytotoxic. To prove this hypothesis, we initially carried out a phase I study to determine the maximum tolerated dose (MTD) and the duration of a mitomycin C infusion with concomitant radiation therapy. Then we focused on its effect in the treatment of liver metastases in patients with adenocarcinoma of the colon.

## 2. Methods

### 2.1. Mitomycin C–radiation regimen

We first conducted a phase I study to determine the MTD of the MMC administered by continuous intravenous infusion while patients with adenocarcinoma of the colon were receiving standard radiation therapy to the site(s) of measurable metastatic lesions. The MMC infusion was started at a dose of 0.8 mg/m$^2$, which was escalated in each group of 3 enrolled cases by 0.2 mg/m$^2$ per day until either unwanted side effects developed or the dose of 1.2 mg/m$^2$ per day was reached which was found to be the MTD for continuous intravenous infusion alone.

### 2.2. Patients on study: phase I trial

Seven patients who failed previous chemotherapy with 5-FU were enrolled between September 1988 and January 1991 in this study approved by the hospitals' IRB; there were 2 patients with palpable abdominal wall metastatic lesions from adenocarcinoma of the colon, 2 with measurable mediastinal and lung metastases from adenocarcinoma of the lung and 3 with well defined metastatic lesion(s) in the liver, one of whom also had measurable pelvic metastases from primary adenocarcinoma of the colon. MMC was delivered diluted in 50 ml normal saline by a portable pump through a port-a-cath (Mediport, Groshong), whose catheter was inserted in the subclavian vein through a standard ambulatory procedure. Patient's CBC, reticulocyte count, serum haptoglobin, GGPT, LDH, SGPT and bilirubin were monitored twice weekly. The infusion was discontinued after 21 days as recommended by Lokich [21], who after a phase I study found prohibitive bone marrow toxicity when the MMC is administered by intravenous infusion beyond 21 days.

### 2.3. Phase II study on mitomycin C–radiation regimen in patients with colon carcinoma metastatic to the liver

After establishing the maximum tolerated dose (MTD) of the MMC by c.i. at 1 mg/m$^2$ per day for 21 days when administered with concomitant radiation therapy, we conducted a small phase II study with this concomitant combined modality regimen in patients with colo-rectal adenocarcinoma metastatic to the liver. Ten patients with measurable metastatic lesions in their liver, but without detectable extra hepatic metastases at the time of their entry, were enrolled in this study at two institutions, University Hospital of Brooklyn (UHB) and Long Island College Hospital-(LICH) over a period of 3 years (1991–1994). The demographic characteristics of the enrolled patients are presented in Table 1. They all had more than 2 lesions in their liver determined by CT scan with contrast or magnetic resonance imaging (MRI). Their tumor size was best monitored by the elevation of their serum LDH which varied between 320 and 1340 units/dl at the start of the treatment. They received radiation therapy (RT) to their whole liver which was planned to be delivered over a period of 3 weeks, 5 days a week in single doses of 180 cGy per session. Whenever indicated, a short boost was administered to a more prominent single lesion to a total dose varying between 300 and 800 cGy.

MMC was infused through a port-a-cath from a portable pump at a rate of 1 mg/m$^2$ per day for 21 days in an ambulatory setting without interruptions unless side effects developed. Patients were monitored for side effects possibly due to early bone marrow suppression, hemolysis, renal insufficiency, hepatic toxicity. WBC differential, reticulocyte count and red cell morphology analysis on their peripheral blood smear were performed every other day. Their serum chemistry and urine analysis were performed once weekly. This included serum haptoglobin, serum bilirubin (direct and total) and serum carcinoembryonic antigen (CEA) as tumor marker that could possibly monitor tumor response to therapy. Three weeks after the completion of the combined modality therapy the response was evaluated by the same method used to measure the liver lesions at their entry to the study (MRI or CT scan with contrast). Then patients were treated for 6–10 months (mean 7.5 months) with calcium leucovorin (200 mg/m$^2$) followed 1 h later by 5-FU (400 mg/m$^2$) i.v. bolus for 5 consecutive days every 4 weeks. A dose adjustment for grade 3 mucositis had to be made on just two occasions; the calcium leucovorin and 5-FU were reduced by 30%.

Table 1

Patients' dermographic characteristics in phase II study

| | |
|---|---|
| Sex | |
| Males | 6 |
| Females | 4 |
| Race | |
| Caucasians | 4 |
| Afro Americans | 3 |
| Hispanics | 2 |
| Asians | 1 |
| Performance status (PS) | |
| 0 | 2 |
| 1 | 6 |
| 2 | 2 |
| Age (years) | 51–74 |

## 3.  Results

### 3.1.  Establishing the maximum tolerated dose

The phase I study was carried out on 7 patients only because at the third escalation of the mitomycin C dose, prohibitive side-effects developed in the single patient entered at that level.

As indicated in Table 2, at the first MMC dose level of 0.8 mg/m$^2$ per day only minor side-effects developed; grade I diarrhea (2–5 loose stools/day) was present in one case after 15 days of continuous i.v. MMC. It responded to loperamide and kaopectate without requiring the treatment to be discontinued. In 2 patients mild leukopenia and granulocytopenia developed on the 16th day of therapy and slowly progressed throughout the last week of therapy; WBC remained above 2500/$\mu$l and the absolute granulocyte count remained above 1800/$\mu$l.

At level two after a first escalation by 0.2 mg/m$^2$ of the daily dose of MMC by continuous infusion, only minor gastrointestinal side-effects developed. One patient had grade I diarrhea and mild oral nucositis (grade I); he developed two superficial escoriations on his lip mucosa that resolved after applying acyclovir ointment while the MMC infusion was completed. One other patient developed grade II oral mucositis with depapillated tongue that presented 4–5 white plaques on its posterior two-thirds and with 3 superficial ulcers on her bucal mucosa. The administration of mycelex troches as well as of acyclovir p.o. permitted the treatment to be continued after a 3-day interruption. All 3 patients at level 2 of the MMC dose developed moderate leukopenia in the last week of treatment (WBC between 1200 and 1950/$\mu$l with absolute granulocyte counts of 1050 to 1425/$\mu$l). They also developed mild anemia with a drop in their hematocrit by 2–5%. Mild thrombocytopenia with platelet counts <140 000 but >100 000 developed in 2 out of 3 patients 5–6 days after the completion of the therapy.

At level three of the MMC dose of 1.2 mg/m$^2$ per day just one patient was enrolled. She was a 58-year-old B/F with metastatic carcinoma of the colon to the abdominal wall with a prominently protruding mass originating in part from her omentum. She had no history of cardiovascular disease or hypertension. After 1 week of therapy she developed grade II diarrhea with 6–10 watery stools/day that responded just in part to loperimide and kaopectate.

Table 2

Side effects developed during the phase I study of MMC CI–RT (related to the MMC dose)

| Mitomycin C dose (mg/m$^2$ per day) | No. of patients | Side effects | Rate/ no. of patients |
|---|---|---|---|
| 0.8 | 3 | Diarrhea grade 1 | 1/3 |
| | | Leukopenia grade 1 | 2/3 |
| | | Anemia grade 1 | 2/3 |
| 1 | 3 | Diarrhea grade 1 | 1/3 |
| | | Oral mucositis grade 1 | 1/3 |
| | | Oral mucositis grade 2 | 1/3 |
| | | Leukopenia grade 1 | 3/3 |
| | | Anemia grade 1 | 3/3 |
| 1.2 | 1 | Diarrhea grade 2 | 1/1 |
| | | Cardiac A-V conduction defect | 1/1 |

At the end of the second week of therapy 30 min after she completed the daily radiation therapy she had a syncopal episode that lasted only 30 s. A complete workup of this episode revealed only the presence of a first degree A-V block in the patient's ECG. This could suggest a higher degree of blockade of her electrical myocardial conduction at the time of syncope. However, mitomycin C has never been previously reported to interfere with the A-V conduction. For this reason a decision was made to restart the patient's MMC infusion after a 24-h interruption. Radiation therapy was continued without interruption.

Several ECGs during the first 2 h of the MMC infusion did not show any changes besides the persistent first degree A-V block. The patient was sent home 1 h after receiving radiation therapy. On her way out she had a second syncopal episode. This time the ECG documented an asystole for a few seconds. The patient recovered within 5 min. During the 30 h period between these two syncopes, the patient also had 6 watery bowel movements; her serum K level remained within normal limits (3.9 then 3.7 mequiv/l). It was decided to discontinue the MMC-RT treatment in this patient for 1 week. Her diarrhea resolved after 48 h of loperimide treatment. The treatment was restarted at a lower MMC dose of 1 mg/m$^2$ per day and it was completed within 12 days without any further incident. It was concluded that a dose of MMC of 1 mg/m$^2$ per day should be considered the MTD for those patients also receiving radiotherapy especially if the radiation field included at least part of their heart.

### 3.2. Mitomycin C continuous infusion–radiation therapy in patients with colon carcinoma metastatic to the liver

We then administered MMC by continuous intravenous infusion at its MTD level of 1 mg/m$^2$ per day for 21 days to 10 consecutive cases of patients with colo-rectal carcinoma metastatic to the liver whose demographic characteristics were previously presented.

Over a period of 2 years we enrolled 10 patients in this study. Each of them had at least two metastatic lesions in their liver located in different lobes (were consequently not resectable) and did not have metastases elsewhere detectable by current radiologic imaging techniques.

The details of their treatment were previously presented in Section 2. All patients received, thereafter, 5-FU 400 mg/m$^2$ by i.v. bolus 1 h after starting a 2 h infusion of calcium leucovorin 200 mg/m$^2$ qd for 5 consecutive days every 4 weeks. Three patients completed the scheduled 10 cycles; one completed 8 months of treatment. Three received 7 cycles, and three received only 6 cycles . However, just one of the cases that received 6 cycles and 2 of those that received 7 cycles refused to continue because of the moderate side-effects they developed 3–5 days following the completion of each cycle represented by grade II diarrhea (5–8 bowel movements/day) with loose stools and/or grade I oral mucositis manifested by superficial escoriations on the tongue and bucal mucosa. The remaining 4 cases stopped treatment because they felt much better to the point of restarting their usual activities and regaining some weight.

The results of treatment (see Table 3) were assessed 3 weeks after the completion of the initial combined modality treatment, then every 4 months for the radiologic imaging tests (CT scan with contrast, MRI or sonogram of the liver) and every month for the serologic tests monitoring disease response (LDH and CEA) as well as for their liver function tests (SGOT, SGPT, GGT and alkaline phosphatase) and their CBC (see Table 4).

Five patients achieved partial response with the reduction of the size of their tumor mass by at least 50% and a corresponding reduction of their LDH. As indicated in Table 4, the

Table 3

Response to therapy in 10 evaluable patients

| Type of response | No. of patients | Duration of response (weeks) | Total mean RT dose (cGy) | Total mean mitomycin dose (mg/m$^2$) |
|---|---|---|---|---|
| Partial response (PR) (reduction of tumor size >50%) | 5 | 48 ± 4 | 2400± | 19.5± |
| Minimal response (MR) (reduction of tumor size >10% < 30%) | 4 | 20 ± 4 | 2500 ± 350 | 20.5 ± 2 |
| Disease progression (Prog.) | 1 | – | 3200 | 21 |

total surface area occupied by the tumor on the liver imaging tests decreased from 124.6 to 24.12 cm$^2$ on day 2 after the concomitant combined modality treatment.

In only 2 out of the 5 cases that achieved PR, the size of their tumor continued to decrease during the administration of the monthly cycles of 5-FU and calcium leucovorin until it reached a steady size after the fourth and fifth cycles, respectively.

Four patients showed only minimal response with a decrease in the total surface occupied by the tumor by less than 25 cm$^2$. The average tumor area decreased from 91.5 to 84 cm$^2$ 3–4 weeks after completion of the combined modality therapy. In one case, the disease progressed while the patient received the same regimen (RT-MMC c.i.).

When we analyzed various serologic parameters that were selected due to their possible correlation with the variations of the tumor size (Table 5), it was found that the best coefficient of correlation (0.88) existed between the LDH serum values and tumor size variations. A lesser correlation (0.56) was seen with the serum CEA values. The patient's liver function tests have varied little while the patient reached maximum response.

Table 4

Clinical and laboratory parameters (related to the type of response)

|  | PR | MR | Disease progression |
|---|---|---|---|
| No. of patients | 5 | 4 | 1 |
| Age (years) | 60.4 | 59.2 | 72 |
| Sex (male/female) | 3/2 | 2/2 | 1/0 |
| PS | 1 (0–2) | 1 (0–2) | |
| Time to dg (months) | 14.8 | 14.25 | 13.5 |
| Total dose of MMC (mg) | 31.3 | 34.2 | 36 |
| Total RT dose (cGy) | 2500 | 2800 | 3000 |
| CEA (μl) | 138.6 | 133.7 | 145 |
| GGPT (μl) | 78.9 | 73.75 | 70 |
| SGOT (μl) | 39.8 | 49.5 | 52 |
| Total bilirubin (mg/dl) | 1.58 | 1.75 | 1.6 |
| LDH (units/dl) | 554 | 1152.5 | 1350 |
| Average tumor surface at start (cm$^2$) | 124.65 | 91.5 | 72 |
| Average tumor surface at MX response (cm$^2$) | 24.12 | 84 | 95 |

Table 5

Monitoring response to therapy

| | PR | | MR | | Correlation coefficient |
|---|---|---|---|---|---|
| | Before Rx | After Rx | Before Rx | After Rx | |
| TS (average cm$^2$) | 123.65 | 24.12 | 91.5 | 84 | |
| CEA ($\mu$l) | 138.6 | 37.5 | 133.7 | 98.2 | 0.56 |
| LDH ($\mu$l) | 554 | 285 | 1152 | 870 | 0.88 |

The duration of the response (Table 6) was significantly greater for patients who achieved PR (48 ± 5 weeks) than for those who had a minimal response (20 ± 4 weeks). Their overall survival from the time of enrollment in this study was more than a year (62 ± 9 weeks). This is greater than twice the survival of patients who achieved only minimal response (29 ± 7 weeks) (see Table 6). The patients whose disease progressed while on therapy survived only 6.5 weeks.

### 3.3.  Side-effects of infusional mitomycin C–radiation regimen

The most common side effects encountered during this limited phase II study of continuous i.v. infusion of mitomycin C and concomitant radiation therapy are listed in Table 7. They are similar to those seen during the phase I study. Diarrhea was encountered in all patients being more severe in 4; it caused hypokalemia in 2, accompanied by mild prerenal azotemia (BUN elevation by 50% to a BUN/creatinine ratio of 20–22:1).

Oral mucositis was mild and rarely seen. In 3 patients it manifested only by superficial escoriations on the lips, dry mouth mucosa and minimal sore throat.

All 10 patients had a drop of their absolute granulocyte count by more than 50% but less than 80% from that at the start of treatment. It occurred between day 23 and 30 from the start of the regimen (2–7 days from the completion of MMC continuous intravenous infusion), never fell below 1000 cells/$\mu$l and recovered to the starting point within 8–14 weeks. Moderate thrombocytopenia, with a drop of the platelet count by more than 25% but less than 50% from the therapy initiation, was noted in 6 cases. The platelet count fully recovered within 4 weeks. Anemia was mild in 3 cases with a drop in the hematocrit of less than 20% from the starting level between the 10th and 22nd day from the completion of the combined modality regimen.

In one case a hemolytic episode was noted in the 20th day of MMC continuous infusion. The patient complained of weakness. Within 24 h his hematocrit fell from 36 to 28% while his indirect bilirubin rose to 1.9 mg/dl. His haptoglobin fell to 5 mg/dl (from the normal of

Table 6

Response duration

| | PR | MR | Disease progression |
|---|---|---|---|
| Mean time to progression (weeks) | 48 ± 4 | 20 ± 4 | |
| Mean survival (weeks) | 62 ± 9 | 29 ± 7 | 6.5 |
| Average decrease in tumor size (cm$^2$) | 100 ± 9 | 7.5 | |

Table 7

Side-effects of the RT-MMC c.i. regimen

| Clinical manifestation | Degree of intensity | No. of patients/ total no. of patients |
|---|---|---|
| Diarrhea | Grade II (5–9 BM/day) | 4/10 |
| Diarrhea | Grade I (2–4 BM/day) | 6/10 |
| Granulocytopenia | Decrease by 50–80% (nadir 1225 ± 240/$\mu$l) | 9/10 |
| Thrombocytopenia | Decrease by 25–50% (nadir 88 ± 16 × $10^3$/$\mu$l) | 6/10 |
| Anemia | Decrease of hematocrit by 10–30% | 3/10 |
| Moderate hemolysis | Decrease of hematocrit by 60% | 1/10 |
| Oral mucositis | Grade II | 1/10 |
| Oral mucositis | Grade I | 3/10 |
| Acute pharyngitis | Erythema + purulent discharge | 3/10 |
| Urinary tract infection | Cloudy urine, hematuria | 2/10 |
| Hypokalemia | Decrease of K < 3.4 mequiv/l | 2/10 |
| Azotemia (pre-renal) | Increase of BUN by 70% | 2/10 |
| SGPT elevation | Increase by >25% | 2/10 |
| GGT elevation | Increase by >25% | 1/10 |
| Alkaline phosphatase elevation | Increase by 20% | 0/10 |
| Serum bilirubin (direct) elevation | Increase by 10% | 1/10 |
| Serum bilirubin (indirect febrile) | Increase by 50% | 1/10 |

90–150 mg/dl). The patient's peripheral smear showed mild anisocytosis and poikilocytosis with a few spherocytes (5%). Two schystocytes were encountered. Mitomycin C was discontinued as soon as these data became available. This corresponded to the last day of the 3 week scheduled course of MMC.

Patient hemolysis resolved within 24 h. His haptoglobin started to rise the next day to 12 mg/dl then returned to 120 mg/m$^2$ within 2 weeks. During this hemolytic episode, the patient did not have any urinary abnormalities (BUN remained at 16 mg/dl while urine analysis was normal).

## 4. Discussion

The study described here was developed from the premise that MMC by continuous intravenous infusion would permit the synchronization of its effect with that of concomitant radiation therapy delivered to a growing tumor. Hence this mode of administration of MMC could better test the hypothesis that mitomycin C, having a higher cytocidal effect on hypoxic cells, is likely to be accompanied by fewer side-effects in view of the fact that the normal tissues surrounding the tumor contain very few or no hypoxic cells at all. This appeared to be the case in the study presented previously which could lead only to preliminary conclusions due to the limited number of patients enrolled.

The therapeutic use of MMC by continuous intravenous infusion could be seen as controversial based on the preliminary experimental studies of Grau and Overgaard [19] that have found that MMC had additive effects when administered 15 min before but not 4 h after radiation therapy administered to a mouse mammary carcinoma in vivo. On the other hand, in a series of experiments at Yale University, Moulder, Rockwell and collaborators showed that regimens combining MMC with radiation are not influenced significantly by the details of the sequence or timing of these treatments. In a simple experimental model, Rockwell et al. [22] have shown that the toxicity of MMC decreased when the drug was given as daily doses. The equivalent of 8.3 $\mu$g/g of body weight for a single dose of MMC was 9.0 $\mu$g/g for 5 daily treatments, 12.4 $\mu$g/g for 10 daily treatments and 18 $\mu$g/g for 20 daily treatments; the decreased toxicity seen with protracted treatments was accompanied by a decrease in antineoplastic efficacy [23] unless the total dose administered was proportionally increased. Still the equivalent increase of 0.56 $\mu$g/g per day between the 10th and 20th day of MMC daily administration is lower than the increase of 0.68 $\mu$g/g per day between the 5th and 10th day of the daily doses suggesting a slightly synergistic effect during the protracted administration of MMC with concomitant radiation. The decision to administer MMC as a continuous i.v. infusion is supported in part in the elegant discussion of this topic by Dr. Sara Rockwell elsewhere in this book [23]. She indicates that at present there are not sufficient data to decide what happens to the ratio between oxygenated and hypoxic cells during the administration of MMC and irradiation. Because of this, it is impossible to decide at present which schema of single doses of MMC is better during a 20–30 day delivery: a single large dose at the beginning or at the end of irradiation or single daily small doses throughout the 20 days of irradiation.

For this reason when Lokich et al. in a pilot clinical trial [21] established the MTD at 1.2 mg/m$^2$ per day over 21 days continuous i.v. infusion, we intuitively decided that the continuous i.v. infusion would be the most appropriate way of administering MMC with concomitant radiation therapy. The MTD for an infusion lasting 21 days was found at 1 mg/m$^2$ per day (see Table 2). The dose limiting side-effect surprisingly was found to be cardiac: a blockade of the AV conduction to the myocardium. This effect was not previously reported as a possible complication of MMC.

The development of diarrhea with accompanying slight decrease in serum potassium level with only a few cases of clinical hypokalemia and pre-renal azotemia noted during the phase II study could have been contributory to the cardiac conduction defect.

When the dose of 1 mg/m$^2$ per day for 21 days was administered to another 10 cases in the phase II study, no other episodes of cardiac arrhythmias were noted. The patients' ventricular ejection fraction was found to be consistently normal; there were no changes after the completion of the combined MMC–radiation therapy. The results of the concomitant MMC by continuous intravenous infusion radiation therapy regimen in patients with liver metastases from colo-rectal carcinoma not amenable to surgical resection, but without other detectable metastases, were encouraging. The 50% partial response rate is comparable with the response rates reported after the administration of FUDR (the 5-FU metabolite resulting from the processing of 5-FU by the hepatocytes) directly in the hepatic artery (HA1) through a catheter inserted at laparatomy [24–26].

Randomized studies comparing intrahepatic artery FUDR infusion with systemic intravenous infusion of FUDR showed [27] a clear advantage for the HAI with response rates varying between 37 and 62% versus 10–19.6% responses seen among patients receiving i.v. FUDR. When 5-FU continuous i.v. infusion was used instead of FUDR, the response rate was of 38%. However, the HAI of FUDR was accompanied in all studies by significant side effects. Chemical hepatitis with elevation of transpeptidases, alkaline phosphatase and bilirubin were reported in various studies with an incidence varying between 50 and 100% [27] related to the duration and intensity of the FUDR infusion. Biliary strictures were seen in 4–20% of cases. There have also been reports of significant and occasionally life threatening biliary sclerosis. The occurrence of gastritis, gastric ulcer, pyloroduodenitis duodenal ulcer and duodenal proliferation lesions with structural distortion and cellular atypia were also reported in 5–15% of cases.

By comparison with these side effects the ones encountered in patients receiving mito-mycin C by continuous i.v. infusion have been modest. Granulocytopenia has been univer-sal with nadir between the 2nd and 7th day from completion of MMC infusion. However, it has been modest and was never accompanied by sepsis. There have been five infectious episodes related to patient's granulocytopenia (three acute pharyngitis and two urinary tract infections) that rapidly resolved with antibiotics.

Mild diarrhea occurred in six patients; it resolved with treatment while the infusion has continued. In 4 patients it was more severe; but just in 2 it occurred before the MMC c.i. completion after the first 2 weeks of MMC administration and was conducive to mild hypo-kalemia and dehydration with pre-renal azotemia. It rapidly resolved after a 48 h continua-tion of the MMC administration and appropriate therapy and diet. The latter permitted the MMC regimen to be restarted and completed. Nausea and occasional vomiting was seen only in patients whose radiation port included part of the stomach and occurred usually after the administration of the daily radiation treatment. The anemia occurring during the radia-tion–mitomycin C infusion regimen was modest and represented a continuation of patients' anemia of chronic disease caused by their malignancy. However, in one case a mitomycin C induced hemolytic episode occurred at the end of patient's 3-week infusion. The presence of schystocytes on the peripheral smear besides that of moderate anisocytosis and poikylocyto-sis was consistent with what is known about the toxicity of mitomcyin C; its ability to cause a process similar to thrombotic thrombocytopenic purpura in adults and the uremic hemo-lytic syndrome in children. Fortunately, in our case, it rapidly reversed after drug discon-tinuation and did not require hemodialysis. This episode, together with the relatively slow recovery of the granulocyte count to normal, are indications that the MMC dose chosen in this study is close to the absolute MTD for a continuous intravenous infusion of MMC and that the hematologic parameters should be monitored daily during the last week of treatment while they can be performed just twice weekly during the first 2 weeks.

Our study also indicated that among the commonly performed serologic tests in patients with metastatic carcinoma of the colo-rectum, the variations in serum LDH better reflect the changes in tumor size and the patients' response to treatment than the variations in serum CEA. A multivariate statistical analysis [24] showed a much better coefficient of correlation for LDH (0.88) than for CEA (0.56).

This observation offers a relatively inexpensive test to monitor patients' response. How-ever, the LDH monitoring of tumor response is not valid in patients that may develop hemolysis, for which we should also be testing, during the third week of the MMC c.i.-RT regimens.

The overall response rate and duration of the response in patients enrolled in the phase II study reported here and treated for unresectable liver metastases of colo-rectal adenocarci-noma are encouraging but are not conclusive due to the small sample size of the study. The duration of the response measured as mean time to progression of 48 ± 4 weeks for patients achieving partial remission is comparable with some of the best results of intrahepatic artery infusion of FUDR [24–26] without being accompanied by the numerous side-effects this methodology has. Thus Kemeny et al. reported a 52% partial response determined by a more then 50% decrease in measurable hepatic lesions in 34 previously untreated patients who received FUDR through a catheter inserted in the hepatic artery [24]. A 32% partial response defined by same criteria using similar methodology was reported by Shepard [25] in a study which enrolled 62 patients while Weiss [26] found a 29% partial response with the same regimen among 21 patients with colon carcinoma with hepatic metastases. Higher response rates of 83 and 88% were reported in early studies by Niederhuber [29] and Balch [30] in which the response was not defined by stringent criteria and there was a selection of cases with a better performance status and fewer detectable metastatic lesions in their liver.

The results of the concomitant radiation therapy–mitomycin C continuous infusion regimen also compare favorably with the results of continuous intravenous infusion of 5-FU with concomitant split course radiation therapy completed at our institution in 1985 [31]; those who entered the study achieved partial response with a median duration of their survival of 45 weeks while the median survival in the MMC-RT study reported here was of 62 weeks. The 5-FU continuous infusion with concomitant radiation trial was remarkable for the fact that the combined modality regimen was administered as a split course for 5 days every 2 weeks. This made this regimen very well tolerated; patients had only moderate nausea and diarrhea and in 3 instances only moderate leukopenia and thrombocytopenia [31]. As in the case of mitomycin C, the administration of 5-FU by continuous infusion during the radiation therapy delivery was found to be preferable to the bolus administration due to the fact that this drug has a short effective plasma half-life [32] and its cytotoxic effect is exercised primarily during the synthetic phase of the cycle. Tumor cells whose DNA synthetic phase can vary from a few minutes to hours benefit from the prolonged exposure to cytotoxic agents when continually infused.

These data on concomitant radiation therapy with continuous infusion mitomycin C, as well as those previously reported with concomitant 5-FU continuous intravenous infusion, compare favorably with the results of prior studies of radiation therapy administered alone to liver metastases with palliative intent. An RTOG study reported by Borgelt et al. [33] indicated that various schema of treatment delivering approximately the same total radiation dose were equally effective and well tolerated (30 Gy delivered as 2 Gy/fraction (Fx) $\times$ 15 or 25.6 Gy delivered as 1.6 Gy/Fx $\times$ 16). The median survival of various groups was around 19 weeks. When later [34] misonidazole was administered concomitantly with radiation, therapy to liver metastases using 21 Gy delivered on 3 Gy/Fx $\times$ 7 a median survival of 29 weeks was found to be practically no different from the median survival of 25 weeks of patients that received radiation therapy alone and had a good performance status [34].

Administration of mitomycin C alone or in combination with other chemotherapeutic agents for the treatment of liver metastases from GI malignancies have led to objective partial responses ranging from 8 to 25%, but survival has been virtually unaffected [35,36].

The fact that all patients enrolled in the study reported here relapsed and 8 out of 10 ultimately progressed in the liver is an indication that further improvements should be sought over the currently tested regimen of MMC by continuous infusion for 21 days and concomitant radiation therapy to the liver involved by unresectable liver metastases.

Further improvement in our previously reported results could possibly be obtained with several approaches.

Firstly one could add a second radiosensitizing drug to mitomcyin C especially one of those that could inhibit DNA repair like the platinum compounds (cisplatin, carboplatin) or those that could promote apoptosis like taxanes (paclitaxel and doxytaxel) or topotecans (topoisomerase inhibitors).

Among all these drugs only cisplatin and irinotecan do not induce significant bone marrow suppression. They could induce, however, a plethora of other side-effects; for this reason, careful phase I studies of the combination of cisplatin or irinotecan with mitomycin continuous infusion will have to be carried out before limited phase II studies could be implemented. These studies are currently in progress at our institutions with some indications that complete remissions could be obtained that may not be followed by local progression in the liver.

The combination of mitomycin infusion with 5-FU infusion is less likely to give synergistic radiosensitizing effect especially due to additive similar toxicity (mucositis, diarrhea, pancytopenia).

Secondly one could improve on the currently tested MMC c.i.-RT regimen by diminishing its toxicity; this could be achieved by administering the radiation therapy and the concomitant mitomycin C continuous intravenous infusion as a split course of 2 10-day cycles with a 2–3 weeks interval between them.

The splitting of the course of irradiation may potentially lead to a decrease of its antineoplastic effect. This decrease could be overcome by administering the radiation therapy on daily split doses (2–3 doses/day) to an increased total daily dose of 200 cGy instead of 150 cGy/day.

The continuous intravenous infusion of mitomycin C with concomitant radiation therapy, through its effective killing of hypoxic cells otherwise preserved after the oxygen dependent radiation cell killing, represents the backbone of future regimens that could ultimately eradicate the malignant cells when confined to areas that could be safely included in irradiation fields.

## Summary

Experimental data indicating that the mitomycin C (MMC) is active against hypoxic cells and enhances RT when administered concomitantly or 6 h prior to RT [19] and our prior pilot study [33] defining the MTD for MMC by CI with concomitant conventional RT led to the present study aiming to test this concomitant combined modality regimen in a phase II protocol enrolling patients with adenocarcinoma of the colo-rectum with multiple non-resectable liver metastases. Ten cases, enrolled over a period of 26 months with minimum observation period of 8 months are so far evaluable. There were 6 males, 4 females aged 51 to 74, performance status 0–2, with more than two lesions and LDH elevation: 320–1340 units (mean 520). They received an average of 2700 cGy to the whole liver while MMC was infused through a port-a-cath from a portable pump at a rate of 1 mg/m$^2$ per day for 21 days in an ambulatory setting. Three weeks later the response was evaluated by MRI or CT. Then patients were treated for 6–10 months (mean 7.5) with calcium. Leucovorin (200 mg/m$^2$) followed 1 h later by 5-FU (400 mg/m$^2$) i.v. bolus for 5 days every 4 weeks. Nausea and vomiting occurred in 4 patients whose RT ports included part of their stomach. Moderate pancytopenia was universal with nadir of granulocytes at $1225 \pm 240\,\mu$l and platelets at $88 \pm 16 \times 10^3/\mu$l. Grade II mucositis developed after 35% of courses. Five patients achieved partial response (PR > 50% reduction in tumor size); 4 had minimal response (MR < 50% size reduction) and in one, lesions remained unchanged (SD = stable disease). The mean time to progression was $20 \pm 4$ weeks for MR and $48 \pm 4$ weeks for PR. The mean survival was of $62 \pm 9$ weeks for patients who achieved PR and was only $29 \pm 7$ weeks for MR patients. Survival correlates best in a multivariate analysis with type of response and LDH level but did not correlate with CEA level or with time from diagnosis. MMC by CI appears to enhance RT effects on liver metastases of patients with colo-rectal cancer and should be further tested in a phase III study.

# References

1. Gray LH, Conger AD, Ebert M, et al. The concentration of oxygen dissolved in tissues at the time of irradiation as a factor in radiotherapy. Br J Radiol 26: 638–648, 1953.
2. Gray LH. Radiobiologic basis of oxygen as a modifying factor in radiation therapy. Am. J. Roentgenol 85: 803–815, 1961.
3. Thomlinson RH, Gray LH. The histologic structure in some human being cancers and the possible implications for radiation therapy. Br J Cancer 9: 539–549, 1955.
4. Chaplin DJ, Olive PL, Daran RF. Intermittent blood flow in a murine tumor. Radiobiological effects. Cancer Res 47: 597–601, 1987.
5. Moulder JF, Rockwell S. Tumor hypoxia, its impact in cancer therapy. Cancer Metast Rev 5: 313–341, 1987.
6. Rockwell S, Maulder JE. Hypoxic fractions of human tumors xenografted into mice. A review. Int J Radiat Oncol Biol Phys 19: 197–202; 1990.
7. Suit HD. Modification of radiation response. Int J Radiat Oncol Biol Phys 10: 101–108, 1984.
8.. Moulder JF, Dutreix J, Rockwell S, et al. Applications of animal tumor data to cancer therapy in humans. Int J Radiat Oncol Biol Phys 11: 913–927, 1988.
9. Teicher BA, McIntesh-Lowe NL, Rose CM. Effect of various oxygenation conditions and Fluosol DA on cancer chemotherapeutic agents. Biomat Arit Cells Artif Organs 16: 533–546, 1988.
10. Morton JD, Porter E., Yabuki H, et al. Effects of a perfluorochemical emulsion on the response of BA 11112 rat rhabdomysarcomas to gutinous low dose rate irradiation. Radiat Res 124: 178–182, 1990.
11. Fisher JJ, Rockwell SW, Martin DF. Perfluorochemicals and hyperbaric oxygen in radiation therapy. Int J Radiat Oncol Biol Phys 12: 95–102, 1986.
12. Rockwell S: Use of hypoxia directed drugs in the therapy of solid tumors. Semin Oncol 19: 29–40, 1992.
13. Rauth AM, Barton B, Lee CPY. Effects of caffeine in L-cells exposed to mitomycin C. Cancer Res 30: 2724–2729, 1970.
14. Rockwell S, Sartorelli AC. Mitomycin C and radiation. In Hill BJ, Belamy AS (Eds), Antitumor Drug-Radiation Interactions. Boca Raton, FL: CRC Press, pp. 125–139, 1990.
15. Rockwell S, Keyes SR, Sartorelli AC. Preclinical studies of porfiromycin as adjunct to radiotherapy. Radiat Res 116: 100–113, 1988.
16. Weissberg JB, Son YH, Papac RJ, et al. Randomized clinical trial of mitomycin C as an adjunct to radiotherapy in head and neck cancer Int J Radiat Oncol Biol Phys 17: 3–9, 1989.
17. Cummings BJ, Keane TG, O'Sullivan B. Epidermoid anal cancer treatment by radiation and 5-fluorouracil with or without mitomycin C. Int J Radiat Oncol Biol Phys 21: 1115–1125, 1991.
18. Thomas G, Dembo A, Fyles A, et al: Concurrent chemoradiation in advanced cervical cancer. Gynecol Oncol 328: 446–451, 1990.
19. Grau C, Overgaard J. Radiosensitizing and cytotoxic properties of mitomycin C in a C3H mouse mammary carcinoma in vivo. Int J Radiat Oncol Biol Phys 20: 265–269, 1991.
20. Von Hazel GA, Kovach JS. Pharmacokinetics of mitomycin C in rabbit and human. Cancer Chemother Pharmacol 8: 189–192, 1982.
21. Lokich J, Peeri J, Frue N, et al. Mitomycin C: phase I study of a constant infusion ambulatory treatment schedule. Am J Clin Oncol: Cancer Clinical Trials 5: 443–447, 1982.
22. Rockwell S, Nierenberg M, Irvin CG. Effects of the mode of administration of mitomycin on tumor and marrow response and on therapeutic ratio. Cancer Treatment Rep 71: 927–934, 1987.
23. Rockwell S. Hypoxia directed drugs; use with irradiation. In: Rosenthal CJ (Ed), Infusion Chemotherapy-Radiation Interaction: Its Biology and Significance for Organ Salvage and Prevention of Second Primary Neoplasms. Oxford: Elsevier, Ch. 8, 1997.
24. Kemeny N, Daly J, Oderman P, et al. Hepatic artery pump infusion: toxicity and results in patients with metastatic colo-rectal carcinoma. J Clin Oncol 2: 595, 1984.
25. Shepard K, Levin B, et al. Therapy for metastatic colo-rectal cancer with hepatic artery infusion chemotherapy using a subcutaneous implanted pump. J Clin Oncol 3: 161, 1985.
26. Weiss GR, Barneck MB, Osteen RT, et al: Long term hepatic arterial infusion of 5-fluorodeoxyuridine for liver metastases using an implantable infusion pump. J Clin Oncol 1: 337, 1983.
27. Niederhuber JE, Grochow LB. Status of infusion chemotherapy for the treatment of liver metastases. Principles Practices Oncol 3: 1–9, 1989.

28. Godfrey K. Simple linear regression. In: Baylar JC III, Mosteller F (Eds), Medical Uses of Statistics. Boston, MA: NEJM Books, 1992.

29. Niederhuber JE, Ensminger W, Gyves J, et al. Regional chemotherapy of colo-rectal cancer metastatic to the liver. Cancer 53: 1336, 1984.

30. Balch CM, Urist MM, Song SJ, McGregor M. A prospective phase II clinical trial of continuous FUDR regional chemotherapy for colo-rectal metastases to the liver using a totally implantable drug infusion pump. Ann Surg 198: 567–578, 1983.

31. Rotman, M., Kuruvilla AM, Choi K, et al. Response of colo-rectal hepatic metastases to concomitant radiotherapy and intravenous infusion 5 fluorouracil. Int J Radiat Oncol Biol Phys 12: 2179–2187, 1996.

32. Seifert P, Baker LH, Reed MI, et al. Comparison of continuously infused 5 Fluorouracil with bolus injection in treatment of patients with colo-rectal adenocarcinoma. Cancer 36: 123–128, 1975.

33. Bargelt BB, Gelber R, Brady LW, et al. The palliation of hepatic metastases: results of the Radiation Therapy Oncology Group pilot study. Int J Radiat Oncol Biol Phys 7: 587–591, 1981.

34. Liebel SA, Pajak TF, Order SE, et al: Hepatic metastases: Results of treatment and identification of prognostic factors (Radiation Therapy Oncology Group report) (Abstr) Int J Radiat Oncol Biol Phys 11(Suppl 1): 116–117, 1985.

35. Daly JM, Kemeny N. Metastatic cancer to the liver. In: DeVita VT, Hellman S, Rosenberg SA (Eds), Cancer - Principles and Practice of Oncology, 5th edn. Lippincott-Raven, pp. 2551–2570, 1997.

36. Kemeny N. The systemic chemotherapy of hepatic metastases. Semin Oncol 10: 148–158, 1983.

37. Rosenthal CJ, Rotman M, Choi KN, Papandreu C. Rapid tumor lysis induced by mitomycin C (MC) administered by continuous infusion (C.I.) with concomitant radiation therapy (RT). A phase I study (Abstract). Proc Am Assoc Cancer Res 32: 391, 1991.

C.J. Rosenthal and M. Rotman (Eds.), *Infusion Chemotherapy–Irradiation Interactions*
© 1998 Elsevier Science B.V. All rights reserved

CHAPTER 10

# Concurrent paclitaxel and radiation therapy for solid tumors

## HAK CHOY

*Center for Radiation Oncology, Vanderbilt Medical Center, TVC B-902, Nashville, TN 37232-5671, USA*

## 1. Introduction

Combinations of chemotherapy and radiotherapy have been used in cancer management for over 25 years. Possible reasons for combining radiation therapy and chemotherapy can be based on several effects: (1) when a chemotherapy agent is present at the time of radiation exposure, the interaction between the two modalities may increase lethal cell damage; (2) chemotherapy may alter the cell's ability to repair sublethal cell damage; (3) chemotherapy may alter cell cycle kinetics such that cells are more susceptible to radiation effects; (4) chemotherapy has intrinsic antitumor activity which may add to the efficacy of radiation without synergistic or enhancing activity [1]. While laboratory studies continue to investigate the interaction of chemotherapy and radiation, clinical trials are being conducted to determine the therapeutic efficacy of concomitant therapy. A number of agents are known to enhance radiation activity including: cisplatin, 5-fluorouracil (5-FU), mitomycin, paclitaxel, hydroxyurea, bleomycin, actinomycin D, and adriamycin. In addition, a recently reported intergroup trial demonstrated a marked survival advantage for patients with advanced nasopharyngeal carcinoma receiving concomitant cisplatin and radiation therapy [2].

The taxanes are a new class of plant-derived antineoplastic compounds which share a unique mechanism of cytotoxic action and significant demonstrable efficacy in a wide variety of malignancies [3–12]. Paclitaxel and docetaxel are the first members of this class to be used in clinical practice. They act by promoting assembly of microtubules and rendering the microtubules resistant to depolymerization [13–15]. Microtubules function not only in mitotic spindle formation, but also in many vital interphase functions of the cell including maintenance of shape, motility, anchorage, mediation of signals between surface receptors and the nucleus, and intracellular transport [16,17]. Consequently, interference of these actions may cause irreversible damage initiating apoptosis and/or resulting in arrest of cells in the $G_2/M$ phases of the cell cycle, the phases with particular sensitivity to radiation [18]. Both actions have the potential to contribute to enhanced radiation effect. Although limited experience in combined modality therapy exists, these attributes provide strong support for the clinical application of taxanes with radiation.

## 2. Preclinical studies

Significant efforts have been focused on the ability of taxanes to potentiate the effects of radiation (Table 1) [19–34]. While support exists for several potential mechanisms of interaction in vitro, cell synchronization appears to be the dominant factor [35–40]. Paclitaxel,

Table 1

In vitro studies on paclitaxel/RT

| Authors | Cell line | Concentration (nM) | Exposure (h) | $G_2/M$ block | Additivity status |
|---------|-----------|---------------------|--------------|---------------|-------------------|
| Choy [21,24] | HL-60 | 30 | 1 | Yes | Supra |
| Tishler [19,20] | G18 | 10 | 24 | Yes | Supra |
| Liebmann [22,30,31] | MCF-7, PC-Sh | 1–10 | 24 | Yes | Add |
| | MCF-7, PC-Sh, A549 | 100–1000 | 24 | Yes | Supra |
| Chang [23] | A549 | | 24 | Yes | Supra |
| | | 10 | 0.5–3 | No | Anta |
| Steren [25,26] | Ovarian | 0.5–50 | 1.5 | No | Supra |
| Hei [27] | C3H | 100 | 24 | No | Add |
| Gupta [28] | U-251 MG | 5 | 24 | Yes | Supra |
| Geard [29] | Siha | 10 | 24 | Yes | Add |
| Stromberg [33] | MCF-7, HT-29 | 2–25 | 24 | No | Add |
| Lokeshwar [34] | PC-3 | 10 | 24 | Yes | Supra |

the prototype taxane, is extremely effective in causing arrest of tumor cells in the $G_2/M$ phase of the cell cycle. After only brief and low level exposure to paclitaxel at concentrations of 30 nM for 1 h, arrest of proliferating cells in $G_2/M$ can be noted starting as early as 4 h and approach a maximum of 70% at 24 h. These concentrations are routinely exceeded by 100 in the plasma and are achievable within the tumor in clinical practice [41]. The fraction of arrested cells increases as a function of both concentration and duration of exposure [42].

Following treatment with paclitaxel and consequent synchronization of tumor cells, enhanced sensitivity to radiation can be demonstrated in many cell lines. In the study by Choy et al., the sensitizer enhancement ratio (SER) was increased to 1.5 (50% greater cell kill at equal doses of radiation after correcting for direct effects of paclitaxel) in HL-60 cells after 1 h exposure at 30 nM [21]. In PC-3 cells with a greater duration of exposure for 24 h at 10 nM paclitaxel, the SER was increased to 1.8 and at 50 nM, the ratio approaches 2.0.

Enhancement of radiation response by taxanes may also occur through additional mechanisms independent of cell cycle synchronization. Recently, Liebmann et al. [29] have shown that the $G_2/M$ cell cycle block alone may not be sufficient for paclitaxel-induced radiation sensitization in other human tumor cells. A good correlation between $G_2/M$ arrest and degree of radiation sensitization, however, was obtained with the other cell lines tested in in vitro studies [26,33].

Several groups have shown that mechanisms other than the paclitaxel-induced cell cycle perturbation must exist, at least in the in vivo setting, by which paclitaxel potentiates cellular radioresponse. Milas et al. addressed a possibility that paclitaxel makes tumor cells more susceptible to radiation-induced apoptosis [45]. There is increasing evidence that various anticancer agents, including radiation [43,44] and chemotherapeutic drugs [45,46], induce apoptosis in tumors and that paclitaxel is capable of inducing a strong apoptotic response in murine tumors, including the MCA-4 tumor [47]. Paclitaxel-induced apoptosis developed mainly from mitotically arrested cells. Because development of apoptosis after paclitaxel treatment depended on mitotic arrest, the pattern of development of apoptosis was similar to the kinetics of mitotic arrest with the difference being that the development of apoptosis lags several hours behind that of mitotic arrest. The apoptotic response induced by paclitaxel persists for about 2 days. In contrast to paclitaxel, radiation-induced apoptosis in

Table 2

In vivo studies on paclitaxel/RT

| Authors | Cell line | Schedule | Growth drug | Delay (days) RT | Combined |
|---------|-----------|----------|-------------|-----------------|----------|
| Jochko [48] | FaDu | Single | 13.6 | 53 | CR |
|  |  | 10-days | 23 | 53 | CR |
| Milas [49] | MCA-4 | Single | 7.2 | 5.7 | 8.4–14.2 |
| Lokeshwar [28] | DUR | 5-days | 9.1 | 12 | 21 |

MCA-4 tumors increased rapidly so that the peak in apoptotic response occurred 4 h after irradiation. Radiation-induced apoptosis rapidly declined, approaching the background level by 12 h after irradiation. The efficacy of radiation in inducing apoptosis in tumors treated with paclitaxel depended on the time when radiation was delivered after paclitaxel administration or whether cells were in mitosis at the time of irradiation. Radiation delivered 1 h after paclitaxel, when only a low percentage of cells were in mitosis, was not more effective in inducing apoptosis than in tumors not treated with paclitaxel. However, when radiation was given 9 or 24 h after paclitaxel, when many cells were in mitosis, there was a significant increase in radiation-induced apoptosis.

Recent in vivo studies (Table 2) [48,49] suggest that mechanisms other than prometaphase arrest may act to provide synergistic interaction between taxoids and radiation. In particular, the manipulation of the oxygen supply has shown that reoxygenation plays a major role in enhancing tumor radioresponse in vivo when combined with paclitaxel [49].

At the present time, we can postulate that paclitaxel enhances the radiation effect in in vitro and in vivo due to cell cycle synchronization, apoptosis, and tumor reoxygenations.

## 3.  Clinical studies

Based on radiation-enhancing effects found in extensive preclinical studies, a large number of clinical trials are underway in the United States. The ideal tumor types for concurrent paclitaxel and radiation are listed in Table 3. In this chapter some of the findings from various clinical trials are discussed by tumor site.

### 3.1.  Primary brain tumors

Chamberlain and his colleagues at the University of San Diego recently reported a single institution phase II trial to observe the safety and efficacy of paclitaxel given at a dose of 175 mg/m$^2$ every 3 weeks as a 3–4 h outpatient infusion to patients with recurrent malignant

Table 3

Tumor types

| | |
|---|---|
| Primary brain | Gastric cancer |
| Head/neck cancer | Pancreatic cancer |
| Lung cancer | Bladder cancer |
| Esophagus | Cervical cancer |

primary brain tumors who had received prior radiotherapy and at least one chemotherapy regimen containing nitrosoureas and who were no longer responding to therapy [50]. Paclitaxel was administered intravenously at a dose of 175 mg/m$^2$ every 3 weeks with necrologic and neuroradiographic evaluation every 8–9 weeks. A median of 6 cycles of paclitaxel (range, 2–12) was administered to 20 assessable patients. Toxicities included partial alopecia ($n = 10$), thrombocytopenia ($n = 4$), paclitaxel administration-dependent bradycardia ($n = 3$), and non-disabling peripheral neuropathy ($n = 1$). No patient developed neutropenia, fever, or sepsis or required cytokine support. Two patients required blood-product support (platelet transfusions in both). Four patients (20%) demonstrated a partial response (PR) and seven (35%) had stable disease (SD) for a total response plus SD rate of 55%. The median time to tumor progression was 6 months (range 2–20). In their study, paclitaxel demonstrated modest efficacy with minimal toxicity in this heavily pretreated cohort of young patients with recurrent primary brain tumors.

Glantz et al. conducted a phase I study of paclitaxel administered weekly by 3-h infusion, concurrent with daily cranial irradiation, as the initial treatment for patients with newly diagnosed primary brain tumors. The treatment protocol was designed to increase the opportunity for a radiosensitizing interaction, to take advantage of the phase-specific properties of paclitaxel, and to permit treatment to proceed entirely on an outpatient basis. The objectives of this study were to establish the maximum-tolerated dose (MTD) of paclitaxel administered in this setting and to identify the toxicities associated with this treatment regimen [51].

Cranial irradiation and intravenous (i.v.) paclitaxel were given concurrently, both beginning on day 1 of treatment and starting within 28 days of diagnostic surgery. Paclitaxel was administered as a 3-h infusion once weekly for 6 consecutive weeks in the outpatient setting. The initial weekly dose of paclitaxel (20 mg/m$^2$) was escalated in cohorts of 3 patients until dose-limiting toxicity was observed. Premedication with dexamethasone (20 mg i.v.), diphenhydramine (50 mg i.v.), and prochlorperazine (10 mg orally) was given 1 h prior to the start of the infusion. No other premedication or anti-emetic therapy was used. Use of hematopoietic growth factors was not allowed. Cranial irradiation (using a linear accelerator with an energy of at least 6 MeV) was administered in 2-Gy fractions, one fraction per day, for 5 consecutive days per week to a total dose of 60 Gy. The initial 40 Gy was given to the area of contrast enhancement on the preoperative magnetic resonance imaging scan, plus a 4-cm margin. The final 20 Gy was given to the enhancing lesion plus a 2-cm margin.

Sixty patients were entered into this study and received at least one course of therapy. The weekly dose of paclitaxel ranged from 20 to 275 mg/m$^2$. Fifty-six patients completed the prescribed course of therapy, and four discontinued treatment after one (3 patients) or two (1 patient) treatments. Four of the 60 patients entered into this study died after receiving 2 or fewer courses of treatment. Death was due solely to disease progression in 3 patients.

Hematologic toxicity was minimal and never required a dose reduction or treatment delay (Table 4). No patient experienced greater than grade 2 anemia or grade 1 thrombocytopenia. One patient developed grade 3 neutropenia 2 days after her sixth course of paclitaxel at 175 mg/m$^2$. Aspiration pneumonia (secondary to a recent stroke) and subsequent sepsis preceded the development of neutropenia in this patient and were the causes of her death. Grade 2 neutropenia was seen in four patients. Most patients (27, 48%) experienced their lowest absolute neutrophil count during week 3 of treatment. The timing of platelet nadirs during therapy was similar. Anemia, although mild, was most common during the last 3 weeks of treatment. Peripheral neuropathy was the dose-limiting toxicity in this study (Table 5). Fourteen of the 56 evaluable patients (25%) developed some degree of neuro-

Table 4

Hematologic toxicity: phase I study of weekly outpatient paclitaxel and concurrent cranial irradiation in adults with astrocytomas

| Dose level (mg/m²/ course) | No. of patients | ANC grade | | | Thrombocytopenia grade | | Anemia grade | | |
|---|---|---|---|---|---|---|---|---|---|
| | | 1 | 2 | 3 | 1 | 2–4 | 1 | 2 | 3,4 |
| 20 | 3 | 0 | 0 | 0 | 0 | 0 | 1 | 0 | 0 |
| 30 | 3 | 0 | 0 | 0 | 0 | 0 | 0 | 0 | 0 |
| 40 | 3 | 0 | 1 | 0 | 0 | 0 | 0 | 1 | 0 |
| 50 | 3 | 0 | 1 | 0 | 0 | 0 | 1 | 0 | 0 |
| 60 | 3 | 0 | 0 | 0 | 0 | 0 | 0 | 2[a] | 0 |
| 70 | 3 | 1 | 0 | 0 | 0 | 0 | 1 | 1 | 0 |
| 80 | 3 | 0 | 0 | 0 | 0 | 0 | 1 | 0 | 0 |
| 90 | 2 | 0 | 0 | 0 | 0 | 0 | 1 | 0 | 0 |
| 100 | 3 | 0 | 0 | 0 | 0 | 0 | 1 | 0 | 0 |
| 110 | 3 | 0 | 0 | 0 | 0 | 0 | 0 | 0 | 0 |
| 135 | 3 | 0 | 0 | 0 | 1 | 0 | 0 | 0 | 0 |
| 150 | 3 | 0 | 0 | 0 | 1 | 0 | 2 | 0 | 0 |
| 175 | 5 | 1 | 0 | 1[b] | 2 | 0 | 1 | 1 | 0 |
| 200 | 4 | 1 | 0 | 0 | 1 | 0 | 4 | 0 | 0 |
| 225 | 3 | 2 | 0 | 0 | 0 | 0 | 1 | 0 | 0 |
| 250 | 6 | 0 | 1 | 0 | 0 | 0 | 4 | 0 | 0 |
| 275 | 3 | 0 | 1 | 0 | 1 | 0 | 2 | 0 | 0 |
| Total | 56 | 5 | 4 | 1 | 6 | 0 | 20 | 5 | 0 |

[a]Secondary to gastrointestinal bleeding in 1 patient.
[b]Patient died of aspiration pneumonia following a stroke. From Ref. [51].

pathy (grade 1 in four patients, grade 2 in eight, and grade 3 in two). All patients with grade 3 neuropathy received 275 mg/m² of paclitaxel. The neuropathy developed during the second (one patient), third (four patients) fourth (seven patients), or fifth (two patients) weeks of treatment, progressed during the remainder of therapy, and continued to progress for 1–3 weeks after treatment had ended. Symptoms included tingling, loss of sensation, and,

Table 5

Non-hematologic toxicity: phase I study of weekly outpatient paclitaxel and concurrent cranial irradiation in adults with astrocytomas

| Dose level (mg/m²/ course) | No. of patients | Cutaneous toxicity grade | | | | Sensory neuropathy grade | | | Pruritus grade | | |
|---|---|---|---|---|---|---|---|---|---|---|---|
| | | 1 | 2 | 3 | 4 | 1 | 2 | 3 | 1 | 2 | 3 |
| 20–150 | 39 | 0 | 0 | 0 | 0 | 0 | 0 | 0 | 0 | 0 | 0 |
| 175 | 5 | 0 | 0 | 0 | 1 | 1 | 2 | 0 | 0 | 0 | 0 |
| 200 | 4 | 0 | 0 | 0 | 0 | 0 | 0 | 0 | 0 | 0 | 0 |
| 225 | 3 | 1 | 1 | 0 | 0 | 1 | 2 | 0 | 0 | 0 | 1 |
| 250 | 6 | 1 | 1 | 1 | 0 | 2 | 3 | 0 | 0 | 1 | 1 |
| 275 | 3 | 0 | 1 | 1 | 0 | 0 | 1 | 2 | 0 | 0 | 1 |
| Total | 60 | 2 | 3 | 2 | 1 | 4 | 8 | 2 | 0 | 1 | 3 |

[a]1, mild; 2, moderate; 3, severe (no formal CALG8 criteria available. From [51].

rarely, mildly painful dysesthesias, beginning in the fingertips and toes and progressing proximally. Fine finger movement (buttoning, tying shoes, manipulating keys) and gait were impaired in both patients with grade 3 neuropathy. In 4 patients (receiving paclitaxel doses of 225, 250 and 275 mg/m$^2$), the neuropathy was also accompanied by severe, at times continuous, pruritus that was undiminished by oral, parenteral, or topical diphenhydramine, dexchlorpheniramine, codeine, morphine, emollients, or soaking.

Reinstitution of increasing daily doses of dexamethasone provided modest relief in 2 patients, and complete resolution was seen in all patients within 4 weeks of the end of therapy. Neuropathic symptoms improved in all patients within 2–4 months of completing treatment and disappeared in all but four. Those four patients continue to report mild numbness in the toes of both feet. Decreased vibratory sensation has persisted in all patients with grade 2 or 3 neuropathy.

Cutaneous toxicity developed in 8 patients and first appeared during weeks 2 (1 patient), 3 (3 patients), 4 (1 patient), 5 (2 patients), or 6 (1 patient). The cutaneous toxicity was grade 1 in 2 patients, grade 2 in 3, grade 3 in 2, and grade 4 in 1 patient. Early skin changes consisted of prominent erythema of the face, hands, and feet, and scattered, painless erythematous, macular lesions on the hands, arms, feet, distal legs, and buttocks. In three patients these lesions coalesced, became vesicular, and in one patient led to ulceration and desquamation. The skin lesions resolved in all patients within 2–4 weeks of discontinuing paclitaxel. No nausea, vomiting, diarrhea, stomatitis, myalgias, or seizures were seen in any patients.

The median survival for patients with glioblastoma multiforme (GBM) was 9.2 months and has not been reached for patients with AAs or astrocytoma. Survival durations for these three groups differ significantly ($P = 0.002$, log-rank test). Within the GBM group, a proportional hazards regression analysis revealed that Karnofsky performance status and age were significant predictors of survival time ($P = 0.03$ and $P = 0.004$, respectively). Paclitaxel dose did not appear to be a significant predictor of survival ($P = 0.66$).

From the 60 patients entered in the study, plasma pharmacokinetic studies were performed on 10 patients receiving paclitaxel doses of 100 mg/m$^2$ (1 patient), 175 mg/m$^2$ (5 patients), 200 mg/m$^2$ (1 patient), 225 mg/m$^2$ (1 patient), and 250 mg/m$^2$ (2 patients). Calculated pharmacokinetic parameters for these patients closely resemble those previously described for women with breast or ovarian cancer receiving 3-h infusions of paclitaxel (Fig. 1). Pharmacokinetic parameters for individual patients were used to calculate AUC and the duration that the plasma paclitaxel concentration exceeded 0.05 $\mu$mol/l (the threshold closely correlated with percentage reduction in granulocytes). The resulting AUCs and durations above 0.05 $\mu$mol/l are very similar to those observed in patients receiving 3-h infusions of paclitaxel for other malignancies. The simulated durations during which plasma concentration of paclitaxel exceeded 0.05 $\mu$mol/l also allowed calculation of expected percent reductions in absolute neutrophil counts. The reductions expected from just the first week's dose of paclitaxel are much greater than those actually observed after all 6 doses administered in this study [52,53].

There are at least several possible explanations for this finding: (1) patients in this study had received no prior chemotherapy; (2) bone marrow or other extraneural tumor involvement is extremely rare in patients with primary brain tumors and was not a factor in reducing tolerance to chemotherapy; (3) the high-dose weekly steroids administered to all patients as part of their premedication regimen may have produced chronic bone marrow stimulations and hastened white blood cell recovery; and/or (4) the weekly schedule of paclitaxel administration may somehow have produced changes in the bone marrow that rendered the

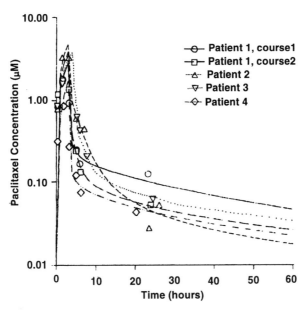

Fig. 1. Concentrations of paclitaxel in the plasma of the four patients studied. Symbols depict actual concentrations measured in the plasma of each patient. Lines represent the complete concentration versus time profiles generated by the patient-specific pharmacokinetic parameters derived for each patient with the pharmacokinetic model described in Section 3.1 [52].

bone marrow less sensitive to the effects of subsequent doses or may have stimulated increasingly rapid recovery of the marrow. The current study does not provide enough data to evaluate these hypotheses directly. Further studies are under way.

A final obvious but incorrect hypothesis would be that a concurrent medication altered the metabolism of paclitaxel. Most patients with brain tumors also receive daily corticosteroids and anticonvulsants which may induce the P-450 enzyme systems primarily responsible for paclitaxel clearance. However, data from the 10 patients studied in this trial do not support altered pharmacokinetics as the major explanation for the unexpectedly mild neutropenia we observed. All pharmacokinetic parameters (particularly AUC and the length of time plasma paclitaxel concentrations remained above 0.05 $\mu$mol/l) in the 10 study patients are nearly identical to those observed in women with other solid tumors who received 3-h paclitaxel infusions at similar doses [54]. Others reported the altered pharmacokinetics of paclitaxel among patients [55,56].

Chang and his colleagues reported in their phase I/II studies that the administration of significantly higher doses of paclitaxel may be possible in brain tumor patients on medications such as corticosteriods or anticonvulsants (AC) [55]. Fetell's study also suggested altered pharmacokinetics in patients receiving anticonvulsant drugs known to induce hepatic microsomal enzymes [56].

Two significant and previously unreported toxicities were observed in our patients. Patchy, erytheramatous skin changes, which developed first on the face and distal extremities and sometimes progressed to involve the proximal arms and legs and, in some cases, the body, were seen in 8 patients. In 3 patients, these lesions progressed to a painful vesicular exfoliate dermatitis. Skin biopsies in 2 patients demonstrated changes consistent with a drug reaction. This drug-related side effect developed in 1 patient receiving a paclitaxel dose of 175 mg/m$^2$.

A second unprecedented, but self-limited, paclitaxel-related side effect was severe pruritus. This developed only in patients who were also experiencing some degree of peripheral neuropathy, and the pruritus is believed to be a manifestation of small fiber peripheral neuropathy. Electophysiologic studies are under way to better characterize this form of paclitaxel-related neuropathy.

A phase II study of weekly paclitaxel and concurrent cranial irradiation for the patients with glioblastoma multiforme has been closed recently and the final survival and toxicity analysis is underway. Meanwhile the Radiation Therapy Oncology Group (RTOG) has initiated another phase II study in primary brain tumor with weekly paclitaxel at a dose of 225 mg/m$^2$ weekly for 6 weeks while patients are receiving cranial irradiation.

## 3.2.  Head and neck cancers

In phase II studies, paclitaxel has demonstrated significant single agent activity in a number of solid tumors including carcinomas of the head and neck. The Eastern Cooperative Oncology Group recently reported the results of a phase II trial of paclitaxel in recurrent and metastatic squamous carcinoma of the head and neck. The overall response rate was 40% with acceptable toxicity [57]. These results have been confirmed by investigators at Ohio State [58].

Flood et al. recently reported the results of a phase I trial of weekly paclitaxel and weekly paclitaxel/cisplatin. The recommended phase II dose of weekly paclitaxel is 30 mg/m$^2$ [59]. With this dose and schedule, toxicity was within acceptable limits.

The Brown University Oncology Group initiated a prospective phase II study using paclitaxel (60 mg/m$^2$) and carboplatin (AUC of 2), each given as a single dose weekly with concurrent conventional fractionated external beam radiotherapy (XRT) [60]. Patients were stratified as either operable or inoperable/unresectable groups. The operable and inoperable groups received 5 weeks (45 Gy) and 8 weeks (72 Gy) of chemoradiotherapy, respectively. Patients in the operable group are evaluated with repeat biopsies after 5 weeks: those with positive biopsy undergo surgery; and those with negative biopsy receive 3 additional weeks of chemoradiotherapy. Sixteen patients (10 operable, 6 inoperable) are evaluable at this time. Eleven patients completed at least 5 weeks of chemoradiotherapy with 5 CRs, 5 PRs and 1 stable disease. Nine patients sustained grade 3 or 4 toxicity. The grade 4 toxicity was as follows: mucositis, 4 patients; neutropenia, 1 patient; anemia, 1 patient; and neuropathy, 1 patient. The first 5 patients developed grade 3–4 toxicity, therefore, the dose of carboplatin was reduced by 50% to AUC of 1. This reduced the toxicity in subsequent patients. In summary, concomitant paclitaxel, carboplatin and XRT yielded excellent clinical responses but produced significant grade 4 toxicity at a paclitaxel dose of 60 mg/m$^2$ and carboplatin AUC of 2. Tolerance to treatment improved markedly after carboplatin was reduced to AUC of 1. The study will continue for necessary accrual.

Murphy and his colleagues at the Vanderbilt Medical Center are conducting a phase II study to evaluate the efficacy and toxicity of paclitaxel and carboplatin as an induction regimen for patients with resectable squamous carcinoma of the larynx [61]. At the completion of three cycles of chemotherapy, patients with a complete or partial response will proceed with definitive radiation therapy. During radiation therapy, patients will receive weekly low-dose paclitaxel as a chemosensitizing agent. At the completion of radiation therapy, patients with residual cervical lymphadenopathy will undergo neck dissection at the discretion of the otolaryngologist. Patients who develop progression of disease at any time during or after treatment will be considered for surgical salvage.

### 3.3. Non-small cell lung cancer (NSCLC)

#### 3.3.1. Clinical experience with paclitaxel and radiation: phase I trials
Phase I and II studies have established the activity of paclitaxel in advanced NSCLC [8,9]. Murphy et al. [8] treated 25 stage III and IV NSCLC patients with paclitaxel (200 mg/m$^2$) administered over 24 h every 3 weeks and achieved 1 CR and 5 PRs, for an overall response rate of 24%. The Eastern Cooperative Oncology Group studied 24 stage IV NSCLC patients who received paclitaxel (250 mg/m$^2$) over 24 h every 3 weeks and observed a response rate of 21% (5 PRs) [9].

Given the promising preclinical findings of paclitaxel's radiosensitizing properties as well as its reported clinical activity in NSCLC, a phase I trial of concurrent paclitaxel and thoracic irradiation in NSCLC patients was initiated.

In the phase I trial of weekly paclitaxel and radiation for stage III non-small cell lung cancer, paclitaxel was initiated at 10 mg/m$^2$ per week with dose escalation of 10 mg/m$^2$ in each successive group of 3 new patients as tolerated [62]. Dose-limiting toxicity was defined as grade 3 or 4 non-hematologic toxicity excluding nausea and vomiting or grade 4 hematologic toxicity according to CALGB expanded common toxicity criteria. Thoracic radiation was administered for 6 weeks with original and boost volumes irradiated sequentially. The dose to the original volume was 40 Gy in 20 fractions of 200 cGy; the boost volume dose was 20 Gy in 10 fractions. Eligible patients had inoperable stage III or stage IV disease limited to previously treated brain metastases.

Twenty-seven patients were accrued to 7 dose levels ranging from 10 to 70 mg/m$^2$ per week. Esophagitis was the principle dose-limiting toxicity of the paclitaxel-radiation combination in lung cancer patients (Table 6). Grade 4 esophagitis with hospitalizations for i.v. hydration and analgesic administration occurred in 2 of 3 patients at 70 mg/m$^2$ per week dose level. In the expanded 60 mg/m$^2$ level, one of 7 patients developed grade 3 esophagitis and 3 patients developed grade 2 esophagitis. Despite an aggregate paclitaxel dose of

Table 6

Non-hematologic toxicity: phase I trial of outpatient weekly paclitaxel and concurrent radiation therapy for advanced non-small cell lung cancer

| Dose (mg/m$^2$) | No. of patients | Toxicity (grade) | | | | | | | | | | | |
|---|---|---|---|---|---|---|---|---|---|---|---|---|---|
| | | Esophagitis | | | | Dermatitis | | | | Myalgias | | | |
| | | 1 | 2 | 3 | 4 | 1 | 2 | 3 | 4 | 0 | 1 | 2 | 3 |
| 10 | 3 | 1 | 2 | 0 | 0 | 2 | 1 | 0 | 0 | 2 | 1 | 0 | 0 |
| 20 | 3 | 2 | 1 | 0 | 0 | 3 | 0 | 0 | 0 | 2 | 1 | 0 | 0 |
| 30 | 3 | 3 | 0 | 0 | 0 | 3 | 0 | 0 | 0 | 2 | 1 | 0 | 0 |
| 40 | 2 | 2 | 0 | 0 | 0 | 3 | 0 | 0 | 0 | 3 | 0 | 0 | 0 |
| 50 | 3 | 2 | 1 | 0 | 0 | 1 | 1 | 1 | 0 | 2 | 1 | 0 | 0 |
| 60 | 7 | 3 | 3 | 1 | 0 | 5 | 2 | 0 | 0 | 5 | 2 | 0 | 0 |
| 70 | 3 | 0 | 1 | 0 | 2 | 1 | 1 | 1 | 0 | 2 | 1 | 0 | 0 |

From Ref. [62].

Table 7

Hematologic toxicity: phase I trial of outpatient weekly paclitaxel and concurrent radiation therapy for advanced non-small cell lung cancer

| Dose (mg/m$^2$) | No. of patients | Hemoglobin (g/dl) | | WBC count ($\times 10^3/\mu l$) | | Platelet count ($\times 10^3/\mu l$) | |
|---|---|---|---|---|---|---|---|
| | | Median | Range | Median | Range | Median | Range |
| 10 | 3 | 11.4 | 10.7–14.4 | 3.6 | 3.2–5.7 | 313 | 265–352 |
| 20 | 3 | 13.8 | 10.8–15.4 | 5.6 | 4.6–8.8 | 179 | 133–301 |
| 30 | 3 | 12 | 11–13.4 | 5.4 | 4.7–6.5 | 348 | 170–374 |
| 40 | 2 | 10.6 | 11.3–9.9 | 3.3 | 2.7–3.9 | 215 | 140–291 |
| 50 | 3 | 9.4 | 8.8–14 | 4.1 | 1.8–5.1 | 161 | 48–198 |
| 60 | 7 | 10.7 | 8.9–12.7 | 3.3 | 2.1–6.3 | 174 | 144–347 |
| 70 | 3 | 11.9 | 10 8–12 8 | 2.6 | 1.2–5.5 | 150 | 144–301 |

From Ref. [62].

210 mg/m$^2$ per 21 days, only 1 patient developed grade 3 neutropenia (Table 7) without fever; and there were no episodes of complete alopecia or neuropathy. There was no apparent added pulmonary toxicity from concurrent therapy. Four of 23 evaluable patients had a complete response (17%) and 13 achieved a partial response (56%), for an overall objective response rate of 73% (95% confidence interval 65–83%). Paclitaxel at 60 mg/m$^2$ per week was recommended as the phase II dose level for further evaluation.

These phase I studies show that treatment with taxane and concurrent radiation is feasible in a wide variety of malignancies. In addition, it would appear that paclitaxel delivered on a 7-day schedule is less toxic than the conventional 21-day schedule. The dose-limiting toxicities from these trials occurred within the radiation field at a rate greater than expected and provide evidence for some degree of interaction between the modalities which warrant phase II evaluation.

### 3.3.2. Phase II study of weekly paclitaxel and radiation therapy for non-small cell lung cancer (NSCLC)

Previously untreated patients with histologically documented inoperable stage IIIA or stage IIIB NSCLC were entered in this study [63]. Patients with direct vertebral body invasion or a malignant or exudative pleural effusion were not eligible. All patients had measurable or assessable disease.

Paclitaxel (60 mg/m$^2$) was administered weekly as a 3-h intravenous (i.v.) infusion in the outpatient setting for 6 weeks. Paclitaxel was usually given at the beginning of the week, prior to the first weekly dose of radiation treatment. Radiation was delivered as 200 cGy fractions 5 days weekly for 6 weeks. The original and boost volumes were irradiated sequentially. Treatment volume and dose were the same as those in the phase I study.

Thirty-three patients entered this study. The age range was 40–80 years and the median age was 68. There were 19 males and 14 females. Twelve patients had stage IIIA disease and 21 had Stage IIIB. The most common histologic type was squamous carcinoma (55%). Most patients had a CALGB performance status of 1.

Of the 33 patients enrolled, 4 were not evaluable. One patient was removed from the study after the discovery of subcutaneous metastatic disease during the first week of treatment. Two patients withdrew from the study during the second week of treatment due to disease progression in 1 patient and the other patient's refusal to receive any additional chemotherapy. One patient developed a hypersensitivity reaction to her first dose of paclitaxel and was not rechallenged. The remaining 29 patients form the basis of this report.

Twenty-seven of 29 patients received all 6 paclitaxel treatments. Two patients received only 5 treatments due to esophagitis. Thus a total of 172 cycles of weekly paclitaxel were administered for the 29 evaluable patients or 99% of the planned paclitaxel doses. Twenty-seven of 29 patients received the planned 60 Gy radiation. Radiation dosage was reduced to 48 and 50 Gy in two patients due to esophagitis.

The complete response rate was 7% (2/29) and the partial response rate was 79% (23/29) for an overall response rate of 86% (95% confidence interval, 68–5%). Three patients had stable disease (10%). One patient had local tumor progression on chest CT scan at completion of treatment.

All subgroups responded favorably and no statistically significant differences were noted with regard to performance status, histology or stage. The response rate was 100% for women and 78% for men. The most frequent histologic subtype in this trial was squamous cell carcinoma. Fourteen of 17 patients with squamous cell carcinomas responded (82%). All 7 patients with adenocarcinoma had at least partial responses (100%). Patients with stage IIIB disease responded equally well as patients with stage IIIA disease.

Esophagitis was the most significant toxicity noted in this study. Six patients (20%) had grade 3 esophagitis (requiring narcotics in order to eat solids). Five patients (17%) had grade 4 esophagitis defined as the requirement for parenteral or enteral support or the need for hospitalization for intravenous hydration. Only one patient required a jejunostomy tube for enteral nutrition to complete therapy and no patient required total parenteral nutrition (TPN). Esophagitis generally began in the final 2 weeks of treatment and resolved within 2 weeks of completing treatment in all patients. Two patients had grade 2 peripheral neuropathy, characterized by numbness and hypesthesia of the hands and feet which resolved within a few weeks of completing treatment. Two patients had significant pulmonary toxicity. These patients had pneumonitis with shortness of breath, hypoxia, and interstitial infiltrates. The pneumonitis improved rapidly with corticosteroids. The only significant hematologic toxicity was grade 3 neutropenia in 2 patients. One patient had a fever that persisted for 4 weeks during treatment as an outpatient without an identified source of infection. One patient had a grade 3 supraventricular tachycardia with a near syncopal episode. No other cardiac toxicity was observed. One patient had a grade 3 hypersensitivity reaction during her first cycle of paclitaxel with hypotension and rash and was not retreated. No patient had grade 3 or 4 nausea, vomiting, or complete alopecia.

The overall median survival time has not yet been reached in this study. At a median followup of 12 months, the overall survival rate was 73% (95% CI 66–6%).

This phase II study of concurrent paclitaxel/RT for patients with stage III NSCLC demonstrated an 86% overall response rate. Responses were noted in all subgroups. There was no statistically significant difference in response rates according to gender, histology, or stage.

Although mean follow-up in this study is just 12 months, our overall response rate is promising and comparable to the most active chemoradiation combinations recently reported, including the 38% response rate observed with radiation alone in the control arm of the Hoosier Oncology Group study [64] or the 45% response rate reported by Perez for locally advanced NSCLC [38]. Our current response rate is also much greater than 20–25% response rate anticipated from paclitaxel as a single agent [16,17]. Thus, the substantial response rate seen with concurrent paclitaxel/RT appears to justify the clinical use of concurrent RT/paclitaxel, and is suggestive, although not conclusive, for a radiation enhancement effect.

### 3.3.3.  Phase II study of weekly paclitaxel, carboplatin and RT for NSCLC

The results from the previous phase II study of weekly paclitaxel and RT demonstrated an 86% overall response rate and 73% 1-year survival [65]. This response rate and survival was very promising and comparable with that reported for the most active platinum-based chemoradiation combinations presently available [66,67]. However 60 mg/m$^2$ weekly for 6 weeks of paclitaxel may not be sufficient to have an impact on microscopic distant metastatic disease. Therefore, concurrent paclitaxel, carboplatin and RT for 7 weeks followed by two additional cycles of paclitaxel and carboplatin is initiated [68,69].

Previously untreated patients with stages IIIA and IIIB non-small cell lung cancer (NSCLC) entered a phase study to evaluate the activity and toxicity of paclitaxel, carboplatin, and concurrent radiation. Patients received paclitaxel (50 mg/m$^2$ weekly) as a 1 h infusion and carboplatin AUC of two per week for 7 weeks with radiation to the primary tumor and regional lymph nodes (44 Gy) followed by a boost to the tumor (22 Gy). In addition to concurrent chemoradiation, patients received an additional two cycles of paclitaxel (200 mg/m$^2$) and carboplatin (AUC 6) every 3 weeks. From March 1995 to February 1996, 23 patients were entered in this study. The overall response rate (complete plus partial responses) was 82%. The major toxicity was esophagitis. 45% of patients ($n = 9$) had grade 3 or 4 esophagitis at the end of concurrent phase. Seven out of 9 patients recovered from the esophagitis within 2 weeks and received the planned additional 2 cycles of standard dose of paclitaxel and carboplatin. Only 1 patient (4%) had grade 4 pneumonitis but also recovered within 2 weeks and received posterior radiation chemotherapy. This response rate was promising and comparable to a previous phase II study [62]. Despite the additional carboplatin given weekly during the concurrent phase of study, the overall toxicity was also comparable to the previous phase II study.

Paclitaxel–carboplatin–RT was safely administered on an outpatient basis. The toxicity was acceptable and compared favorably with other regimens currently used. Several new studies using a weekly schedule of paclitaxel administration are under way.

### 3.3.4.  Phase II study of weekly paclitaxel–carboplatin and hyperfractionated RT for NSCLC

A third phase II study was designed to build on our own experiences of using systemic chemotherapy as a radiation sensitizer by combining paclitaxel with carboplatin along with hyperfractionated chest radiation therapy [70].

This is a prospective phase II study to determine the response rate, toxicity, and survival rate of concurrent weekly paclitaxel, carboplatin, and hyperfractionated radiation therapy (paclitaxel–carboplatin–HFX RT) followed by two cycles of adjuvant paclitaxel and carboplatin for locally advanced unresectable non-small cell lung cancer (NSCLC). The weekly paclitaxel and carboplatin regimen was designed to optimize the radiosensitizing properties of paclitaxel during the concurrent phase of treatment.

Thirty-two patients with unresectable stage IIIA and IIIB NSCLC from Vanderbilt Cancer Center Affiliate Network (VCCAN) institutions were entered onto the study from June of 1996 until February 1997. Weekly intravenous (i.v.) paclitaxel (50 mg/m$^2$ per 3 h) and weekly carboplatin (AUC 2) plus concurrent hyperfractionated chest RT (1.2 Gy bid,

69.6 Gy) were delivered for 6 weeks followed by two cycles of paclitaxel (200 mg/m$^2$) and carboplatin (AUC 6). Twenty-two patients were evaluable for response. One patient achieved a complete response (4.5%) and 16 patients achieved a partial response (72.7%) for an overall response rate of 77%. Twenty-three patients were evaluable for response. Esophagitis was the principal toxicity. Grade 3 or 4 esophagitis occurred in 8 patients (34%). There were 13% grade 3 and 13% grade 4 pulmonary toxicities. Weekly paclitaxel, carboplatin, plus concurrent hyperfractionated RT was a well tolerated outpatient regimen. The response rate from this regimen is encouraging and appears to be at least equivalent to more toxic chemoradiation trials. These findings warrant further clinical evaluation of weekly paclitaxel–carboplatin/HFX RT in phase III trials.

## 3.4. Esophageal cancer

Cisplatin is generally considered the most active standard agent for esophageal cancer. Single agent activity is 25–35% [71]. Cisplatin is also a potent radiosensitizer, making cancer cells more sensitive to radiation therapy [72].

Paclitaxel has demonstrated single agent activity comparable to cisplatin. In an ongoing trial at M.D. Anderson and Memorial Sloan Kettering, 42 patients with esophageal cancer have been treated with paclitaxel with a 30% response rate [73]. Paclitaxel appears to be active against both adenocarcinoma and squamous cell carcinoma of the esophagus (9 of 29 evaluable patients with adenocarcinoma have had a partial response and 3 of 11 evaluable patients with squamous cell carcinoma have had a partial response). Paclitaxel was combined with cisplatin and radiation as preoperative therapy for esophageal cancer.

Meanwhile Safran initiated a phase II study [74] of neoadjuvant paclitaxel (60 mg/m$^2$ per day) and cisplatin (25 mg/m$^2$ per day) on days 1, 8, 15 and 22 with concurrent radiation 40 Gy. Five patients have entered this study (mean age 68, range 43–83 years) Three patients had squamous cell carcinoma and 2 had adenocarcinoma. One patient had celiac adenopathy and 1 had mediastinal adenopathy upon entry. Four patients have completed neoadjuvant chemoradiation, while 1 patient had grade 3 neutropenia, and 1 patient had grade 4 neutropenia and grade 2 esophagitis. All 4 patients had objective radiographic responses. Two patients underwent complete resection. One patient was unresectable because metastatic disease outside of the radiation port was detected at laparotomy. One patient had no residual tumor by endoscopy and biopsy but refused surgery. These ongoing studies demonstrate a high response rate of esophageal cancer to combined modality treatment with paclitaxel, cisplatin, and radiation therapy.

Blanke and his colleagues at Vanderbilt University conducted a phase II study [75] of preoperative chemotherapy with cisplatin and paclitaxel concomitantly with radiotherapy followed by esophagectomy. Postoperatively, chemotherapy with paclitaxel, 5-FU, and high dose leucovorin. The objectives of the study were to establish the activity of this regimen in combined modality treatment of patients with esophageal cancer and to evaluate whether paclitaxel adds to the demonstrated activity of our previous regimen. The preliminary analysis revealed 17% pathological complete response.

## 3.5. Role of concurrent paclitaxel and RT for pancreatic and gastric cancer

A phase I study of paclitaxel–RT for patients with gastric and pancreatic cancer. was initiated by the Clinical Oncology Group-Rhode Island (COGRI) [76]. Eligible patients in-

Table 8

Paclitaxel dosage levels: paclitaxel and concurrent radiation for locally advanced pancreatic and gastric cancer: a phase I study

| Dosage level | Paclitaxel ($mg/m^2$/week) | No. of gastric cancer patients | No. of pancreatic cancer patients |
|---|---|---|---|
| 1 | 30 | 4 | 6 |
| 2 | 40 | 3 | 3 |
| 3 | 50 | 6 | 6 |
| 4 | 60 | 3 | 3 |

From Ref. [76].

cluded those with residual postoperative disease, involved/close margins, recurrent disease after resection, or unresectable disease. Paclitaxel was given by weekly 3-h i.v. infusion for 6 weeks with 30–50 Gy (Table 8). Patients with pancreatic cancer received a boost to a maximum of 62 Gy with two additional courses of paclitaxel. Twenty-one patients were entered; 18 patients completed treatment. One patient had a hypersensitivity reaction, 1 patient had grade 4 neutropenia, and 2 had abdominal pain. Dose-limiting toxicity was abdominal pain with MTD of 50 $mg/m^2$ per week (Table 9). Three of 11 patients (27%) with measurable disease have had partial responses; 5 of 6 patients (83%) without measurable disease remain progression-free at a median followup of 9 months. Only 3 of 13 (23%) tumors had p53 mutations by single-stranded conformational polymorphism (SSCP) analysis. Since p53 gene mutations do not predict response to paclitaxel–RT in NSCLC, the p16 cell cycle control gene was evaluated in these neoplasms. Seven of 13 (54%) tumors had deletions or mutations of p16 gene. Strikingly, p16 alterations were associated with highly aggressive tumors, including both cases of linitus plastica. Six of 7 (86%) patients with p16 alterations had rapid tumor progression. Paclitaxel–RT is a promising new regimen for locally advanced gastric and pancreatic carcinoma.

At the Vanderbilt Medical Center, investigators are currently studying paclitaxel-based neoadjuvant chemoradiation in patients with potentially resectable adenocarcinoma of the pancreatic head under the auspices of a phase I/II clinical trial. This study is based on the 30% response rate recently reported in a phase I Brown University study involving patients with unresectable pancreatic cancer using this regimen [76]. In order to obtain more precise pretreatment staging information and more accurately assess therapy response, pre- and

Table 9

Dose-limiting toxicities: paclitaxel and concurrent radiation for locally advanced pancreatic and gastric cancer: a phase I study

| Dose level ($mg/m^2$/week) | No. of patients | Grade abdominal pain | | | | Grade nausea/anorexia | | | |
|---|---|---|---|---|---|---|---|---|---|
| | | 1 | 2 | 3 | 4 | 1 | 2 | 3 | 4 |
| 30 | 10 | 1 | 2 | 0 | 0 | 2 | 0 | 0 | 0 |
| 40 | 6 | 1 | 1 | 0 | 0 | 3 | 3 | 0 | 0 |
| 50 | 12 | 0 | 3 | 0 | 0 | 5 | 1 | 1 | 0 |
| 60 | 6 | 0 | 1 | 2* | 0 | 1 | 0 | 3* | 0 |

[a]One patient had both grade 3 nausea and abdominal pain. From Ref. [76].

post-chemoradiation 18FDG-PET scans have been undertaken in all patients. Despite modest reductions in tumor dimensions as measured by CT scans performed before and after paclitaxel-based chemoradiation, 18FDG-PET scanning demonstrated marked chemoradiation-induced reductions in tumor cell activity, correlating with histologic evidence of significant tumor cell destruction in resected specimens. While these results are dramatic, associated benefits in local control or long-term survival remain to be established.

### 3.6.   Bladder cancer

Results of an Eastern Cooperative Oncology Group (ECOG) phase II trial using paclitaxel at a dose of 250 mg/m$^2$ by 24-h continuous infusion every 21 days with granulocyte-colony stimulating factor (G-CSF) support showed an objective response rate of 42% as first-line treatment among 26 patients with advanced transitional cell carcinoma (TCC) [77]. The complete clinical response rate of 27% confirms paclitaxel as one of the most active single-agents for the treatment of TCC; however, toxicity was significant with grade 3–4 granulocytopenia in 23% and an 8% incidence of febrile neutropenia despite use of G-CSF. Lower dose paclitaxel which does not require growth-factor support has not yet been compared to dose-intense therapy in a randomized trial.

Preclinical in vitro studies have revealed cytotoxic synergy between cisplatin and paclitaxel in human ovarian cancer cells (HOCC) [78]. Although the exact mechanism for the interaction is not known, investigators have suggested that paclitaxel may either increase intracellular cisplatin accumulation, reduce repair of cisplatin–DNA adducts, or paclitaxel may potentiate the cytotoxicity of cisplatin through its microtubule stabilizing properties. Preliminary results of a phase II study of paclitaxel followed by cisplatin in patients with advanced TCC showed a response rate of 72% with median survival of 12 months [79].

The Radiation Therapy Oncology Group(RTOG) proposes to undertake a phase I study of radiation therapy for locally advanced unresectable TCC of the bladder with concurrent cisplatin 70 mg/m$^2$ on days 1, 22, and 43 plus escalating doses of paclitaxel. The initial dose of paclitaxel will be 20 mg/m$^2$. Patients will be treated in cohorts of three. If no dose-limiting toxicity is identified, the dose level will be increased by 10 mg/m$^2$. Dose escalation will continue until the maximum tolerated dose (MTD) is reached.

## References

1.   Nias AH. An Introduction to Radiobiology. New York: Wiley, p. 168, 1990.
2.   Al Sarraf M, LeBlanc M, et al. Superiority of chemo radiotherapy vs radiotherapy in patients with locally advanced nasopharyngeal cancer. Preliminary results of intergroup randomized study (abstr. 882). Proc Am Soc Clin Oncol 15: 313, 1996.
3.   McGuire WP, Rowinsky EK, Rosenshein NB, et al. Taxol. Intern Med 111: 273, 1989.
4.   Holmes F, Walters R, Theriault R, et al. Phase II trial of Taxol, an active drug in metastatic breast cancer. J Natl Cancer Inst 83: 1797, 1991.
5.   Reichman B, Seidman A, Crown J, et al. Paclitaxel and recombinant human granulocyte-colony-stimulating factor as initial chemotherapy for metastatic breast cancer. J Clin Oncol 11: 1943, 1993.
6.   Seidman A, Crown J, Reichman B, et al. Lack of cross-resistance of Taxol (T) with anthracycline (A) in the treatment of metastatic breast cancer (MBC) (abstr.). Proc Am Soc Clin Oncol 12: 63, 1993.
7.   Gelmon K, Nabholtz JM, Bontebal M, et al. Randomized trial of two doses of Taxol in metastatic breast cancer after failure of standard therapy (abstr.). Proc 8th NCI-EORTC Symp on New Drugs in Cancer Therapy, Vol. 8, p. 198, 1994.

8. Murphy WK, Fossella FV, Winn RJ, et al. Phase II study of Taxol in patients with untreated non-small cell lung cancer. J Natl Cancer Inst 85: 384–388, 1993.

9. Chang A, Kim K, Glick J, et al. Phase II study of Taxol, merbarone, and piroxantrone in stage IV non-small cell lung cancer; the Eastern Cooperative Oncology Group (ECOG) results. J Natl Cancer Inst 85: 388–393, 1993.

10. Forastiere AA, Neuberg D, Taylor S, et al. Phase II evaluation of Taxol in advanced head and neck cancer: an Eastern Cooperative Oncology Group trial. J Natl Cancer Inst Monogr 15: 181, 1993.

11. Roth BJ, Breicer R, Einhorn LH, et al. Paclitaxel in previously advanced transitional cell carcinoma of the urothelium: a phase II trial of the Eastern Cooperative Oncology Group (ECOG) (abstr.). Proc Am Soc Clin Oncol 13: 230, 1994.

12. Ajani J, Ilson D, Daugherty K, et al. Activity of Taxol in patients with squamous cell carcinoma and adenocarcinoma of the esophagus. J Natl Cancer Inst 86: 1086, 1994.

13. Schiff PB, Fant J, Horwitz S. Promotion of microtubule assembly in vitro by Taxol. Nature 22: 665–667, 1979.

14. Parness J, Horwitz S. Taxol binds to polymerized tubulin in vitro. J Cell Biol 91: 479–487, 1981.

15. Manfredi J, Parness J, Horwitz S. Taxol binds to cellular microtubules. J Cell Biol 94: 688–696, 1982.

16. Wilson L. Microtubules as drug receptors: pharmacological properties of microtubule protein. Ann N Y Acad Sci 253: 213, 1975.

17. Carney D, Crossin K, Ball R, et al. Changes in the extent of microtubule assembly can regulate initiation of DNA synthesis. Ann N Y Acad Sci 466: 919, 1986.

18. Sinclair WK, Morton RA. X-ray sensitivity during the cell generation cycle of cultured Chinese hamster cells. Radiat Res 29: 450–474, 1966.

19. Liebmann J, Cook JA, Teague D, et al. Taxol mediated radiosensitization in human tumor cell lines. Proc Am Assoc Cancer Res 34: 349, 1993.

20. Chang A, Keng P, Sobel S, Gu CZ. Interaction of radiation (XRT) and Taxol. Proc Am Assoc Cancer Res 34: 364, 1993.

21. Choy H, Rodriguez FF, Koester S, et al. Investigation of Taxol as a potential radiation sensitizer. Cancer 71: 3774–3778, 1993.

22. Steren A, Sevin BU, Perras J, et al. Taxol sensitizes human ovarian cancer cells to radiation. Gynecol Oncol 48: 252–258, 1993.

23. Steren A, Sevin BU, Perras J, et al. Taxol as a radiation sensitizer: a flow cytometric study. Gynecol Oncol 50: 89–93, 1993.

24. Hei TK, Hall EJ. Taxol, radiation, and oncogenic transformation. Cancer Res 53: 1368–1372, 1993.

25. Liebmann J, Cook JA, Fisher J, et al. Changes in radiation survival curve parameters in human tumor and rodent cells exposed to paclitaxel (Taxol). Int J Radiat Oncol Biol Phys 29: 559–564, 1994.

26. Tishler RB, Schiff PB, Geard CR, Hall EJ. Taxol: a novel radiation sensitizer. Int J Radiat Oncol Biol Phys 22: 613–617, 1992.

27. Stromberg JS, Lee YJ, Armour EP, et al. Lack of radiosensitization after paclitaxel treatment of three human carcinoma cell lines. Cancer 75: 2262–2268, 1995.

28. Lokeshwar BL, Ferrell SM, Block NL. Enhancement of radiation response of prostatic carcinoma by Taxol: therapeutic potential for late–stage malignancy. Anticancer Res 15: 93–98, 1995.

29. Gupta N, Hu L, Fan PD, Deen DF. Effect of Taxol and radiation on brain tumor cell lines. Proc Am Assoc Cancer Res 35: 647, 1994.

30. Geard CR, Jones JM. Radiation and Taxol effects on synchronized human cervical carcinoma cells. Int J Radiat Oncol Biol Phys 29: 565–569, 1994.

31. Liebmann J, Cook JA, Fisher J, et al. In vitro studies of Taxol as a radiation sensitizer in human tumor cells. J Natl Cancer Inst 86: 441–446, 1994.

32. Minarik L, Hall EJ. Taxol in combination with acute and low dose rate irradiation. Radiother Oncol 32: 124–128, 1994.

33. Tishler RB, Geard CR, Hall EJ, Schiff PB. Taxol sensitizes human astrocytoma cells to radiation. Cancer Res 52: 3495–3497, 1992.

34. Choy H, Rodriguez F, Wilcox B, et al. Radiation sensitizing effects of Taxotere (RP 56976). Proc Am Assoc Cancer Res 33: 500, 1992.

35. Choy H, Rodriguez F, Koester S, et al. Investigation of Taxol as a potential radiation sensitizer. Cancer 71: 3774–3778, 1993.

36. Geard CR, Jons JM, Schiff PB. Taxol and radiation. J Natl Cancer Inst 15: 89–94, 1993.

37.  Tishler R, Schiff PB, Geard C, et al. Taxol: a novel radiation sensitizer. Int J Radiat Oncol Biol Phys 22: 613–617, 1992.
38.  Liebmann J, Cook J, Fisher J, et al. In vitro studies of Taxol as a radiation sensitizer in human tumor cells. J Natl Cancer Inst 86: 441–446, 1994.
39.  Minarik L, Hall E. Taxol in combination with acute and low dose rate irradiation. Radiother Oncol 32: 124–128, 1994.
40.  Geard C, Jones J. Radiation and Taxol on synchronized human cervical carcinoma cells. Int J Radiat Oncol Biol Phys 29: 565–569, 1994.
41.  Holmes F, Walters R, Theriault R, et al. Phase II trial of Taxol, an active drug in the treatment of metastatic breast cancer. J Natl Cancer Inst 83: 1797–1805, 1991.
42.  Schiff PB, Fant J, Auster LA. Effects of Taxol on cell growth and in vitro microtubule assembly. J Supramol Struct (Suppl 2): 328–335, 1978.
43.  Stephens L, Ang K, Schultheiss T, et al. Apoptosis in irradiated men tumors. Radiat Res 127: 308–316, 1991.
44.  Stephens L, Hunter N, Ang K, et al. Development of apoptosis irradiated murine tumors as a function of time and dose. Radiat Res 135: 75–80, 1993.
45.  Milas L, Hunter N, Kurdoglu B, et al. Apoptotic death of mitotically arrested cells in murine tumors treated with Taxol. Proc Am Assoc Cancer Res 35: 314, 1994.
46.  Meyn R, Stephens L, Hunter N, et al. Induction of apoptosis in murine tumors by cyclophosphamide. Cancer Chemother Pharmacol 33: 410–414, 1994.
47.  Milas L, Hunter, N, Mason K, et al. Enhancement of tumor radioresponse of a murine mammary carcinoma by paclitaxel. Cancer Res 54: 3506–3510, 1994.
48.  Joschko MA, Webster LK, Groves J, et al. Radiation enhancement by Taxol in a squamous carcinoma of the hypopharynx (FaDu) in nude mice. Proc Am Assoc Cancer Res 35: 647, 1994.
49.  Milas L, Hunter NR, Mason KA, et al. Enhancement of tumor radioresponse of a murine mammary carcinoma by paclitaxel. Cancer Res 54: 3506–3510, 1995.
50.  Chamberlain MC, Kormanik P. Salvage chemotherapy with paclitaxel for recurrent primary brain tumors. J Clin Oncol 13: 2066–2071, 1995.
51.  Glantz M, Choy H, Kearns M, et al. Phase I study of weekly outpatient paclitaxel and concurrent cranial irradiation in adults with astrocytomas. J Clin Oncol 14: 600–609, 1996.
52.  Glantz MJ, Choy H, Kearns CM, et al. Paclitaxel disposition in plasma and central nervous systems of humans and rats with brain tumors. J Natl Cancer Inst 87: 1077–1081, 1995.
53.  Glantz M, Choy H, Kearns CM, et al. Weekly outpatient paclitaxel and concurrent cranial irradiation in adults with brain tumors: preliminary results and promising directions. Semin Oncol 22 (Suppl 12): 26–32, 1995.
54.  Glantz M, Choy H, et al. Weekly paclitaxel with and without concurrent radiation therapy: toxicity, pharmacokinetics, and response. Semin Oncol 23(Suppl 16): 128–135, 1996.
55.  Chang S, Schold C, Spence A, et al. Preliminary report. North American Brain Tumor Consortium (abstr #276). Proc Am Soc Clin Oncol 15:153, 1996.
56.  Fetell, MR, Grossman, SA, Fisher, J, et al. Pre-irradiation paclitaxel in glioblastoma multiforme (GBM): efficacy, pharmacology, and drug interaction (abstr. 275). Proc Am Soc Clin Oncol 15: 153, 1996.
57.  Forastiere AA, Neuberg D, Taylor SG, et al. Phase II evaluation of Taxol in advanced head and neck cancer: an Eastern Cooperative Oncology Group trial (abstr. 893). Proc Am Soc Clin Oncol 12: 277, 1993.
58.  Thorton D, Singh K, Putz B, et al. A phase II trial of Taxol in squamous cell carcinoma of the head and neck (abstr. 933). Proc Am Soc Clin Oncol 13: 288, 1994.
59.  Flood WA, Lee DJ, et al. A phase I study of weekly paclitaxel and cisplatin concurrent with postoperative radiation therapy for treatment of high risk patients with squamous cell cancer of the head and neck(abstr. 885). Proc Am Soc Clin Oncol 15: 314, 1996.
60.  Chougule P, Wehbe T, Leone L, et al. Concurrent Taxol, carboplatin, and radiotherapy in advanced head and neck cancer: a phase II study (abstr. 899). Proc Am Soc Clin Oncol 15: 317, 1996.
61.  Murphy B. A pilot study of larynx preservation using induction carboplatin and Taxol followed by radiation therapy with surgical salvage. Vanderbilt Medical Center Protocol HN-9, 1996.
62.  Choy H, Akerley W, Safran H, et al. Phase I trial of outpatient weekly paclitaxel and concurrent radiation therapy for advanced non-small cell lung cancer. J Clin Oncol 12: 2682–2686, 1994.
63.  Choy H, Safran H. Preliminary analysis of a phase II study of weekly paclitaxel and concurrent radiation therapy for locally advanced non-small cell lung cancer. Semin Oncol 22: 55–57, 1995.

64.   Ansari R, Tokars R, Fisher W, et al. A phase III study of thoracic irradiation with or without concomitant cisplatin in locoregional unresectable non-small cell lung cancer (NSCLC): a Hoosier Oncology Group (H.O.G.) protocol (abstr.). Proc Am Soc Clin Oncol 10: 241, 1991.

65.   Choy H, Akerley W, Safran H, et al. Phase II trial of weekly paclitaxel and concurrent radiation therapy for locally advanced non-small cell lung cancer. American Society of Clinical Oncologists Annual Meeting, 1996, submitted.

66.   Albain K, Rusch V, Crowley J, et al. Concurrent cisplatin/etoposide (PE) + chest radiation (CRT) followed by surgery for stages 3A(N2) and 3B non-small cell lung cancer: completed analysis of SWOG-8805 (abstr.). Proc Am Soc Clin Oncol 13: 1120, 1994.

67.   Strauss GM, Herndon JE, Sherman DD, et al. Neoadjuvant chemotherapy and radiation followed by surgery in stage IIIA non-small cell carcinoma of the lung: report of a cancer and leukemia group B phase II study. J Clin Oncol 10: 1237–1244, 1992.

68.   Choy H, Akerley W, Safran H, et al. Combination trial of paclitaxel, carboplatin, and concurrent radiation therapy for locally advanced non-small cell lung cancer. Semin Oncol 23(Suppl 16): 117–119, 1996.

69.   Choy H, King T, Akerley W, et al. Paclitaxel, carboplatin, and concurrent radiation in the treatment of patients with advanced non-small cell lung cancer. Semin Radiat Oncol 7: 15–18, 1997.

70.   Choy H, Devore RD, Hande KR, et al. Preliminary analysis of a phase II study of Taxol, carboplatin, and radiation therapy for locally advanced inoperable hyperfractionated non-small cell lung cancer. Semin Oncol, 1997, in press.

71.   Ajani JA. Contributions of chemotherapy in the treatment of carcinoma of the esophagus: results and commentary. Semin Oncol 21: 474–482, 1994.

72.   Turrisi AT. Platinum combined with radiation therapy in small cell lung cancer: focusing like a laser beam on crucial issues. Semin Oncol 21: 36–32, 1994.

73.   Ajani JA, Ilson D, Dougherty K, et al. Paclitaxel is active against carcinoma of the esophagus. Report of a phase II trial. Proc Am Soc Clin Oncol 13: 192, 1994.

74.   Safran H, King T, Hesketh P, et al. A phase II study of neo-adjuvant paclitaxel, cisplatin and radiation therapy followed by esophagectomy (abstr. 512) . Proc Am Soc Clin Oncol 15: 218, 1996.

75.   Blanke C, Chiappori A, Epstein BE, et al. A phase II study of neoadjuvant paclitaxel and cisplatin with radiotherapy followed by surgery and postoperative paclitaxel with 5-FU and leucovorin in patients with locally advanced esophageal cancer. Proc Am Soc Clin Oncol, 1997, in press.

76.   Safran H, Choy H, Sikov W, et al. Phase I study of paclitaxel and concurrent radiation for locally advanced gastric and pancreatic cancer. J Clin Oncol 15: 901–907, 1996.

77.   Roth BJ, Dreicer R, Einhorn LH, et al. Significant activity of paclitaxel in advanced transitional cell carcinoma of the urothelium: a phase II trial of the Eastern Cooperative Oncology Group. J Clin Oncol 12: 2264–2270, 1994.

78.   Jekunen A, Christen R, Shalinsky D, Howell SB. Synergistic interaction between cisplatin and Taxol in human ovarian carcinoma cells in vitro. Proc Am Assoc Cancer Res 34: 298, 1993.

79.   Murphy BA, Johnson DR, Smith J, et al. Phase II trial of paclitaxel and cisplatin for metastatic or locally unresectable urothelial cancer. Proc Am Soc Clin Oncol 15: 617, 1996.

C.J. Rosenthal and M. Rotman (Eds.), *Infusion Chemotherapy–Irradiation Interactions*
1998 Elsevier Science B.V.

CHAPTER 11

# The paclitaxel module: phase I and pharmacokinetic study of 96 h paclitaxel

## WYNDHAM H. WILSON

*The Medicine Branch, Division of Clinical Sciences, National Cancer Institute, Building 10,*
*Room 12-N-226, 9000 Rockville Pike, Bethesda, MD, 20892, USA*

## 1. Introduction

Paclitaxel (Taxol[R]) is one of two recently approved agents which belong to the new taxane class of drugs. Taxanes, in contrast to *Vinca* alkaloids, promote polymerization, and in mammalian cells, low concentrations of paclitaxel produce significant increases in microtubule number, resulting in the mitotic arrest of dividing cells and inhibition of motility [1,2]. Clinically, a variety of drug schedules have been studied including 3, 6, 24, 72 and 120 h infusions [3–6]. With all schedules, reversible hematopoietic toxicity is usually dose-limiting although mucositis may be dose-limiting with prolonged infusion schedules [6,7]. Other toxicities which are seen include myalgia, neuropathy, alopecia, hypersensitivity reactions and cardiac arrhythmias.

Paclitaxel is of considerable clinical interest because of its activity against a number of solid tumors including breast, ovarian and non-small cell lung cancers [5,8,9]. Although most clinical trials have tested 3 or 24 h infusion schedules, the optimal administration time has yet to be clearly determined [10]. Indeed, pre-clinical studies strongly suggest that the activity of paclitaxel is schedule dependent and most cytotoxic to cells in mitosis [11]. In both colon and breast cancer cell lines, for example, increasing the duration of exposure to paclitaxel markedly increases cytotoxicity (A. Fojo, pers. commun.). Like other phase-specific agents, paclitaxel cytotoxicity reaches a plateau at a specific drug concentration; above that concentration, cytotoxicity is highly dependent on exposure time [11]. Longer drug exposure times may also partially overcome multidrug resistance (mdr-1), a mechanism which is present in a number of cancers including breast cancer and lymphomas [12]. Several recent clinical trials also suggest that longer infusions of paclitaxel may be more effective than shorter ones in metastatic breast cancer, and a randomized trial of 3 versus 96 h paclitaxel in metastatic breast cancer is presently underway to test this observation [13].

There has been interest in the radiosensitizing effect of paclitaxel based on results from several preclinical studies. In an astrocytoma cell line, Tishler et al. demonstrated that paclitaxel had a sensitizer enhancement ratio (SER) of 1.8, and subsequent studies have shown similar effects in a number of cell types including ovarian and leukemia cells [14–16]. The radiosensitizing effect of paclitaxel, like the cytotoxic activity, also appears to be schedule dependent. Experimentally, only minimal radiosensitization was seen in tumor cells exposed to paclitaxel for less than 12 h, whereas prolonged exposure for up to 72 h produced progressively greater radiosensitization [17]. Based on these results, the Radiation Oncology

Branch of the National Cancer Institute has begun a clinical trial to examine the radiation sensitizing effect of a 120 h continuous infusion of paclitaxel for the treatment of locally advanced head and neck cancer.

Because of the preclinical evidence suggesting that paclitaxel is a schedule dependent drug, we were interested in developing a prolonged infusion schedule of paclitaxel. Thus, we performed a clinical phase I study to define the toxicity, maximum tolerated dose and pharmacokinetics of a continuous 96 h infusion of paclitaxel.

## 2. Phase I study of 96 h paclitaxel

We conducted a phase I/II trial of 96 h continuous infusion paclitaxel in 42 patients with relapsed or refractory lymphoma, non-small cell lung cancer, and refractory metastatic breast cancer as previously reported (Table 1) [7]. In the phase I portion, paclitaxel dose levels ranged from 120 to 160 mg/m$^2$ over 96 h. Infusions were administered through a central venous device and no patients received premedications to prevent hypersensitivity reactions; subsequent doses of paclitaxel were reduced for hematopoietic toxicity as previously reported [7].

Twelve patients were entered into the phase I portion of the study and received 73 cycles of paclitaxel administered at three different dose levels (Table 2). Dose-limiting toxicity was reached at 160 mg/m$^2$ where 3 patients experienced grade 4 granulocytopenia and 2 experienced grade 3 mucositis. Six patients were entered at the next lower dose level of 140 mg/m$^2$. On the first cycle at this dose level, 3 patients developed grade 4 granulocytopenia and 2 developed grade 3 mucositis. Of relevance was that 2 of the patients who experienced increased toxicity also had liver metastases; both had grade 3 mucositis and grade 4 granulocytopenia. In contrast, among the 3 patients without liver metastases, none had grade 3 mucositis and only one had grade 4 granulocytopenia. Furthermore, an analysis of all patients at this dose level revealed that 69% of all dose reductions occurred in the cycles administered to the 2 patients with liver disease, and a relationship between liver disease, high paclitaxel steady state serum concentration and delayed drug clearance was subsequently confirmed by pharmacokinetic analysis. The phase II dose of paclitaxel was determined to be 140 mg/m$^2$ in patients without liver metastases based on the acceptable toxicity profile at

Table 1

Phase I paclitaxel

| Patient characteristics | No. (%) |
| --- | --- |
| Total patients | 12 |
| Sex (female) | 8 (67) |
| Median age (years) | 47 |
| Range | 23–71 |
| Median performance status | 1 |
| Range | 1–3 |
| Tumor histologies | |
| Breast cancer | 6 (50) |
| Lymphoma | 5 (42) |
| Lung cancer | 1 (8) |
| Median prior regimens | 2 |
| Range | 1–4 |

Table 2

Phase I paclitaxel dose escalation and toxicities

| Dose level[a] (mg/m$^2$) | Patient no. | Toxicity grade[b] | | | | | | | | |
|---|---|---|---|---|---|---|---|---|---|---|
| | | Mucositis | | | | Granulocytopenia | | | | |
| | | 0 | 1 | 2 | 3 | 0 | 1 | 2 | 3 | 4 |
| 120 | 3 | 2 | 1 | – | – | – | – | – | 3 | – |
| 140 (MTD) | 6 | 2 | 1 | 1 | 2 | 1 | 0 | 0 | 2 | 3 |
| 160 | 3 | – | – | 1 | 2 | – | – | – | – | 3 |

[a]Total dose administered over 96 h. No G-CSF was administered.
[b]Acute toxicity on cycle one only. Toxicity grade based on Cancer Therapy Evaluation Program (CTEP) National Cancer Institute schedule.

this dose, whereas in patients with liver metastases, the recommended phase II dose was determined to be 105 mg/m$^2$.

An additional 34 patients with refractory breast cancer were treated at the phase II dose(s) of paclitaxel, and 32 of these were included in the analysis of toxicity; 2 patients withdrew from study before toxicity data could be obtained and were not included. Although no premedications were administered to prevent hypersensitivity reactions, none were observed in 227 cycles of therapy. Peripheral neuropathy, myalgias, arthralgias, diarrhea, and nausea and vomiting were infrequent and mild.

In order to assess the hematological and mucosal toxicity of paclitaxel, the first 11 patients did not receive granulocyte-colony stimulation factor (G-CSF). Once tolerance to the phase II dose of paclitaxel was demonstrated, the subsequent 21 patients received G-CSF on all cycles of paclitaxel to determine if hematopoietic toxicity could be reduced and paclitaxel dose-intensity increased. Patients who received G-CSF, compared to those who did not, had a significantly lower incidence of granulocytopenia, 22 versus 44% of cycles, respectively ($P_2 = 0.001$), but no difference in incidence of febrile neutropenia, 6 versus 9% of cycles, respectively. There was no difference between these groups in incidence of thrombocytopenia, mucositis or deaths on study. The dose-intensity of paclitaxel, however, was 17% greater in patients who received G-CSF, compared to those patients who did not ($P_2 = 0.005$), but there was no difference in response rate between the two groups.

Four patients died during the first cycle of therapy and were counted as treatment failures. Three patients had extensive pulmonary disease with radiographic evidence of diffuse (lymphangitic) involvement and all died in pulmonary failure within the first 3 weeks of therapy. The fourth patient developed sepsis secondary to *Escherichia coli* bacteremia during the first week of therapy, and died with irreversible lactic acidosis and multiorgan failure. Although she had extensive liver replacement by tumor, she had normal liver synthetic function prior to treatment.

## 3. Pharmacology and pharmacodynamics of 96 h paclitaxel

In 25 patients, blood samples for paclitaxel measurement were drawn at 48, 72 and 96 h after the start of the paclitaxel infusion, on the first cycle of therapy, and paclitaxel plasma

Table 3

Pharmacokinetics of 96 h paclitaxel in patients without hepatic metastases

| Total paclitaxel dose (mg/m$^2$) | Patient no. | Mean ± standard error | | | |
|---|---|---|---|---|---|
| | | $C_{ss}$[a] ($\mu$M) | $P_2$ | Clearance (ml/min per m$^2$) | $P_2$ |
| 120 | 3 | 0.053 ± 0.003 | | 473 ± 20.3 | |
| 140 (MTD) | 7 | 0.060 ± 0.003 | 0.0067 | 487 ± 29.0 | 0.41 |
| 160 | 3 | 0.077 ± 0.003 | | 430 ± 20.0 | |

[a]Mean of the values from 48, 72 and 96 h for each patient on cycle 1.

concentrations were measured by high performance liquid chromatography as previously described [18]. A separate plasma standard curve with concentrations of 0.05–1.0 $\mu$M paclitaxel was performed with each set of samples. The limit of quantitation was 0.05 $\mu$M, recovery was >90%, and the coefficient of variation was 6%. The clearance of paclitaxel was determined by the formula: Clearance = infusion rate/$C_{ss}$, where $C_{ss}$ is the steady state plasma concentration calculated from a mean of three samples for each patient collected at 48, 72 and 96 h.

Steady state concentrations ($C_{ss}$) of paclitaxel were reached in plasma by 48, h and did not significantly change over the duration of the 96 h infusion ($P_2 = 0.99$). $C_{ss}$ increased in proportion to paclitaxel dose ($P_2 = 0.0067$) and showed no evidence of dose-dependent clearance within the narrow dose range of this study ($P_2 = 0.41$) (Table 3). At the phase II dose of paclitaxel (140 mg/m$^2$), the 7 patients without metastatic liver involvement in whom paclitaxel pharmacokinetics was measured had a mean (±SE) paclitaxel $C_{ss}$ of 0.06 ± 0.003 $\mu$M. In contrast, paclitaxel clearance was significantly lower in patients with liver metastases (Table 4). The extent of liver involvement was estimated by CT as none (–), modest (+) (≤2 cm masses) or extensive (++) (>2 cm masses or diffuse involvement) and found to inversely correlate with paclitaxel clearance. Thirteen patients with no liver involvement had a mean clearance (ml/min per m$^2$) of 471 compared to 9 patients with extensive involvement who had a clearance of 336 ($P_2 = 0.0022$). Spearman correlations between liver function tests and clearance also demonstrated a moderate correlation (Table 5). Of the serum markers, the AST level was the best predictor of decreased paclitaxel clearance, and correlated with the presence of liver metastases; 7/9 patients with extensive liver involvement had ≥1.5-fold AST elevation compared to 0/16 with modest or no liver involvement ($P_2 < 0.0001$; Fisher's exact test)). Based on these findings, we developed an algorithm to

Table 4

Clearance of 96 h paclitaxel in patients ± hepatic metastases

| Hepatic[a] metastases | No. of patients | Paclitaxel clearance (ml/min per m$^2$) (mean ± standard error) | $P_2$ |
|---|---|---|---|
| – | 13 | 470.9 ± 17.4 | |
| + | 3 | 324.7 ± 41.2 | 0.0022 |
| ++ | 9 | 335.6 ± 38.2 | |

[a]Extent of liver involvement by tumor: –, none; +, ≤2 cm masses; ++, >2 cm masses or diffuse involvement.

Table 5

Correlation between hepatic function and paclitaxel clearance[a]

| Liver function | $r$ | $r^2$ | $P_2$ |
|---|---|---|---|
| Total bilirubin | −0.42 | 0.18 | 0.035 |
| AST | −0.51 | 0.26 | 0.0094 |
| ALT | −0.38 | 0.14 | 0.06 |
| Alkaline phosphatase | −0.40 | 0.16 | 0.05 |

[a]Spearman correlation.

reduced the starting dose of paclitaxel whereby patients who had either extensive liver involvement by CT (++) or a $\geq$1.5-fold elevation of AST received a reduced dose of 105 mg/m$^2$. The dose of paclitaxel was slowly increased if there was no significant toxicity at the lower doses.

There was a significant pharmacodynamic correlation between paclitaxel $C_{ss}$ and granulocyte and mucosal toxicity (Table 6). Patients with grade 4 granulocytopenia had significantly higher paclitaxel $C_{ss}$ compared to patients with $\leq$ grade 3 ($P_2 = 0.011$), as did patients with severe mucositis compared to those with mild or no mucositis ($P_2 = 0.0043$). Of interest was the finding that both mucosal and granulocyte toxicity were significantly more severe in patients with $C_{ss}$ above a threshold of 0.07 $\mu$M. Of 11 patients with paclitaxel $C_{ss}$ > 0.07 $\mu$M, 10 (91%) had grade 4 granulocyte and 8 (73%) had $\geq$ grade 3 mucosal toxicity. By comparison, only 5 of 14 (36%) patients with paclitaxel $C_{ss} \leq 0.07$ $\mu$M had grade 4 granulocyte toxicity ($P_2 = 0.012$) and none had grade 3 or 4 mucosal toxicity ($P_2 = 0.0002$). The fact that 45% of patients with paclitaxel $C_{ss}$ > 0.07 $\mu$M also received G-CSF, compared to only 21% of patients with $C_{ss} \leq 0.07$ $\mu$M, further emphasizes the degree of granulocyte toxicity associated with high $C_{ss}$.

In this study, we did not measure cerebral spinal fluid (CSF) concentrations of paclitaxel. However, three patients who developed brain metastases but were responding in peripheral sites of disease were continued on paclitaxel based on both clinical and experimental evidence that the central nervous system is a sanctuary site. Rowinsky et al. was unable to detect paclitaxel in the cerebrospinal fluid of one patient (limit of detection; 0.05 $\mu$M) who had a serum level of 2.74 $\mu$M at the end of a 24 h infusion [19]. Lesser et al. was also unable to

Table 6

Pharmacodynamics of 96 h paclitaxel

| Toxicity grade | No. of patients | Paclitaxel $C_{ss}$ ($\mu$M) (mean ± standard error) | $P_2$[a] |
|---|---|---|---|
| *Granulocyte* | | | |
| 0–3 | 9 | 0.062 ± 0.005 | 0.011 |
| 4 | 16 | 0.084 ± 0.005 | |
| | | | |
| *Mucosal* | | | |
| 0 | 7 | 0.060 ± 0.007 | |
| 1–2 | 9 | 0.072 ± 0.006 | 0.0043 |
| 3–4 | 9 | 0.093 ± 0.005 | |

[a]Statistical tests: granulocyte toxicity, Wilcoxon rank sum; mucosal toxicity, Kruskal-Wallis test.

detect [³H]paclitaxel by autoradiography in the brain, spinal cord, and dorsal root ganglia of rats, but found homogeneous distribution in other major organs [20]. These studies suggest that paclitaxel does not accumulate in the normal tissues or fluids of the CNS, although concentrations may be higher in areas where the blood–brain barrier has been disrupted by tumor.

## 4. Comparison of 3, 24 and 96 h paclitaxel

The maximum tolerated dose of 140 mg/m$^2$ identified for the 96 h schedule is significantly lower than that described in phase I trials of 3 and 24 h infusion schedules where MTDs range from 210 to 250 mg/m$^2$ [21,22]. These differences appear related to schedule-dependent toxicity. Previous trials in ovarian cancer comparing 3 and 24 h infusion schedules established that higher doses of paclitaxel (175 mg/m$^2$) are better tolerated on the 3 h schedule with less granulocytopenia than on the 24 h schedule [23,24]. The incidence and severity of mucositis is similarly affected by schedule. In a phase I trial of paclitaxel administered over 24 h in refractory acute leukemias, grade 3/4 mucositis was dose-limiting at 315 mg/m$^2$, double the dose at which mucositis was dose-limiting on the 96 h infusion schedule [19]. The incidence of hypersensitivity reactions is also affected by schedule. In three trials in which no premedications to prevent hypersensitivity reactions were administered, severe reactions were observed in 16–18% of patients receiving paclitaxel over 3 h, compared to a 2% incidence during 24 h infusions [25]. In the 96 h trial, no hypersensitivity reactions occur, even though premedications were not administered.

In our phase II study, 16 (48%) of 33 heavily pretreated patients with doxorubicin and/or mitoxantrone refractory breast cancer responded to paclitaxel. These results compare favorably with two recent phase II studies of paclitaxel in patients with stage IV breast cancer who had either received no prior therapy for metastatic disease or had received one prior regimen (including adjuvant therapy) [5,26]. In both studies, paclitaxel was administered at a starting dose of 250 mg/m$^2$ over 24 h. In one study of 14 patients, there were 2 CRs and 6 PRs (57% RR), and in another study of 26 patients, 2 achieved CRs and 13 achieved PRs (62% RR). However, 24 h infusional paclitaxel has shown a significantly lower response rate in doxorubicin-refractory and/or heavily pretreated patients. In a trial of 51 patients who had received a median of three prior regimens for stage IV breast cancer, Seidman et al. reported a partial response rate of 22% with no CRs [27]. By contrast, 96 h paclitaxel was quite effective in a similar patient group. There are several potential explanations for these different results. First, our patients had received less prior treatment than those of Seidman et al., a median of two as compared to three regimens, and, therefore, may have had less resistant disease. However, 73% of the present patients had not responded to prior doxorubicin or mitoxantrone (primary refractory), compared to only 43% of the patients treated by Seidman et al. Furthermore, in our patient population, the number of prior regimens was not predictive of response to paclitaxel. A second factor which may explain the higher response rate in our trial is the prolonged infusion schedule. The hypothesis that paclitaxel is a schedule dependent drug is supported by two recent clinical trials which examined the activity of 96 h paclitaxel in patients with breast cancer who had failed 1 or 3 h infusion schedules. In one study of 26 patients who had failed short infusions, 7 (26.9%) achieved major objective responses, lasting a median 6 months, when paclitaxel was administered over 96 h [28]. These clinical results support the preclinical findings that the activity of paclitaxel is schedule dependent.

Table 7

Comparative pharmacokinetics of 3, 24 and 96 h paclitaxel infusions

| Dose (mg/m$^2$) | Infusion schedule (h) | Infusion rate (mg/m$^2$/h) | Patient no. | Mean | |
|---|---|---|---|---|---|
| | | | | End infusion concentration[a] ($\mu$m/l) | clearance (ml/min per m$^2$) |
| 135[b] | 3 | 45 | 7 | 2.54 | 295 |
| 135[b] | 24 | 5.6 | 2 | 0.23 | 364 |
| 140 | 96 | 1.5 | 7 | 0.08 | 487 |

[a]Equivalent to peak concentration.
[b]Data summarized from Huizing et al. [24].

In the present study, there was a proportional relationship between dose and $C_{ss}$, and no evidence of dose-dependent clearance over the narrow dose range of this study. Prior work, however, suggests that paclitaxel clearance is dose-dependent and capacity limited. Kearns et al. measured the pharmacokinetics of 3 h infusions of paclitaxel over doses ranging from 135 to 300 mg/m$^2$ and found that as the dose increased, clearance fell [29]. Comparison of the pharmacokinetics of 175 mg/m$^2$ paclitaxel administered over 3 or 24 h showed that paclitaxel clearance increased from 212 to 393 ml/min/m$^2$ as the rate of drug delivery decreased from 58 to 7 mg/m$^2$ per h [24]. A similar increase in clearance rate is seen when the infusion rate of 135–140 mg/m$^2$ of paclitaxel decreases from 45 to 1.5 mg/m$^2$ per h (Table 7).

An important finding of the present study, and confirmed by subsequent investigators, is the association between metastatic liver disease and paclitaxel clearance [28]. In the present study, even modest hepatic involvement significantly increased the steady state concentration of paclitaxel and lead to increased toxicity. Clinically, however, the affect of hepatic involvement on clearance is primarily a problem with prolonged infusion schedules because of the narrow therapeutic index compared with short infusion schedules.

We found a significant association between paclitaxel $C_{ss}$ and clinical toxicity. For both mucosal and granulocyte toxicity, most patients with $C_{ss}$ above a 0.07 $\mu$M threshold had significant toxicity while those patients with concentrations below this level had only moderate toxicity. Although the association between $C_{ss}$ and toxicity had not been previously described, Longnecker et al. reported a "rough association" between the degree of leukopenia and paclitaxel area under the curve (AUC) [30]. In a four arm pharmacodynamic study of paclitaxel administered at 135 or 175 mg/m$^2$ over 3 or 24 h, Huizing et al. found no relationship between AUC or peak concentration of paclitaxel and toxicity [24]. However, a correlation was found between granulocyte toxicity and the duration of paclitaxel plasma concentrations above a threshold of 0.1 $\mu$M, a threshold concentration which is close to that identified in our study (i.e., 0.07 $\mu$M) [24]. This suggests that the cytotoxicity of paclitaxel is more dependent on the duration of exposure above a threshold level than on the AUC (or peak level). Seidman et al. recently reported very similar pharmacodynamic results to those found in the present study [28].

## 5. Conclusions

Both preclinical and clinical studies have demonstrated the cytotoxic schedule dependency of paclitaxel. This schedule dependency has also been shown in vitro for its radiosensitizing effects, and suggests that when considering a clinical trial of paclitaxel as a radiosensitizer, a prolonged infusion schedule should be considered. Clinically, paclitaxel has shown very clear pharmacodynamic relationships with both granulocyte and mucosal toxicity, principally with prolonged infusion schedules. In addition, its clearance is quite dependent on both the infusion rate and presence of hepatic disease, and these factors should be considered when selecting both the dose and schedule of paclitaxel.

## References

1. Schiff PB, Fant J, Horwitz SB. Promotion of microtubule assembly in vitro by Taxol®. Nature (London) 22: 665–667, 1979.
2. Schiff PB, Horwitz SB. Taxol® stabilizes microtubules in mouse fibroblast cells. Proc Natl Acad Sci USA 77: 1561–1565, 1980.
3. Kris MG, O'Connell JP, Gralla RJ, et al. Phase I trial of Taxol® given as a 3-hour infusion every 21 days. Cancer Treatment Rep 70: 605–607, 1986.
4. Wiernik PH, Schwartz EL, Strauman JJ, et al. Phase I clinical and pharmacokinetic study of Taxol®. Cancer Res 47: 2486–2493, 1987.
5. Holmes FA, Walters RS, Theriault RL, et al. Phase II trial of Taxol®, an active drug in the treatment of metastatic breast cancer. J Natl Cancer Inst 83: 1797–1805, 1991.
6. Spriggs DR, Tondini C. Taxol® administered as a 120 hour infusion. Invest New Drugs 10: 275–278, 1992.
7. Wilson WH, Berg SL, Bryant G, et al. Paclitaxel in doxorubicin-refractory or mitoxantrone-refractory breast cancer: a phase I/II trial of 96-hour infusion. J Clin Oncol 12: 1621–1629, 1994.
8. McGuire WP, Rowinsky EK, Rosenshein NB, et al. Taxol: A unique antineoplastic agent with significant activity in advanced ovarian epithelial neoplasms. Ann Intern Med 111: 273–279, 1989.
9. Georgiadis MS, Schuler BS, Brown JE, et al. Paclitaxel by 96-hour continuous infusion in combination with cisplatin: a phase I trial in patients with advanced lung cancer. J Clin Oncol 15: 735–743, 1997.
10. Arbuck SG. Paclitaxel. What schedule? What dose? J Clin Oncol 12: 233–236, 1994.
11. Lopes NM, Adams EG, Pitts TW, Bhuyan BK. Cell kill kinetics and cell cycle effects of taxol on human and hamster ovarian cell lines. Cancer Chemother Pharmacol 32: 235–242, 1993.
12. Lai GM, Chen YN, Mickley LA, Fojo A. P-glycoprotein expression and schedule dependence of adriamycin cytotoxicity in human colon carcinoma cell lines. Int J Cancer 49: 696–703, 1991.
13. Holmes FA, Trissel LA, Boehnke-Michaud L, Hortobagyi GN. Extended stability paclitaxel for prolonged infusion in metastatic breast cancer: convenient, less toxic and effective. Proc Am Soc Clin Oncol, 1997, in press.
14. Tishler RB, Schiff PB, Geard CR. Taxol. A novel radiation sensitizer. Int J Radiat Oncol Biol Phys 22: 613–617, 1992.
15. Steren A, Sevin BU, Perras J, et al. Taxol sensitizes human ovarian cancer cells to radiation. Gynecol Oncol 48: 252–258, 1993.
16. Milas L, Hunter NR, Mason KA, et al. Enhancement of tumor radioresponse of a murine mammary carcinoma by paclitaxel. Cancer Res 54: 3506–3510, 1994.
17. Liebman JE, Cook JA, Lipschultz C, et al. Cytotoxic studies of paclitaxel in human tumour cell lines. Br J Cancer 68: 1104–1109, 1993.
18. Jamis-Dow C, Klecker R, Sarosy G. Taxol steady-state levels and toxicity after a 250 mg/m$^2$ dose in combination with granulocyte colony stimulating factor (G-CSF), (Abstr. G-8). Second Natl Cancer Inst Workshop on Taxol and Taxus, 1992.
19. Rowinsky EK, Burke PJ, Karp JE, et al. Phase I and pharmacodynamic study of Taxol® in refractory acute leukemias. Cancer Res 49: 4640–4647, 1989.

20.  Lesser GJ, Grossman SA, Eller S, Rowinsky EK. Distribution of $^3$H-Taxol® in the nervous system (NS) and organs of rats (abstr. 441). Proc Am Soc Clin Oncol 12: 160, 1993.

21.  Wiernik PH, Schwartz EL, Einzig A, et al. Phase I trial of Taxol® given as a 24-hour infusion every 21 days: responses observed in metastatic melanoma. J Clin Oncol 5: 1232–1239, 1987.

22.  Schiller JH, Tutsch K, Arzoomian R. Phase I trial of a 3 hour Taxol® infusion plus or minus granulocyte-colony stimulating factor (G-CSF) (abstr.). Proc Am Soc Clin Oncol 12: 166, 1993.

23.  Swenerton K, Eisenhauer E, ten Bokkel Huinink W, et al. Taxol® in relapsed ovarian cancer: high vs. low dose and short vs. long infusion: a European-Canadian study coordinated by the NCI Canada Clinical Trials Group (abstr.). Proc Am Soc Clin Oncol 12: 256, 1993.

24.  Huizing MT, Keung ACF, Rosing H, et al. Pharmacokinetics of paclitaxel and metabolites in a randomized comparative study of platinum-pretreated ovarian cancer patients. J Clin Oncol 11: 2127–2135, 1993.

25.  Arbuck SG, Canetta R, Onetto N, Christian MC. Current dosage and schedule issues in the development of paclitaxel (Taxol®). Semin Oncol 20(Suppl 3): 31–39, 1993.

26.  Reichman BS, Seidman AD, Crown JPA, et al. Paclitaxel and recombinant human granulocyte-colony stimulating factor as initial chemotherapy for metastatic breast cancer. J Clin Oncol 11: 1943–1951, 1993.

27.  Seidman AD, Norton L, Reichman BS, et al. Preliminary experience with paclitaxel (Taxol®) plus recombinant human granulocyte-colony stimulating factor in the treatment of breast cancer. Semin Oncol 20: 40–45, 1993.

28.  Seidman AD, Hockhauser D, Gollub M, et al. Ninety-six-hour paclitaxel infusion after progression during short taxane exposure: a phase II pharmacokinetic and pharmacodynamic study in metastatic breast cancer. J Clin Oncol 14: 1877–1884, 1996.

29.  Kearns C, Gianni L, Vigano A, et al. Non-linear pharmacokinetics of Taxol® in humans (abstr. 341). Proc Am Soc Clin Oncol 12: 135, 1993.

30.  Longnecker SM, Donehower RC, Cates AE, et al. High-performance liquid chromatographic assay for Taxol® in human plasma and urine and pharmacokinetics in a phase I trial. Cancer Treatment Rep 71: 53–59, 1987.

C.J. Rosenthal and M. Rotman (Eds.), *Infusion Chemotherapy–Irradiation Interactions*

135

CHAPTER 12

# Paclitaxel by protracted infusion with concomitant radiation therapy: phase I study

## C. JULIAN ROSENTHAL[1–4], HASSAN AZIZ[3], HITENDRA RAMBHIA[1,3], KWAN CHOI[4] and MARVIN ROTMAN[2–4]

[1]*Othmer Cancer Center and Departments of* [2]*Medicine, and* [3]*Radiation Oncology, Long Island College Hospital, 339 Hicks Street, Brooklyn, NY 11201, USA, and* [4]*State University of New York, Health Science Center at Brooklyn, 450 Clarkson Avenue, Brooklyn, NY 11203, USA*

## 1. Introduction

Paclitaxel (Taxol-Bristol-Meyers Squibb Company, Princeton, NJ) is known since the early experimental work of Schiff et al. [1,2] to promote the formation of tubulin dimers and to stabilize cytoplasmic microtubules enhancing their rate of assembly and preventing their depolymerization. These changes led to the arrest of a high percentage of cells at the $G_2/M$ phase of the cycle, which explains the enhancement of in vitro radiosensitivity of several cancer cell lines after treatment with paclitaxel [3]. These experimental observations led to the early clinical observations of paclitaxel as radiation sensitizer [4] and to its more systematic study in phase I/II studies by Choi et al. [5,6] and more recently by at least another four teams of investigators [7–10].

### 1.1. Preclinical studies of paclitaxel–radiation interaction

The preclinical studies recently published by Hoffman and Rodeman [8] convincingly proved on cultured lines of normal fibroblasts as well as of squamous cell carcinoma cells from a head and neck carcinoma (the HTB43 line), the enhancing effect of their exposure to paclitaxel (5 or 10 nmol/l) for 24 h to radiation cytotoxicity (2 Gy). The cells were seeded 24 h later in Dulbecco's modified Eagle's medium at a constant cell density of 30 000 cells/25 cm². A significant inhibition of cell growth in a colony formation assay that determine the survival fraction at 2 Gy ($SF_2$) was noted. The growth rate of normal fibroblasts was reduced by 70–80% while that of the HTB43 cells was reduced by 95%.

Similar results were reported in earlier studies by Lopes et al. [11] on human ovarian cell lines and Tishler et al. on human astrocytoma cell lines [12]. These in vitro experimental data led to initial phase I clinical studies that tested a weekly schedule of 3 h intravenous delivery of paclitaxel concomitantly with radiation therapy [5,6].

### 1.2. Studies of paclitaxel weekly administration during radiation therapy

Choy established the MTD for the weekly administration of paclitaxel with radiation in patients with lung cancer at 60 mg/m² [6] with dose limiting toxicities represented by esophagitis and neutropenia while a more recent study performed in inpatients with head and neck cancer [8] established the weekly paclitaxel MTD at 40 mg/m$^2$ with dose limiting toxicity again represented by mucositis. However, previously mentioned experimental studies [12] revealed that the radiation enhancing effect of paclitaxel correlated with the degree of mitotic arrest which peaked and persisted at greater than 95% after at least 16 h of incubation. Further loss of clonogenicity was noted with more prolonged incubation, while a paclitaxel dose as little as 1 nmol/l was found sufficient to induce radiosensitization in several cell lines [12,13]. Higher doses did not lead to enhanced cytotoxicity in proliferating cells. Paclitaxel cytotoxicity reaches a plateau at a certain concentration above which it becomes highly dependent on exposure time [11]. Longer drug exposure times could also overcome multidrug resistance a process that was found to be triggered by taxanes.

### 1.3. Study of paclitaxel continuous intravenous administration

The above mentioned observations led us [7] and others [9,10] to look at improving the clinical radiosensitizing effect of paclitaxel through its administration by continuous infusion at a low dose.

Preliminary results of a phase I study reported by Wilson et al. in 1994 [14] showed that over a period of 96 h the total dose of paclitaxel that can be administered by continuous infusion (140 mg/m$^2$) was moderately lower than the total paclitaxel dose tolerated when it was delivered over a period of 3 and 24 h infusion (210–240 mg/m$^2$); however, this lower dose led to objective responses in many cases that relapsed after shorter intravenous infusions of paclitaxel (for 3 or 24 h).

### 1.4. Rationale of current study

We postulated that the dose of paclitaxel that could be administered with concomitant radiation therapy over a 96-h period could be higher than the dose of weekly paclitaxel previously administered by Choy [5] and Hoffman [8] and may lead to better results because the prolonged exposure time to a steady paclitaxel level could increase cytotoxic effect against neoplastic cells.

The results of a limited phase I study that aimed at defining the feasibility, side effects and the maximum tolerated dose of a concomitant combined administration of paclitaxel by continuous intravenous infusion and radiation therapy to recurrent or metastatic malignant lesions using a split schema of administration of 5 day cycles every 2 weeks are presented here.

## 2. Methods

### 2.1. Paclitaxel–radiation therapy regimen

Paclitaxel (Bristol Myers Squibb) was administered by continuous i.v. infusion dissolved in 1000 ml normal saline (NS) over 96 h at a rate of 42 cm$^3$/h starting at a dose of 80 mg/m$^2$ per 96 h. If no significant side effects were noted, the dose was escalated after 5 cycles at each dose level. For the first two levels, the escalation was of 20 mg/m$^2$ per 96 h; it was only 10 mg/m$^2$ per 96 h thereafter.

Diphenhydramine (25 mg) was administered intravenously before the start of paclitaxel infusion then q 8 h throughout the administration of paclitaxel.

Cimetidine (300 mg) was administered intravenously 1 h before starting paclitaxel then q 24 h × 4 for each cycle.

Radiation therapy (RT) was administered in fractions of 200 cGy per daily session for lesions located on limbs and head and neck areas and in fractions of 180 cGy for lesions located in the pelvis, abdomen, chest. RT was delivered for 5 consecutive days starting 2 h after the beginning of paclitaxel infusion and ending on the 5th day 2 h before the completion of the 96 h infusion.

The cycles of concomitant paclitaxel by continuous infusion and RT were administered every 14 days with occasional delays by 1 week if the absolute granulocyte count (AGC) was <2000/$\mu$l or the platelet count was <120 000/$\mu$l.

G-CSF (Neupogen-Amgen) at a dose of 7.5 $\mu$g/kg was administered subcutaneously (s.c.) daily between cycles starting 24 h after the completion of the paclitaxel infusion and ending 24 h before the next cycle of paclitaxel or whenever the AGC was >10 000/$\mu$l.

## 2.2. Patients on study

Twenty-six cycles of the combined concomitant paclitaxel–radiation therapy regimen were administered to 5 patients with advanced metastatic disease with various histology whose characteristics are schematically presented in Table 1.

There were 4 females and 1 male; their age varied between 46 and 71 and all but one had received one prior chemotherapy regimen following their initial diagnostic workup and surgical treatment. Only 1 patient with lymphoma received prior radiation therapy to a site (left axilla) relatively distant from the site of active disease that received radiation therapy while enrolled in the current study.

There were 2 patients with recurrent metastatic infiltrating ductal carcinoma of the breast. Both had large recurrent lesions on the chest wall scared after previous surgical resection of the primary breast tumor; patient G.H. underwent simple mastectomy 1 year before she developed the 7 × 5 cm chest wall recurrence while also having distant metastases in her bones and liver. In patient F.J. the chest wall recurrence (8 × 3 cm) developed 6 years

Table 1

Patients' characteristics

| Patient | Sex | Race | Age | Histologic. diagnosis | Metastasis | Serologic parameters | Prior surgery | Prior CT | Prior RT (cGy) |
|---------|-----|------|-----|----------------------|------------|---------------------|---------------|----------|----------------|
| J.S. | M | B | 52 | Squamous cell lung | Cervical mass | – | Radical neck | 0 | 0 |
| G.H. | F | B | 54 | Breast carcinoma | Chest wall | Ca15–3: 126 | Simple mastectomy | CAF | 0 |
| S.L. | F | W | 71 | Lymphoma | Pelvis | LDH: 385 $\mu$/dl | None | CHOP | 2500 |
| N.K. | F | B | 46 | Ovarian carcinoma | Pelvis | Ca125: 245 | Laparotomy TAH with BSO | Carbo-cytox. | 0 |
| F.J. | F | B | 70 | Breast carcinoma | Chest wall | Ca15–3: 280 | Modified radical mastectomy | CMF | 0 |

after she underwent modified radical mastectomy followed by cyclophosphamide–
methotrexate–5 fluorouracil (CMF) combination adjuvant chemotherapy.

One patient had sero mucinous adenocarcinoma of the ovary with a $10 \times 8$ cm recurrent
mass in the pelvis 2 years after total abdominal hysterectomy with bilateral salpingo-
ophorectomy for stage III carcinoma of the ovary which was followed by six cycles of carboplatin–cyclophosphamide chemotherapy.

One patient had stage II squamous cell carcinoma of the right upper lobe of the lung and
a recurrent $12 \times 5$ cm right cervical mass 3 years after glossectomy and radical neck dissection for squamous cell carcinoma of the base of the tongue.

Finally, a fifth patient had a recurrent non-Hodgkin's large cell diffuse lymphoma with a
$14 \times 12$ cm pelvic mass 2 years after being brought to clinical complete remission following
cyclophosphamide, doxorubicin (hydroxy-adriamycin), oncovin and prednisone (CHOP)
combination chemotherapy.

All but one patient (J.S.) had serologic monitors of their tumor size that also reflected
their response to treatment: Ca15–3 for the two cases of breast cancer, Ca-125 for the ovarian cancer patient, LDH for the patient with lymphoma.


## 3. Results

### 3.1. Determination of maximum tolerated dose

As can be seen in Table 2, three times the paclitaxel dose was increased in increments of
20 mg/m² per 96 h cycle. A fourth increment was of only 10mg/m² per 96 h above the dose
level of 140 mg/m² per 96 h.

At the first two levels of the paclitaxel (PTL) infusion dose, patients complained occasionally of paresthesias (see Table 3). These were represented by "pins and needles" sensations on the tips of their fingers and some of their toes lasting 2–3 days during the week
following the administration of paclitaxel.

Patients receiving 120 mg/m² over 96 h (second dose escalation) presented a moderate
degree of leukopenia (with the median nadir of the absolute granulocyte count (AGC) of
$900 \pm 700$ cells/$\mu$l) and mild thrombocytopenia (median platelet nadir at $105 \times 10^3/\mu$l) and

Table 2

Administration of paclitaxel(PTL) by continuous infusion in escalating doses

| PTL dose (mg/m² per 96 h) | No. of cycles | Patient | RT sites | RT dose (cGy/cycle) |
|---|---|---|---|---|
| 80 | 5:3 | J.S. | Neck mass | 1000 |
|  | 2 | G.H. | Anterior chest | 900 |
| 100 | 5:3 | G.H. | Anterior chest | 900 |
|  | 2 | J.S. | Neck mass | 900 |
| 120 | 5:3 | S.L. | Pelvis | 900 |
|  | 2 | N.K. | Pelvis | 900 |
| 140 | 6:3 | S.L. | Pelvis | 900 |
|  | 3 | F.J. | Anterior chest | 900 |
| 150 | 5:3 | F.J. | Anterior chest | 900 |
|  | 2 | N.K. | Pelvis | 900 |

Table 3

Major toxicities at escalating doses of paclitaxel (PTL) (percentage of cycles administered)

| PTL dose (mg/m$^2$ per 96 h) | Leukopenia | | Thrombocytopenia | | Paresthesias | Mucositis | Fever (>101°F) |
|---|---|---|---|---|---|---|---|
| | AGC <500/$\mu$l | Median nadir (×10$^3$/$\mu$l) | Platelets <60000/$\mu$l | Median nadir (×10$^3$/$\mu$l) | | | |
| 80 | 0/5 | 2.2 ± 1.1 | 0/5 | 136 ± 35 | Gr. I 1/5 20) | 0/5 | 0/5 |
| 100 | 0/5 | 1.4 ± 0.9 | 0/5 | 115 ± 24 | Gr. I 3/5 (60) | 0/5 | 0/5 |
| 120 | 0/5 | 0.9 ± 0.7 | 0/5 | 105 ± 21 | Gr. I 4/5 (80) Gr. II 1/5 (20) | 0/5 | 0/5 |
| 140 | 1/6 (16.5) | 0.7 ± 0.5 | 2/6 (33) | 86 ± 16 | Gr. I 4/6 (66) Gr. II 2/6 (33) | Gr. I 2/6 (33) | 0/6 |
| 150 | 2/5 (40) | 0.6 ± 0.4 | 2/5 (40) | 72 ± 18 | Gr. II 3/5 (60) Gr. III 2/5 (40) | Gr. II 2/5 (40) Gr. III 2/5 (40) | 3/5 (60) |

consistently developed paresthesias in their distant extremities. In one occasion paresthesia persisted throughout the interval between cycles of paclitaxel (grade II).

At the dose of 140 mg/m$^2$ per 96 h (third escalation) patients' thrombocytopenia and especially neutropenia were more significant. The median nadir of patients' granulocyte count was of 700 ± 500/$\mu$l; at this level we started prophylaxis for potential infections with cyprofloxacillin 500 mg p.o. bid, diflucan 200 mg p.o. qd and acyclovir 400 mg p.o. ×5/day. The WBCs recovered to normal by the 12–13th day of the cycle without the administration of growth factors. Patients' platelet count at 140 mg/m$^2$ per 96 h level reached a median nadir of 86 000 ± 16 000/$\mu$l and was not accompanied by any bleeding dyscrasia. At the same level all patients developed paresthesias in their distant extremities. After two of the cycles of paclitaxel the paresthesias were unrelentless (grade II) despite administration of thiamine.

At the same dose level after two of the cycles of paclitaxel administered with concomitant radiation therapy to the chest wall and in one occasion also to the neck, patients developed mild mucositis (grade I) manifested with mild dysphagia for solid food for 3–4 days and transient sore throat without fever.

At the next escalation of the paclitaxel dose (150 mg/m$^2$ per 96 h) patients developed more severe neutropenia with median nadir of the AGC of 600 ± 400/$\mu$l. After two cycles the granulocyte count was lower than 500/$\mu$l (230 and 340, respectively) and it took longer to recover to normal in the 19th and 20th day of the cycle, respectively. Febrile neutropenia occurred after 3 of the 5 cycles despite the administration of prophylactic anti-infectious therapy as for patients with neutropenia entered at the previous paclitaxel level. In one occasion patient also had rigors and positive blood and urine cultures for *Escherichia coli*. This patient was hospitalized for 1 week with urosepsis from which she rapidly recovered after 1 week of timentin i.v. infusion therapy.

Thrombocytopenia at the 150 mg/m$^2$ per 96 h level of paclitaxel was just mild with median nadir counts at 72 000 ± 18 000$\mu$l and rapid recovery (within 5 days).

All patients complained of paresthesias after all cycles of paclitaxel at 150 mg/m$^2$ per 96 h After two cycles paresthesias were severe in the patients' feet not allowing them to sleep at night for 3–5 nights in the week following the paclitaxel administration (grade III paresthesias).

Table 4

Response to therapy paclitaxel (PTL)–RT regimen

| Patient | Histology | Total RT dose (cGy) | Total PTL dose (mg/m$^2$) | Tumor size (cm) Before Rx | Tumor size (cm) After Rx | Serologic monitor | Before Rx | After Rx |
|---------|-----------|---------------------|---------------------------|---------------------------|--------------------------|-------------------|-----------|----------|
| J.S. | Squamous cell lung | 4800 | 440 | $12 \times 5$ | $3 \times 2$ | – | | |
| G.H. | Breast carcinoma | 4500 | 460 | $7 \times 5$ | 0 | Ca15–3: | 126 | 72 |
| S.L. | Lymphoma | 5400 | 780 | $14 \times 12$ | $5 \times 3$ | LDH | 385 | 290 |
| N.K. | Ovarian carcinoma | 4500 | 790 | $10 \times 8$ | $3 \times 1$ | Ca125: | 245 | 95 |
| F.J. | Breast carcinoma | 4500 | 720 | $8 \times 3$ | 0 | Ca15–3: | 280 | 45 |

After three of the cycles at 150 mg/m$^2$ per 96 h dose, patients also developed mild dysphagia for solid food and had moderate diarrhea (3–5 stools/day) that resolved within 3 days after administration of loperimide and kaopectate and appropriate diet.

Based on these toxicity data and aiming at a safe administration of the paclitaxel by continuous intravenous infusion and concomitant radiation therapy, we decided that a dose of paclitaxel of 130 mg/m$^2$ per 96 h with the concomitant delivery of a dose of radiation therapy of 180 cGy per daily session for 5 days in cycles repeated every 2 weeks represented the maximum tolerated dose (MTD). Granulocytopenia with a blood count less than 500/$\mu$l and grade II paresthesias with unrelentless sensations of painful foot numbness were the dose limiting toxicities at the 140 mg/m$^2$ per 96 h and at 150 mg/m$^2$ per 96 h.

### 3.2. Preliminary clinical responses

While the design of the reported study was exclusively that of a phase I dose finding protocol, a look at the tumor response to the administered antineoplastic therapy is of interest because it is suggestive of noticeable antineoplastic activity (Table 4). In two patients with metastatic breast carcinoma, the chest wall mass disappeared after 5 cycles of therapy. In the other 3 patients with malignant tumors of various histologies, ovarian cancer, squamous cell cancer of lung and neck and malignant large cell diffuse lymphoma, a reduction of the irradiated masses by more than 70% was noted. There were, however, no parameters to help us measure the contribution of the paclitaxel infusion to the effect of irradiation on these masses.

## 4. Discussion

The phase I study reported here was designed to determine the MTD of a concomitant radiation therapy and paclitaxel intravenous infusion based on previous investigations that have shown that paclitaxel acts as one of the most effective radiosensitizers so far tested in preclinical studies and that paclitaxel administration by continuous intravenous infusion is clinically feasible.

### 4.1. Paclitaxel concentration and exposure time dependent radiation sensitization

Among the in vitro studies that reported radiation sensitization by paclitaxel, Tischler et al.

[3] found a concentration dependent interaction between paclitaxel and radiation in an astrocytoma cell line (G-18). This interaction was found to be dependent on the paclitaxel exposure time; the sensitizing enhancing ratio of paclitaxel at 1 nmol/l was found to be 1.2 while at 10 nmol/l it rose to 1.8. Choy et al. [5,12] reported similar findings in a human leukemic cell line (HL-60). Using a somewhat different approach, Steren et al. showed [15] by flow cytometry an enhancement of radiation effect after paclitaxel exposure in several human ovarian cancer cell lines. Treatment with paclitaxel 48 h before radiation had greater effect than same treatment administered only 24 h before radiation. Proliferating cells were found to be more sensitive than confluent cells. Of interest is the fact that, in one cell line, paclitaxel, at a concentration of 5 nmol/l, despite not having effect on the cell cycle, had radiation sensitization effect with a sensitization enhancement ratio of 2.3. This suggests that the interaction between paclitaxel and radiation is not exclusively based on the cell cycle effects of this drug.

These studies and those previously mentioned of Hoffman [8] and Lopes [11] clearly indicated a potential advantage for radiosensitization by a continuous intravenous administration of paclitaxel as compared to its administration as a bolus or as a short infusion.

Previously reported clinical phase I studies of paclitaxel by continuous infusion in protracted periods helped us decide at what level to start the paclitaxel dose in the currently reported study of concomitant radiation therapy and continuous infusion paclitaxel. Wilson et al. [14] found that a dose of 140 mg/m$^2$ is the maximum tolerated dose when delivered over a 96-h period; the dose limiting toxicities were neutropenia and mucositis. In another study by Spriggs and Tondini [16], a 120 h schedule for continuous intravenous infusion of paclitaxel administered every 3 weeks was investigated. At 36 mg/m$^2$ per day (180 mg/m$^2$ per 5 days), 50% of patients developed grade 4 leukopenia and mucositis; the dose of 30 mg/m$^2$ per day for 5 days was recommended for further testing.

In choosing the schedule of continuous intravenous infusion of paclitaxel to be administered with concomitant radiation we preferred the 96 h schedule delivered every 2 weeks to the 120 h schedule delivered every 3 weeks because of the known decreased biologic effect related to the length of the interval between cycles of irradiation in patients receiving split courses of radiation therapy.

## 4.2. MTD of paclitaxel 96 h intravenous infusion–radiation therapy regimens

The data presented here indicate that the MTD for paclitaxel by intravenous infusion over 96 h administered concomitantly with a split course of daily standard radiation was reached at 130 mg/m$^2$ (32.5 mg/m$^2$ per day). At a dose immediately above this value, grade 4 granulocytopenia and severe paresthesias occurred.

## 4.3. Side effects of the radiation–paclitaxel 96 h i.v. infusion regimen

Overall, the toxicities induced by the radiation–paclitaxel 96 h continuous intravenous infusion were mild and rapidly reversible (see Table 3).

Paresthesias of distant extremities represented by "pins and needles" sensations and numbness were reported practically by all patients and developed after 80% of all cycles of the radiation–paclitaxel c.i. (RT-PTL c.i.) regimen. Protracted numbness of the feet intermittently painful and causing occasional erythromelalgia of the toes and fingers or severe nocturnal feet pain disrupting patients' sleep was reported after a few cycles at the last two levels of the paclitaxel dose escalation (150 and 140 mg/m$^2$ per 96 h) and just on one occasion at a lower level of 120 mg/m$^2$ per 96 h.

This more severe grade 2 peripheral neuropathy resolved slowly within 2–6 months after completion of the whole regimen; it was treated with thiamine 100 mg. p.o. tid; in the case of erythromelalgia or foot pain we also administered Tegretol (carbamazepine) tbs 200 mg p.o. bid.

Mild to moderate leukopenia developed as expected after all cycles of paclitaxel. Its degree of intensity was related to the total paclitaxel dose. The median nadir of granulocytes was $2.2 \times 10^3$ cells/$\mu$l after 80 mg/m$^2$ per 96 h of paclitaxel, $1.4 \times 10^3$ cells/$\mu$l after 100 mg/m$^2$ per 96 h, $0.9 \times 10^3$ cells/$\mu$l after 120 mg/m$^2$ per 96 h and $0.7 \times 10^3$ cells/$\mu$l after 140 mg/m$^2$ per 96 h of paclitaxel. Grade 4 neutropenia with granulocyte counts lower than 500/$\mu$l occurred only once at 140 mg/m$^2$ per 96 h dose level and twice at 150 mg/m$^2$ per 96 h. On three occasions the leukopenia was accompanied by fever just at the highest dose level tested. The fever was due to sepsis on just one occasion. The nadir of granulocyte counts occurred between the 9th and 11th day of each cycle and was followed by a rapid recovery before day 14 of the cycle. On just one occasion, at the highest dose level tested, the recovery occurred within 21 days and required the postponement of the following cycle of RT-PTL c.i. regimen.

Thrombocytopenia has been less significant; although present after all cycles, it was never more severe than grade 2, recovered promptly within 12 days from the start of each cycle and was never accompanied by clinical manifestations like petecchiae, ecchymoses or overt bleeding.

Mucositis of the esophagus manifested with moderate dysphagia occurred on three occasions all in patients receiving radiation to the neck or chest wall. Mucositis of the oropharynx and bowel manifested with sore throat, cheilitis and grade II diarrhea (2–5 bowel movements/day with watery stools) occurred after only two cycles at the highest dose level tested. Milder diarrhea occurred occasionally at lower doses of paclitaxel.

A correlation between the increase in the intensity of the side effects developed during and after the administration of 96 h infusion has been with the increase in the dose of paclitaxel delivered; similar correlation was reported also by others only for the protracted infusion of paclitaxel [14].

### 4.4.  *Pharmacokinetics of paclitaxel continuous intravenous infusion*

The above mentioned finding is at variance with the observations made in patients receiving short infusions of paclitaxel over 1 or 3 h, for which it has been convincingly demonstrated that the drug pharmacokinetics are non-linear [17–19]. This non-linearity indicates that dose-normalized concentrations versus time profiles are not superimposable and a disproportional relationship exists between changes in the dose and the resulting peak concentrations and the area under the curve (AUC) of drug concentration. The non-linear pharmacokinetic processes in the case of paclitaxel can be described by the Michaelis–Menton kinetics model [19,20]. Estimates can be generated for the parameters: $V_{max}$ (the maximum process rate) and $K_m$ (the concentration or amount associated with one-half $V_{max}$). At concentrations below $K_m$, like the ones administered in the currently reported study, the process approximates a proportional or linear rate. As the concentration exceeds $K_m$ and the maximum rate ($V_{max}$) is approached, the process proceeds at increasingly disproportional rates. In these conditions, for instance, as the paclitaxel dose is increased from 135 to 175 mg/m$^2$ both the peak plasma paclitaxel concentration and the AUC increase at a much steeper rate by 80 and 70%, respectively, while the dose of the 3 h infusion increased only by 30%.

These paclitaxel kinetics following the Michaelis–Menton model explains why it is generally easier to adjust the dose of the drug to the intensity of the occurring side effects without significantly compromising the paclitaxel efficacy in patients receiving protracted (96 h and above) intravenous infusions than in those receiving short 1 or 3 h infusions.

These pharmacokinetics data also suggest that an even longer infusion of paclitaxel could permit an easier adjustment of the total dose administered to the patients' renal function due to its direct relationship with the variations of the drug AUC and to the intensity of the side effects they develop.

## 5.   Future directions

We and others [21] are currently in the process of testing the administration of paclitaxel by continuous infusion over the entire course of standard radiation therapy administration testing the hypothesis that this could further improve the synergistic antineoplastic effect of radiation therapy and concomitant intravenous infusion of paclitaxel which could lead to improved survival data. This regimen has become feasible since containers made of paclitaxel non-degrading material became available for the portable ambulatory pumps. The dose limiting toxicity has not yet been reached in these studies in which the starting dose has been low at 3 and 4 mg/m$^2$ per day.

## 6.   Conclusions

The study reported here showed the feasibility of the continuous paclitaxel intravenous infusion administration with concomitant radiation therapy as a split course with 96 h cycles repeated every 2 weeks and determined its MTD. Future investigations will determine how this schedule of administration, permitting the delivery of a relatively high total dose of paclitaxel, will compare with a lower dose of paclitaxel administered by continuous infusion throughout the whole standard (non-split) course of radiation therapy.

### Summary

Paclitaxel the first taxane used for its antineoplastic effect against many solid tumors due to its binding to the $\beta$ subunit of tubulin was also found to enhance the cytotoxic effects of ionizing radiation in vitro [3] (this effect could occur in the absence of morphologic changes in microtubules at lower drug concentrations still capable of arresting cells in G2/M phase, the most radiosensitive phase of the cell cycle. Previous reports suggested that a continuous intravenous infusion (c.i.) of paclitaxel of 140 mg/m$^2$ over 96 h leads to a steady state concentration in the serum of approximately $109 \pm 019 \,\mu$M [14]. We decided to determine the effect of a 96 h infusion of paclitaxel while administered concomitantly with RT in patients with lymphoma or with measurable metastatic lesions from ovary, breast and lung primary tumors, that were not previously irradiated. Here, we report the results of this phase I study. Paclitaxel was administered in doses escalating from 80 mg/m$^2$ in 20 and 10 mg increments each 5 cycles. RT was delivered at a dose of 180 cGy for 5 consecutive days while pacli-taxel was running. G-CSF (7.5 $\mu$/kg) was administered s.c. daily starting 48 h after the pa-clitaxel infusion. The cycle of RT with concomitant paclitaxel was restarted usually on day 14 or 21 from the prior cycle as soon as AGC was stable at >2500/$\mu$l while the patient was off G-CSF for at least 2 days. A 150 mg/m$^2$ per 96 h paclitaxel we encountered grade 4 neutropenia in 2/5 cycles (AGC < 100/$\mu$l) and grade 3 mucositis in two cases in whom the esophagus was tangentially irradiated. At 140 mg/m$^2$ over 96 h granulocytopenia was still significant (AGC 700 ± 500/$\mu$l) and after one cycle the AGC dropped under 500/$\mu$l (grade 4 neutropenia); in two cases severe paresthesias were also reported. No hypersensitizing reac-tion was registered while patients received daily i.v. cimetidine 300 mg, benadryl (25 mg i.v. PB q 8 h) and dexamethasone (20 mg p.o.) 12 and 6 h before paclitaxel administration. It is concluded that the MTD for paclitaxel administered as a 96 h continuous i.v. infusion with concomitant RT is 130 mg/m$^2$. This regimen can be repeated every 14 days if G-CSF is also administered 48 h after completion of paclitaxel. The pharmacokinetics of the pacli-taxel continuous intravenous infusion are reviewed.

## References

1.   Schiff PB, Fant J, Horwitz SB. Promotion of microtubule assembly in vitro by Taxol. Nature 277: 665–667, 1979.
2.   Schiff PB, Horwitz SB. Taxol stabilizes microtubules in mouse fibroblast cells. Proc Natl Acad Sci USA 77: 1561–1565, 1980.
3.   Tischler RB, Geard R, Hall EJ, et al. Taxol sensitizes human astrocytoma cells to radiation. Cancer Res 52: 3495–3492, 1992.
4.   Tischler RB, Schiff PB, Geard CR, et al. Taxol: a novel radiation sensitizer. Int J Radiat Oncol Biol Phys 22: 613–617, 1992.
5.   Choy H, Rodriguez FF, Koester S, et al. Investigation of Taxol as a potential radiation sensitizer. Cancer 71: 3774–3778, 1993.
6.   Choy H, Akerley W, Safron H, et al. Phase I trial of outpatient weekly paclitaxel and concurrent radiation therapy for advanced non small cell lung cancer. J Clin Oncol 12: 2682–2686, 1994.
7.   Rambhia H, Aziz H, Rotman M, Rosenthal CJ. Paclitaxel 96 h i.v. infusion with concomitant radiation therapy - phase I study (abstr 1535). Proc Am Soc Cancer Oncol 14: 473, 1995.
8.   Hoffman W, Rodeman HP, Balka C, et al. Paclitaxel in simultaneous radiochemotherapy of head and neck cancer: preclinical and clinical results. Semin Oncol 24(Suppl 2): 72–77, 1997.
9.   Vokes EE, Stupp R, Haraf D, et al. Hydroxyurea with continuous infusion paclitaxel, 5 fluorouracil and concomitant radiotherapy for poor prognosis head and neck cancer. Semin Oncol 22(Suppl 6): 47–52, 1995.
10.  Rosenthal DI, Carbone DP. Taxol plus radiation for head and neck cancer. J Infus Chemother 5: 46–54, 1995.
11.  Lopes NM, Adams EG, Pitts TW, et al. Cell kill kinetics and cell cycle effects of Taxol on human and hamster ovarian cell lines. Cancer Chemother Pharmacol 32: 235–242, 1993.
12.  Choy H, Browne MJ. Paclitaxel as a radiation sensitizer in non small cell lung cancer. Semin Oncol 22(Suppl 6): 70–74, 1995.
13.  Lieberman J, Cook JA, Fisher J, et al. In vitro studies of Taxol as radiation sensitizer in human tumor cells. J Natl Cancer Inst 86: 441–446, 1994.
14.  Wilson WH, Berg SI, Bryant G, et al. Paclitaxel in doxorubicin-refractory or mitoxantrone - refractory breast cancer: a phase I/II trial of 96 h infusion. J Clin Oncol 12: 1621–1629, 1994.
15.  Steren A, Sevin BU, Perras J, et al. Taxol as radiation sensitizer: a flow cytometric study. Gynecol Oncol 50 (Suppl 1): 89–93, 1993.
16.  Spriggs DR, Tondini C. Taxol administered as a 120 hour infusion. Invest New Drugs 10: 275–278, 1992.

17.   Gianni L, Kearns CM, Giani A, et al. Non Linear pharmacokinetics and metabolism of paclitaxel and its pharmacokinetic/pharmacodynamic relationships in humans. J Clin Oncol 13: 180–190, 1995.

18.   Sonnichsen DS, Hurwitz CA, Pratt CB, et al. Saturable pharmacokinetics and paclitaxel pharmacodynamics in children with solid tumors. J Clin Oncol 12: 532–538, 1994.

19.   Kearns CM, Gianni L, Egorin MJ. Paclitaxel pharmacokinetics and pharmacodynamics. Semin Oncol 22(Suppl 6): 16–23, 1995.

20.   Ludden TM. Nonlinear pharmacokinetics clinical implications. Clin Pharmacokinet 20: 429–446, 1991.

21.   Rosenthal DI, Okani O, Truelson JM, et al. Intensive radiation therapy concurrent with up to 7 week continuous infusion paclitaxel for locally advanced solid tumors: phase I study. Semin Oncol 24(Suppl 2): 81–84, 1997.

C.J. Rosenthal and M. Rotman (Eds.), *Infusion Chemotherapy–Irradiation Interactions*

# CHAPTER 13

# Doxorubicin as radiation potentiator: concurrent doxorubicin and radiation therapy interaction and its clinical applications

LI-TEH WU

*Department of Medicine, Long Island College Hospital, 339 Hicks Street, Brooklyn, NY 11201, USA*

## 1. Doxorubicin, mechanism of cytotoxicity

Doxorubicin has been one of the most commonly used anti-neoplastic agents for many years. The mechanism of its cytotoxic activity remains controversial. Although DNA single-strand breaks (ssb) and double-strand breaks (dsb) caused by inhibition of topoisomerase II have been accepted by most investigators as the most important mechanism [1], doxorubicin was also shown to inhibit helicase [2], which separates double strand DNA into single strand DNA before replication. Doxorubicin also interferes with topoisomerase independent DNA unwinding and inhibits DNA synthesis [3]. The concentration of doxorubicin required to inhibit these enzymes can be easily achieved clinically. As other quinones, doxorubicin can mediate free radical formation including superoxide anion, hydroxyl radical, and others. Damage induced by these free radicals to DNA, lipid membrane, and proteins was thought to be the main cause of cardiac toxicity [4]. More recent laboratory data suggest free radical formation may play an important role in its antineoplastic activity [5,6]. Furthermore, doxorubicin has high affinity for phospholipid and affect cell membrane directly and causes cytotoxicity without entering cells [7].

## 2. Interaction between doxorubicin and radiation

The effect of doxorubicin and radiation on cells seems to be similar. Radiation causes ssb and dsb in DNA. Double-strand breaks are most closely correlated with radiation cyto-toxicity [8]. Damage to lipid membrane and other macromolecules may contribute to its cytotoxic effects . The repair of radiation induced DNA damage is responsible for the treatment failure in human cancers. Watring et al. had demonstrated in the early 1970s that doxorubicin made a radiation survival curve shift to the left in tissue culture [9]. The left shift was mainly due to a decrease in the width of the shoulder [10]. Depending on the cell lines, either the repair of radiation-induced sublethal damage is inhibited or inde-pendent classes of damage are created by doxorubicin [11]. DNA unwinding and helicase are required in the repair of sublethal damage, including dsb rejoining and repair replica-tion, which are affected by doxorubicin [12,13]. The net effect of the combination of doxorubicin and radiation is either synergistic or additive. Multicellular spheroids, which resemble human cancer more closely than regular tissue culture, have demonstrated a synergistic effect between doxorubicin and radiation. In this particular situation, oxygen consumption by cells in the outer layers is inhibited by doxorubicin and permits oxygen tension increase in previously hypoxic inner layer cells which makes them more radiation sensitive [14,15].

Both radiation and doxorubicin can produce apoptosis and cells with defects in apoptosis, such as p53 inactivation, were shown to be resistant to both radiation and doxorubicin [16]. This may imply that cancer cells resistant to doxorubicin will be resistant to radiation and vice versa. But there are reports demonstrating that doxorubicin resistant cell lines exhibit variable radiation responses. Actually some of the cell lines showed significant increase in radiation sensitivity [17–19] and others showed that the degree of doxorubicin resistance could be reduced by pre-radiation [20].

## 3. Concurrent doxorubicin and radiation, early clinical experience

While laboratory evidence supporting that doxorubicin given right before or throughout radiation was either synergistic or additive was confirmed, clinical trials of this combination began shortly after. In the early trials, Chan et al. demonstrated that doxorubicin, either 40 mg/m$^2$ every 3 weeks or 13 mg/m$^2$ each week with concurrent radiation was safe and effective in lung cancer and ovarian cancer [9,21,22]. Eleven out of 35 lung cancer patients achieved complete response and another 12 had partial response. Toxicity to skin and esophagus occurred with higher dose of doxorubicin and progressive bowel fibrosis occurred in patients received pelvic radiation. EKG change occurred in one patient who received radiation to more than 50% of heart volume. Subsequently, concurrent doxorubicin containing chemotherapy and radiation has been applied to many different types of cancer, specially in soft tissue sarcoma.

## 4. Concurrent doxorubicin and radiation, in soft tissue sarcoma

Because soft tissue sarcoma is moderately sensitive to doxorubicin and radiation, combination of both agents may offer synergistic effect. Doxorubicin has been given intravenously or intraarterially, pre-operatively or post-operatively. This subject has been extensively reviewed in Dr. Toma's chapter. A recent publication from Kempe et al. showed pre-operative intravenous doxorubicin containing chemotherapy and concurrent radiation for synovial sarcoma made all patients able to undergo limb-sparing surgery. Local recurrence occurred in only 1 out of 14 treated patients after a median followup of 37 months [23]. Eilber et al. reported intraarterial doxorubicin and radiation before surgery for high grade soft tissue sarcoma. Only 5% of patients required amputation as compared with 22% in historical control. The local recurrence rate was 8–14% [24]. More recently, a Southeastern cancer study group reported 66 patients undergoing neoadjuvant intraarterial infusion of doxorubicin 30 mg/24 h for 3 days and radiation. Sixty patients were able to have limb sparing surgery, but wound complication occurred in 41% of patients. Distant metastasis still occurred, but the local control rate was 98.5% [25].

## 5. Concurrent doxorubicin and radiation, in thyroid carcinoma

Another cancer where concurrent doxorubicin and radiation has made a major difference is anaplastic thyroid carcinoma. Anaplastic giant and spindle cell carcinoma is one of the most lethal cancers in human. Most tumors are unresectable at presentation. Only a handful of patients have achieved local control with aggressive radiation and chemotherapy. The median survival usually is less than 4 months. Kim et al. treated 19 patients with anaplastic giant and spindle cell thyroid carcinoma with weekly doxorubicin 10 mg/m$^2$ 1.5 h before hyperfractionated radiation. Eighty-four percent achieved complete response and most of them remained free of local recurrence. The median survival was 1 year and most of the deaths were from distant metastasis. This treatment was very well tolerated and the main toxicities were transient pharynesophagitis, tracheitis and skin reaction at the radiated field. No patients experienced cardiac or other systemic toxicity, such as hair loss and reduction of blood counts. No long term toxicity was seen in this group of patients either [26]. The author has treated a patient with anaplastic thyroid carcinoma who required an emergent tracheostomy shortly after presentation with a rapidly enlarging neck mass. Modified Kim's regimen, i.e., doxorubicin 10 mg/m$^2$ weekly plus cisplatin 20 mg/m$^2$ per day for 5 consecutive days monthly and concurrent radiation, was used. This patient had a complete response and has remained disease free for more than 3 years. Mucositis and skin breakdown at the neck were the significant acute toxicities. The tracheostomy was successfully closed without stricture. Kim's group also applied their regimen on well-differentiated papillary and follicular thyroid carcinoma relapsed locally after surgery and radioiodine treatment. A 91% complete response rate and 77% 2 year local tumor control rate were achieved [26].

## 6. Toxicities of the concurrent treatment

Experimentally and clinically, addition of doxorubicin to radiation increases radiation's antineoplastic effect. It is expected that this combination will cause more toxicities to normal tissue, specially to the intestine and heart when radiation is applied to the abdomen or thorax [21,27]. It has been demonstrated that even sequential treatment with doxorubicin applied before radiation can cause more radiation pneumonitis [28]. Doxorubicin, by itself, can cause cardiomyopathy. But its cardiac toxicity is significantly increased in patients who had received previous mediastinal radiation, even in the remote past. This recall phenomenon of latent radiation damage by doxorubicin was demonstrated in small intramyocardial vessels by endomyocardial biopsies [29,30]. The same radiation recall phenomenon has been observed in other tissues, such as skin and lung, in human and experimental animals [31]. To reduce the doxorubicin cardiac toxicity, Legha et al. used continuous infusion of doxorubicin over 48–96 h. Patients were able to take a much higher cumulative dose of doxorubicin, 660 mg/m$^2$ versus 470 mg/m$^2$ with standard bolus schedule. Significant pathological changes at endomyocardial biopsy were seen only in patients received previous mediastinal radiation. Antitumor activity of the continuous infusion of doxorubicin was not compromised [32].

## 7. Continuous infusion of doxorubicin with concurrent radiation

To take this approach one step further, Rosenthal et al. has pioneered 5-day continuous infusion of doxorubicin at 12 mg/m$^2$ per day with concurrent radiation in a variety of cancers. Doxorubicin was given every 3–4 weeks. Radiation was given each time doxorubicin was administered. The plateau doxorubicin serum concentration was 60 ng/ml. The maximal tolerated cumulative dose was 840 mg/m$^2$. Four out of 11 patients with soft tissue sarcoma in the extremities or trunk achieved complete response and another 4 achieved partial response and the remaining 3 were in stable disease. All had doxorubicin and some had radiation before. The total dose of radiation required to achieve response was 15–30 Gy which was far lower than the usual 60 Gy when radiation was used alone. Complete response was also seen in patients who failed previous radiation. Response has been quite durable. Three complete responders remained free of disease for more than 3 years. None of the responders had a relapse at the radiated site despite the low dose of radiation [33]. In addition, Stark et al. reported that with the same 5 days continuous infusion of doxorubicin and radiation, repeated every 3–4 weeks for 3 cycles, 4 out of 8 patients with hepatoma limited to liver achieved partial response. The total dose of radiation to the liver was between 25 and 28 Gy. Median duration of response was 36 weeks [34]. Acute toxicities are alopecia, moderate mucositis with dysphagia or diarrhea, skin erythema, transient elevation of liver function test, and grade 2–3 myelosuppression. Decrease in ventricular ejection fraction and pulmonary fibrosis only occurred in one patient who received 45 Gy radiation to the mediastinum [33].

## 8. Conclusions

The synergistic effect between doxorubicin and radiation has been demonstrated in several cancers that are most difficult to treat, as has been discussed here. Although toxicity of this combination may be higher, it has been manageable. With the advance of continuous infusion of doxorubicin, its safety and efficacy have been further improved. WR 2721 and ICRF 187 have been approved for clinical use. Incorporating these chemotherapy and radiation protectors to the concurrent doxorubicin and radiation therapy might eliminate most of the side-effects and make this treatment applicable to more cancers in future clinical trials.

## References

1. Pommier Y. DNA topoisomerase I and II in cancer chemotherapy: update and perspectives. Cancer Chemother Pharmacol 32: 103, 1993.
2. Bachur NR, Yu F, Johnson R, et al. Helicase inhibition by anthracycline anticancer agents. Mol Pharmacol 41: 993, 1992.
3. Fornari FA, Randolph JK, Yalowich JC, et al. Interference by doxorubicin with DNA unwinding in MCF-7 breast tumor cells. Mol Pharmacol 45: 649–656, 1994.
4. Doroshow JH, Locker GY, Myers CE, et al. Enzymatic defenses of the mouse heart against reactive oxygen metabolites: alterations produced by doxorubicin. J Clin Invest 65: 128, 1980.
5. Sinha BK, Mimnaugh EG, Rajagopalan S, et al. Adriamycin activation and oxygen free radical formation in human breast tumor cells: protective role of glutathione peroxidase in adriamycin resistance. Cancer Res 49: 3844, 1989.
6. Taylor SD, Davenport LD, Speranza MJ, et al. Glutathione peroxidase protects cultured mammalian cells from the toxicity of adriamycin and paraquat. Arch Biochem Biophys 305: 600, 1993.
7. Tritton TR, Yee G. The anticancer agent adriamycin can be actively cytotoxic without entering cells. Science 217: 248, 1982.

8.  Radford IR. Evidence for a general relationship between the induced level of DNA double-strand breakage and cell killing after x-irradiation of mammalian cells. Int J Radiat Biol 49: 611, 1986.

9.  Watring WG, Byfield JE, Lagasse LD, et al. Combination adriamycin and radiation therapy in gynecologic cancers. Gynecol Oncol 2: 518–526, 1974.

10. Bistrovic M, Nagy Z, et al. Interaction of adriamycin and radiation in combined treatment on mouse L-cells. Eur J Cancer 14: 411–414, 1978.

11. Belli JA, Piro AJ. The interaction between radiation and adriamycin damage in mammalian cells. Cancer Res 37: 1624–1630, 1977.

12. Lee YC, Byfield JE, Bennett LR. X-ray repair replication in L1210 leukemic cells. Cancer Res 34: 2624–2633, 1974.

13. Bonner JA, Lawrence TS. Doxorubicin decreases the repair of radiation induced DNA damage. Int J Radiat Biol 57: 55–64, 1990.

14. Durand RE. Adriamycin: a possible indirect radiosensitizer of hypoxic tumor cells. Radiology 119: 217–222, 1976.

15. Durand RE, Vanderbyl SL. Sequencing radiation and adriamycin exposures in spheroids to maximize therapeutic gain. Int J Radiat Oncol Biol Phys 17: 345–350, 1989.

16. Lowe SW, Bodis S, McClatchey A, et al. p53 status and the efficacy of cancer therapy in vivo. Science 266: 807–810, 1994.

17. Belli JA. Interaction between radiation and drug damage in mammalian cells. Radiat Res 119: 88–100, 1989.

18. Belli JA, Harris JR. Adriamycin resistance and radiation response. Int J Radiat Oncol Biol Phys 5: 1231–1234, 1979.

19. Zhang Y, Sweet KM, Sognier MA, et al. Interaction between radiation and drug damage in mammalian cells. Radiat Res 132: 105–111, 1992.

20. Sognier MA, Zhang Y, Eberle RL, et al. Sequestration of doxorubicin in vesicles in a multi-drug-resistant cell line. Biochem Pharmacol 48: 391–401, 1994.

21. Chan PYM, Bffield, JE, Lemkin SR, et al. Coincident adriamycin and X-ray therapy in bronchogenic carcinoma: response and cardiotoxicity. Am Soc Clin Oncol 17: 276, 1976.

22. Byfield JE, Watring WG, Lemkin SR, et al. Adriamycin: a useful adjuvant drug for combination with radiation therapy. Am Soc Clin Oncol 16: 253, 1975.

23. Kampe CE, Rosen G, Eilber F, et al. Synovial sarcoma. Cancer 72: 2161–2169, 1993.

24. Eilber FR, Giuliano A, Huth J, et al. Neoadjuvant chemotherapy, radiation, and limited surgery for high grade soft tissue sarcoma of the extremity. Recent concepts in sarcoma treatment. In: Proc Int Symp Sarcomas. Tarpon Springs, FL, 1987. Dordrecht: Kluwer, 1988.

25. Wanebo HJ, Temple WJ, Popp MB, et al. Preoperative regional therapy for extremity sarcoma. A tricenter update. Cancer 75: 2299–2306, 1995.

26. Kim JH, Leeper RD. Treatment of locally advanced thyroid carcinoma with combination doxorubicin and radiation therapy. Cancer 60: 2372–2375, 1987.

27. Phillips TL, Wharam MD, Margolis LW. Modification of radiation injury to normal tissue by chemotherapeutic agents. Cancer 35:1678–1684, 1975.

28. Mah K, Keane TJ, Van-Dyk J, et al. Quantitative effect of combined chemotherapy and fractionated radiotherapy on the incidence of radiation induced lung damage. Int J Radiat Oncol Biol Phys 28: 563–74, 1994.

29. Phillip TL, Fu KK. Quantification of combined radiation therapy and chemotherapy effects on critical normal tissues. Cancer 37: 1186–1200, 1976.

30. Billingham ME, Bristow MR, Glastein E, et al. Adriamycin cardiotoxicity: endomyocardial biopsy evidence of enhancement by irradiation. Am J Surg Pathol 1: 17, 1977.

31. Vegesna V, Withers HR, McBride WH, et al. Adriamycin induced recall of radiation pneumonitis and epilation in lung and hair follicles of mouse. Int J Radiat Oncol Biol Phys 23: 977–981, 1992.

32. Legha SS, Benjamin RS, Mackay B, et al. Reduction of doxorubicin cardiotoxicity by continuous intravenous infusion. Ann Int Med 96: 133–139, 1982.

33. Rosenthal CJ, Rotman M. Concomitant continuous infusion adriamycin and radiation: evidence of synergistic effects in soft tissue sarcomas. In: Rotman M, Rosenthal CJ (Eds), Concomitant Continuous Infusion Chemotherapy and Radiation. Berlin: Springer, pp. 271–280, 1991.

34. Stark RS, Rosenthal CJ, Rotman M. Infusion adriamycin and radiation in hepatoma. In: Rotman M, Rosenthal CJ (Eds), Concomitant Continuous Infusion Chemotherapy and Radiation. Berlin: Springer, pp. 281–284, 1991.

# SECTION II

## ORGAN SALVAGE AFTER TREATMENT WITH IRRADIATION AND CONCOMITANT INFUSION CHEMOTHERAPY IN LOCALLY ADVANCED MALIGNANT TUMORS

*"The pen is mightier than the sword! The case for prescriptions rather than surgery."*

Marvin Kitman

C.J. Rosenthal and M. Rotman (Eds.), *Infusion Chemotherapy–Irradiation Interactions*

# CHAPTER 14

# Is organ salvage in advanced disease possible?

## MAURICE TUBIANA

*The Centre Antoine Béclère, 45 rue des Saints-Pères, 75006 Paris, France*

## 1. Introduction

Improvement of long term survival remains the goal of therapeutic research; however another important objective is to improve the quality of life. Towards this aim, preservation of organ function is essential in a large number of cancer sites such as the anus, rectum, bladder, upper respiratory and digestive tract, esophagus, and breast. Even in tumor types with low long term survival, avoidance of mutilation is beneficial if the survival rate is not lowered and treatment sequelae are acceptable.

This introductory chapter intends to show that organ preservation is feasible in a fair proportion of patients (from 1/3 to 2/3), even in advanced cancers, without jeopardizing survival. However, this can only be done using elaborate strategies that vary in relation to cancer types, which is discussed in the other chapters in this section. This overview is limited to a few general considerations in the light of personal experience and a few recent studies.

The main hazard of conservative treatment is lack of local control since residual disease and local recurrence can originate metastatic dissemination [1,2].

## 2. The contribution of radiotherapy and chemotherapy to local control

Local control in small tumors is relatively easy to achieve with conservative surgery and radiotherapy (RT) and/or combination of RT + chemotherapy (CT). In patients with bulky tumors, recurrence at the site of previous tumor involvement occurs frequently. The tumor resection is often macroscopically or microscopically incomplete when, in order to avoid mutilation, surgery is not radical. The combination with other therapeutic modalities becomes mandatory and in particular when surgery has been associated with CT alone or when the dose of RT has been too low.

An error which is frequently made is to overestimate the impact of CT and the significance of complete remission (CR). A high radiation dose remains necessary even when induction CT has achieved a CR. A CR means only that the tumor is not clinically or radiologically detectable; it may still contain many hundred millions of cells. A simple calculation will illustrate the respective role of RT and CT in the local control of a tumor [3]. Let us consider a tumor of 100 g in which 1% of the tumor cells are clonogenic. If the radiosensitivity of the tumor is within the average range ($D_{50}$ of the cells equal to 2 Gy), the tumor control dose (TCD) is approximately 60 Gy in 30 fractions. When the number of cells is

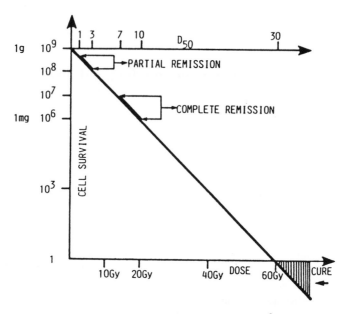

Fig. 1. Proportion of surviving cells in an irradiated tumor containing $10^9$ clonogenic tumor cells. The dose is expressed either in the number of lethal dose 50% (upper horizontal scale) or in gray, assuming that the lethal dose 50% is equal to 2 Gy. It is seen that after a partial remission, the proportion of surviving cells is so high that the dose which is necessary for producing a tumor control is only slightly reduced. A complete remission means only that the tumor is not clinically detectable, it may still contain a high number of cells.

reduced by half after CT, which corresponds to a partial remission, the dose needed is 58 Gy; it is still 54 Gy if 90% of the tumor cells have been killed which corresponds to a marked regression of the tumor size under CT. It is only when CT has achieved a complete remission of the tumor (residual tumor mass smaller than 100 mg) that RT given to eradicate the remaining subclinical disease can be reduced to 20 $D_{50}$ (40 Gy) (Fig. 1, Table 1). If the tumor is radioresistant ($D_{50} = 3$ Gy under fractionated irradiation with dose per fraction equal to 2 Gy), the corresponding doses are 90, 87, 81, and 60 Gy, respectively. For radio-

Table 1

Tumor dose which is required for the control of a tumor containing $10^9$ clonogenic tumor cells when radiotherapy is used alone or when it is delivered following one or several courses of chemotherapy which have produced a partial or a complete remission

|  | Tumor control dose (Gy) | |
|  | $D_{50}$: 2 Gy | $D_{50}$: 3 Gy |
| --- | --- | --- |
| RT used alone | 60 | 90 |
| CT has induced partial remission | | |
| Cell kill 50%58 | 87 | |
| Cell kill 90% | 54 | 81 |
| CT has induced complete remission ($10^{-3}$) | 40 | 60 |
| (residual tumor $\leq 10$ mg) | | |

Table 2

Recurrence rate in para-aortic lymph nodes in patients with supradiaphragmatic HD

| RT | CT = O (%) | CT = VLB (%) | CT = H + MOPP (%) |
|---|---|---|---|
| O | 19 | 12 | 8 |
| + | 3 | | 1 |

From Tubiana et al. [4]. Comparison of the recurrent rate in para-aortic lymph nodes in four series of patients with Hodgkin's disease Stages I + II treated either by supradiaphragmatic irradiation, the same irradiation plus vinblastine (VLB) or MOPP, or extended radiotherapy (mantle field + para-aortic irradiation). Eighteen hundred patients were included in these three consecutive controlled clinical trials.

resistant tumors, the TCD can be reduced below the dose tolerated by the normal tissues only when CT produces a complete remission.

However, this reasoning is overoptimistic because it assumes that the radiation tolerance dose is not reduced by the toxic effect induced by CT. Most drugs cause some damage to the normal tissues located in the irradiated volume and a combination of CT and RT can improve the local control of the tumor only when the cumulative toxicity of drugs and radiation allows the delivery of a radiation TCD to the residual tumor.

A few clinical data can help estimate the relative contribution of CT and RT for those patients in whom the tumors are both chemosensitive and radiosensitive. The cumulative effect of the two modalities on the malignant tissues can be assessed by comparing the incidence of local recurrence in the irradiated lymph-node areas in patients treated by RT alone or by combination of CT + RT within the three EORTC clinical trials on early-stage Hodgkin's disease (HD) (Table 2) [4]. In each of these three trials, the relapse rate was approximately halved in patients treated by CT + RT, from approximately 8% in patients treated by RT alone to 4%. This difference is statistically significant ($P = 0.0017$), but is not very large, even for this very chemosensitive tumor. The respective effectiveness of RT and CT given alone can be approximately assessed for para-aortic lymph nodes in patients with supradiaphragmatic HD. When a lymphangiogram does not detect the presence of neoplastic disease in these sites, which means that the maximum tumor mass is less than 200 mg, several therapeutic strategies have been followed during the past three decades, and a comparison of the incidence of relapse in this region can give an estimate of the efficacy of the various treatments. When patients were treated only by supradiaphragmatic irradiation, the incidence of relapse in this untreated nodal area was equal to 19%; in the other arm of the trial, in which patients received the same RT followed by a course of non-aggressive mono-CT, the incidence of relapse was 12% [4]. When supradiaphragmatic RT is combined with aggressive multiple CT by MOPP, the incidence is 8%; when this area receives a so-called prophylactic irradiation without CT, it is equal to 3% [5]; and finally, following the combination of CT and prophylactic irradiation, it is approximately 1%. However, it should be emphasized that Hodgkin's disease is a tumor which is both highly chemosensitive and radiosensitive [6]. Therefore these results cannot be extrapolated to most solid tumors. The association of CT and RT often provides such a small gain in survival that it is not significant in controlled clinical trials including a few hundred patients and can be evidenced only by meta-analyses. For example, in patients with non-small cell lung cancer, it was a meta-analysis carried out in 1995 on over 9000 patients which demonstrated a 4% reduction in mortality in patients treated by RT + CT as compared to patients treated by RT alone [7].

Two meta-analyses were carried out in order to analyze the data provided by the association of CT and RT in patients with head and neck cancers. In the Munro meta-analysis [8], which gathered 54 trials, the reduction of mortality was equal to 6.5% in patients treated by RT + CT as compared to those treated by RT alone; however this reduction was higher in those treated by concurrent administration of the two therapeutic modalities than in those receiving neo-adjuvant CT (12 and 3.7%, respectively). This lower effectiveness of neo-adjuvant CT is in accordance with previous data showing the poorer effectiveness of sequential administration of CT and RT as compared to concurrent or alternating administration [3,9]. In the El-Sayed meta-analysis [10], which grouped 42 trials, a significant reduction in mortality was observed only when RT and CT were administered simultaneously; it was equal to 20%. However, these two meta-analyses were criticized for methodological reasons [11].

In patients with small cell lung cancer, a meta-analysis of 13 trials demonstrated an increase in the survival rate from 8.9 to 14.3% in patients who received RT in addition to CT [12]. The relative smallness of these gains can be explained by the correlation between radiosensitivity and chemosensitivity. An important finding, made a decade ago, was the correlation between the responses of a tumor to drugs and radiation. For example, in the study of Ensley et al. [13], out of 42 patients who initially responded to CT, only one subsequently did not respond to RT, whereas out of 18 patients who failed to respond to CT, only one responded to RT thereafter.

## 3.  The example of breast cancer

Breast cancer is one of the most frequent cancers and certainly one of the first for which conservative treatment has been investigated. Furthermore, its natural history has been extensively studied and the impact of lack of local control on probability of metastatic dissemination has been quantified. The studies carried out with adjuvant CT provide useful quantitative information. The CMF regimen in breast cancer reduces by about 30% the incidence of distant metastases in premenopausal women with breast cancer [14]. An analysis with a simulation mathematical model of the metastasis appearance curve in treated and controlled patients showed that the maximum number of cells in the occult metastases which are controlled by the CT is approximately $10^6$ [15]. These clinical data are consistent with experimental results which showed that control of colonies of more than $10^6$ cells is extremely difficult to achieve with CT alone [16]. Assuming that the proportion of clonogenic cells is $10^{-3}$, this result means that the proportion of surviving tumor cells after completion of six cycles of CMF is $10^{-3}$. This corresponds to a radiation dose equal to 10 $D_{50}$.

In patients with breast cancer, the comparison of the incidence of local-regional recurrence in patients treated by surgery alone, or by surgery followed by postoperative RT, enables the efficacy of RT to be estimated. In order to take into account the indicators which are related to the incidence of local relapse, such as the histological grade or the number of involved axillary nodes, a multivariate analysis must be carried out. The results show that in over three-quarters of the patients, the local-regional residual disease is controlled by RT (10-year recurrence rates 30 and 6%, respectively in patients without or with postoperative RT) [17].

The addition of adjuvant CT further reduces this incidence, but its relative effectiveness is limited. In the NSABP trial [18], in patients with axillary lymph node involvement, a local recurrence occurred in 36% of the patients treated by surgery + CT, whereas in the group treated by conservative surgery + CT + RT this incidence was much lower, approximately 2%. However, the contribution of CT is not negligible. In patients without axillary lymph node involvement treated by surgery + RT a local recurrence was observed in 9% of patients. This subset of patients is not comparable to the subset of patients with axillary involvement treated by CT + RT in whom the incidence was only 2%; nevertheless the higher recurrence rate in the group treated by RT without CT strongly suggests that CT had been able to increase the rate of local control of the residual tumor foci.

In the Danish breast cancer controlled trials [19], the incidence of local-regional recurrence was slightly but not significantly lower in the group treated by RT + adjuvant CT than in the group treated by RT alone (7 versus 12% in premenopausal, 12 versus 17% in postmenopausal patients). In a more recent Danish trial [20]the local recurrence rate was significantly lower in patients treated by RT + CMF than in patients treated by CT alone (7 versus 24% in premenopausal, 5 versus 25% in postmenopausal patients). In patients with inflammatory breast cancer [21], the 4-year local recurrence rate was significantly higher in patients treated by RT alone (45 Gy plus a boost of 20 Gy to the tumor) than in those treated by RT (45 + 15 Gy) plus CT (53 versus 32%). However, this local recurrence rate was not further diminished when a more aggressive CT regimen was administered. These data suggest that inflammatory breast cancer is less radiosensitive and more chemosensitive than the other types of breast cancer; this may be due to a more rapid cell proliferation.

In summary, although CT is much less effective than RT for local control, it can still play a role towards this aim. When the treatment is initiated with CT, these figures also show that, unless the tumor is extremely radiosensitive, it is safer to deliver the maximum tolerated radiation dose, in particular when the tumor has not rapidly shrunk under CT.

The correlation between radio and chemoresponsiveness strongly suggests that the effect of CT on a tumor can be used as a short term predictor for the efficacy of RT. It was immediately felt that the prediction would be of great value when the aim of the combination of CT and RT is to avoid a mutilating treatment of the primary tumor. This strategy was explored in several protocols in which CT was initiated first [22]. Its validity was confirmed by a recent controlled trial carried out at the Institut Curie. The aim of this study was to assess a potential advantage in survival by neoadjuvant as compared to adjuvant chemotherapy. Four hundred and fourteen patients with T2-T3 N0-N1 M0 breast cancer were randomized to receive either four cycles of neoadjuvant chemotherapy (cyclophosphamide, doxorubicin, 5-fluorouracil), followed by local-regional treatment (group I) or four cycles of adjuvant chemotherapy after primary irradiation ± surgery (group II). Surgery was limited to those patients with a persisting mass after irradiation, and aimed to be as conservative as possible. Three hundred and ninety patients were evaluable. The local-regional treatment began with a dose of 54 Gy over 6 weeks. It was followed by surgery for patients with a residual mass or by a boost of up to 75–80 Gy for patients without palpable mass. The results of this trial were reported in two articles [23,24]. In the two groups of the study, despite the relatively large size of the tumors, a 5-year rate of breast conservation was achieved in about two-thirds of the patients. There were no differences between the two groups. A slight but significant survival advantage was observed in the neoadjuvant group at 5 and 7 years of followup; however the current followup is still too short to allow a definite conclusion. During the first months the rate of breast conservation was higher in the neoadjuvant group than in the group where only RT was carried out prior to surgery and CT afterwards. This was due to a higher proportion of complete remission at the completion of

CT + RT. However, later, due to local recurrence, the breast conservation rate became identical showing that the timing of CT had no impact on local control.

Another interesting result of the trial was the significant prognostic value of response to CT [24]. Two hundred patients were included in the neoadjuvant group and 195 were evaluable for response to two cycles of primary CT. A small but non-significant survival advantage was observed for patients whose tumors shrank by $\geq 50\%$ after two cycles ($P = 0.16$); however, the difference in local recurrence-free rates approached significance (78 versus 67%, $P = 0.06$) in favor of responding patients which suggests that chemosensitive tumors are also radiosensitive. The distant relapse-free rates were identical in the two groups, showing that the probability of control of occult metastases by CT was not increased in chemosensitive patients. The 7-year preservation rate was 73% for responders versus 54% for non-responders. These data show that there is a clear impact of the response to two cycles on the rate of local control and confirm the existence of a correlation between chemo and radiosensitivity.

However, there was a non-negligible incidence of local recurrence among patients who were treated by CT + RT without surgery when a complete remission had been achieved after CT. These data emphasize the dubious significance of complete remission. They show also that, in order to maintain a high survival rate, surgery should be performed early in case of local recurrence or when the response is too small, or paradoxically when it is too rapid, which indicates a rapid proliferation rate. These conclusions are consistent with those provided by studies on cancers of other sites.

## 4. Conservative treatment of upper respiratory and digestive tract (URDT) cancers

The preservation of the larynx in patients with cancers of the URDT is another important goal as long as the morbidity of the treatment is not excessive and overall survival is not compromised.

The Veteran Affairs (VA) controlled trial, published in 1991, showed that organ preservation is achieved in about one-third of patients with primary tumors of the larynx treated by induction CT, while two-thirds of those who were still alive at 3 years had retained functional larynges [25]. Despite a slightly lower incidence of distant metastases there was no improvement in survival or in local disease control. The conclusions of other studies on larynx cancer were similar [26–28].

Recent data (EORTC) of a randomized trial on cancer of the hypopharynx concur with these conclusions [29]. This randomized trial compared in patients with cancers of the pyriform sinus immediate surgery followed by postoperative radiation (RT) with, in another arm, induction chemotherapy followed by RT. Patients with T2-T4 and N0, N1, N2a, or N2b disease were eligible. Induction chemotherapy consisted of up to three cycles of the very effective combination of cisplatin 100 mg/m$^2$ followed by infusion of fluorouracil (1000 mg/m$^2$ per day) on days 1–5. Patients were endoscoped after every cycle; patients achieving a clinical CR received 70 Gy to the primary site and both sides of the neck (50 Gy to all areas and boost of 20 Gy to involved sites).

Patients randomly allocated to immediate surgery, and those failing to achieve a CR to induction chemotherapy, underwent a total laryngectomy and partial pharyngectomy with a neck dissection as indicated by the original presentation of the tumor. Among patients randomized to receive CT, the 3- and 5-year estimates of preserved, functional larynges were 28 and 17%, respectively. If patients whose deaths were due to metastatic disease or unrelated to cancer, but who maintained a functional larynx are included as successful organ preservation, these rates rise to 42 and 35%, respectively. Among patients with CR following cycles of CT and surviving at 5 years, the proportion of functional larynx at 5 years was 58%. Thus, organ preservation is achievable even in cancers with a prognosis as poor as that of hypopharynx. Induction CT followed by RT can now be accepted as a standard treatment because it allows preservation of the larynx in a significant minority of patients with otherwise equivalent outcomes. At 3 years, survival was superior in the CT group, however the difference had vanished at 5 years but distant relapse rates were statistically less frequent (0.04) in patients who had received CT.

The results of this study are important because of the usually poor clinical status of patients with hypopharynx cancer and the risks involved in salvage surgery. However, survival was not improved and this strategy is not totally satisfactory. In this French EORTC study, induction CT was used mainly as a predictive test. It is noteworthy that this timing did not lower survival in patients in whom CR was not observed despite a 2–3 month delay in the beginning of an effective treatment and despite the probable initiation of a tumor repopulation. However, we have shown in previous papers that for tumors which are not chemosensitive, the delay caused by induction CT may compromise local control by RT or even by surgery. Moreover, in the Munro meta-analysis [8] on RT + CT which is discussed above, the long-term survival is clearly smaller in patients treated by neo-adjuvant CT than in patients treated by concurrent administration of RT + CT. Merlano [9] has shown a higher survival in patients treated by alternating RT plus CT than in patients in whom modalities were performed sequentially.

Furthermore, the article strategy assumes that organ preservation is achievable only in patients with CR whereas the breast cancer study discussed above shows that it is possible also in patients with only partial response [23,24]. Another drawback is that responsive patients receive only two cycles of CT in this study and only four in the Curie Institute breast trial. Hyperfractionated accelerated RT, alternating CT + RT or concurrent administration of CT and RT should be explored [3,9,30], but in this other strategy the first cycles of CT cannot be used as a predictive test. Obviously tests able to distinguish earlier responsive from non-responsive patients would represent a marked progress, but this is a challenging endeavor [31].

## 5.  Other sites

Different approaches have been used for other cancer sites. In bladder carcinoma, for example, in several studies the treatment begins with a trans-urethral resection of as much of the primary tumor as is judged safe. Thereafter a combined or concurrent CT + RT is carried out with an early cystectomy for patients whose tumor is not responding [32]. This strategy has two advantages: early resection of the bulk of the tumor and early inception of radio-chemotherapy. But it cannot select the non-responsive patients for whom total cystectomy should be performed. Thus with this strategy, besides tumor regression, other predictive tests have to be explored [31].

In advanced anal cancer, RT + CT or RT alone are carried out first, up to maximal tolerated doses. Radical surgery is performed only in patients in whom the tumor is not controlled [33].

These few data show that organ salvage is possible even in advanced cancer. Until now combined modality therapy has been able to save organs, but was unable to significantly improve cure rate in any of the trials although meta-analyses were able to detect a small survival advantage. Clearly, in the future, the goal of increasing the proportion of patients with functional organs should not be separated from that of improving the cure rate. Concurrent or alternating administration of RT + CT may play a role towards this aim [34].

In conclusion, even in advanced cancers an organ preservation strategy does not jeopardize survival when patients are carefully followed up. Early extended surgery in non-responsive tumors maximize cure rates. The tumor's response to induction CT provides crucial information but delays effective treatment on chemoresistant tumors. Other predictors of tumor response, in particular tumor cell proliferative rate [24], molecular biological characteristics of the tumor as given by immunostaining may provide useful predictors and should be assessed [31,35]. Some authors even suggest that the question of testing for drug sensitivity in vitro should be reopened as resistance in vitro and in vivo seems to be correlated [36]. Whatever the technique used, the aim is to identify rapidly non-responsive tumors. Approaches that allow intensive CT for control of metastatic disease and curative RT dose should be devised and tested. In several early studies, the radiotherapy dose was often relatively small (40 Gy). It is now generally accepted that the maximum tolerated dose should be given. However, this is not sufficient since when the two modalities are given sequentially the length of the treatment becomes a problem [1,3]. Timing, also, is important [37]. It is conceivable that early administration of both RT and CT might improve the therapeutic results because they avoid proliferation and tumor repopulation. Concomitant or alternating RT + CT and accelerated hyperfractionated RT should therefore be explored.

## Summary

Preservation of organ function has become one of the main aims of treatment in oncology, even for advanced disease. Its main hazard is lack of local control. However, experience gained over the past few years shows that for most tumors, in order to avoid a rate of local recurrence higher than after radical surgery, high dose radiotherapy and chemotherapy should be associated with conservative surgery. For chemoresistant or radioresistant tumors, these combination treatments remain less effective than radical surgery and therefore it would be helpful to identify those resistant tumors as early as possible.

In several trials, the response to neoadjuvant chemotherapy may serve this purpose, and in cancers of the breast or the upper respiratory and digestive tracts, the survival rates with this approach are as good as those achieved with radical surgery. However, this strategy delays surgery and radiotherapy which might be detrimental, particularly for chemoresistant tumors. This is why other pointers of tumor response to chemotherapy should be investigated. Their introduction would allow concurrent or alternating administration of radiotherapy and chemotherapy which are probably more effective than sequential administration. A comparison of conservative treatments used in various cancer sites shows that the strategy probably should be adapted to the cancer site.

Conservation of organ function appears to be achievable for most cancer sites but only on a relatively small, although variable, proportion of patients. The goal of research should be both to increase this proportion and also to take advantage of the combined treatment for increasing the survival rate.

## References

1. Tubiana M. The role of local treatment in the cure of cancer. Eur J Cancer 12: 2061–2069, 1992.
2. Leibel SA, Scott CB, Mohinddin M, et al. The effect of locoregional control on distant metastatic dissemination in carcinoma of the head and neck: results of an analysis from the RTOG database. Int J Radiat Oncol 21: 549–556, 1991.
3. Tubiana M. The role of radiotherapy in the treatment of chemosensitive tumors. Int J Radiat Oncol Biol Phys 16: 763–774, 1989.
4. Tubiana M, Henry-Amar M, Hayat M, et al. The EORTC treatment of early stages Hodgkin's disease. Int J Radiat Oncol Biol Phys 10: 197–210, 1984.
5. Carde P, Burgers JMV, Henry-Amar M, et al. Clinical stages I and II Hodgkin's disease: a specifically tailored therapy according to prognostic factors. J Clin Oncol 6: 239–252, 1988.
6. Tubiana M. The combination of radiotherapy: a review. Int J Radiat Biol 55: 497–511, 1989.
7. Non-small cell lung cancer collaborative group. Chemotherapy in non-small cell lung cancer: a meta-analysis using updated data on individual patients from 52 randomized clinical trials. Br Med J 311: 899–909, 1995.
8. Munro AJ. An overview of randomized controlled trials of adjuvant chemotherapy in head and neck cancers. Br J Cancer 71: 83–91, 1995.
9. Merlano M, Vitale V, Rosso R, et al. Treatment of advanced squamous cell carcinoma of the head and neck with alternating chemotherapy and radiotherapy. N Engl J Med 327: 1115–1121, 1992.
10. El-Sayed S, Nelson N. Adjuvant and adjunctive chemotherapy in the management of squamous cell carcinoma of the head and neck region: a meta-analysis of prospective and randomized trials. J Clin Oncol 14: 838–847, 1996.
11. Pignon JP, Bourhis J, Domenge C. Meta-analysis of chemotherapy in head and neck cancer: individual patient data versus literature data. Br J Cancer 72: 1062, 1995.
12. Pignon JP, Arriagada R, Ihde DC, et al. A meta-analysis of thoracic radiotherapy for small-cell cancer. N Engl J Med 327: 1618–1624, 1990.
13. Ensley JF, Jacobs JR, Weaver A, et al. Correlation between response to cis-platinum combination and subsequent radiotherapy in previously untreated patients with advanced squamous cell cancers of the head and neck. Cancer 54: 811–814, 1984.
14. Bonadonna G, Valagussa P, Rossi A, et al. Ten-year experience with CMF-based adjuvant chemotherapy in resectable breast cancer. Breast Cancer Res Treatment 5: 95–115, 1985.
15. Guiguet M, Koscielny S, Valleron AJ, Tubiana M. Estimation par un modèle de simulation de la taille maximale des nodules métastatiques guéris par une thérapie adjuvante. In: Jacquillat C, Weil M, Khayat D (Eds), Neo-adjuvant chemotherapy, Colloque INSERM, Vol. 137. Paris: J Libbey, pp. 825–833, 1986.
16. Steel GC. The search for therapeutic gain in the combination of radiotherapy and chemotherapy. Radiother Oncol 11: 31–53, 1988.
17. Tubiana M, Sarrazin D. The role of post-operative radiotherapy in breast cancer. In: Ariel JM, Cleary JB (Eds), Breast Cancer: Diagnosis and Treatment. New York: McGraw Hill, pp. 280–299, 1987.
18. Fisher B, Bauer M, Marolese R, et al. Five-year results of a randomized clinical trial comparing total mastectomy and segmental mastectomy with or without radiation in the treatment of breast cancer. N Engl J Med 312: 665–673, 1985.
19. Overgaard M, Syrak Hansen P, Rose C, et al. Postmastectomy radiotherapy and adjuvant systemic treatment in high-risk breast cancer patients (abstr.). Eur J Cancer 30A(Suppl 2): S28, 1994.
20. Dombernowsky P, Hansen M, Mouridsen HT, et al. Randomized trial of adjuvant CMF + radiotherapy (RT) vs CMF alone vs CMF + tamoxifen (TAM) in pre- and menopausal stage II breast cancer (abstr.). Eur J Cancer 30A(Suppl 2): S28, 1994.
21. Rouesse J, Friedman S, Sarrazin D, et al. Primary chemotherapy in the treatment of inflammatory breast carcinoma: a study of 230 cases from the Institut Gustave-Roussy. J Clin Oncol 4: 1765–1771, 1986.
22. Touboul E, Buffet L, Lefranc JP et al. Possibility of conservative local treatment after combined chemotherapy and preoperative irradiation for locally advanced non-inflammatory breast cancer. Int J Radiat Oncol Biol Phys 34: 1019–1028, 1996.
23. Scholl SM, Fourquet A, Asselain B, et al. Neo-adjuvant versus adjuvant chemotherapy in premenopausal patients with tumours considered too large for breast preserving surgery: preliminary results of a randomized trial: S6. Eur J Cancer 30A: 645–652, 1994.

24.  Scholl SM, Pierga JY, Asselain B, et al. Breast tumour response to primary chemotherapy predicts local and distant control as well as survival. Eur J Cancer 31A: 1969–1975, 1995.
25.  The Department of Veteran Affairs Laryngeal Cancer Study Group. Induction chemotherapy plus radiation compared with surgery plus radiation in patients with advanced laryngeal cancer. N Engl J Med 324: 1685–1690, 1991.
26.  Demard F, Chauvel P, Schneider M, et al. Induction chemotherapy for larynx preservation in laryngeal and hypopharyngeal cancers. In: Johnson JT, Didolkar MS (Eds), Head and Neck Cancer. Vol III, Amsterdam: Excerpta Medica, pp. 3–11, 1993.
27.  Karp DD, Vaughan CW, Carter R, et al. Larynx preservation using induction chemotherapy plus radiation therapy as an alternative to laryngectomy in advanced head and neck cancer. a long-term follow-up report. Am J Clin Oncol 14: 273–279, 1991.
28.  Pfister DG, Strong EW, Harrison L, et al. Larynx preservation with combined chemotherapy and radiation therapy in advanced but resectable head and neck cancer. J Clin Oncol 9: 850–859, 1991.
29.  Lefebvre JL, Chevalier D, Luboinsky B, et al. Larynx preservation in pyriform sinus cancer: Preliminary results of a European organisation for research and treatment of cancer phase III trial. J Natl Cancer Inst 88: 890–899, 1996.
30.  Yu L, Vikram B, Malamud S et al. Chemotherapy rapidly alternating with twice-a-day accelerated radiation therapy in carcinoma involving the hypopharynx or esophagus: an update. Cancer Invest 13: 567–572, 1995.
31.  Shipley WV. Translational research in bladder cancer. Int J Radiat Oncol Biol Phys 35: 411–412, 1996.
32.  Orsatti M, Curotto A, Canobbio L, et al. Alternating chemo-radiotherapy in bladder cancer - a conservative approach. Int J Radiat Oncol Biol Phys 33: 173–178, 1995.
33.  Allal A, Kurtz J, Pipard G, et al. Chemoradiotherapy versus radiotherapy alone for anal cancer. A retrospective comparison. Int J Radiat Oncol Biol Phys 27: 59–66, 1995.
34.  Vikram B, Malamud S, Siverman P, et al. A pilot study of chemotherapy alternating with twice a day accelerated radiation therapy as an alternative to cystectomy in muscle infiltrating (Stages $T_2$ and $T_3$) cancer of the bladder: preliminary results. J Urol 151: 602–604, 1994.
35.  Tester W, Porter A, Asbell S, et al. Combined modality program with possible organ preservation for invasive bladder cancer: Results for RTOG protocol 85–12. Int J Radiat Oncol Biol Phys 25: 783–790, 1993.
36.  Carbone DP, Minna J. Chemotherapy for non-small lung cancer. Br Med J 311: 889–891, 1995.
37.  Buchholtz TA, Austin-Seymour MM, Moe RE, et al. Effect of delay in radiation in the combined modality treatment of breast cancer. Int J Radiat Oncol Biol Phys 26: 23–35, 1993.

C.J. Rosenthal and M. Rotman (Eds.), *Infusion Chemotherapy–Irradiation Interactions*
© 1998 Elsevier Science B.V. All rights reserved

# CHAPTER 15

# Preservation of structure and function in epidermoid cancer of the anal canal

B.J. CUMMINGS

*Department of Radiation Oncology, University of Toronto, Toronto, Canada and Department of Radiation Oncology, Princess Margaret Hospital, 610 University Avenue, Toronto, ON M5G 2M9, Canada*

## 1. Introduction

The ideal treatment of cancer leads to cure without loss of normal function. The acceptance of radiation-based treatment protocols has brought this ideal nearer for patients with epidermoid cancer of the anal canal. When surgery was the principal treatment, conservation of anorectal function was possible only in the minority of patients who presented with small superficial cancers amenable to local resection. Although radiation therapy was recognized in a few centers as being capable of eradicating many anal cancers without excessive toxicity, which of itself could lead to loss of function [1], the majority of patients underwent surgery designed to remove the primary cancer and adjacent lymph nodes. The procedure most frequently performed was abdominoperineal resection, with its attendant interference with function and associated psycho-social disabilities [2]. The development of effective combinations of radiation and cytotoxic chemotherapy and the acceptance of such combinations as primary treatment for anal cancer has led to the cure of many patients without the need to sacrifice anorectal function. This chapter addresses the current status of the quest for the ideal treatment for epidermoid cancer of the anal canal.

## 2. Preservation of anorectal anatomy and function

Preservation of gross anatomical relationships does not always equate to maintenance of normal function. Whenever a cancer at any site regresses due to the effects of radiation, the site of the cancer is marked by varying degrees of fibrosis, and specialized tissues destroyed by the cancer are not reconstituted. Furthermore radiation, with or without concomitant chemotherapy, itself has deleterious effects on normal tissues [3]. The severity of these effects varies with the dose and the volume irradiated [4]. Host factors, such as age and coincidental illness or previous damage to the organs and tissues irradiated, also affect the long term outcome after radiation therapy. Thus, while normal anatomical relationships in the pelvis can be preserved by successful treatment of anal cancer by radiation with or without chemotherapy, it has also been found that the degree to which function is preserved varies and is frequently less than the ideal.

The greatest attention has, understandably, been given to preservation of anorectal function. As with other organs, function of the anorectum is multi-faceted and involves not only continence but also frequency and pattern of defecation, presence of discharge and/or bleeding, and various degrees of loss of integrity of the anorectal mucosa and underlying tissues, ranging from anal fissures to ulcers and necrosis. Other pelvic organs and tissues are also affected by radiation therapy. Changes may be seen in the perianal skin, the ovaries and vagina, the prostate and testes, small bowel, the urinary bladder, major blood vessels, and the pelvic framework. Even this list is incomplete, but the complexity of establishing the degree to which normal function is preserved is apparent.

## 3. Analysis of results reported in studies of anal preservation

The measurement and reporting of the results of treatment for anal cancer are often uneven, as they are for most malignancies. Reports stress rates of survival and of control of the primary tumor and regional nodes. Reference is often made to major treatment-associated morbidity, particularly when the management of toxicity requires surgical intervention, but lesser degrees of injury, or injuries not amenable to surgery, are not well described. Discussions of function are generally confined to descriptive and/or subjective parameters. More objective measures, such as physiological, radiological and histological assessments are rare and usually appear only as case reports in the literature relating to the treatment of anal cancer.

The presentation of actuarial rates of damage and prospective studies of function are uncommon. Many reports do include the local tumor recurrence-free rate, which gives a reasonably reliable measure of the preservation of structure (although it does not make allowance for all potential losses of structural integrity, such as that which may be associated with, for example, a recto-vaginal fistula which persists despite eradication of the anal cancer which led to the fistula; and care must be taken to establish that the recurrence-free rate is that due to radiation or radiation and chemotherapy, and excludes secondary control gained by ablative surgery for recurrence). The colostomy-free rate provides a measure of preservation of function but it must be recognized that that rate is a composite of one or more possible outcomes: (i) local recurrence managed by means other than colostomy, (ii) freedom from major treatment related morbidity requiring colostomy, (iii) successful closure of a colostomy opened prior to treatment, or for temporary management of treatment toxicity. It is evident that local tumor control does not equate with preservation of anorectal function, nor vice versa. The assessment of preservation of function of other pelvic organs may be equally complex.

Commentators have generally correlated variations in late functional outcome with the dose and technique of radiation used. This to some extent may be justified by the close similarities in chemotherapy doses and schedules from study to study, in contrast to the many variations in radiation parameters. However, it is highly probable that there are significant interactions between radiation and cytotoxic drugs, especially when they are delivered concurrently, and these interactions require further study both in the laboratory and the clinic [5].

Various combinations of radiation therapy coupled with infusions of cytotoxic drugs have proven capable of eradicating epidermoid anal cancer. The most effective combinations studied are radiation, 5-fluorouracil (5-FU) with or without mitomycin C, and radiation, 5-FU and cisplatin.

## 4. Anal preservation with radiation and 5-FU with or without mitomycin C

Two randomized trials have demonstrated that radiation, 5-FU and mitomycin C are superior to identical doses and schedules of protracted radiation delivered without concurrent chemotherapy. The United Kingdom Coordinating Committee on Cancer Research (UKCCCR) trial randomized 577 patients to receive 45 Gy in 20 or 25 fractions over 4–5 weeks, or the same regimen combined with 5-FU (1000 mg/m$^2$ for 4 days or 750 mg/m$^2$ for 5 days) by continuous infusion during the first and last weeks of radiation treatment, and mitomycin C (10 mg/m$^2$) on day 1 of the first course [6]. Six weeks after radiation, those whose cancer had regressed by 50% or more received boost radiation, 15 Gy in 6 fractions, or 25 Gy in 2.5 days by interstitial implant. Those with less or no response underwent surgery. Although the 3-year overall survival rates were not significantly different (65% combined modality, 58% radiation only, $P = 0.25$), the risk of dying from anal cancer was reduced in those who received combined modality therapy (28 versus 39%, $P = 0.02$). Furthermore, the local failure rate at 3 years was 61% in the 285 patients who received radiation, but only 39% in the 292 patients who were treated by radiation and chemotherapy ($P < 0.0001$). Local failure was defined as the presence of cancer and/or surgery involving the formation of a colostomy for any reason. Of the 81 patients who received radiation and chemotherapy and who had residual or recurrent loco-regional cancer, 49 underwent colostomy as part of management of the recurrence. A further 10 had a colostomy for morbidity (the same number underwent colostomy for morbidity after radiation alone), and a pretreatment colostomy could not be closed in 7 and 3 had a colostomy for other reasons. A colostomy-free rate was not given by the authors, but the crude proportion of those undergoing colostomy, based on the number of patients initially randomized to combined modality treatment, is 24% (69 of 292). No other information on organ function, including that of the anorectum in those whose primary cancer was controlled, was provided. The authors note that a quality-of-life study was conducted as part of the trial and that more detailed data on treatment side-effects will be presented.

The European Organization for the Research and Treatment of Cancer (EORTC) conducted a trial of similar design in which 110 patients with relatively advanced cancers were treated [7]. Radiation therapy consisted of 45 Gy in 5 weeks. Six weeks later patients in whom there was complete clinical response received a boost of 15 Gy by external beam or interstitial implant; 20 Gy was given for partial response; surgery was performed if there was no response, or for later persistent or recurrent cancer. One half of the patients were randomized to receive concomitant chemotherapy in the form of a continuous infusion of 5-FU (750 mg/m$^2$ per 24 h) for 5 days in the first and fifth weeks of radiation, with a single dose of mitomycin C 15 mg/m$^2$ on the first day of radiation only. The 3-year local tumor control rate was approximately 65% for the patients who received combined modality treatment, and 55% for those treated by radiation alone ($P = 0.02$). The corresponding colostomy-free rates were about 75% and 45% ($P = 0.003$). Severe late side effects to the anorectum or adjacent skin and soft tissue were tabulated. More anal ulcers were noted in the patients treated by combined modalities, but otherwise the pattern of toxicity was similar. The 3-year severe toxicity-free rate in each group was about 65%. Analysis also showed that, in this study, by 3 years after treatment only about 30% of the patients were surviving free of local recurrence, severe side effects or colostomy. As with the UKCCCR trial, despite the improved likelihood of local tumor control with combined modality therapy, the overall survival rate was not significantly better than that achieved with radiation alone.

While these two trials demonstrate that the delivery of short infusions of 5-FU and bolus injections of mitomycin C concurrently with split course radiation produces higher local tumor control rates than split course radiation alone, no direct comparison with radical uninterrupted radiation has been undertaken. Several studies of single course radical radiation alone reported local control, survival and major toxicity rates similar to those obtained with combined modality treatment in the trials described earlier [1]. For example, Newman et al. [8] described 72 patients, treated for the most part with 50 Gy in 20 fractions in 4 weeks. Local tumor control was achieved in 76% (55 of 72), and the 5-year actuarial survival rate was 66%. Anorectal function was reported to have been lost due to colostomy for complications in only 2 patients, so that 94% of those in whom the primary cancer was eradicated by radiation retained some measure of anal function. However, at least 4 of those cured were reported to have had incontinence and/or anal stricture, and 8 others had mild to moderate proctitis.

The choice of drugs to combine with radiation has been examined in several studies. The addition of both 5-FU and mitomycin C to radiation led to better results than did the addition of 5-FU alone in a randomized trial conducted by the Radiation Therapy Oncology Group (RTOG) and the Eastern Cooperative Oncology Group (ECOG) [9]. Two hundred and ninety-one patients who were treated with 45–50.4 Gy in 5–5.5 weeks received 5-FU ($1000$ mg/m$^2$ per 24 h) by continuous intravenous infusion for 96 h, starting on day 1 and again on day 29 of radiation. Of these, 146 also received mitomycin C ($10$ mg/m$^2$) by intravenous bolus injection on day 1 and day 29. Biopsies from the site of the primary tumor 6 weeks after treatment were positive in 15% of patients in the radiation plus 5-FU arm compared to 8% in those who received both 5-FU and mitomycin C ($P = 0.14$). Those with positive biopsies were treated with a salvage regimen that consisted of 9 Gy in 5 treatments in 1 week, a further 96 h infusion of 5-FU, and cisplatin ($100$ mg/m$^2$) intravenously over 6 h on day 2 of radiation. The estimated 4-year local failure rates were 34% in the 5-FU arm and 16% in the 5-FU plus mitomycin C group ($P = 0.0007$). The colostomy rates were 22% and 9% ($P = 0.0025$). The overall survival rates were 67% and 76% ($P = 0.18$), however disease-free survival significantly favored the 5-FU, mitomycin C and radiation combination (51% versus 73%, $P = 0.0002$). Apart from the colostomy rates, little information was provided about functional outcome.

Unexpectedly, the very low colostomy rates obtained by RTOG/ECOG in the trial just described were not reproduced in a later phase II trial with a higher radiation dose of 59.6 Gy over 8.5 weeks, incorporating a 2-week rest period, but including two courses of 5-FU and mitomycin C as before [10]. In the 47 patients entered on this study, the 2 year colostomy rate was 30%, compared with only 7% in the previous trial. The colostomies were required for uncontrolled primary cancer. The patients had not been followed sufficiently long at the time of the report to allow adequate assessment of late toxicity, and no other details on function were given. The possible effects of protracted or split course radiation programs on the control of anal cancer have been discussed elsewhere [11]. The effects of split course radiation on function are not easy to predict. Prolongation of the overall duration of radiation will not protect against damage to so-called "late responding" tissues, but reduction in the severity of the acute reaction may lower the risk of residual damage from the acute changes.

## 5. Anal preservation with radiation and 5-FU and cisplatin combination

Infusions of 5-FU combined with either bolus injections or infusions of cisplatin have also been used to treat anal epidermoid cancers. Wagner et al. [12] reported treating 51 patients with a two-phase program of pelvic radiation and chemotherapy. In the first phase, external beam radiation of approximately 35 Gy tumor dose in 3 weeks was coupled with 5-FU (1000 mg/m$^2$ per 24 h) by continuous infusion over days 1–4, and cisplatin (25 mg/m$^2$) by bolus injection on days 2–5. Eight weeks after external radiation, the second phase which involved an interstitial implant was delivered. The local tumor was controlled in about 90%. Late complications requiring medical treatment only occurred in 16% (8 of 51) and 3 patients (6%) needed surgery for toxicity. Rich et al. [13] treated patients with external beam doses of from 45 to 55 Gy in 4–6 weeks, sometimes supplemented by interstitial radiation. Chemotherapy consisted of either a continuous infusion of 5-FU alone (250–300 mg/m$^2$ per day) for 5 or 7 days/week, or continuous infusions of 5-FU (250 mg/m$^2$ per day for 5 days/week) and cisplatin (4 mg/m$^2$ per day for 5 days/week). The actuarial local control rate at 2 years in those who received 5-FU and cisplatin with radiation was 85%, compared to 75% after 5-FU alone with radiation. No patients experienced toxicity requiring surgery, but the authors noted that nearly all had occasional rectal bleeding, and 3 of 18 (17%) had bleeding, pain, and tenesmus managed medically. Efforts have been made to combine 5-FU and cisplatin with higher doses of radiation, 59.4 Gy in 33 fractions over 8.5 week, with a 2-week split [14]. In that study only 72% (13 of 18) achieved complete response, and there was significant acute morbidity. No data relating to function were presented. Whether the combination with radiation of 5-FU and cisplatin should supplant 5-FU and mitomycin C will be resolved only by comparative trials.

## 6. Anal function after radiation–chemotherapy combination

There have been few detailed studies of impairment of function short of that for which surgery was necessary. An analysis of outcome in patients treated at the Princess Margaret Hospital (PMH) has shown that some degree of post-treatment dysfunction is common, or stated conversely, that after radiation and chemotherapy completely normal function is rare. The degree of dysfunction was greater in patients who had larger primary tumors. This was not due to variation in radiation dose since the doses given were identical for both large and small tumors. It is presumably related to the more extensive initial local damage and reparative fibrosis associated with larger tumors. An interim analysis of the PMH data is shown in Table 1. In addition to the indices shown, all women who were previously menstruating suffered radiation-induced menopause. All patients noted some degree of perianal irritation, either ongoing or intermittent, presumably due to loss of the normal lubricating function of perianal cutaneous glands. In several patients, proctitis and rectal urgency were so severe that they were unable to return to employment or suffered other serious dislocation of social relationships. Actuarial analyses of the functional deficits outlined in Table 1 are not yet

Table 1

Moderate grade late toxicity after radiation, 5-FU with/without mitomycin C (interim analysis)

| | Grade 2[a] % (no.) | Grade 3[a] % (no.) | Overall |
|---|---|---|---|
| Skin atrophy/telangiectasia/ subcutaneous fibrosis[b] | 65 (81) Mild | 15 (19) Marked | 80 ($n = 125$)[c] |
| Rectal urgency/frequency/ incontinence/bleeding[b] | 57 (71) >5 movements/day; Some incontinence; Bleeding >3/week[b] | 4 (5) Required surgery | 61 ($n = 125$)[c] |
| Dyspareunia | 47 (21) Discomfort | 42 (19) Unable to tolerate intercourse | 89 ($n = 45$)[d] |

[a]Grading based on RTOG/EORTC scales [15].
[b]One or more of symptom group present.
[c]$N = 125$ patients with primary cancer controlled for at least 2 years by radiation, 5-FU with/without mitomycin C.
[d]$N = 45$ women sexually active prior to treatment.

available. However, the onset of all changes appears to be early, within a few months of treatment, and may be progressive in severity.

It is probable that the extent of functional disability can be reduced by attention to the technical aspects of the radiation therapy delivered, including the total dose, fractional daily dose, orientation of external radiation beams, and the volume treated by interstitial therapy [1]. In particular, avoiding beams tangential to the perineum and reducing the daily radiation dose to below 2 Gy appear to be beneficial. For smaller anal cancers, up to about 3–4 cm in size, combining drugs such as 5-FU and mitomycin C with total radiation doses of no more than 45–50 Gy in 5–6 weeks will control 90% or more and carries a lower risk of serious dysfunction than higher radiation doses [1]. There are no data on whether higher doses of chemotherapy would allow a further decrease in radiation dose.

In clinical trials the combination of mitomycin C, 5-FU and radiation has proved capable of eradicating from 60 to 85% of epidermoid anal cancers, depending on the initial stage mix, and is now the reference treatment regimen. Claims of similar control rates are made for 5-FU, cisplatin and radiation but have not yet been confirmed in large numbers of patients. Ninety-five percent or more of the patients treated successfully with radiation and chemotherapy have not required a colostomy, but more detailed analysis of non-randomized studies suggests that some level of anorectal dysfunction is common and that other pelvic tissues are also affected adversely by drug and radiation combinations. The inclusion of quality-of-life and functional assessments in future studies will help identify the ideal treatment regimen.

## References

1.   Cummings BJ. Anal cancer: radiation, with and without chemotherapy. In: Cohen AM, Winawer SJ, Friedman MA, Gunderson LL (Eds), Cancer of the Colon, Rectum and Anus. New York: McGraw-Hill, pp. 1025–1042, 1995.

2.   Williams NS, Johnston D. The quality of life after rectal excision for low rectal cancer. Br J Surg 70: 460–462, 1983.

3.   Fajardo LF. Pathology of Radiation Injury. Masson, USA, 1982.

4.   Vaeth JM, Meyer JL (Eds). Radiation tolerance of normal tissues. Front Radiat Ther Oncol 23: 1989.

5.   Steel GG. The search for therapeutic gain in the combination of radiotherapy and chemotherapy. Radiother Oncol 11: 31–35, 1988.

6.   UKCCCR Anal Cancer Trial Working Party. Epidermoid anal cancer: Results from the UKCCCR randomized trial of radiotherapy alone versus radiotherapy, 5 fluorouracil and mitomycin C. Lancet 348: 1049–1054, 1996.

7.   Bartelink H, Roelofsen F, Bosset JF, et al. Radiotherapy with concomitant chemotherapy superior to radiotherapy alone in the treatment of locally advanced anal cancer: results of a phase III randomized trial of the EORTC Radiotherapy and Gastrointestinal Tract Cooperative Groups (abstr.). Int J Radiat Oncol Biol Phys 36(Suppl): 210, 1996.

8.   Newman G, Calverley DC, Acker BD, et al. The management of carcinoma of the anal canal by external beam radiotherapy, experience in Vancouver 1971–1988. Radiother Oncol 25: 196–202, 1992.

9.   Flam M, John M, Pajak TF, et al. Role of Mitomycin in combination with Fluorouracil and radiotherapy, and of salvage chemoradiation in the definitive nonsurgical treatment of epidermoid carcinoma of the anal canal: results of a Phase III randomized Intergroup study. J Clin Oncol 14: 2527–2539, 1996.

10.  John M, Pajak T, Flam M, et al. Dose escalation in chemoradiation for anal cancer: preliminary results of RTOG 92–08. Cancer J Sci Am 2: 205–211, 1996.

11.  Cummings BJ. Anal canal cancer - to split or not to split? Cancer J Sci Am 2: 194–196, 1996.

12.  Wagner JP, Mahe MA, Romestaing P, et al. Radiation therapy in the conservative treatment of carcinoma of the anal canal. Int J Radiat Oncol Biol Phys 29: 17–23, 1994.

13.  Rich TA, Ajani JA, Morrison WH, et al. Chemoradiation therapy for anal cancer: radiation plus continuous infusion of 5-fluorouracil with or without cisplatin. Radiother Oncol 27: 209–215, 1993.

14.  Martenson JA, Lipsitz SR, Wagner H, et al: Initial results of a Phase II trial of high dose radiation therapy, 5-Fluorouracil, and cisplatin for patients with anal cancer. (E4292): an Eastern Cooperative Oncology Group Study. Int J Radiat Oncol Biol Phys 35: 745–749, 1996.

15.  Perez CA, Brady LW. Late radiation morbidity scoring system (RTOG, EORTC). In: Perez CA, Brady LW (Eds), Principles and Practice of Radiation Oncology, 2nd edn. Philadelphia, PA: JB Lippincott, pp. 53–55, 1992.

C.J. Rosenthal and M. Rotman (Eds.), *Infusion Chemotherapy–Irradiation Interactions*
173

CHAPTER 16

# Infusional chemoradiation in the conservation management of rectal cancer

## TYVIN A. RICH

*Department of Radiation Oncology, Box 383, University of Virginia Health Sciences Center, Charlottesville, VA 22903, USA*

## 1. Introduction

The standard surgical approach for low lying cancer of the rectum has been extirpation with in continuity removal of the anal/rectal complex and the creation of a permanent colostomy. Recent attempts to limit surgery have employed anal sphincter sparing approaches with coloanal anastomosis and local excision. Along with these newer surgical approaches external irradiation has been used both before and after excision. The results of differing sequences of irradiation combined with chemotherapy and surgery are addressed.

## 2. Conservation surgery and post-operative irradiation alone or combined with chemotherapy

The notion that limited surgery and XRT can be substituted for radical surgery in the management of operable rectal cancer is gaining wider acceptance. One approach currently being tested is limited surgery with post-operative irradiation since this sequence has been standard practice for a long time. One of the strongest reasons for continuing this treatment sequence is that the cancer can be pathologically staged. This provides an assessment of the risk of local regional recurrence based on the level of tumor penetration and the involvement of the lymph nodes. Additional factors that predict for local recurrence are the extent of lymphatic and blood vessel invasion, and perineural invasion.

Patient selection for conservation therapy is based on clinical, anatomic, and pathologic factors. The location of the primary rectal cancer for the newer conservation approaches is usually in the lowest rectal segment measured from the dentate line to the first rectal valve of Houston (<8 cm). Here the abdominoperineal resection (APR) has been the standard operation and it can usually achieve negative margins of normal tissue along three directions of tumor spread (upward, downward, and around) [1]. Margins along the lumen of the rectum may be 2–3 cm [2], whereas radial tumor infiltration frequently results in surgical margins of only 6–9.0 mm in patients undergoing APR and low anterior resection [3–6]. The close radial margins are inversely correlated with the extent of tumor penetration through the bowel wall and up to 85% with positive radial margins may later experience pelvic recurrence [5]. These data are consistent with pathologic assessments of extramural tumor extension, which have been incorporated into a modification of the Dukes' staging, and have been found to predict for pelvic recurrence after surgery [7–9]. In addition to high pathologic stage and positive margin status, other pathologic factors predicting for high local recurrence after surgery are high tumor grade, the presence of lymphatic invasion, and colloid tumor histology [7,10].

In patients selected for conservation treatment, tumor diameter <3 cm is one of the single most important clinical parameters used in selection. In a review of over 750 patients treated with a conservative surgical approaches, 85% had tumor diameters <3 cm [11]. Generally, tumor size has not been identified as a strong prognostic factor in operable rectal cancer, but it is practical to select patients with small tumors for limited surgery. Tumors arising <12 cm above the anal ring are also selected for these alternative procedures since they are relatively accessible [12]. Tumors that are small and mobile have also been accurately staged by digital rectal exam (DRE) based on assessments of mobility and bowel wall penetration [13]. DRE based staging is also correlated with 5-year survival differences between mobile and fixed-tethered lesions [14]. Clinical DRE staging has been augmented recently by endoscopic or endorectal ultrasound (EUS), computed tomography (CT), or magnetic resonance imaging (MRI). EUS has been found to be 85–93% accurate in demonstrating the degree of transmural tumor extension. EUS describes five layers of the normal rectal wall and tumor extension within and through the muscle wall can be readily determined. Lymph node staging by EUS is controversial since universally accepted criteria for nodal positivity do not exist [15,16]. Nodal size is usually not helpful [17], while some consider round and echo-poor perirectal structures to be indicative of tumor involvement [16]. A proposed TNM staging based on EUS follows the AJC rectal cancer classification: a stage uT1 lesion is a cancer confined to the submucosa; stage uT2, a lesion that invades into but not through the muscularis propria; stage uT3, a lesion that invades into the perirectal fat; and stage uT4, a lesion that invades into an adjacent organ or structure (prostate, bladder, or sacrum) [18,19]. For nodal staging, uN1 implies there are features consistent with nodal involvement.

Other staging methods such as CT and MRI of the abdomen and pelvis can be helpful in assessing the presence of extramural tumor [15] and in revealing high pelvic and paraortic nodal involvement, and liver metastasis. Similarly, MRI with endorectal coils can determine transmural extension but it is no better than EUS or CT in detecting lymph node involvement [20].

Local excision alone for selected low rectal cancers results in local recurrence rates ranging from 0 to 27% [21]. This procedure alone may cure a majority of properly selected patients, while in the minority that ultimately fail locally, radical surgery with the creation of a permanent colostomy can be done if the disease recurs. Alternatively, a different treatment philosophy could be to offer adjuvant irradiation to all patients after local excision to maximize anal and rectal preservation. An "up-front" treatment approach may thus reduce the overall need for colostomy, but at a price of over treatment. Conservation surgery followed by postoperative XRT results in local control rates >90% and high survival rates. Prospective phase I–II trials have been done in an effort to understand the toxicity, limitations, efficacy, and functional results of various combinations of limited surgery and radiotherapy [12,22–25]. One of the largest series is a prospective study from UTMDACC for patients with stages T1, T2, and T3 disease who refused radical surgical excision [26]. Forty-six patients were treated with transanal, Kraske, transphincteric, or abdomino-sacral operations and postoperative XRT. Local failure occurred in one of 31 T1/T2 patients with follow-up ranging from 30 to 43 months. In staged T3 patients 20% (3/15) failed locally probably because these higher staged patients had less adequate clearance of disease; three patients had positive margins on final pathologic sections. For all patients in this series, the average tumor margin was 3 mm and the average tumor size was 3 cm. This series supports the use of limited excision and postoperative XRT as an alternative to APR for the patients with T1 and T2. Patients with pathologically staged T3 disease, those having compromised resection margin, or those with uT3, N1 staged tumors have a higher risk for local recurrence and possibly require higher doses of radiotherapy.

## 3. Pre-operative irradiation alone or combined with chemotherapy followed by conservation surgery

One logical rationale for preoperative irradiation of operable rectal cancer is to reduce tumor bulk in order to facilitate surgical resection. Surgery may be made more effective if wider cancer free margins are obtained around low-lying cancers. Several non-randomized and randomized studies have shown that preoperative irradiation significantly reduces local recurrence [27,28] and recently a large Swedish co-operative study shows that pre-operative irradiation alone improves survival [29]. These results have led to preoperative irradiation being used as a sole modality or combined with infusional chemoradiation for patients with operable and locally advanced rectal cancer [28,30–32]. Although the optimal preoperative chemoradiation schedule for rectal cancer patients is not known, the acute and late toxicity are key measurements of outcome that need to be examined carefully in the newer treatment schedules. In the pre-operative infusional chemoradiation program at M.D. Anderson Cancer Center, protracted infusional 5-fluorouracil (5-FU) chemoradiation was given to patients with staged T3, T4, and recurrent disease rectal cancers. Over 130 patients were treated with intermittent protracted 5-FU infusional chemoradiation in dosages of 300 mg/m$^2$ for 5 days/week allowing for 5-FU to be administered with each irradiation dose [28,31,32]. The external beam dose was 45 Gy in 25 fractions over 5 weeks and boost irradiation doses were given with intraoperative electron beam (IORT) to non-responding patients when there was major operative adherence or documented residual disease at the time of resection. In 77 patients with clinical T3 disease, operable rectal cancer was confirmed with an endoscopic ultrasound in 58 (75%). All patients completed infusional chemoradiation without interruption but three needed a brief hospital admission for the management of acute toxicity consisting of dehydration associated with diarrhea. Treatment response was scored histopathologically and was either complete or microscopic residual in 47 patients (61%). Although this clinical complete response rate is high, up to 50% of complete clinical responders can have microscopic residual in the resected specimen so that surgical resection was routinely performed [33]. Conservation surgery which spared the anal/rectal complex was performed in two-thirds. Local control was obtained in 96% after preoperative infusional chemoradiation; surgery was performed in two of three patients failing locally which resulted in an overall local control rate of 99% (76 of 77). Survival was better in those with a good treatment response compared to those with residual disease; patients with node negative specimens did only slightly better than those with involved lymph nodes. Preoperative 5-FU infusional chemoradiation is highly effective in tumor down staging and the responding patient has a better outcome. Treatment toxicity was also found to be acceptable with <5% suffering severe acute, or late effects. In comparison, preoperative biomodulated bolus 5-FU regimes are associated with lower pathologic complete response rates (even with the use of a higher irradiation dose) and with higher toxicity rates compared to those treated with infusional chemoradiation.

In more advanced patients (tethered T3 or T4 tumors), or in those with pelvic recurrence after surgery, the same infusional 5-FU chemoradiation protocol was used in 79 patients [30,32]. Poorly responding patients were also treated in a dedicated EB-IORT facility where boost doses could be administered to areas of residual disease. Local control in these patients was higher for those with T4 primaries compared to those with recurrent disease after surgery, local control 96% and ~70%, respectively. The pathologic treatment response was again found to predict treatment response to infusional chemoradiation where those that responded had better survival [33–32]. Another interesting finding was that in about half of the patients with recurrent disease the surgeon performed a sphincter-saving procedure which did not compromise survival [30]. These data suggest that pre-operative infusional chemoradiation is highly effective for patients with advanced rectal cancer.

The use of adjuvant infusional chemoradiation up to doses of 45 Gy have shown that these doses are well tolerated and that there is most likely room to push the irradiation dose higher with concurrent chemotherapy. Studies with kinetic and genetic markers may be of some help in the future for selection of patients for this more intensive therapy.

## 4. Non-operative infusional chemoradiation

Based on the successes with infusional chemoradiation in organ preserving treatment of anal, esophageal, and now rectal cancers, and because of the high activity seen with 5-FU infusional chemoradiation in the pre-operative treatment of rectal cancer, a non-surgical management for adenocarcinoma of the distal rectum may be possible for selected patients. There are some preliminary data on radical external beam irradiation alone for rectal cancer patients that provide further support for this approach. An accelerated irradiation schedule of 52 Gy (axis dose) in 20 fractions over 4 weeks has been used in the radical management of operable rectal cancer [34]. In patients with mobile tumors, local control was obtained in 31%, while those with partially fixed or fixed cancers, the local control rate was only 13%, and 3%, respectively. Although many of these rectal cancers regress slowly, this radio responsiveness did not equate to cure since 31% of the complete responders with mobile cancers (18/48) later recurred. These patients require very close followup between the radiation oncologist and the surgeon and allowed surgical salvage in about half the patients who recurred [35,36]. These data suggest that even more patients who refuse surgery or have a marginal medical status for anesthetic can be cured with infusional chemoradiation.

In the pre-operative infusional 5-FU chemoradiation program at M.D. Anderson Cancer Center, a few patients were treated without surgical resection and one such patient is illustrated in Fig. 1. This patient had an excellent clinical response to infusional chemoradiation but refused surgery that required a permanent colostomy. This anecdotal case and the finding of a ~30% complete clinical response with the chemoradiation used to treat her, suggests that there are patients that may be cured with relatively modest doses of chemoradiation. A potentially tantalizing hypothesis is that there may be a future role for a non-operative management for operable rectal cancer patients. The paradigm for this approach is already established with infusional chemoradiation for anal cancer patients. In this regard, another observation supporting the use of radical infusional chemoradiation for selected rectal cancer patients is that the incidence of late complications after this therapy is very low. This

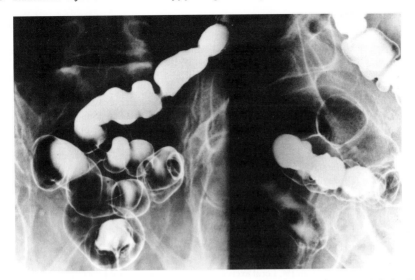

Fig. 1. Posterior and lateral radiographs of a patient treated with 60 Gy and concurrent 5-FU infusion for an ultrasound stage T3 N0 rectal cancer. The patient refused to have an abdomino-perineal resection. After 7 years of follow up examinations there is no evidence of recurrence. The bowel and bladder function are normal.

finding is also supported by the radiobiologic knowledge that the use of small daily doses of cytotoxic therapy of both fractionated irradiation and infusional chemoradiation may likely result in low levels of late effects suggesting that late effects are "spared with protracted treatment" [37]. This observations is consistent with the results of a randomized postoperative rectal adjuvant trial showing that late effects were also very low. These results indicate the need for further studies of the best "fractionation" patterns of both agents in combined modality programs.

*References*

1. Curley SA, Roh MS, Rich TA. Surgical therapy and early rectal carcinoma. Hematol Oncol Clin North Am 3: 87–102, 1989.
2. Wolmark N, Fisher B. An analysis of survival and treatment failure following abdominoperineal and sphincter-saving resection in Dukes' B and C rectal carcinoma. Ann Surg 204: 480–489, 1986.
3. Chan KW, Boey J, Wong SKC. A method of reporting radial invasion and surgical clearance of rectal carcinoma. Histopathology 9: 1319–1327, 1985.
4. Quirke P, Durdey P, Dixon MF, Williams NS. Local recurrence of rectal adenocarcinoma due to inadequate surgical resection. Histopathological study of lateral tumor spread and surgical excision. Lancet 996–999, 1986.
5. Quirke P, Scott N. The pathologist's role in the assessment of local recurrence in rectal carcinoma. Surg Oncol Clin North Am 1: 1–17, 1992.
6. Rich TA, Terry NHA, Meistrich M, et al. Pathologic, anatomic, and biologic factors correlated with local recurrence of colorectal cancer. Semin Radiat Oncol 3: 13–19, 1993.
7. Rich T, Gunderson LL, Lew R, et al. Patterns of recurrence of rectal cancer after potentially curative surgery. Cancer 52: 1317–1329, 1983.
8. Gunderson LL, Sosin H. Areas of failure found at reoperation (second or symptomatic look) following "curative surgery" for adenocarcinoma of the rectum. Cancer 34: 1278–1292, 1974.
9. Eker R. Some prognostic factors for carcinoma of the colon and rectum. Acta Chir Scand 126: 636–656, 1963.

10.  Minsky BD, Mies C, Rich TA, et al. Colloid carcinoma of the colon and rectum. Cancer 60: 3103–3112, 1987.

11.  Rich TA. Radiotherapy for early rectal cancer. In: Levin B (Coord Ed), Proc 30th Annu MD Anderson Clin Conf. Austin, TX: University of Texas Press, pp. 167–175, 1988.

12.  Enker WE, Paty PB, Minsky BD, Cohen AM. Restorative or preservative operations in the treatment of rectal cancer. Surg Oncol Clin North Am 1: 57–69, 1992.

13.  Nichols RJ, Mason AY, Morson BC. The clinical staging of rectal cancer. Br J Surg 69: 404–409, 1982.

14.  Duncan W. Adjuvant radiotherapy in rectal cancer: the MRC trials. Br J Surg (Suppl): s59–s66, 1985.

15.  Grabbe E, Lierse W, Winkler R. The perirectal fascia: morphology and the use in staging of rectal cancer. Radiology 149: 241–246, 1983.

16.  Wong WD, Orom WJ, Jense LL. Preoperative staging of rectal cancer with endorectal ultrasonography. Perspect Colon Rect Surg 3: 315–334, 1990.

17.  Hinder JM, Chu J, Bokey EL, et al. Use of transrectal ultrasound to evaluate direct tumor spread and lymph node status in patients with rectal cancer. Aust N Z J Surg 60: 19–23, 1990.

18.  Hildebrandt U, Feifel G. Preoperative staging of rectal cancer by intrarectal ultrasound. Dis Colon Rectum 28: 24–26, 1985.

19.  American Joint Committee, Staging Manual, AJC Classification, 1990.

20.  Chan TW, Kressel HY, Milestone B, ET AL. Rectal carcinoma: staging at MR imaging with endorectal surface coil. Radiology 181: 461–467, 1991.

21.  Graham RA, Garnsey L, Jessup JM. Local excision of rectal carcinoma. Am J Surg 160: 306–312, 1992.

22.  Rich TA, Weiss DR, Mies C, et al. Sphincter preservation in patients with low rectal cancer treated with radiation therapy with or without local excision or fulguration. Radiology 156: 527–531, 1985.

23.  Summers GE, Mendenhall WM, Copeland EM III. Update on the University of Florida experience with local excision and postoperative radiation therapy for the treatment of early rectal carcinoma. Surg Oncol Clin North Am 1: 25–130, 1992.

24.  Wood WC, Willett CG. Update of the Massachusetts General Hospital experience of combined local excision and radiotherapy for rectal cancer. Surg Oncol Clin North Am 1: 131–136, 1992.

25.  Jessup JM, Bothe A Jr, Stone MD, et al. Preservation of sphincter function in rectal carcinoma by a multimodality treatment approach. Surg Oncol Clin North Am 1: 137–145, 1992.

26.  Ota DM, Skibber J, Rich TA. M.D. Anderson Cancer Center experience with local excision and multimodality therapy for rectal cancer. Surg Oncol Clin North Am 1: 147–152, 1992.

27.  Frykholm GJ, Glimelius B, Pahlman L. Preoperative or postoperative irradiation in adenocarcinoma of the rectum: final treatment results of a randomized trial and an evaluation of late secondary effects. Dis Colon Rectum 36: 564–572, 1993.

28.  Rich TA, Skibber JM, Ajani JA, et al. Preoperative infusional chemoradiation therapy for stage T3 rectal cancer. Int J Radiat Oncol Biol Phys 32: 1025–1029, 1995.

29.  Swedish Rectal Cancer Trial. Improved survival with preoperative radiotherapy in resectable rectal cancer. N Engl J Med 336: 980–987, 1997.

30.  Lowy AM, Rich TA, Skibber JM, et al. Preoperative infusional chemoradiation, selective intraoperative radiation, and resection for locally advanced pelvic recurrence of colorectal adenocarcinoma. Ann Surg 223: 177–185, 1996.

31.  Shumate CR, Rich TA, Skibber JM, et al. Preoperative chemotherapy and radiation therapy for locally advanced primary and recurrent rectal carcinoma. A report of surgical morbidity. Cancer 71: 3690–3696, 1993.

32.  Weinstein GD, Rich TA, Shumate CR, et al. Preoperative infusional chemoradiation and surgery with or without an electron beam intraoperative boost for advanced primary rectal cancer. Int J Radiat Oncol Biol Phys 32: 197–204, 1995.

33.  Meterissian S, Skibber J, Rich T, et al. Patterns of residual disease after preoperative chemoradiation in ultrasound T3 rectal carcinoma. Ann Surg Oncol 1: 111–116, 1994.

34.  Brierley JD, Cummings BJ, Wong CS, et al. Adenocarcinoma of the rectum treated by radical external radiation therapy. Int J Radiat Oncol Biol Phys 31: 255–259, 1995.

35.  Rich TA, Gunderson LL. Radical nonoperative management of early rectal cancer [editorial]. Int J Radiat Oncol Biol Phys31: 677–678, 1995.

36.  Rich TA. Treatment of low rectal cancer with conservation surgery and radiotherapy. Front Radiat Ther Oncol 27: 118–129, 1993.

37.  Rich TA. Chemoradiation or accelerated fractionation: basic considerations. J Infus Chemother 1: 2–8, 1992.

C.J. Rosenthal and M. Rotman (Eds.), *Infusion Chemotherapy–Irradiation Interactions*

179

# Treatment of advanced bladder carcinoma with concomitant infusion of 5-fluorouracil and irradiation

HASSAN AZIZ and MARVIN ROTMAN

*Department of Radiation Oncology, State University of New York Health Science Center at Brooklyn, Brooklyn, NY and Long Island College Hospital, Long Island, NY, USA*

## 1. Introduction

In the United States, each year there is constant increase in the incidence and death rates resulting from bladder carcinoma. The estimated incidence of bladder carcinoma has increased from 49 400 in 1990 to 54 500 in 1997 [20,33]. Similarly, death rates increased from 9700 to 11 000 during the same period. While the increase in the incidence of bladder carcinoma may represent the urbanization of the population, the unchanging death rates depict the inefficacy of present conventional treatments, for advanced bladder carcinoma.

The 5-year survival rate in muscle-invading advanced bladder carcinoma with radical cystectomy is poor, i.e., in the range of 26–40% [19,21]. In addition, radical cystectomy is emotionally devastating due to loss of vital organs such as bladder and prostate, the need for urinary diversion, and impotence. The result of pre-operative radiation and radical cystectomy, although better by 10–15% [3,6], still means debilitating side-effects from loss of vital organs. Planned post-operative irradiation is not popular due to increased complication rate [17].

In the United States, traditionally, radiation alone with curative intent has been reserved for only those patients with advanced bladder carcinoma who are deemed medically unfit for surgery. In Europe, however, the primary modality for the treatment of advanced bladder cancer in many centers is irradiation. The 5-year survival rate with radiation alone in the treatment of muscle-invading bladder carcinoma is comparable to that obtained with radical cystectomy; however, it is still regarded as poor, i.e., in the range of 20–38% [12,17,23]. However, observations made with curative irradiation of bladder involved with advanced carcinoma (T3a, T3b) by Blandy et al. [5] and Goodman et al. [10] were exceptionally rewarding as downstaging to p$^0$ gave the basis for bladder preservation. Blandy et al. [5] reported a series of patients with advanced bladder cancer who received curative irradiation. The survival rate among patients who achieved p$^0$ status was 56% at 5 years with preservation of their bladder, with cystectomy being reserved for those who had either failed or recurred. These findings meant that, if by using an additional modality such as a radio-sensitizing agent, such as 5-fluorouracil (5-FU), further downstaging to p$^0$ could be obtained, then survival would increase with more preservation of the bladder.

In 1958, Heidelberger [11], using rodent tumors and tissue cultures, demonstrated the effectiveness of 5-FU as a radiosensitizer. However, it was Stein and Kaufman [34] who in 1968 first used 5-FU as a radiosensitizer with pre-operative irradiation in the treatment of bladder carcinoma. Rotman et al. [28] have treated a series of patients with advanced bladder carcinoma using concomitant infusion of 5-FU and irradiation, with curative intent aiming at higher cure rates and greater numbers of bladder preservation rates.

## 2. Materials and methods

From 1980 to 1990, Rotman et al. [28] included a series of 25 patients either with muscle-invading carcinoma or patients with poor prognostic factors scheduled to be treated curatively with concomitant 5-FU infusion and radiation at the State University of New York, Health Science Center at Brooklyn. Twenty of the 25 patients (80%) were males and 5 (20%) were females. The median age of these patients was 72 years with a range of 45–95. To ensure localized disease only, all patients had undergone computed tomography of pelvis and abdomen, chest radiograph, blood chemistries, intravenous pyelograms, and liver function tests. All patients were staged according to the Jewett Marshall System [13], but later staging was changed to the American Joint Committee TNM System [4].

Twenty-two of 25 (88%) patients had transitional cell carcinoma. Of these, only two (9%) had Grade 2 disease; the rest or 20 (91%) were diagnosed with either Grade 3 or 4 disease. Three of the 25 patients (12%) had squamous cell carcinoma. According to the TNM Staging System [4], 1 patient had Stage I and 7 patients had Stage T2 carcinoma. The numbers of Stages T3a, T3b, and T4a carcinomas were 9, 6 and 2, respectively (Table 1). Most of these patients not only had high grade and high stage tumors, but also other poor prognostic features. Eight of 25 patients (32%) were shown to have more than 50% involvement of the bladder. Seven of 25 patients (28%) had between 25% and 50% of the circumferential wall of the bladder involved with tumor, while 10/25 (40%) had hydronephrosis. Sixteen of 25 patients (64%) on cystoscopy were shown to have residual disease after transurethral resection of the tumor (Table 2).

All patients first received radiation to the entire pelvis via four-field technique on the 4 MV linear accelerator to a dose equal to 4140 cGy or 5040 cGy given in 4.5–5 weeks. This was followed by boost dose to the bladder using a skip arc technique giving another 2000 to 2500 cGy with total dose to the bladder being 6500 cGy. Concomitant infusion of 5-FU was given at a dose of 1000 mg/m$^2$ per 24 h for 120 h in weeks 1, 4 and 7 or 2, 5 and 8 of radiation treatment. In addition, 9% of patients received mitomycin given as a 10-mg intravenous bolus on day 1 of the first week of radiation therapy.

Table 1

Irradiation and concomitant infusion of 5-FU mitomycin ± staging in carcinoma of the bladder

|  | Stage TNM | | | | |
| --- | --- | --- | --- | --- | --- |
|  | T1 | T2 | T3a | T3b | T4a |
| No. of patients | 1/25 | 7/25 | 9/25 | 6/25 | 2/25 |
| % | 4.0 | 28.0 | 36.0 | 24.0 | 8.0 |

Table 2

Irradiation and concomitant infusion of 5-FU and mitomycin ± prognostic factors in carcinoma of the bladder

| | Prognostic factors | | | | | | | | |
|---|---|---|---|---|---|---|---|---|---|
| | Histology | | Transitional cell carcinoma | | Extent of involvement | | | | |
| | | | | | >50% | 25–50% | <25% | Hydro- | Gross |
| | SCC[a] | TCC[a] | II | III, IV | | | | | |
| No. of patients | 3/25 | 22/25 | 2/22 | 20/22 | 8/25 | 7/25 | 10/25 | 8/25 | 16/25 |
| % | 12[b] | 88 | 9 | 91 | 32 | 28 | 40 | 32 | 64 |

[a]SCC, squamous cell carcinoma; TCC, transitional cell carcinoma.
[b]Excluded from analysis of survival.

## 3.  Results

### 3.1.  Response

Three patients who were diagnosed with squamous cell carcinoma were excluded from the evaluation of the response and survival rates. The remaining 22 patients with transitional cell carcinoma were evaluated for response and survival. To evaluate response, all patients underwent cystoscopy and biopsy 4–6 weeks after completion of treatment.

In the group of patients with Stages T1 and T2, 6 of 8 (75%) had an initial complete response (Table 3). In the higher stages, i.e., Stages T3a, T3b, and T4a, 10/14 (71%) achieved complete response. In both groups of patients the initial complete response rate was 73%. Further, three patients who had superficial disease and positive urinary cytology were aggressively treated with repeated TUR and instillations of mitomycin or BCG and also became free of disease. Thus, the overall total complete response, including both initial and late response, was 19/22 (86%).

### 3.2.  Survival

Two patients who had developed measurable metastatic disease, either during or soon after completion of treatment, were excluded from evaluation of response, leaving 20 patients for

Table 3

Irradiation and concomitant infusion of 5-FU mitomycin ± response in carcinoma of the bladder

| | Complete pathological response | | | | |
|---|---|---|---|---|---|
| | Initial | | | With TUR and intravesical BCG/mitomycin T3a, T3b, T4a | Overall complete response |
| | T1, T2 | T3a, T3b, T4a | Total | | |
| No. of patients | 6/8 | 10/14 | 16/22 | 3/14 | 19/22 |
| % | 75 | 71 | 86 | 21 | 86 |

Table 4

Irradiation and concomitant infusion of 5-FU and mitomycin C ± survival in carcinoma of the bladder

|  | Stages | | |
|---|---|---|---|
|  | T1, T2 | T3a, T3b[a], T4a | All stages |
| No. of patients | 6/8 | 5/12 | 11/20 |
| % 5-year survival[b] | 80 | 41 | 55 |

[a]Two patients excluded due to development of distant metastases during treatment.
[b]Calculated by life table method.

the analysis of survival. The adjusted 5-year survival for the patients with Stages T1 and T2 was satisfactory at 80%, while the survival in the advanced stages, i.e., T3a, T3b, and T4a was 41% (Table 4). The difference in survival rates between the early stages and advanced stages was further confirmed by comparing the survival of Stages T2 and T3a. The minimum survival of Stage T2 was 72 months, as compared to a mean survival of 52 months for Stage T3a patients ($P \leq 0.001$). The adjusted overall 5-year survival for all tumor stages was 55%. The effect of grade and hydronephrosis on survival rates could not be confirmed due to disproportionate numbers of patients in each sample of patients. The number of patients with low grade was only 2 compared to 18 with high grade. The presence of hydronephrosis only showed a trend towards a poor prognosis ($P = 0.22$).

### 3.3. Complications

RTOG/ECOG Complication Grading System was employed to evaluate complications arising in this series of patients. The incidence of high grade complications was low, as compared to low grade complications. Twenty-one of the 22 patients (95%) developed grade I/II diarrhea treated with conservative management. Nine of 21 patients (43%) developed Grade II cystitis, while 2/22 (9%) had Grade III hematuria. Only one patient exhibited Grade IV toxicity. The incidence of mucositis as low as Grade I/II mucositis was seen in only three of 22 patients (13%). Hematological complications were also less common as only 2 of 22 patients (9%) required reduction of dose of 5-FU due to WBC being below 2.5. The rate of late complications was low. Two patients of 22 (9%) had recurrent symptoms of cystitis and dysuria. Both patients responded to treatment. One patient who had developed symptoms of proctitis with chronic rectal bleeding and thrombocytopenia had required colectomy.

### 3.4. Pattern of failure

From both groups of patients (the superficial and deep muscle-invading group) a total of 11/20 patients (55%) have died. Most of these patients, however, died from the deep muscle-invading (T3a, T3b and T4a) group. Three patients died of intercurrent disease, while one died from regional disease. All patients who died of metastatic disease died within 2 years.

Preservation of bladder was achieved in the majority of patients. Of the 9 patients who survived, 7 retained their bladders and only 2 underwent salvage cystectomy. The majority of patients (70%) who died of metastatic or intercurrent disease also retained their bladders.

## 4. Discussion

In the treatment of advanced bladder carcinoma conventional treatments given either with radical cystectomy or with planned pre- or post-operative irradiation, all have failed to yield a worthwhile 5-year survival rate. With radical cystectomy the reported 5-year survival is in the range of 26–40% [19,21] with significant patients still dying from distant metastases which could be as high as 40–50% [22,27] in a period of the first 2 years. Patients submitted to pre-operative irradiation and cystectomy may have a better survival by about 10–15% [3,6], but still many patients with profound disability with loss of vital organs. Planned, post-operative radiation following radical cystectomy has only added to the pre-existing morbidity of the patient [17].

The results of treatment of advanced bladder carcinoma with irradiation alone is also not encouraging, ranging between 20 and 38% [12,17,25]. Treatment of advanced bladder carcinoma with radiation given as primary modality, however, has an important advantage over radical cystectomy, as patients obtaining full pathological response to p° may preserve their bladders. This was amply demonstrated by Blandy et al. [5] in England where a series of Stage T2, T3 patients were treated with curative dose of radiation. A 5-year survival rate of 56% was obtained in patients who achieved complete pathological response to p°, as compared to 17.5% for those patients who did not achieve complete response and required cystectomy. Trials by RTOG, utilizing misonidazole as radiosensitizer [25] and high LET radiation such as neutron [24] was also without benefit. The use of hyperfractionated radiation [26], although initially promising, did not achieve appreciably better results.

Following conventional treatment about 40–50% of patients with muscle-invading bladder carcinoma will die with metastatic disease [22,27] within 2 years and a substantial number will remain with local disease. This underscores the necessity for effective chemotherapy for both micrometastases, clinically persistent disease, and for radiosensitization to enhance the local effect. A host of single agents are active against transitional cell carcinoma of the bladder, the response rate varying from 15 to 50%. The most active cytotoxic agent are cisplatinum, methotrexate, 5-FU, doxorubicum and vinblastine. These single agents have variable response rates depending on factors such as heterogeneity of tumors, patients and inaccurate staging. Combined with each other or with radiation will enhance the effect considerable.

There are mainly two main varieties of combined chemotherapy available against transitional carcinoma of the bladder. These may be either cisplatinum-based or may be based on cisplatinum and methotrexate. Using cisplatinum-based combination of CISCA (cisplatinum, cyclophosphamide and adriamycin) the Memorial group reported 13 complete and partial responses in 28 evaluated patients (46%). At the M.D. Anderson Hospital, the use of CISCA in advanced bladder carcinomas produced a complete clinical response rate of 48%. In the group of combination-based cisplatinum and methotrexate, two most efficacious regimens are M-VAC and MCV. M-VAC (methotrexate, vinblastine, adriamycin and cisplatinum) developed at the Memorial Sloan Kettering Hospital [31] in a series of locally advanced bladder carcinomas produced a complete response rate of 48%. At the University of Chicago [31] with the use of M-VAC, complete clinical response rate was 32%. At the Mayo Clinic and at Massachusetts General Hospital, using MCV (methotrexate, cisplatinum and vinblastine) a complete response rate of 52% and 50%, respectively, was obtained [32]. In the treatment of advanced bladder carcinoma at Massachusetts General Hospital [14], two upfront courses of MCV are being given before concomitant cisplatinum bolus and irradiation. The multidrug chemotherapy is often too toxic and its effect not sustained. Scher et al. in 1989 [30] showed that after obtaining complete clinical response when treated with multidrug chemotherapy, a substantial number of patients, i.e., up to 40%, had residual disease in the bladder as demonstrated by cystectomy.

In order to enhance the local control in advanced bladder carcinoma to achieve better survival and bladder preservation, Rotman et al. [28] investigated the use of concomitant infusion of 5-FU and, irradiation in the treatment of advanced bladder carcinoma. The selection of 5-FU was based on its known radiosensitizing effect and its activity against bladder carcinoma. The reported response rate of 5-FU in bladder carcinoma as a single agent is reported to be 19% [32] with tolerable gastro-intestinal and hematological toxicities.

Heidelberger et al. in 1958 [11] first described greater effect of radiation and 5-FU when used together in certain rodent tumors, as compared to when these modalities were used alone. In 1961, Bagshaw et al. [2] and Vermund et al. in 1964 [36] confirmed the radiosensitizing effect of 5-FU using tissue culture. More specifically, Woodruff et al. in 1963 [38] demonstrated the radiosensitizing effect of 5-FU on the transitional cell carcinoma of the bladder. In 1968, Stein and Kaufman [34] showed enhanced tumor regression in surgically treated bladders. In 1971, Vietti et al. [37], using mouse leukemia cells, again not only demonstrated the radiosensitizing effect of 5-FU, but also showed its relationship to time of administration. It was Byfield et al. [7], however, who discussed prerequisites for the administration of 5-FU as a radiosensitizer. These authors showed that 5-FU radiosensitization is a post-radiation phenomenon and that 5-FU must be available to the cells for 24 h after each exposure of radiation, requiring constant, slow infusion. The exact mechanism of 5-FU radiosensitization is not known. However, it is thought that the cellular presence of 5-FU may inhibit the de novo synthesis of DNA by binding thymidine synthetase. A defective RNA synthesis may also occur as a result of its being taken as an RNA precursor nucleotide. Vietti et al. [37] further hypothesized that the presence of 5-FU may also inhibit the repair of sub-lethal damage-producing radiation, thus further radiosensitizing the tumor cells.

In early studies, Moertel et al. [18] and Lo et al. [15] used bolus 5-FU and radiation in the treatment of unresectable gastrointestinal and head and neck carcinomas. 5-FU was given by bolus until myelosuppression had occurred. Interrupted treatments, lack of clinical benefit and myelotoxicity led to a steady decline in the use of bolus 5-FU. Studies by Byfield et al. [7] later explained the importance of 5-FU being given as infusion, to reduce its toxicity and to obtain better clinical control. Byfield et al. [7] defined radiosensitization as "a state of cellular condition that develops gradually in 24 h or more of continuous 5-FU exposure after each radiation exposure".

Further support for the use of 5-FU as infusion is derived from the studies of Chabner et al. [8] and Lockich [16] in which they studies pharmacodynamics of cytotoxic agents. Most cytotoxic agents are active in the DNA synthetic phase of the cell cycle and have a short plasma half-life, meaning that exposure of the drug will be limited to a small fraction of the cell cycle. With continuous infusion chemotherapy, there would be prolonged exposure to the drugs. Seifert et al. [29a], after conducting a randomized trial, confirmed the usefulness of chemotherapeutic agents being given as infusion.

The results of treatment with this group of patients with their host of poor prognostic factors seem satisfactory. Although most of the patients in our series presented with bulky infiltrating disease, 6/25 patients had more than 50% of the bladder involved, 8/25 had hydronephrosis, and 16/25 had gross residual disease following TURBT; their complete response rate (urine cytology negative) within 6 months was 62.5%. The final complete response rate of 86% was achieved after three patients underwent further treatment with transurethral resection and intravesical BCG or mitomycin. It is noteworthy that in our series, a prior transurethral resection was not required to achieve a similar complete response rate as was mentioned by Shipley et al. [32]. Russel et al. [29] using 5-FU infusion and a concomitant radiation dose of 4000 cGy, demonstrated a complete response rate of 76%. It appears that the complete response rate obtained with the use of infusion 5-FU and concomitant radiation is twice that of irradiation alone when compared to p° of the preoperative series. Bladder preservation, a major goal of our study, was achieved in the majority (17/20) of patients. Salvage cystectomy was necessary in only two cases.

In this study, the 5-year survival rate for the patients with superficial tumors (T and T2) was 80%. The survival at 5 years for deep muscle-invading tumor (T3a, T3b, and T4a) was 40%. The survival for the superficial group of tumors, with the presence of other poor prognostic features was regarded as satisfactory. However, the survival of 40% in the latter group was disappointingly low in spite of the fact that high complete local response was achieved in these patients. Since the vast majority of patients died of metastatic disease within a period of 2 years, it is assumed that the reason for lower survival in the deep muscle-invading group of patients was due to the presence of micrometastases at the time of presentation. Recently, there has been a renewed interest in the use of intra-arterial infusion. Eapen et al. [9], through bilateral hypogastric arteries, used infusion of cisplatinum at 3 weeks prior to radiation and concomitantly again during the first week of radiation. The results are promising with 90% control rate at 2 years and some increase in survival rate.

Another new approach to improve local control and survival is being tried in Rome [1]. Early results of this trial were presented at a recent International Meeting in Rome and also at the ASTRO meeting in Los Angeles. Arcangelli et al. [1] reported on a phase 1–2 trial where a series of invasive bladder carcinomas were treated either with or without two upfront courses of MCV (methotrexate, cisplatinum and vinblastine). This was followed by concomitant continuous infusion of cisplatinum and continuous infusion of 5-FU. Radiation consisted of three 100-cGy fractions per day, 5 days per week for a total dose of 5000 cGy in 4.5 weeks. A further consolidative dose of 2000 cGy was also given in 1 week if required due to residual disease. During radiation both 5-FU and cisplatinum were infused through separate tubing using cisplatinum at 6 mg/m$^2$ per day and 5-FU at 200 mg/m$^2$ per day. Thirty-four patients were evaluated, obtaining a complete response rate of 91%. Serious high grade toxicity was uncommon, while low grade toxicity was common.

## 5.   Conclusions

The experience with the continuous concomitant infusion of 5-FU with radiation therapy in the treatment of advanced bladder carcinoma has been encouraging. The 5-year survival rate of 80% in T1 and T2 bladder carcinoma with bladder preservation is an excellent result. However, the rate of 5-year survival in deep muscle-invading tumors (T3a, T3b, and T4a) is not satisfactory at 41%, due to the presence of micrometases at the time of diagnosis. However, bladder preservation was achieved in the majority of patients. Efforts are being made [1,14] to improve the survival in advanced bladder carcinoma with new adjuvant multi-drug chemotherapy such as MCV. Long-term results of such trials are awaited.

## References

1. Arcangeli G, Tirindelli Danesi D, Mecozi A, et al. Combined hyperfractionated irradiation and protracted infusion chemotherapy in invasive bladder cancer with conservative intent. Phase I study. Int J Radiat Oncol Biol Phys 36: 314, 1996.

2. Bagshaw MA. Possible role of potentiators in radiation therapy. Am J Roentgenol 85: 822, 1961.

3. Batata MA, Chu FCH, Hilaris BS, et al. Preoperative whole pelvis versus true pelvis irradiation and/or cystectomy for bladder cancer. Int J Radiat Oncol Biol Phys 7: 1349, 1981.

4. Beahrs OH, Henson DE, Hutter DE, Myers MH (Eds). American Joint Committee on Cancer Manual for Staging of Cancer, 3rd edn. Philadelphia, PA: JB Lippincott, 1983.

5. Blandy JP, England HR, Evans SJ, et al. T3 bladder cancer; the case for salvage cystectomy. Br J Urol 52: 506, 1980.

6. Bloom HJ, Hendry WF, Wallace DM, et al. Treatment of T3 bladder cancer. Controlled trial of preoperative radiotherapy and radical cystectomy versus radical radiotherapy. Second report and review (for the Clinical Trial Group Institute of Urology). Br J Urol 54: 136, 1982.

7. Byfield JE, Chan P, Seagren SL. Radiosensitization of 5-FU: molecular origins and clinical scheduling implications (abstr.). Proc Am Assoc Cancer Res 18: 74, 1977.

8. Chabner B. Pharmacologic Principles of Cancer Treatment, Vol. 3. Philadelphia, PA: WB Saunders, p. 14, 1982.

9. Eapen L, Stewart D, Danjoix D, et al. Intra-arterial cisplatin and concomitant radiation for locally advanced bladder cancer. J Clin Oncol 7: 230–233, 1989.

10. Goodman GB, Hislop TG, Elwood JM, et al. Conservation of bladder function in patients with invasive bladder cancer treated by definitive irradiation and selective cystectomy. Int J Radiat Oncol Biol Phys 7: 569, 1982.

11. Heidelberger C, Greisbach L, Montag B, et al. Studies in fluorinated pyrimidine II. Effects of transplanted tumor. Cancer Res 18: 305–317, 1958.

12. Hope-Stone HF, Blandy JP, Oliver RTD, et al. Radial radiotherapy and salvage cystectomy in the treatment of invasive carcinoma of the bladder. In: Oliver RTD, Hendry WF, Bloom HJ (Eds), Bladder Cancer Principles of Combination Therapy. London: Butterworths, pp. 127–138, 1981.

13. Jewett HJ, Strong GH. Infiltrating carcinoma of the bladder: relation of depth of penetration of the bladder wall to incidence of local extension and metastases. J Urol 55: 366, 1946.

14. Kaufman DS, Shipley WU, Griffin PP, et al. Selective bladder preservation by combination treatment of invasive bladder cancer. N Engl J Med 329: 1377, 1993.

15. Lo TCM, Wiley AL, Ausfield FJ, et al. Combined radiation therapy and 5-fluorouracil for advanced squamous cell carcinoma of the oral cavity and oropharynx: a randomized study. Radiology 126: 229, 1976.

16. Lockich JJ. Infusion chemotherapy for cancer. Curr Concepts Oncol 6: 3, 1984.

17. Miller LS, Johnson DE. Megavoltage irradiation for bladder cancer: alone, postoperative or preoperative? Genitourinary Cancer 10: 771, 1973.

18. Moertel CG, Childs DS, Reitemeier RJ, et al. Combined 5-fluorouracil and supervoltage radiation therapy of locally unresectable gastro-intestinal cancer. Lancet ii: 865, 1969.

19. Montie JE, Straffon RA, Stewart BH. Radical cystectomy without radiation therapy for carcinoma of the bladder. J Urol 131: 477, 1984.

20. Parker SL, Tong T, Bolden S, Wingo PA. Cancer statistics, 1997. Cancer J Clin 47: 5–27, 1997.

21. Poole-Wilson DS, Barnard RJ. Total cystectomy for bladder tumors. Br J Urol 43: 16, 1971.

22. Prout GR, Griffin PP, Shipley WU. Bladder carcinoma as a systemic disease. Cancer 43: 2532, 1979.

23. Quilty PM, Duncan W. Primary radical radiotherapy for T3 transitional cell cancer of the bladder. An analysis of survival and control. Int J Radiat Oncol Biol Phys 12: 853, 1986.

24. RTOG 77–05/81–10. Phase I, II study comparing the value of neutrons alone, mixed beam and preoperative mixed beam in bladder carcinoma. Philadelphia, PA: RTOG.

25. RTOG 81–05. Phase I/II study on the value of combining misomidazole and radiotherapy in the treatment of bladder cancer. Philadelphia, PA: RTOG.

26. RTOG 83–08. Randomized phase II study to evaluate hyperfractionated radiation for locally advanced carcinoma of the bladder. Philadelphia, PA: RTOG.

27. Raghavan D, Shipley WU, Garnick MB, et al. Biology and management of bladder cancer. N Engl J Med 322: 1129, 1990.

28.   Rotman M, Aziz H, Porrazzo M, et al. Treatment of advanced transitional cell carcinoma of the bladder with irradiation and concomitant 5-fluorouracil infusion. Int J Radiat Oncol Biol Phys 18: 1131, 1990.

29.   Russel KJ, Boileau MA, Ireton RC, et al. Transitional carcinoma of the urinary bladder; histologic clearance with combined 5-FU chemotherapy and radiation therapy. Preliminary results of bladder preservation study. Radiology 167: 845, 1988.

29a.  Seifert P, Baker CH, Reed ML, et al. Comparison of continuously infused 5-FU with bolus injection in treatment of patients with colo-rectal carcinoma. Cancer 36: 123–128, 1975.

30.   Scher H, Hess H, Sternberg C, et al. Neo-adjuvant chemotherapy for invasive bladder cancer. Experience with M-VAC regimen. Br J Urol 64: 250, 1989.

31.   Shipley WU, Kaufman D, Griffin P, et al. Radio-chemotherapy for invasive carcinoma of the bladder. In: Vaeth JM (Ed), Radiotherapy/Chemotherapy Interaction in Cancer Therapy. Front Radiat Ther Oncol. Basel:, Karger 26: p. 142, 1992.

32.   Shipley WU, Coombs LJ, Eienstein AB Jr, et al. National Bladder Cancer Collaborative Group. Cisplatin and full dose irradiation for patients with invasive bladder carcinoma: a preliminary report of tolerance and local response. J Urol 132: 899, 1984.

33.   Silverberg BS, Lubera JA. Cancer statistics. Cancer J Clin: 9–26, 1990.

34.   Stein JJ, Kaufman JJ. Treatment of carcinoma of bladder with special reference to use of preoperative radiation therapy combined with 5-fluorouracil. Am J Roentgenol 102: 519, 1968.

35.   Van der Werf-Messing BHP, Friedal GH, Menon RS, et al. Carcinoma of the urinary bladder T3NxMo treated by preoperative irradiation followed by simple cystectomy. Int J Radiat Oncol Biol Phys 8: 1849, 1982.

36.   Vermund H, Hodget J, Ausfield FJ. Effects of combined radiation and chemotherapy on transplanted tumors in mice. Am J Roentgenol 85: 559–567, 1961.

37.   Vietti J, Eggerding F, Valeriote F. Combined effect of radiation and 5-fluorouracil on survival of transplanted leukemia cells. J Natl Cancer Inst 47: 865, 1971.

38.   Woodruff MW, Murphy WT, et al. Further observations on use of combination 5-fluorouracil and supervoltage irradiation therapy in the treatment of advanced carcinoma of bladder. J Urol 90: 747, 1963.

# CHAPTER 18

# Combined modality therapy for patients with cancer of the esophagus

HAYTHEM ALI and MUHYI AL-SARRAF

*Providence Cancer Center, Southfield, MI 48075, USA*

## 1. Introduction

Esophageal carcinoma is a disease of middle aged men in most of the western world. In the United States, the incidence in African American males is 6 times higher than in European Americans. Differences in incidence vary geographically, while incidence is 4:100 000 among European Americans, it is 100:100 000 in some parts of China and in Iran. The incidence has doubled among African American males since 1950 but has remained stable among European Americans. In the United States and other developed countries, alcohol and tobacco abuse is the major etiological factor. In other less developed countries micronutrient deficiency in the staple diet of the population is the main culprit. Other less common but noteworthy syndromes associated with esophageal carcinomas, include Barrets esophagus, Plummer Vincent syndrome and Tylosis [35]. In recent years there has been a shift in the histological picture from that of squamous cell carcinoma to adenocarcinoma, which is similar to the change seen in the histology of lung carcinoma. This shift may be related to a change in the type of carcinogen exposure following the popularity of filtered and lighter brands of cigarettes.

The traditional treatment modality for patients with potentially curable disease has been surgical resection. This represents 40–50% of candidates who are potentially operable. The surgeon is able to resect all visible disease in about 60–70% of the cases which means that about 20–25% of patients will be eligible to have curative resection. The rest will need some form of definitive or adjuvant therapy other than surgery. Surgical treatment is difficult because of the awkward position of the esophagus making access hard. This difficulty translates into a high mortality rate, ranging from 3–10%, and morbidity rate, ranging from 20–50%. Surgical complications include local recurrence, anastomotic leaks, aspiration pneumonia and loss of physiologic integrity. Survival statistics show that the median survival of surgical patients is about 9 months, the 2-year survival is about 10% and the 5-year survival about 5%.

If surgery was not possible, the traditional approach has been to give radiation therapy with curative intent [38,39]. The results seen with curative radiation therapy are modest with a median survival of about 9 months, a 2-year survival of 10% and a 5-year survival of 5%. It is important to note that most radiation therapy trials have patients who are otherwise unresectable or inoperable with many medical problems, and a direct comparison with the surgical population is probably incorrect. These poor results have initiated further investigation to improve the natural history of this disease. Previous observations had shown that locoregional failure occurred in as high as 40–50% of autopsy specimens of patients dying of esophageal cancer following surgery. Therefore, delivering higher intensity local treatment, to control locoregional failure rates in order to improve overall survival rate have been investigated. Many trials reported on the results of radiotherapy given either pre- or post-operatively. Radiation as adjuvant therapy was the subject of a randomized trial conducted by the EORTC [1] in the late 1970s in which 208 patients were randomized to surgery versus preoperative radiation therapy. The addition of preoperative irradiation, significantly decreased the incidence of loco-regional recurrence. But did not impact survival, with a median survival of 12 months for both groups, and a 5-year survival of 20% for the surgery only patients, and 14% for the combined arm. This fact underscored the importance of distal control to improve survival in esophageal cancer treatment. Teniere et al. [2] reported on randomized trial of surgery alone versus postoperative radiotherapy, the combined arm resulted in significant decrease in loco-regional recurrence as was reported with preoperative irradiation therapy in the EROTC trial. Many single agent chemotherapy agents show moderate activity in esophageal carcinoma, and have been used as palliative treatment for patients with metastatic disease. Most of these agents have response rates in the 15% range in patients with metastatic or recurrent esophageal cancers. The best activity seen using 5-fluorouracil (5-FU), cisplatin, mitomycin, vindisine, and lately paclitaxel. Combination chemotherapy has also been advocated with the most widely used being 5-FU based combinations with cisplatin or mitomycin. These combinations have been widely accepted as standard chemotherapy when treating esophageal carcinoma. Usually the 5-FU is given as intravenous continuous infusion for 96–120 h. Other combinations, incorporating *Vinca* alkaloids and bleomycin with cisplatin based combination, have also been studied and show less impressive results. The availability of paclitaxel in recent years and its promising activity as a single agent holds promise for its use in combination with other agents that have shown good activity in esophageal carcinoma.

## 2. Multimodality therapy

Multimodality therapy has its advantages and disadvantages. Theoretic benefits of combination chemo-radiation therapy include increased local control, and the possibility of decreasing distant metastasis. Local control may be achieved by sensitization of hypoxic cells to radiotherapy mimicking the effects of oxygen [3], the ability of some chemotherapeutic agents to kill hypoxic cells enhancing the effects of radiation therapy locally [3], and the use of concurrent chemotherapy halting repopulation between radiation fractions. On the other hand, disadvantages of combination modality therapy is the high incidence of side effects requiring intensive patient care. Recent developments in oncological supportive care, more effective management of chemo-radiation side effects, and improved antibiotics are important in achieving the best survival results with minimal mortality or long term morbidity. When looking at the patterns of failure in patients who received curative radiation, one notices that local recurrence is the number one pattern of failure but interestingly 35–50% of these patients also fail distally. The use of chemotherapeutic agents as radiotherapy sensitizers augments the local effect of irradiation, and achieves a better distant control of the disease.

## 3.  Pre-operative chemotherapy

In an attempt to control distant metastasis and improve survival, a number of studies explored the use of chemotherapy in the preoperative setting in order to improve the results of surgery. Kelsen et al. [4] tested a combination of cisplatin, bleomycin and vindesine preoperatively and achieved a median survival of 16 months and a 5-year survival of 18%. This combination chemotherapy given preoperatively produced the same response rate, rate of resectability, median survival, and overall survival, as preoperative radiation therapy when compared in a randomized trial [5]. Many phase II trials using cisplatin based chemotherapy showed an improvement in median survival (16–28 months), and overall survival over those achieved historically by surgery alone [6–12]. Randomized trials [13–15] investigating preoperative chemotherapy failed to show a statistically significant survival advantage over surgery alone in patients with esophageal cancers.

## 4.  Pre-operative chemo-radiotherapy and surgery

Many non-randomized studies were conducted in the early 1980s to study the effectiveness of combined modality therapy (Table 1) [16–21,36,37]. The Wayne State University group studied two 5-FU infusion combinations: 5-FU with mitomycin [17] and 5-FU with cisplatin [18], both given concurrently with radiation therapy of 3000 cGy given in 15 fractions and followed by surgical resection. The median survival of these patients was 18 months. The interesting finding in these studies was that of the 70–75% of patients who were able to undergo surgery, about 24% achieved a complete pathological response, and this finding was the strongest predictor of future survival in the study group. Later studies by the Radiation Therapy Oncology Group (RTOG) [21], and the Southwest Oncology Group (SWOG) [19], investigated the combination of 5-FU and cisplatin, concurrent with irradiation preoperative, the combination produced a complete pathological response rate of 27 and 25%, respectively. Forestiere et al. [9] studied a more complex preoperative chemo-radiotherapy, which included a 21-day continuous infusion of 5-FU with two 5-day periods of continuous infusion cisplatin and vinblastin in a 21-day intensive therapy with radiation given in a dose of 3750 cGY that was later intensified to 4500 cGY. The regimen achieved a 5-year survival of 35% and a complete pathological response rate similar to those achieved earlier by the Wayne State group. Randomized phase III trials comparing surgery with or without preop-

Table 1

Phase II pilot studies of preoperative chemo-radiotherapy

| Authors | No. of patients | Agents | Radiation (cGy) | Median (months) | Survival (%) | |
|---|---|---|---|---|---|---|
| | | | | | 3 years | 5 years |
| Franklin et al. [17] | 30 | FM | 3000 | 18 | 30 | |
| Leichman et al. [18] | 21 | PF | 3000 | 18 | | |
| Urba et al. [20] | 24 | F | 4900 | 11 | | 33 |
| Foriester et al. [16] | 43 | PFV | 3750–4500 | 29 | | 34 |
| Poplin et al. [19] | 113 | PF | 3000 | 12 | 16 | |
| Syedel et al. [21] | 41 | PF | 3000 | 13 | 8 | |

Table 2

Phase II pilot studies of preoperative chemo-radiotherapy

| Authors | No. of patients | Agents | Radiation (cGy) | Median (months) | Survival (%) | |
|---|---|---|---|---|---|---|
| | | | | | 2 years | 5 years |
| Urba et al. [24] | 100 | PFV | 4500 | 18 | 42 | |
| | | Surgery | | 18 | 39 | |
| Le Price et al. [23] | 86 | PF | 2000 | | | 19 |
| | | Surgery | | | | 14 |
| Walsh et al. [22] | 113 | PF | 4000 | 16 | 37 | |
| | | Surgery | | 11 | 26 | |

erative chemoradiotherapy (Table 2) [22–24] failed to show a significant survival advantage in either group.

## 5.  Total chemo-radiotherapy

In earlier studies of neoadjuvant chemo-radiation therapy performed at Wayne State University, surgical resection might not significantly improve survival. Because of the consistent observation that a complete pathological response was a strong predictor of survival, efforts were focused on achieving better survival rates with chemo-radiation alone. A phase II pilot study reported from Wayne State University [25] with the combination of 5-FU, and cisplatin given concurrently with 5000 cGy of radiotherapy, and mitomycin, plus bleomycin given as adjuvant therapy, resulted in a median survival of 22 months. These results were compared to historical counterparts at the same institution that achieved a median survival of 18 months after neoadjuvant chemoradiation followed by surgery. Several studies have been reported without the use of bleomycin which was responsible for a high incidence of pulmonary toxicity. These studies employed either 5-FU and mitomycin or 5-FU and cisplatin using radiation therapy ranging from 4000 to 6000 cGY and achieving 2-year survival rates of 20–41% (Table 3) [26–30] which are comparable if not better than traditional surgical survival statistics. These trials paved the way for more extensive phase III trials.

Chemoradiation was compared to curative radiation alone in phase III prospective ran-

Table 3

Phase II pilot studies of preoperative chemo-radiotherapy

| Authors | No. of patients | Agents | Radiation (cGy) | Median (months) | Survival (%) | |
|---|---|---|---|---|---|---|
| | | | | | 2 years | 5 years |
| Leichman et al. [25] | 20 | PFMB | 5000 | 22 | | |
| Coia et al. [27] | 57 | FM | 6000 | 18 | | 18 |
| John et al. [28] | 30 | PFM | 4140–5040 | 15 | 29 | |
| Chan et al. [26] | 21 | PF | 4000–5000 | 13 | 0 | |
| Seitz et al. [30] | 35 | PF | 5600–6000 | 17 | 41 | |
| Richmond et al. [29] | 25 | PF | 4000 | 12 | 37 | |

Table 4

Phase II pilot studies of preoperative chemo-radiotherapy

| Authors | No. of patients | Agents | Radiation (cGy) | Median (months) | Survival (%) | |
|---|---|---|---|---|---|---|
| | | | | | 2 years | 5 years |
| Sischy et al. [34] | 118 | FM | 6000 | 14.8 | | |
| | | | 6000 | 9.1 | | |
| Herskovic et al. [33] | 123 | PF | 5000 | 14.1 | 38 | 30 |
| and Al-Sarraf et al. [31] | | | 6400 | 9.3 | 10 | 0 |
| Araujo et al. [32] | 59 | FM | 5000 | | 38 | 16 |
| | | | 5000 | | 22 | 6 |

domized trials (Table 4) [31–34]. In a recent intergroup study reported by Herskovic et al. [33], 123 patients were randomized to chemo-radiotherapy versus radiotherapy alone. In the combined group, the chemotherapy was two courses of cisplatin and 5-FU given concurrently with 5000 cGy, followed by two additional courses of the same chemotherapy. In the standard group, total radiotherapy of 6400 cGy was given. The patients in the chemoradiotherapy group had a 2-year survival of 38%, as compared to 10% in the radiation only group, and the median survival was 14 and 9 months, respectively. This led to an early closure of this trial, because of the statistical survival advantage shown in the chemo-radiation group. In a recent followup to the study, the investigators [31] reported survival advantage for continuous accrual in the chemoradiation group after the closure of the randomized trial, and 5-year survival of the original randomized group of chemo-radiotherapy of about 30%. Other studies collaborate these results reported by the Eastern Cooperative Oncology Group (ECOG) [34], which showed a survival advantage for the group receiving concurrent 5-FU and mitomycin and radiotherapy over radiation therapy alone. In a study by Araujo et al. [32] using the same combination of the ECOG study but with 5000 cGy, the differences in 2-year and 5-year survival were not significant. This is may be due to the small number of patients included in this randomized trial.

The toxicity profile of combined modality therapy is high when compared to a single modality. In the study reported by Herskovic and colleagues, 68% of patients in the chemoradiation group experienced side effects with one treatment related fatality, while only 28% of the radiation only group experienced any side-effects. When one reviews the side-effect profile of combined modality therapy, we recognize that hematological complications cause most of the toxicity, and 20% represented life-threatening complications. In our view the development of hematological stimulating factors and good supportive care will control side-effects and improve the results of combined modality therapy.

## 6. Conclusions

The combination of radiation therapy and chemotherapy is superior to radiation therapy alone in patients with locally advanced esophageal cancers. The therapeutic advantage are improved median survival, overall survival, local control, and distant metastasis, with tolerable and acceptable toxicities. Chemo-radiotherapy followed by planned surgery is probably better than surgery alone. This still need to be proved by a phase III randomized trial. Conclusions regarding the role of surgery after chemo-radiotherapy need to answered in the near future.

## References

1. Gignous M, Roussel A, Paillot B, et al. The value of preoperative radiotherapy in esophageal cancer: results of a study of the EORTC. World J Surg 11: 426–432, 1987.
2. Teniere P, Hay JM, Fingerhut A, et al. Postoperative radiation therapy dose not increase survival after curative resection for squamous cell carcinoma of the middle and lower esophagus as shown by a multicenter controlled trial. Gynecol Obstet 173: 123–130, 1991.
3. Tannock I. Treatment of cancer with radiation and drugs. J Clin Oncol 14: 3156–3174, 1996.
4. Kelson DP, Hillaris B, Coonley CJ, et al. Cisplatin, vindisine and bleomycin chemotherapy for locoregional and advanced esophageal carcinoma. Am J Med 75: 45–652, 1983.
5. Kelson DP, Minsky B, Smith M. preoperative therapy for esophageal cancer, a randomized comparison of chemotherapy vs radiation. J Clin Oncol 8: 1352–1361, 1990.
6. Kelsen DP, Hilaris B. Coonley C, et al. Cisplatin, vindesine and bleomycin combination chemotherapy of local-regional and advanced esophageal carcinoma. Am J Med 75: 645, 1983.
7. Kelsen DP, Fein R, Coonley C, et al. Cisplatin, vindesine and mitoguazone in the treatment of esophageal cancer. Cancer Treatment Rep 70: 255, 1986.
8. Kies M, Rosen S, Tsang T, et al. Cisplatin and 5-fluorouracil in primary management of squamous esophageal cancer. Cancer 60: 2156, 1987.
9. Schlag P, Herrmann R, Raeth V, et al: Preoperative chemotherapy in esophageal cancer. A phase II study. Acta Oncol 27: 811, 1988.
10. Vignoud J, Visset J, Paineau J, et al. Preoperative chemotherapy in squamous cell carcinoma of the esophagus: clinical and pathological analysis, 48 cases. Ann Oncol 1: 45, 1990.
11. Ajani JA, Ryan B, Rich TA, et al: Prolonged chemotherapy for localized squamous carcinoma of the esophagus. Eur J Cancer 28A: 880, 1992.
12. Wright CD, Mathisen JD, Wain JC, et al. Evolution of treatment strategies for adenocarcinoma of the esophagus and gastroesophageal junction. Ann Thorac Surg 58:1574, 1994.
13. Ilson D, Kelsen D. Management of esophageal cancer. Oncology 10: 1385–1402, 1996.
14. Roth JA, Pass HI, Fanagan MM, et al. Randomized clinical trial of preoperative and post operative adjuvant chemotherapy with cisplatin, vindisine and bleomycin for carcinoma of the esophagus. J Thor Cardiovasc Surg 96: 242–248, 1988.
15. Schlag P. Preoperative chemotherapy in localized squamous cell carcinoma of the esophagus: results of a prospective randomized trial. Eur J Cancer 27:76, 1991.
16. Forastiere A, Orringer M, Perez-Tamayo C, et al. Preoperative chemoradiation followed by trans-hiatal esophagectomy for carcinoma of the esophagus: final report. J Clin Oncol 11: 1118–1123, 1993.
17. Franklin R, Steiger Z, Vaishampayan G, et al. Combined modality therapy for esophageal squamous cell carcinoma. Cancer 51: 1062–1071, 1983.
18. Leichman L, Herskovic A, Leichman C, et al. Preoperative chemotherapy and radiation therapy for patients with cancer of the esophagus; a potentially curative approach. J Clin Oncol 2: 75–79, 1984.
19. Poplin E, Fleming T, Leichman L, et al. Combined therapies for squamous cell carcinoma of the esophagus ( SWOG-8037). J Clin Oncol 5: 622–628, 1987.
20. Urba S, Orringer M, Perez-Tamayo C, et al. Concurrent preoperative chemotherapy with radiation therapy in localized esophageal adenocarcinoma. Cancer 69: 285–291, 1992.
21. Seydel HG, Leichman L, Byhardt R, et al. Preoperative radiation and chemotherapy for localized squamous cell carcinoma of the esophagus: a RTOG study. Int J Radiat Oncol Biol Phys 14: 33–35, 1988.
22. Walsh T, Noonan N, Hollywood D, et al. A comparison of multimodality therapy and surgery for esophageal adenocarcinoma. N Engl J Med 335: 462–467, 1987.
23. Le Price E, Etienne P, Meunier B, et al. A randomized trial of chemotherapy and radiation  therapy  and surgery vs surgery for localized squamous cell carcinoma of the esophagus. Cancer 73: 1779, 1994.
24. Urba S, Orringer M, Turrisi A, et al. A randomized trial comparing trans-hiatal esophagectomy to preoperative concurrent chemoradiation followed by esophagectomy in locoregional esophageal carcinoma. Proc Am Soc Clin Oncol 14: 199, 1995.

25. Leichman L, Steiger Z, Seydel H, et al. Nonoperative therapy for squamous cell carcinoma of the esophagus. J Clin Oncol 5: 365–370, 1987.
26. Chan A, Wong A, Arthur K, et al. Concomitant 5 fluorouracil infusion, mitomycin C and radical radiation therapy in Esophageal squamous cell carcinoma. Int J Radiat Oncol Biol Phys 16: 59–65, 1989.
27. Coia L, Engstrom P, Paul M, et al. Long term results of infusional 5-FU, mitomycin C and radiation as a primary management of esophageal carcinoma. Int J Radiat Oncol Biol Phys 20: 29–36, 1991.
28. John MJ, Flam MS, Mowry PA, et al. Radiotherapy alone and chemoradiation for nonmetastatic esophageal carcinoma. Cancer 63: 2397–2403, 1989.
29. Richmond J, Seydel H, Bea Y, et al. Comparison of three treatment strategies for esophageal carcinoma within a single institution. Int J Radiat Oncol Biol Phys 13: 1617–1620, 1987.
30. Seitz J, Giovannini M, Padaut-Casana J, et al. Inoperable nonmetastatic squamous cell carcinoma of the esophagus managed by concomitant chemotherapy (5-FU, cisplatin) and radiation therapy. Cancer 66: 214–219, 1990.
31. Al-Sarraf M, Martz K, Herskovic A, et al. Progress report of combined chemoradiotherapy verses radiotherapy alone in patients with esophageal cancer: an intergroup study. J Clin Oncol 15: 227–284. 1997.
32. Araujo M, Souhami L, Gil R, et al. A randomized trial comparing radiation therapy versus concomitant radiation therapy and chemotherapy in carcinoma of the thoracic esophagus. Cancer 67: 2258–2261, 1991.
33. Herskovic A, Martz K, Al-Sarraf M, et al. Combined chemotherapy and radiotherapy compared with radiotherapy alone in patients with cancer of the esophagus. N Engl J Med 326: 1593–1598, 1992.
34. Sischy B, Rayn L, Haller D, et al. Interim report of EST 1282 Phase III protocol for evaluation of combined modalities in the treatment of patients with carcinoma of the esophagus, stage I and II. Proc Am Soc Clin Oncol 9: 105, 1990.
35. Blot W. Esophageal cancer trends and risk factors. Semin Oncol 21: 403–410, 1994.
36. Bates B, Detterbeck F, Bernard S, et al. Concurrent radiation therapy and chemotherapy followed by esophagectomy for localized esophageal carcinoma. J Clin Oncol 14: 156–163, 1996.
37. Forastiere A, Orringer M, Perez-Tamayo C, et al. Concurrent chemotherapy and radiation therapy followed by trans-hiatal esophagectomy for loco-regional cancer of the esophagus. J Clin Oncol 8: 119–127, 1990.
38. Smalley R, Gunderson L, Reddy K, et al. Radiotherapy alone in esophageal carcinoma: current management and future directions of adjuvant, curative and palliative approaches. Semin Oncol 21: 467–473, 1994.
39. Recht A. The role of radiation therapy in treating patients with potentially resectable carcinoma of esophagus. Chest 107: 233–240, 1995.

C.J. Rosenthal and M. Rotman (Eds.), *Infusion Chemotherapy–Irradiation Interactions*
© 1998 Elsevier Science B.V. All rights reserved

# Head and neck cancer. The North American experience: moving towards organ preservation

SAMUEL G. TAYLOR

*Rush University and the Cancer Center, Illinois Masonic Medical Center,
901 West Wellington, Chicago, IL 60657, USA*

There is no one aspect of the biology of head and neck cancer that is uniquely North American or European and, given modern day communications, it is impossible to separate the contributions to head and neck cancer management based on the continental origin of the investigators. This discussion focuses on the use of chemotherapy to facilitate organ preservation in head and neck squamous cell carcinoma management with important contributions from both sides of the Atlantic.

Much of the current attention given to treatment approaches that emphasize organ preservation originates from the VA laryngeal preservation study [1]. This innovative study asked the question whether selecting patients to undergo radiation without surgery based on the degree of cytoreduction by neo-adjuvant chemotherapy, was equivalent to surgical management of all patients. The origins of the concepts that led to this investigation came from three fundamental observations.

The first important observation was that responders to induction chemotherapy had a better subsequent survival over non-responders following standard regional therapy of surgery and/or radiation therapy. While this observation was made during the 1970s, the impact of it was not felt until the Wayne State investigators described a combination of cisplatin and 5-fluorouracil (5-FU) infusion that had two to three times the complete response rate of any other regimen [2]. Previous combination regimens had complete response rates in 5–25% of patients. The initial report of a 54% complete response rate with cisplatin and 5-FU neo-adjuvant chemotherapy did not make the program when initially submitted to the American Society of Clinical Oncology (ASCO) [3]. The dramatic improvement in outcome of complete responders is shown in Fig. 1 [4]. This observation is still interpreted by some as evidence for chemotherapy effectiveness in improving overall survival of treated patients. It has been convincingly shown, however, in several randomized trials that while chemotherapy responders do better than non-responders, the overall outcome is the same as that of patients receiving regional therapy alone [5,6]. The reason is the often neglected fact that non-responders to chemotherapy have a much worse survival than the control group – only 6 months median survival for partial responders, based on the Wayne State data [4]. Thus, induction chemotherapy appears to primarily select the good prognosis patients without affecting outcome.

The next step was to selectively treat those patients who had achieved a good response to

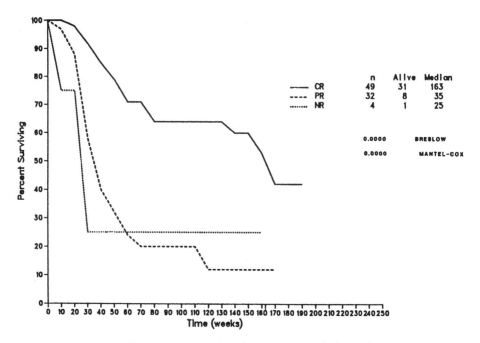

Fig. 1. Response to chemotherapy versus survival.

chemotherapy with radiation alone. This idea was originally described by Ervin et al. from Boston, who also had noted the excellent outcome of chemotherapy responders with a regimen of cisplatin, methotrexate and bleomycin [7]. Jacobs et al. then championed the use of the Wayne State regimen for organ preservation in a pilot study that included multiple sites [8].

The third rationale for exploring the selection of patients to avoid surgery based on chemotherapy responsiveness also had roots with the Wayne State investigators. Ensley et al. correlated radiation responsiveness with chemotherapy responsiveness [9]. Collecting data on subsequent response to radiation of patients who had either a partial response or no response to radiation, they found a direct correlation between chemotherapy responsiveness and subsequent radiation sensitivity (Table 1).

With this background, the VA Laryngeal Preservation Study compared immediate surgery, with laryngectomy followed by radiation, to a program of selectively treating responders to induction chemotherapy with radiation alone, avoiding laryngectomy [1]. Response to chemotherapy was defined as at least 50% tumor shrinkage after 2 cycles of chemotherapy. Eighty-five percent of patients with Stage III and IV laryngeal cancer responded after 2 cycles, but due to death during treatment (5 patients) and other unspecified reasons (5 patients), only 131 patients (79%) underwent radiation without initial laryngectomy. Thirty-three of these patients (20%) required salvage laryngectomy [10]. Ultimately 66% of 79 surviving patients treated with initial induction chemotherapy survived without undergoing laryngectomy. This is only 31% of the original patient population.

One disturbing observation from the VA Study was the slightly (not significant) inferior survival of the treatment arm undergoing the laryngeal preservation approach. Radiation with surgical salvage does not achieve the same survival results as initial surgical treatment

Table 1

Radiation therapy response predicted by induction chemotherapy: impact of adding concomitant cisplatin to radiation [9,14]

| Response to induction chemotherapy | Response to radiation alone | | |
|---|---|---|---|
| | CR (%) | PR (%) | NR (%) |
| PR (*n* = 42) | 52 | 45 | 3 |
| NR (*n* = 18) | 6 | 0 | 94 |
| | Response to radiation and cisplatin | | |
| NR (*n* = 13) | 46 | 54 | 0 |

Abbreviations: CR, complete response; PR, partial response; NR, no response.

of laryngeal cancers [11]. Also meta-analysis of neo-adjuvant chemotherapy programs have failed to identify any disease-free survival benefit from induction chemotherapy programs [12]. While the worst patients prognostically (the non-responders to chemotherapy) were offered surgery and removed from the larynx preservation protocol in the VA study, it is not surprising that a combination of neo-adjuvant chemotherapy (which does not improve survival) plus radiation with surgical salvage (an inferior treatment) to all but the worst prognostic groups of patients would result in a worse survival, albeit with some patients (31%) alive with a preserved larynx.

Part of the reason for the failure to achieve a better survival in the VA study has been the decision to treat partial responders to the chemotherapy with radiation alone. While partial responders to induction chemotherapy may respond to subsequent radiation, their long-term disease control is terrible as shown by the Wayne State investigators. Lefébvre et al. have achieved a favorable survival outcome with the approach in hypopharynx cancers of offering radiation alone to only complete responders to induction chemotherapy. The disadvantage of this approach was being able to offer organ-sparring treatment to only 54% of patients [13]. If the VA study had treated only complete responders to chemotherapy with laryngeal preservation, such as Jacobs et al. had originally advocated, they would have been able to preserve the larynx in only 64% of patients, but might have improved survival [1].

These considerations question the rationale for using current neo-adjuvant chemotherapy programs for organ preservation. There are two major disadvantages: (1) not all patients can be offered organ preservation (only responders); and (2) survival is not altered (or may be worse).

Another approach is to combine chemotherapy with radiation as a radiation sensitizer. Ensley et al. have again shown that non-responders to induction chemotherapy can be converted to radiation responders by giving cisplatin with the radiation (Table 1) [14]. Using cisplatin with radiation followed by adjuvant cisplatin and 5-FU has markedly improved disease control and survival of nasopharyngeal carcinoma [15]. The survival benefit was so significant that the study was stopped prematurely (2 year survival 55% versus 80%, $P = 0.0007$). The role of the adjuvant cisplatin/5-FU treatment in the survival benefit is not clear. Nasopharynx cancers are not benefitted by combined neo-adjuvant and post-radiation adjuvant cisplatin/5-FU infusion [16]. The adjuvant cisplatin/5-FU program of the RTOG was 3 cycles at 80% dosage compared to the adjuvant study that gave 4 cycles at full dose.

Table 2

Timing of chemotherapy for organ preservation

---

Induction chemotherapy
  – Selects a subgroup for organ preservations based on chemotherapy response
  –Survival may be compromised

Concomitant chemotherapy
  – All patients included
  – Regional control shown to be better
  – Survival may be improved

---

Unless one speculates that giving less chemotherapy after regional treatment is somehow better, the major reason for the survival benefit in the RTOG study seems to be the use of cisplatin, given simultaneously with radiation.

While the RTOG trial studied an inoperable cancer (nasopharynx), the conclusion from their studies, supported by a recent meta-analysis [12], is that the greatest impact from chemotherapy in disease control is with its simultaneous use with radiation. The benefits of using simultaneous chemotherapy and radiation treatment (Table 2) include: (1) all patients are included; (2) regional disease control is improved over regional treatment (radiation) [17] or induction chemotherapy followed by radiation [18,19]; and (3) a favorable (rather than worse) survival impact may be achieved [12]. The rest of this chapter concentrates on current directions being explored with the use of simultaneous chemotherapy and radiation regimens.

Three directions in the investigation of combined chemotherapy and radiation are occurring. All need to address the potentially increased toxicity and complexity of treatment required by this approach. The first direction is the pursuit of optimal single agent treatment. The advantage of this approach is the limited regional toxicity that usually allows continuous radiation therapy. The chemotherapy drugs are used primarily as radiation sensitizers, with limited impact on hematogenous metastasis. In addition to cisplatin [20,21], mitomycin C [22] and 5-FU [23–25] have recently been reported. With the exception of using cisplatin at a very low dose, which resulted in only one-third of patients achieving a complete response [20], these trials have achieved improved regional control and cause specific survival (Table 3) [21–25]. Improvement in overall survival has been more elusive.

The most dramatic regional control, however, has come from the use of intra-arterial cisplatin during radiation [26]. High doses of cisplatin can be given (150 mg/m$^2$ weekly) with systemic sodium thiosulfate rescue [27]. Combining this with radiation has achieved a 92% complete response rate at the primary site out of 90 patients treated for unresectable Stage III or IV cancers. The 2-year survival was 51%, with 25% dead of disease and the remaining dead of other causes. New drugs with substantial single agent activity such as the taxanes and drugs with interesting radiation sensitizing properties, such as gemcitabine, are currently undergoing clinical trials with radiation.

The use of more active drug combinations with radiation causes significantly more toxicity and requires innovative approaches with more complex supportive measures to administer. The increased toxicity from combined chemotherapy and radiation has been managed by (1) planning radiation treatment breaks to allow for normal tissue recovery, or (2) using aggressive supportive measures with uninterrupted radiation. The second approach also uses reduced chemotherapy and radiation exposure.

Table 3

Recent randomized trials of concomitant chemotherapy and radiation, testing single drug therapy

| Ref. | Drug | No. of patients | | % Disease-free survival (P) | | % Survival (P) | |
|------|------|---------|-------|---------|-------|---------|-------|
|      |      | Control | Chemo | Control | Chemo | Control | Chemo |
| [21] | DDP 50 mg qw[a] | 44 | 39 | 41 (<0.01) | 65 | NA | |
| [22] | MMC 15 mg/m$^2$ day 3 | 58 | 55 | 47 (<0.03) | 67 | 41 (NS) | 56 |
| [25] | 5-FU 1.2 g/m$^2$ | 87 | 88 | NA (0.057) | NA | 25 months (0.08) | 33 months |
| [24] | 5-FU 250 mg/m$^2$ qod | 277 | 300 | 25 months (0001) | 60 months | 38 months (<0.001) | 85 months |
| [23] | 5-FU 10 mg/kg days 1–3, then 5 mg/kg qod[b] | 66 | 68 | NA | | 15 (0.006) | 36 |

Abbreviations: DDP, cisplatin; MMC, mitomycin C; 5-FU, 5-fluorouracil; NA, not available; NS, not significant.
[a]High risk, post-operative patients.
[b]Study published 1970.

Byfield first described planned weekly breaks in radiation to allow high-dose 5-FU exposure, with radiation only given with the chemotherapy [28]. Taylor first used this approach with combined cisplatin and 5-FU infusion [29]. The program of interrupted radiation schedules has been severely criticized, based on the well-known inferior results achieved when treatment breaks are used with radiation alone. Nevertheless, trials comparing standard radiation [17] or neo-adjuvant chemotherapy and standard radiation [18,19] to combined chemotherapy and radiation with planned breaks, have shown the superiority of this approach. Leyvraz et al. have indeed found that treatment with combined chemotherapy and radiation can actually be delivered over a shorter duration, more intensively, with planned breaks for radiation rather than unplanned breaks that require more prolonged interruptions [30].

Taylor et al. have recently reviewed their single institutional experience with this regimen in 78 patients with a median 8 years followup [31]. One hundred percent of patients responded to this treatment. They observed a 39% failure rate in Stage IV disease patients. None of 16 Stage III patients failed at any site. From the perspective of organ preservation, their best local control was with tongue cancers (16 patients) and glottic larynx (7 patients), in which none recurred locally and only one failed in the neck. Perhaps the most interesting observation from this long term followup, however, was that the rate of deaths from other causes in patients who were cancer-free was strongly related to T stage (P = 0.002), but not N stage or overall stage (Table 4). Deaths from other causes in this study tended to occur later than deaths from cancers and so were not felt to be directly treatment related. The association with T stage would suggest tumor destruction of the primary site may make patients with large primaries susceptible to aspiration or other difficulties that may lead to shortened survival.

Adelstein et al. have delivered the same chemotherapy with radiation, but gave the radiation with a single prolonged (4–8 weeks) break while giving the chemotherapy during a total of 2 of the 7 weeks of radiation [32]. This schedule is being tested in a cooperative

Table 4

Relation between T, N and AJC stage and rate of death from other cancers (DOC)

| T stage | % DOC (P = 0.0015) | N stage | % DOC (P = 0.555) | AJC stage | % DOC (P = 0.765) |
|---------|--------------------|---------|-------------------|-----------|-------------------|
| T0–2    | 11                 | N0–1    | 43                | III       | 38                |
| T3      | 22                 | N2      | 33                | IV        | 31                |
| T4      | 68                 | N3      | 43                |           |                   |

group setting. The advantage of these treatment programs is the use of active drug combinations with radiation. Not only does regional disease appear to be better controlled, but the incidence of distant disease is as low as with neo-adjuvant therapy [19].

Vokes et al. have used a similar schedule of every other week 5-FU infusion and radiation, but added hydroxyurea instead of cisplatin. Hydroxyurea causes less nephrotoxicity, but more mucositis. It is an active radiation sensitizer, but not an active anti-neoplastic agent against head and neck cancer. They combined this with induction chemotherapy and de-bulking surgery [33]. They have questioned the role of surgery, however [33]. In a newer program they are adding cisplatin and avoiding surgery [34].

The third approach, becoming more popular at several centers, is to increase the intensity of radiation by combining chemotherapy with multiple daily fractions of radiation. As both chemotherapy and multiple daily radiation fractions target rapidly proliferating cells, the benefit of this approach is unclear and toxicity can be substantial. Table 5 lists several phase II studies of cisplatin or cerboplatin with twice daily radiation. The short term survival is promising, but not clearly better than using these agents with single daily radiation fractions. A randomized comparison, with the same chemotherapy in both arms, would be very interesting.

To this reviewer, the most provocative report over the last several years is the one by Laccourreye et al. describing the use of chemotherapy alone to treat T1-3N0 well-differentiated glottic squamous cell carcinomas [40]. They used predominantly a 6-day course of

Table 5

Combined platinum regimens with twice daily radiation in treatment of head and neck cancer

| Treatment dose and schedule | No. of patients by stage | %CR | % Survival | Ref. |
|-----------------------------|--------------------------|-----|------------|------|
| DDP 100 mg/m$^2$ day 1, 22, 43 RT 1.8 Gy qd × 6 weeks with 1.6 Gy qd boost during weeks 5,6 | 22IV | 64 | 69 at 2 years | [35] |
| DDP 100 mg/m$^2$ day 1, 22, 43 RT 1.1 Gy bid to 68–74 Gy | 5III, 25IV | NA | 67 at 19 months | [36] |
| DDP 20 mg/m$^2$ days 1–5, 29–33 RT 1.2 Gy bid to 72–76.8 Gy | 1III, 4III, 47IV | 73 | 62 at 3 years | [37] |
| DDP 15–20 mg/m$^2$ CI days 1–5, 29–33 RT 1.6 Gy bid to 64–70.4 Gy | 3III, 17IV | 80 | 59 at 3 years | [38] |
| CBP 60 mg/m$^2$ days 1–5, 29–33 RT 1.6 Gy bid to 64–67 Gy | 15IV | 80 | 73 at 10 months | [39] |

Abbreviations: DDP, cisplatin; RT, radiation therapy; CBP, carboplatin; CR, complete response; NA, not available.

Table 6

Treatment of T1–3NO laryngeal carcinoma with extended chemotherapy alone, following complete clinical response [40]

|  | No. of patients | % Local failures | % DOD[a] | % 5-year survival |
|---|---|---|---|---|
| Extended chemotherapy | 21 | 29[a] | 0 | 95 |
| Conservation surgery/RT | 37 | 3 | 10 | 86 |

[a]All managed with conservation surgery or radiation. DOD, dead of disease.

cisplatin 20 mg/m$^2$ per day and 5-FU 1 mg/m$^2$ per day continuous infusion every 3–4 weeks for 4–11 cycles (mostly 5–7 cycles). Patients who had achieved a clinical complete response, defined as disappearance of all evidence of tumor by exam and CT scan with normal cord and arytenoid mobility and multiple negative biopsies, were offered either further courses of chemotherapy alone (21 patients), radiation (2 patients) or partial laryngectomy (35 patients). While local recurrences were more frequent after extended chemotherapy alone (29 compared to 3%, $P = 0.002$), the meticulous followup of patients allowed partial laryngectomy or radiation to be used in all local recurrences, preserving speech and swallowing in these patients. Five-year survival was 95% with extended chemotherapy, with one second primary and one dead of other causes. This compared favorably to the locally treated patients who had an 86% 5-year survival, with four dead of disease or unknown cause, one dead from radiation complications and one from a second primary (Table 6). This report puts new life into neo-adjuvant programs or perhaps intra-arterial cisplatin [27]. The suggestion is to use chemotherapy in earlier stage disease, to offer treatment with less long-term toxicities than either surgery or radiation can offer. Such approaches, however, would require careful followup, a difficulty task in this patient population.

In conclusion, organ preservation is being achieved today most reliably with combined radiation and chemotherapy programs. More recent regimens using chemotherapy with multiple daily radiation fractions are toxic and need to be done in controlled trials. Reports of successful management of early stage patients, who achieve complete responses to chemotherapy, with chemotherapy alone are most provocative and need further exploration.

## References

1.   Department of Veterans Affairs Laryngeal Cancer Study Group. Induction chemotherapy plus radiation compared with surgery in patients with advanced laryngeal cancer. N Engl J Med 24: 1685–1690, 1991.

2.   Rooney M, Kish J, Jacobs J, et al. Improved complete response rate and survival in advanced head and neck cancer after three-course induction therapy with 120-hour 5-FU infusion and cisplatin. Cancer 55: 1123–1128, 1985.

3.   Al Sarraf M, Drelichman A, Peppard S, et al. Adjuvant cisplatinum and 5-fluorouracil 96 hour infusion in previously untreated epidermoid cancers of the head and neck. Proc Am Soc Clin Oncol 22: 428, 1981.

4.   Jacobs JR, Weaver A, Ahmed K, et al. Proto-chemotherapy in advanced head and neck cancer. Head Neck Surg 10: 93–98, 1987.

5.   Taylor SG IV, Applebaum E, Showel JL, et al. A randomized trial of adjuvant chemotherapy in head and neck cancer. J Clin Oncol 3: 672–679, 1985.

6.   Brunin F, Rodriguez J, Jaulerry C, et al. Place de la chimiothérapie néoadjuvante dans le traitement des tumeurs, avancées de la tete et cou. Résultats de deux essais thérapeutiques randomisés effectués a l'Institut Curie sur 208 patients. Bull Cancer 79: 893–904, 1992.

7.   Ervin TJ, Weichselbaum RR, Fabian RL, et al. Advanced squamous cell carcinoma of the head and neck. A preliminary report of neo-adjuvant chemotherapy with cisplatin, bleomycin and methotrexate. Arch Otolaryngol Head Neck Surg 110: 241–245, 1984.

8.   Jacobs C, Goffinet DR, Goffinet L, et al. Chemotherapy as a substitute for surgery in the treatment of advanced resectable head and neck cancer. A report from the Northern California Oncology Group. Cancer 60: 1178–1183, 1987.

9.   Ensley JF, Jacobs JR, Weaver A, et al. Correlation between response cisplatinum-combination chemotherapy and subsequent radiotherapy in previously treated patients with squamous cell cancers of the head and neck. Cancer 54: 811–814, 1984.

10.  Wolf G, Hong W, Fisher S, et al. Larynx preservation with induction chemotherapy and radiation in advanced laryngeal cancer: final results of the VA Laryngeal Cancer Study Group Cooperative Trial. Proc Am Soc Clin Oncol 12: 277, 1993.

11.  Kramer S, Gelber RD, Snow JB, et al. Combined radiation therapy and surgery in the management of advanced head and neck cancer: final report of 73–03 of the Radiation Therapy Oncology Group. Head Neck Surg 10: 19–30, 1987.

12.  El-Sayed S, Nelson N. Adjuvant and adjunctive chemotherapy in the management of squamous cell carcinoma of the head and neck region: a meta-analysis of prospective and randomized trials. J Clin Oncol 14: 838–847, 1996.

13.  Lefébvre J-L, Chevalier D, Luboinski B, et al. Larynx preservation in pyriform sinus cancer: preliminary results of a European Organization for Research and Treatment of Cancer Phase III trial. J Natl Cancer Inst 88: 890–899, 1996.

14.  Ensley J, Ahmad K, Kish J, et al. Improved responses to radiation and concurrent cisplatinum in patients with advanced head and neck cancer that fail induction chemotherapy. Proc Am Soc Clin Oncol 8: 168, 1989.

15.  Al-Sarraf M, LeBlanc M, Giri PG, et al. Superiority of chemo-radiotherapy vs radiotherapy in patients with locally advanced nasopharyngeal cancer. Preliminary results of intergroups (0099) (SWOG 8892, RTOG 8817, ECOG 2388) randomized study. Proc Am Soc Clin Oncol 15: 313, 1996.

16.  Chan AT, Teo PM, Leung TW, et al. A prospective randomized study of chemotherapy adjunctive to definitive radiotherapy in advanced nasopharyngeal carcinoma. Int J Radiat Oncol Biol Phys 33: 761–763, 1995.

17.  Merlano M, Vitale V, Rosso R, et al. Treatment of advanced squamous cell carcinoma of the head and neck with alternating chemotherapy and radiotherapy. N Engl J Med 327: 1115–1121, 1992.

18.  Adelstein DJ, Sharon VM, Earle AS, et al. Simultaneous versus sequential combined technique therapy for squamous cell head and neck cancer. Cancer 65: 1685–1691, 1990

19.  Taylor SG IV, Murthy AK, Vannetzel J-M, et al. Randomized comparison of neo-adjuvant cisplatin and fluorouracil infusion followed by radiation versus concomitant treatment in advanced head and neck cancer. J Clin Oncol 12: 385–395, 1994.

20.  Haselow RE, Warshaw MG, Oken MM, et al., Radiation alone versus radiation with weekly low-dose cisplatinum in unresectable cancer of the head and neck. In: Fee WE Jr, Goepfert H, Johns ME, et al. (Eds), Head and Neck Cancer, Vol II. Philadelphia, PA: BC Decker, pp. 279–281, 1990.

21.  Bachaud JM, David JM, Boussin G, Daly N. Combined postoperative radiotherapy and weekly cisplatin infusion for locally advanced squamous cell carcinoma of the head and neck: preliminary report of a randomized trial. Int J Radiat Oncol Biol Phys 20: 243–246, 1991.

22.  Haffty BG, Son YH, Sasaki CT, et al. Mitomycin C as an adjuvant to postoperative radiation therapy in squamous cell carcinoma of the head and neck: results from two randomized trials. Int J Radiat Oncol Biol Phys 27: 241–250, 1993.

23.  Ansfield FJ, Ramirez G, Davis HL Jr, et al. Treatment of advanced cancer of the head and neck. Cancer 25: 28–82, 1970.

24.  Sanchiz F, Milla A, Torner J, et al. Single fraction per day versus two fractions per day versus radiochemotherapy in the treatment of head and neck cancer. Int J Radiat Oncol Biol Phys 19: 1347–1350, 1990.

25.  Browman GP, Cripps C, Hodson DI, et al. Placebo-controlled randomized trial of infusional fluorouracil during standard radiotherapy in locally advanced head and neck cancer. J Clin Oncol 12: 2648–2653, 1994.

26.  Robbins KT, Kumar P, Weisman RA, et al. Phase II trial of targeted supradose cisplatin and concomitant radiation therapy for patients with Stage III-IV head and neck cancer. Proc Am Soc Clin Oncol 15: 323, 1996.

27. Robbins KT, Storniolo AM, Kerber C, et al. Phase I study of highly selective supradose cisplatin infusions for advanced head and neck cancer. J Clin Oncol 12: 2113–2020, 1994.
28. Byfield JE, Sharp TR, Frankel SS, et al. Phase I and II trial of five-day infused 5-fluorouracil and radiation in advanced cancer of the head and neck. J Clin Oncol 2: 406- 413, 1984.
29. Taylor SG IV, Murthy AK, Showel JL, et al. Improved control in advanced head and neck cancer with simultaneous radiation and cisplatin/5-FU chemotherapy. Cancer Treatment Rep 69: 938- 939, 1985.
30. Leyvraz S, Pasche P, Bauer J, et al. Rapidly alternating chemotherapy and hyperfractionated radiotherapy in the management of locally advanced head and neck carcinoma: four year results of phase I/II study. J Clin Oncol 12: 1876–1885, 1994.
31. Taylor SG IV, Marthy AK, Griem KL, et al. Concomitant cisplatin/5-FU infusion and radiation in advanced head and neck: eight year analysis. Head Neck: 1997, in press.
32. Adelstein DJ, Kalish LA, Adams GL, et al. Concurrent radiation therapy and chemotherapy for locally unresectable squamous cell head and neck cancer: an Eastern Cooperative Oncology Group pilot study. J Clin Oncol 11: 2136–2142, 1993.
33. Vokes EE, Kies M, Haraf DJ, et al. Induction chemotherapy followed by concomitant chemoradiotherapy for advanced head and neck cancer: impact on the natural history of the disease. J Clin Oncol 13: 876–883, 1995.
34. Vokes EE, Haraf DJ, Mick R, et al. Intensified concomitant chemotherapy with and without filgratin for poor-prognosis head and neck cancer. J Clin Oncol 12: 2351–2359, 1994.
35. Harrison LB, Pfister DG, Fass DE, et al. Concomitant chemotherapy - radiation therapy followed by hyperfractionated radiation therapy for advanced resectable head and neck cancer. Int J Radiat Oncol Biol Phys 21: 703–708, 1991.
36. Fontanesi J, Beckford NS, Lester EP, et al. Concomitant cisplatin and hyperfractionated external beam irradiation for advanced malignancy of the head and neck. Am J Surg 162: 393–396, 1991.
37. Glanzmann C, Litolf UM. Followup data of our pilot study on concomitant hyperfractionated radiotherapy and cisplatinum (CDDP) in patients with advanced cancer of the head and neck. Strahlenther Onkol 168: 453–456, 1992.
38. Kanstens JH, Schaurkowski P, Li L, et al. Definitive radiochemotherapy in advanced head and neck cancer: a followup report of accelerated fractionated irradiation and a pilot study of mucositis prevention. Onkologie 15: 156–159, 1992.
39. Schuabel T, Zamboglou N, Kolotas C, et al. Phase I study of hyperfractionated accelerated radiation and simultaneous carboplatin therapy for advanced head and neck carcinomas. Strahlenther Onkol 168: 318–321, 1992.
40. Laccourreye O, Brasnu D, Bassot V, et al. Cisplatin-fluorouracil exclusive chemotherapy for T1–3N0 glottic squamous cell carcinoma complete clinical responders: five-year results. J Clin Oncol 14: 2331–2336, 1996.

C.J. Rosenthal and M. Rotman (Eds.), *Infusion Chemotherapy–Irradiation Interactions*

# CHAPTER 20

# Preserving the head and neck anatomy while eradicating neoplastic cells: the European experience

## MARCO MERLANO[1] and GIANMAURO NUMICO[2]

[1]*Medical Oncology Department, S. Croce Hospital, Cuneo, Italy and* [2]*Medical Oncology Department, Istituto Nazionale per la Ricerca sul Cancro, Genova, Italy*

## 1. Introduction

In past years, a major effort has been made in the field of head and neck cancer treatment, in order to enhance loco-regional disease control and to reduce the occurrence of distant metastases. Technological development, basic research and pharmacological investigation have stimulated the design of combined modality approaches and trials of integrated surgery, radiation therapy and chemotherapy have been performed.

European and American researchers have both studied integrated treatments and important advances have been made.

Although survival has always been the primary end-point of clinical investigation, a deeper consciousness of the importance of quality of life has gained place. In fact, the impact of treatment on quality of life is often dramatic, especially when the long survival span of many treated head and neck cancer patients is considered. In this light, strategies aiming at reducing treatment morbidity and at preserving organ function have been developed.

Organ preservation has the utmost importance in head and neck cancer treatment, considering the physiological and psychological value of functions such as swallowing, phonation and speech.

Conservative surgical approaches and radiotherapy achieve both optimal local control and organ preservation in early stage head and neck cancer; as for the treatment of other solid neoplasms such as breast cancer and soft tissue sarcomas limited tumor resections and organ function sparing surgery have become the rule when diagnosis is performed at an early stage of disease.

In more advanced stages, aggressive and demolitive surgery is very often the only choice offered to patients. In the case of surgery refusal or in the case of patients unsuitable for surgical approaches due to medical conditions, radiation therapy is currently given. A direct comparison between surgery and radiation is still lacking, since a prospective randomized trial has never been performed. We consequently do not know whether radiation therapy, while achieving the end-point of organ preservation, could be comparable with surgery in terms of survival.

The new active chemotherapy regimens, together with the better knowledge about the interactions between drugs and radiation, allowed the development of chemo-radiotherapy combinations which, at least for advanced, unresectable head and neck cancer, have been shown to give promising results and have been selected as possible alternatives to mutilating surgery.

Several trials assessing the role of combined chemo-radiation have been performed in the past decades. This chapter summarizes the European experience dealing with the organ and function preserving potential of such treatment approaches in advanced head and neck cancer.

## 2. Induction chemotherapy

Among the several methods of combining chemotherapy and radiotherapy, induction chemotherapy has been the most popular in the past. The possibility of inducing major tumor shrinkage has led to the enthusiastic expectation that the use of induction chemotherapy could result in substantial survival improvements in comparison with radiotherapy alone in locally advanced, unresectable, head and neck cancer. Furthermore, its apparently easy and safe application caused widespread and often unjustified use [1]. Table 1 summarizes the

Table 1

European trials of induction chemotherapy

| First author | No. of patients | Sites of primary | Chemotherapy regimen | Courses | Response rate (CR %) |
|---|---|---|---|---|---|
| Richard [2] | 112 | Oral cavity, oropharynx | Vcr, B (i.a.) | – | 46 (7)T |
| Hill [3,4] | 208 | All sites | Vcr, B, M, F, L | 2 | 66(34) |
| Merlano [5] | 55 | All sites | Vbl, B, M | 4 | 52 (13) |
| Jaullery [6] | 46 | All sites | C, B, Vds, M | 2 | 50 (10) T |
|  | 60 | All sites | C, F, Vds | 3 | 70 (22) T |
| Frustaci [7] | 52 | Oral cavity, oropharynx | C, B (i.a.) | – | 90 (26) |
| Recondo [8] | 54 | All sites | C, B, F | 2–3 | 59 (13) |
| Cognetti [9] | 152 | All sites | C, Vcr, B, M | 2–3 | 63 (18) |
| Grau [10] | 72 | Oral cavity | C, B | 2 | 80 (13) |
| Mazeron [11] | 55 | Oral cavity oropharynx | C, F, B, M, L | 3 | 49 (7) |
| Domenge [12] | 83 | Oropharynx | C, F | 3 | 57 (19) |
| Paccagnella [13] | 118 | All sites | C, F | 4 | 49 (31) |
| Licitra [14] | 68 | Oral cavity | C, F | 3 | 79 (31) |
| Pinnarò [15] | 44 | All sites | C, F | 3 | 57 (27) |
| Di Blasio [16] | 35 | All sites | C, F | 3–5 | 69 (37) |
| Fonseca [17] | 79 | All sites | C, F | 4 | 78 (49) |
| Thyss [18] | 108 | All sites | C, F | 3 | 86 (35) |
| Shneider [19] | 39 | All sites | C, F, L | 3 | 82 (42) |
| Demard [20] | 71 | Larynx, hypopharynx | C, F | 3 | 82 (52)T |
| De Andrés [21] | 49 | All sites | C, F | 3 | 92 (27) |
|  | 46 |  | Cb, F | 3 | 76 (20) |
| Gregoire [22] | 83 | All sites | Cb, F | 2–3 | 33 (14) |
| Depondt [23,24] | 150 | All sites | Cb, F | 3 | 63 (31)T |

CR, complete response rate; Vcr, vincristine; Vbl, vinblastine; Vds:, vindesine; B., bleomycin; C, cisplatin; Cb, carboplatin; M, methotrexate; L, L-folinic acid; T., response assessed on the primary tumor.

results of the majority of the European phase II and phase III studies in which an integrated approach consisting of induction chemotherapy followed by loco-regional treatment was evaluated. Even though the huge methodological heterogeneity of these trials is confusing, there was a high complete response rate was observed in treatment-naive head and neck cancer patients, especially when a cisplatin-containing regimen was employed. The response rate ranges from 33 to 92%, with a complete response rate of 7–52%. The sensitivity of head and neck squamous-cell tumors to cisplatin-based chemotherapy combinations encouraged the planning of clinical prospective trials comparing induction chemotherapy followed by surgery and/or radiation with loco-regional treatment alone.

Notwithstanding the promising results of uncontrolled, pilot trials, however, European randomized trials aiming at demonstrating a survival benefit for chemo-radiotherapy combinations when compared with a control group, failed to show any statistically significant survival difference (Table 2).

In reviewing randomized trials on integrated chemo-radiotherapy combinations, a methodological issue should be stated: due to the poor prognosis of advanced head and neck cancer, only a slight survival benefit can be obtained with experimental treatments and, consequently, quite a large number of patients is required in order to reach a reliable statistical power. In the case of small studies, results are often not statistically reliable, especially when negative, because the non-significant $P$ value does not exclude that a difference between the two treatment groups really exists. The probability of obtaining a statistically significant difference if the two treatments are truly different is low with small studies. Results of such studies are rather to be considered indeterminate. For this reason only sufficiently large studies should be taken into account when evaluating the cost/benefit ratio of integrated treatments; otherwise one may be confused by contradictory results of many small, inconclusive studies.

Among the European studies comparing neo-adjuvant chemotherapy with loco-regional treatment alone, the one conducted by Paccagnella et al. [13] showed an improved survival for the experimental group, although the benefit seemed to be limited to the subgroup of

Table 2

European randomized trials of induction chemotherapy followed by loco-regional treatment compared with loco-regional treatment alone

| First author | No. of patients | Site of primary | Survival | Loco-regional control | Metastatic disease control |
|---|---|---|---|---|---|
| Richard [2] | 222 | Oropharynx oral cavity | ↑ | = | = |
| Arcangeli [25] | 142 | Oropharynx oral cavity maxillary antrum | ↑ | = | = |
| Domenge [12] | 166 | Oropharynx | = | = | = |
| Paccagnella [13] | 237 | All sites (no larynx) | = | = | ↑ |
| Jaullerry [6] | 208 | All sites | = | = | ↑ |
| Depondt [23,24] | 300 | All sites (no nasopharynx) | = | ↑ | = |
| Mazeron [11] | 131 | Oropharynx oral cavity | = | = | = |

inoperable patients; authors concluded that induction chemotherapy could be useful in the subset of patients who, having more advanced disease, take no advantage from surgery. Although this observation could reflect a truly existing difference between the chemotherapy effects in inoperable (more advanced) and in operable (less advanced) patients, it should be said that this stratification was not performed a priori and therefore the relevance of the conclusion must be considered statistically weak. When the entire patient group was considered, however, no differences in survival or in loco-regional relapse rate were evident, while a significant reduction in terms of distant recurrences was seen in patients undergoing induction chemotherapy (9 versus 14% at 2 years); a similar reduction in terms of distant metastasis rate was shown in another randomized trial [6].

It might be supposed that induction chemotherapy is really effective in preventing the occurrence of metastatic disease. However, due to the low incidence of distant spread as a first event in head and neck cancer, this effect (a 5% difference in the Paccagnella study) does not translate into an effect on overall survival. Demonstrating a survival benefit in favor of neo-adjuvant chemotherapy would probably require larger studies.

Thus, it is reasonable to expect that in more advanced local disease (such as the inoperable patient group of the Paccagnella study), the benefit offered by induction chemotherapy, if any, may be more evident.

Loco-regional control seems not to be influenced by the induction chemotherapy approach, although in the trial conducted by Depondt et al. [23,24] an increased rate of nodal recurrence was shown, in comparison with the control group. An explanation of the apparent worse loco-regional control in the neo-adjuvant chemotherapy group could be the 6–9 weeks delay in the application of loco-regional treatment. Similar results were shown by our group [26] in a recently performed multivariate analysis on 273 patients treated in two consecutive randomized trials according to 4 treatment approaches: standard radiation therapy, alternating chemo-radiotherapy with either the VBM combination (vinblastine, bleomycin, methotrexate) or the cisplatin–5-fluorouracil combination and induction VBM followed by radiation. A significantly increased risk of death was found for the group of patients treated with the neo-adjuvant approach, in comparison to the radiotherapy-only group. Moreover recently, two literature-based meta-analyses [27,28] suggested similar conclusions. A large meta-analysis based on individual data, conducted by the investigators at the Gustave Roussy Institute, in Paris, is in progress and hopefully will provide definitive information about the use of induction chemotherapy.

All these findings taken together seem to suggest that an indiscriminate use of induction chemotherapy may be detrimental and should be discouraged outside clinical trials; probably this practice should even no longer be object of prospective clinical investigation.

The negative results of randomized studies on neo-adjuvant chemotherapy can be viewed as a consequence of the theoretical principle that underlies the interaction between drugs and radiation when they are employed in a temporal sequencing. In this approach the benefit should arise from "spatial cooperation", meaning an independence between chemotherapy, which acts on systemic disease, and radiotherapy, which provides local antineoplastic activity; drugs and radiation exert their action upon different targets, thus producing an independent additive effect. The results of the sequential use of chemotherapy and radiation at best reflect the sum of the efficacies of the single modalities used. Using such a combination, the best results should be achieved when the best (= most active) chemotherapy regimen is combined with the best loco-regional treatment, for no synergistic properties of the two modalities are of interest.

When induction chemotherapy is applied in the treatment of solid neoplasms character-ized by high rates of distant failures, such as lung cancer, a survival benefit can be demon-strated [29,30]. Advanced unresectable head and neck cancer has a low rate of distant me-tastases and death is usually due to the lack of loco-regional control. Therefore induction chemotherapy before definitive radiotherapy is probably not better than radiotherapy alone. In this setting, a synergistic activity between drugs and radiation upon the loco-regional site is probably more desirable.

## 3.  Induction chemotherapy as organ preserving strategy

Despite its limits, induction chemotherapy has been chosen for organ preserving approaches in larynx and hypopharynx cancers [31]. Analysis of trials on the neo-adjuvant approach revealed that head and neck cancer responsive to chemotherapy, definitively responds to radiotherapy and this observation opened an additional opportunity for combined treatments targeted at organ preservation. Patients who are candidates for radical mutilating surgery (total laryngectomy ± partial pharyngectomy) undergo two or three courses of a cisplatin-based chemotherapy. Responding patients (complete ± partial responders) are considered suitable for definitive radiation therapy while non-responding patients (patients with no change or disease progression) are treated with salvage surgery followed by radiation ther-apy.

At least partial primary tumor shrinkage is considered the necessary condition for a suc-cessful organ-preserving treatment. Neck dissection can be performed at the end of the chemo-radiation program in case of "bulky" initial disease or in case of residual disease, without interfering with larynx function. As mentioned above, regimens with the highest activity in head and neck cancer (namely the cisplatin–5-fluorouracil combination) can achieve a response rate ranging from about 50 to 90%, with a 15–50% complete response rate. The consequence is that a large proportion of patients suitable for total laryngectomy (approximately one-half to two-thirds when partial and complete responders are considered) can be scheduled for the larynx preserving approach.

The major concern with this strategy is obviously related to its impact on survival: is there any therapeutic disadvantage in avoiding radical surgery? In particular, does the late application of loco-regional treatment worsen loco-regional control? In a multivariate analy-sis performed by investigators at the National Cancer Institute Regina Elena in Rome, on a population of 152 head and neck cancer patients treated with induction chemotherapy be-fore loco-regional treatment, the clinical complete response rate to chemotherapy was the strongest predictor of survival [9]. Thus, at least the population of responders should theo-retically not be penalized; but what about non-responders?

Another concern relates to the feasibility of surgery upon chemotherapy-treated tissues: does induction chemotherapy make salvage surgery a difficult and dangerous approach? Does the tumor shrinkage produced by drugs increase the morbidity of surgical procedures?

Two recently published randomized trials, one American [32,33] and one European [34], have addressed these important questions. The American trial compared induction chemo-therapy and radiation with radical surgery, in patients with laryngeal cancer facing total la-ryngectomy. The European trial compared the same treatment approaches in patients with hypopharyngeal cancer. Thus, the information provided by the two studies are somehow complementary. Although a comparison between the two studies is biased by the different

Table 3

Comparison between the two randomized trials on larynx preservation: the EORTC trial [34] and the Department of Veteran Affairs Laryngeal Study Group (VALSG) trial [32,33]

|  | Trial | |
| --- | --- | --- |
|  | EORTC | VALSG |
| *Methods* | | |
| Site of primary | Hypopharynx | Larynx |
| CT regimen | Cisplatin–5-FU | Cisplatin–5-FU |
| No. of courses | 3 | 3 |
| Eligibility for RT | CR | PR or CR |
| No. of patients | 202 | 332 |
| *Results*[a] | | |
| RR (RC) (%)[b] | 86 (54) | 83 (36) |
| Larynx preserved (%) | 57 | 64 |
| Loco-regional recurrence[c] | = | ↑ |
| Distant recurrence[c] | ↓ | ↓ |
| 3-year survival (%) | 57 | 53 |
| 3-year survival with larynx (%) | 28 | 31 |

[a]Numbers refer to the results of the induction chemotherapy group.
[b]Response to the last completed chemotherapy course.
[c]The comparison between the induction chemotherapy group and the control group is represented: =, no difference; ↑, increased; ↓, decreased.

methods of presenting results and especially in evaluating the larynx preserving potential of the induction chemotherapy approach, Table 3 summarizes the main features of the two trials.

In the European trial, 202 patients with resectable stage II–IV hypopharynx cancer (pyriform sinus and aryepiglottic fold), candidates for demolitive surgery requiring total laryngectomy, were randomized to receive either immediate loco-regional treatment (surgery + radiotherapy) or chemotherapy (cisplatin–5-fluorouracil) prior to loco-regional treatment. In the experimental group, loco-regional treatment consisted of radiotherapy alone for patients achieving complete response after two or three chemotherapy courses. Non-complete responders after the third cycle and patients with progressive disease at the first and second cycle underwent surgery and postoperative radiotherapy.

Fifty-four percent of the patients receiving induction chemotherapy had a complete response at the primary site and could undergo organ-sparing definitive radiotherapy. Eight patients relapsed after organ-sparing treatment, and required salvage laryngectomy. At 3 years, 28% of the patients randomized to the induction chemotherapy group were alive with a functional larynx in place. Indeed, very similar figures were shown in the VALSG study (31%). Overall 5-year survival of the two treatment groups was similar (30 versus 35%) as was similar the 5-year disease-free survival (25 versus 27%). Loco-regional failures in the experimental group were as frequent as regional relapses in the control group. On the contrary, induction chemotherapy significantly reduced the development of distant failures (25 versus 36%); this finding is in line with the trials discussed above on induction chemotherapy and it is evident also in the VALSG study. In that study, however, organ-sparing treatment was associated with a higher incidence of loco-regional relapses. The choice of giving definitive radiotherapy also to partial responders obviously translated into a larynx preservation rate (64%) higher than the complete response rate (36%). Whether this choice was responsible of the lower locoregional control shown in the VALSG study for the experimental group in comparison with the immediate surgery group, is a matter of debate.

A further important finding common to both studies was that a similar time to wound healing and a similar incidence of wound infections were detected for salvage surgery following induction chemotherapy in comparison with immediate surgery; induction chemotherapy does not negatively affect surgical morbidity and mortality. Thus, both studies underline that salvage surgery is a safe option in case of non response to chemotherapy.

One can conclude that neo-adjuvant chemotherapy does not compromise survival of this patient population while achieving good figures of larynx preservation.

Considering the findings of these two studies, what could be the future perspectives for organ preservation in head and neck cancer?

First, we have to understand the precise role of neo-adjuvant chemotherapy. In fact two alternatives are possible:

1. . The achievement of a complete response to neo-adjuvant chemotherapy is the key point to select patients for whom organ preservation is suitable. In this case our future target will be to increase the complete response rate to induction chemotherapy through new regimens and/or new drugs.
2. Being well known that response to radiotherapy correlates with response to chemotherapy, induction chemotherapy plays the role of a sort of "in vivo" chemosensitivity test. In this case our goal is to reduce the length and intensity of neo-adjuvant chemotherapy, in order to lower chemotherapy related morbidity and to shorten the delay before loco-regional treatment.

There are not yet answers to these questions. Perhaps increasing the complete response rate could be useful for a more cautious selection of patients in whom radiotherapy may be effective. In fact, partial responders include both patients with most tumor cell clones sensible to chemotherapy (and radiotherapy) and patients with a good balance between sensible and resistant clones. This latter group is probably under-treated by radiotherapy alone. The VALSG analysis, showing that partial responders to neo-adjuvant chemotherapy do poorly compared to non-responders (i.e. resected), support this hypothesis. Consequently, to increase the complete response rate to chemotherapy and to give up organ preservation in partial responders could be the best policy. Whether the cost-benefit ratio of intensifying induction chemotherapy is suitable is an open question.

## 4.   Concurrent chemo-radiotherapy regimens

As already seen, there is increasing evidence that chemotherapy followed by definitive radiotherapy does not jeopardize the cure rates when compared to immediate surgery ± radiation, while achieving the end-point of larynx preservation. However, induction chemotherapy does not improve survival with respect to loco-regional treatment alone. For this reason, even though it could be a useful clue for organ preservation, it must not be considered the best treatment for advanced head and neck cancer.

The main concern that can still be raised about its use as a larynx preserving strategy, is that chemotherapy is used mainly as a predictive test for the selection of patients to be treated with definitive radiotherapy, thus avoiding radical surgery. Since randomized trials have failed to disclose benefit of induction chemotherapy followed by radiation as compared with radiation alone, the need for aggressive multidrug chemotherapy regimens, when the sole target is the selection of patients for organ preservation, is questionable. Moreover, radiotherapy could also be of benefit in patients not responding to cisplatin and 5-fluorouracil (who are usually not offered larynx preservation). Therefore, the problem is to increase the rate of organ preservation while increasing the overall survival over surgery ± radiotherapy.

As mentioned above, the sequential administration of chemotherapy and radiotherapy strives for "spatial cooperation", with chemotherapy applied for the control of metastatic or micro-metastatic disease and radiotherapy for the eradication of loco-regional disease. The concomitant application of drugs and radiation, on the other hand, has the potential to achieve "local cooperation". Since most head and neck cancers recur locally, and loco-regional disease is the usual cause of death, this type of cooperation is more relevant than "spatial cooperation", when the goal of increasing long-term survival is looked for.

Emerging clinical data seem to favor a strict temporal association between these two therapeutic modalities [35].

The first European randomized trials comparing radiotherapy alone with concurrent chemo-radiation in advanced, inoperable head and neck cancer (Table 4) applied drugs as radiation sensitizers along with radiotherapy. Bleomycin and 5-fluorouracil, two drugs tested as single-agent chemotherapy, are not clearly effective per se in head and neck cancer, showing a low response rate when employed in an advanced stage setting. Thus, the expected result of their combination with radiotherapy is a certain degree of enhancement of radiotherapy local effects and not a true additive effect between two independent cytotoxic strategies. Such a potentiation of radiation antineoplastic activity could also be obtained by applying a more aggressive radiotherapy schedule, as is clearly shown by the study of Sanchiz et al. [39]: standard 60 Gy radiotherapy along with single-agent 5-fluorouracil is similar to hyperfractionated 70 Gy radiotherapy alone and both groups give better results when compared to standard 60 Gy radiation. A similar equivalence between concurrent chemo-radiation treatments and radiotherapy alone was also demonstrated in the two trials using

Table 4

Randomized studies of concurrent CT + RT

| First author | No of patients | Control group | CT regimen | Results |
|---|---|---|---|---|
| Vermund [36] | 222 | RT (70 Gy) | Bleomycin | = |
| Eschwege [37] | 224 | RT (70 Gy) | Bleomycin | = |
| Gupta [38] | 313 | RT | Methotrexate | ↑ DFS<br>= survival |
| Sanchiz [39] | 892 | 1) RT (60 Gy)<br>2) HF-RT (70 Gy) | 5-Fluorouracil (c.i.) | ↑ survival<br>(vs RT; = vs HF-RT) |
| Wendt [40] | 235 | RT (70Gy)<br>Accelerated<br>split course | Cisplatin, 5-fluorouracil,<br>leucovorin | ↑ local control<br>↑ survival |
| Merlano [41,42] | 157 | RT (70 Gy) | Cisplatin, 5-fluorouracil<br>(i.v. bolus) | ↑ local control<br>↑ survival |

RT, radiotherapy; HF-RT, hyperfractionated radiotherapy; DFS, disease-free survival.

bleomycin; moreover local toxicity to skin and mucosas appeared to be significantly worsened.

It is with the advent of multi-agent chemotherapy that concurrent chemo-radiation has shown its potential benefit over radiotherapy alone. As already observed, the introduction of poly-chemotherapy regimens led to impressive objective response rates up to more than 90%, including a large proportion of complete responses (Table 1). Indeed head and neck cancer was shown to be a chemosensitive tumor, thus suitable for the combined action of both drugs and radiation.

In 1988 our group published the results of a randomized phase III trial which was designed to assess the best method of combining drugs and radiation [5]. In that study, advanced stage, inoperable head and neck cancer patients were treated either with four courses of induction VBM (vinblastine, bleomycin, methotrexate) followed by continuous course 60 Gy radiation, or with the same regimen alternated with three 20 Gy radiation splits. The latter treatment group produced significantly more complete responses and resulted in a significant survival advantage [43], although a significant increase in mucosal toxicity, most likely due to a negative interaction between radiotherapy and methotrexate, was evident.

A direct comparison between neo-adjuvant chemotherapy and concurrent chemoradiation has been performed in another randomized trial [44], in which 267 patients were randomized to neo-adjuvant VBM (2 courses) followed by 60 Gy radiation and then to 2 other courses of the same chemotherapy regimen, or to an alternating VBM/radiotherapy program. The design of the alternating chemo–radiotherapy aim was very similar between the two studies; the two studies differed only in the neo-adjuvant chemo-radiation group (2 chemotherapy courses before and 2 after radiotherapy in the SECOG I trial, 4 chemotherapy courses before radiotherapy in the Genova trial). There were also minor differences in the chemotherapy regimen: the English investigators used methotrexate in a 24-h infusion instead of in a 2-h infusion. Moreover, the SECOG I trial was a two by two factorial study, designed to investigate the addition of 5-fluorouracil to the VBM regimen. This trial failed to show a survival advantage for the synchronous treatment group, although a disease-free advantage was evident; mucosal toxicity was greater; 5-fluorouracil was shown to add some benefit to the VBM scheme without worsening local toxicity.

The encouraging results obtained in one study prompted us to compare the alternating program with radiation given with a standard fractionation scheme up to a dose of 70 Gy [41,42]. In the second study, however, a cisplatin–5-fluorouracil chemotherapy regimen was chosen due to the high activity shown in head and neck cancer, the property of radiation sensitizers of both cisplatin and 5-fluorouracil and the high rate of mucosal toxicity encountered using a methotrexate-containing regimen. Chemotherapy consisted of cisplatin (20 mg/m$^2$ per day, days 1–5) and 5-fluorouracil (200 mg/m$^2$ per day i.v. bolus days 1–5), after cisplatin administration. Courses were repeated every 21 days and were alternated with three radiotherapy courses (20 Gy each, 2 Gy per fraction, one daily fraction) up to a total radiation dose of 60 Gy. The chemotherapy schedule was modified from the original Al-Sarraf regimen (cisplatin 100 mg/m$^2$ day 1 and 5-fluorouracil 1000 mg/m$^2$ per day continuous i.v. infusion days 1–5) in order to avoid 5-fluorouracil-induced mucositis and to allow the out-patient administration of the entire treatment.

The alternated chemo-radiation program resulted in a significant survival advantage in comparison with standard radiation. It must be underlined that the survival benefit observed in the multimodal treatment arm resulted mainly from a gain in loco-regional control, while the overall incidence of metastatic disease seemed to be unaffected by the addition of active drugs to the radiation program. In contrast with the results obtained with induction chemo-therapy, in which drugs achieved distant disease control at best, this concurrent regimen was shown to be locally active, thus significantly affecting patients survival. Local toxicity was shown to be not greater than that produced by radiotherapy alone and treatment could be performed entirely on an out-patient basis, in most cases.

## 5. Concurrent chemo-radiotherapy and organ preservation

No randomized studies have been published dealing with the larynx preservation potential of combined chemo-radiation regimens. Two European pilot experiences, however, which include patients with resectable advanced disease, have been reported. The first was conducted by Leyvraz et al. [45] and tested a very intensive treatment consisting of accelerated hyperfractionated radiotherapy (2 Gy three times daily on days 1–3, 11–12, 29–31, 39–40, up to a total dose of 60 Gy), alternating with a cisplatin–5-fluorouracil regimen (cisplatin 100 mg/m$^2$ per day 1; 5-fluorouracil 1000 mg/m$^2$ per day continuous infusion on days 1–3, for 2 courses administered on days 8–10 and 36–38). Ninety-one patients were evaluated; most of them had oropharynx cancer (50%) and 76% of the entire patient population was judged resectable. Despite a high treatment-related mortality (5.5%) and a high rate of severe mucositis, the overall response rate was impressive (95.6%) and the complete response rate was as high as 69.2%. Four-year progression-free survival and overall survival were 30 and 40%, respectively. Among the 69 resectable patients, 72% achieved a complete response and 64% were spared mutilating surgery.

This trial highlighted the possibility of sparing major surgery for primary sites other than larynx or hypopharynx and suggested that the high complete response rate achieved with a concurrent chemo-radiation regimen could translate into a high organ preservation rate.

The second trial using concurrent chemo-radiation for organ preservation in head and neck cancer has been conducted in Italy [46] and accrued 40 patients eligible for total laryngectomy ± pharyngectomy. Patients were treated with a concomitant program consisting of standard fractionated radiation therapy (70 Gy) along with cisplatin (20 mg/m$^2$ per day days 1–4) and 5-fluorouracil (200 mg/m$^2$ per day i.v. bolus days 1–4), or carboplatin (75 mg/m$^2$ per day days 1–4) and 5-fluorouracil (1000 mg/m$^2$ per day continuous i.v. infusion days 1–4). Eighty-three percent of the evaluable patients had a complete response on the primary tumor and the larynx preservation rate was 70%. Local toxicity related to this treatment was severe but manageable, with 55% of the patients having a grade III mucositis, no grade IV mucositis and no treatment-related deaths.

The question of the best strategy for larynx preservation in advanced head and neck cancer is the subject of two ongoing EORTC randomized clinical trials, which, in the next few years, will provide the scientific and the medical community with important information: (1). Does concomitant chemo-radiotherapy add something in comparison to neo-adjuvant chemotherapy followed by radiotherapy for larynx preservation? (2) Is radiation alone a safe method for larynx preservation? and (3) Does radiotherapy affect surgical morbidity?

The first trial (EORTC 24954) compares the induction chemotherapy strategy with the alternating chemo-radiation program as developed at the National Institute for Cancer Research in Genova. The latter regimen has been considered suitable for study in an organ preservation trial for its demonstrated survival benefit over the radiotherapy only treatment and for its low local toxicity rate.

Operable patients with larynx (T3-T4) and hypopharynx (T2-T4) squamous cell carcinoma (N0-N2b) are randomized to a control group of induction chemotherapy or to the alternating chemo-radiation program. In the experimental group, salvaged surgery is planned for non-complete responders while in the induction chemotherapy group both partial and complete responders are given two more chemotherapy courses and definitive irradiation. Due to the unreliability of response evaluation in irradiated tissues and to the possible surgical impairment, two options are offered to investigators: evaluation and eventual surgery 2 months after the completion of radiotherapy or after 40 Gy and two chemotherapy courses have been administered.

A second trial (EORTC 22954) has been designed for the comparison of radiotherapy alone (70 Gy with standard fractionation) with a concomitant chemo-radiation treatment consisting of continuous course radiotherapy with cisplatin (100 mg/m$^2$ given on days 1, 22 and 43). Also, in this trial, response evaluation and salvage surgery can be performed 2 months after the end of treatment or after 40–50 Gy have been administered.

The planned accrual is of 300 patients in each trial in a 4-year period. The primary endpoint will be survival with a functional larynx.

A further large larynx preservation trial is ongoing and is coordinated by the Mario Negri Institute, in Italy. This randomized trial is designed to compare immediate total laryngectomy versus a concomitant chemo-radiotherapy program ± salvage surgery in resectable T3-T4, N0-N3 larynx cancer patients. The experimental arm consists of standard fractionated radiotherapy (weeks 1–7) with carboplatin (75 mg/m$^2$ per day days 1–4) and 5–fluorouracil (1000 mg/m$^2$ per day continuous i.v. infusion days 1–4), administered for three courses on weeks 1, 5, 9. This trial is scheduled to accrue 450–500 patients in 3 years and the main end-points are survival, larynx preservation rate and quality of life.

## 6.  Conclusions

Organ preservation is still an open field of investigation in Europe as well as in USA. With current knowledge, the question of whether immediate demolitive surgery (total laryngectomy ± partial pharyngectomy) should still be considered the standard for advanced larynx and hypopharynx cancers is difficult to answer. Only two published randomized trials are available and data cannot be considered conclusive. The only things we can say are that:

- neo-adjuvant chemotherapy followed by radiotherapy achieves good figures of larynx preservation and does not apparently impair salvage surgery;
- the non-surgical approach does not have an evident detrimental impact on patient survival;
- organ preservation can be extended to head and neck regions other than larynx. Many other critical points must still be answered;
- which patients can safely spare surgery: only complete responders or all the objective responders (partial and complete responders)?
- is the Al-Sarraf regimen the best chemotherapy to be employed?
- what role can be played by the combination of chemotherapy and radiotherapy? Could this approach reduce the rate of patients still requiring demolitive surgery while increasing overall survival?

A number of on-going clinical trials should contribute to answer to these questions in the near future. However, two risks are evident: the first is that organ preservation becomes a

standard approach before solid scientific evidence exists as happened for neo-adjuvant chemotherapy during the past decade; the second is that the ongoing trials will not be able to
enroll enough patients for adequate statistical power.

Therefore it must be stressed that organ preservation is still an experimental approach,
and its routine use must be considered inappropriate. It only can be considered a feasible
option when performed for selected patients and in centers with good cooperation between
surgeons, radiation therapists and medical oncologists; in such centers a carefully planned
program of induction chemotherapy, response evaluation, administration of definitive radiation to responders and timely radical surgery for non-responders can be a safe alternative
to immediate surgery.

Further, it is even more important that researchers contribute to multi-institutional, well
designed, cooperative trials rather than designing their own small size trials, which will sat-
isfy their pride, but have few opportunities to reach an adequate statistical power and to give
useful information to the medical community.

## Summary

Organ preservation has gained great importance in head and neck cancer treatment due to
the physiological and psychological role of organs such as the larynx and tongue. While in
early stages radiotherapy and conservative surgery achieve superb results, in advanced stage
disease demolitive surgery is often the only choice offered to patients. Integrated chemoradiotherapy programs have been developed in recent years in order to overcome the need for
surgery. Induction chemotherapy followed by definitive radiation has been until recently the
most popular integrated approach, due to the high response rate achieved by very active
chemotherapy combinations in untreated, squamous cell, head and neck cancer. However,
randomized trials failed to show any survival improvement when compared to radiotherapy
alone. Neo-adjuvant chemotherapy was used for organ preservation strategies in head and
neck cancers requiring total laryngectomy, for the possibility of selecting patients suitable
for definitive radiotherapy. Two large larynx preservation trials have been conducted, one in
the US and one in Europe) and both showed that induction chemotherapy does not jeopardize survival while achieving good figures for larynx preservation. The concomitant administration of active chemotherapy regimens and radiation therapy seems promising in advanced, unresectable head and neck cancer and some groups have already reported pilot
experiences of organ preservation. Trials assessing the impact of such treatments on survival
and on organ preservation in a randomized fashion are in progress and will be able to give
important information in the near future.

## References

1.  Harari PM. Why has induction chemotherapy for advanced H&N cancer become a U.S. community stan-
    dard of practice? Proc 4th Int Conf Head and Neck Cancer, Toronto 98, 1996.
2.  Richard JM, Kramar A, Molinari R, et al. Randomised EORTC Head and Neck Cooperative Group trial of
    preoperative intra-arterial chemotherapy in oral cavity and oropharynx carcinoma. Eur J Cancer 27: 821–
    827, 1991.
3.  Hill BT, Price LA, MacRae K. Importance of primary site in assessing chemotherapy response and 7-year
    survival data in advanced squamous-cell carcinomas of the head and neck treated with initial combination
    chemotherapy without cisplatin. J Clin Oncol 4: 1340–1347, 1986.

4.   Hill BT, Price LA. Lack of survival advantage in patients with advanced squamous-cell carcinomas of the oral cavity receiving neoadjuvant chemotherapy prior to local therapy, despite achieving an initial high clinical complete remission rate. Am J Clin Oncol 17: 1–5, 1994.

5.   Merlano M, Rosso R, Sertoli MR, et al. Sequential versus alternating chemotherapy and radiotherapy in stage III-IV squamous cell carcinoma of the head and neck: a phase III study. J Clin Oncol 6: 627–632, 1988.

6.   Jaullery C, Rodriguez J, Brunin F, et al. Induction chemotherapy in advanced head and neck tumors: results of two randomized trials. Int J Radiat Oncol Biol Phys 23: 483–489, 1992.

7.   Frustaci S, Barzan L, Caruso G, et al. Induction intra-arterial cisplatin and bleomycin in head and neck cancer. Head Neck Surg 13: 291–297, 1991.

8.   Recondo G, Cvitkovic E, Azli N, et al. Neoadjuvant chemotherapy consisting of cisplatin and continuous infusions of bleomycin and 5-fluorouracil for advanced head and neck cancer. Cancer 68: 2109–2119, 1991.

9.   Cognetti F, Pinnaro P, Ruggeri EM, et al. Prognostic factors for chemotherapy response and survival using combination chemotherapy as initial treatment of advanced head and neck squamous cell cancer. J Clin Oncol 7: 829–837, 1989.

10.  Grau JJ, Estapé J, Blanch JL, et al. Neoadjuvant and adjuvant chemotherapy in the multidisciplinary treatment of oral cancer stage III or IV. Oral Oncol, Eur J Cancer 32B: 238–241, 1996.

11.  Mazeron JJ, Martin M, Brun B, et al. Induction chemotherapy in head and neck cancer: results of a phase III trial. Head Neck Surg 14: 85–91, 1992.

12.  Domenge C, Coche-Dequeant B, Wibault P, et al. Randomized trial of neoadjuvant chemotherapy before radiotherapy in oropharyngeal carcinoma. Proc 4th Int Conf Head and Neck Cancer, Toronto 99, 1996.

13.  Paccagnella A, Orlando A, Marchiori C, et al. Phase III trial of initial chemotherapy in stage III or IV head and neck cancers: a study by the Gruppo di Studio sui Tumori della Testa e del Collo. J Natl Cancer Inst 86: 265–272, 1994.

14.  Licitra L, Grandi C, Cavina R, et al. Surgery versus primary chemotherapy and surgery in operable cancers of the oral cavity: interim report of a randomized study. Proc 4th Int Conf Head and Neck Cancer, Toronto 99, 1996.

15.  Pinnarò P, Cercato MC, Giannarelli D, et al. A randomized phase II study comparing sequential versus simultaneous chemo-radiotherapy in patients with unresectable locally advanced squamous cell cancer of the head and neck. Ann Oncol 5: 513–519, 1994.

16.  Di Blasio B, Barbieri W, Bozetti A, et al. A prospective randomized trial in resectable head and neck carcinoma: loco-regional treatment with and without neoadjuvant chemotherapy. Proc Ann Meet Am Soc Clin Oncol 13: 279, 1994.

17.  Fonseca E, Cruz JJ, Gomez A, et al. Neoadjuvant chemotherapy with cisplatin and 5-fluorouracil, both in continuous 96-hour infusion, in the treatment of locally advanced head and neck cancer. Am J Clin Oncol 17: 6–9, 1994.

18.  Thyss A, Schneider M, Santini J, et al. Induction chemotherapy with cis-plutinum and 5-fluorouracil for squamous cell carcinoma of the head and neck. Br J Cancer 54: 755–760, 1986.

19.  Shneider M, Etienne MC, Milano G, et al. Phase II trial of cisplatin, fluorouracil, and pure l-folinic acid for locally advanced head and neck cancer: a pharmacokinetic and clinical survey. J Clin Oncol 13: 1656–1662, 1995.

20.  Demard F, Chauvel P, Santini J, et al. Response to chemotherapy as justification for modification of the therapeutic strategy for pharyngolaryngeal carcinomas. Head Neck Surg 12: 225–231, 1990.

21.  De Andrés L, Brunet J, Lopez-Pousa A, et al. Randomized trail of neoadjuvant cisplatin and fluorouracil versus carboplatin and fluorouracil in patients with stage IV-MO head and neck cancer. J Clin Oncol 13: 1493–1500, 1995.

22.  Gregoire V, Beauduin M, Humblet Y, et al. A phase 1–11 trial of induction chemotherapy with carboplatin and fluorouracil in locally advanced head and neck squamous cell carcinoma: a report from the UCL - Oncology Group, Belgium. J Clin Oncol 9: 1385–1392, 1991.

23.  Gehanno P, Depondt J, Peynegre R, et al. Neoadjuvant combination of carboplatin and 5-FU in head and neck cancer: a randomized study. Ann Oncol 3(Suppl 3): S43–S46, 1992.

24.  Depondt J, Gehanno P, Martin M, et al. Neoadjuvant chemotherapy with carboplatin/5-fluorourscil in head and neck cancer. Oncology 50(Suppl 2): 23–27, 1993.

25.  Merlano M, Vitale V, Benasso M, et al. Multivariate analysis of 273 pts with SCC-HN treated in two randomized trials of alternating chemotherapy and radiotherapy (abstr.). Proc Am Soc Clin Oncol 294: 1995.

26.  Arcangeli G, Nervi C, Righini R, et al. Combined radiation and drugs: the effect of intra-arterial chemotherapy followed by radiotherapy in head and neck cancer. Radiother Oncol 1: 101–1017, 1983.

27.  Munro AJ. An overview of randomized controlled trials of adjuvant chemotherapy in head and neck cancer. Br J Cancer 71: 83–91, 1995.

28.  EI-Sayed S, Nelson N. Adjuvant and adjunctive chemotherapy in the management of squamous cell carcinoma of the head and neck region: a meta-analysis of prospective and randomized trials. J Clin Oncol 14: 838–847, 1996.

29.  Dillman RO, Herdon J, Seagren SL, et al. Improved survival in stage III non-small-cell lung cancer: seven-year follow-up of Cancer and Leukemia Group B (CALGB) 8433 trial. J Natl Cancer Inst 88: 1210–1215, 1996.

30.  Sause WT, Scott C, Taylor S, et al. Radiation Therapy Oncology Group (RTOG1 88 08 and Eastern Cooperative Oncology Group (ECOG) 4588: preliminary results of a phase III trial in regionally advanced, unresectable non-small-cell lung cancer. J Natl Cancer Inst 7: 198–205, 1995.

31.  Lefebvre JL, Bonneterre J. Current status of larynx preservation trials. Curr Opin Oncol 8: 209–224, 1996.

32.  The Department of Veterans Affairs Laryngeal Study Group. Induction chemotherapy plus radiation compared with surgery plus radiation in patients with advanced laryngeal cancer. N Engl J Med 324: 1685–1690, 1991.

33.  Spaulding MB, Fisher SG, Wolf GT, and the Department of Veterans Affairs Cooperative Laryngeal Cancer Study Group. Tumor response, toxicity, and survival after neoadjuvant organ-preserving chemotherapy for advanced laryngeal carcinoma. J Clin Oncol 12: 1592–1599, 1994.

34.  Lefebvre JL, Chevalier D, Luboinsky B, et al. Larynx preservation in pyriform sinus cancer: preliminary results of a European Organisation for Research and Treatment of Cancer phase III trial. J Natl Cancer Inst 88: 890–899, 1996.

35.  Merlano M, Benasso M, Cavallari M, et al. Chemotherapy in head and neck cancer. Oral Oncol, Eur J Cancer 30B: 283–289, 1994.

36.  Vermund H, Kaalhus O, Winther F, et al. Bleomycin and radiation therapy in squamous cell carcinoma of the upper aero-digestive tract: a phase III clinical trial. Int J Radiat Oncol Biol Phys 11: 1877–1886, 1985.

37.  Eschwege F, Sancho-Garnier H, Gerard JP, et al. Ten-year results of randomized trial comparing radiotherapy and concomitant bleomycin to radiotherapy alone in epidermoid carcinomas of the oropharynx: experience of the European Organization for Research and Treatment of Cancer. Natl Cancer Inst Monogr 6: 275–278, 1988.

38.  Gupta NK, Pointon RCS, Wilkinson PM. A randomised clinical trial to contrast radiotherapy with radiotherapy and methotrexate given synchronously in head and neck cancer. Clin Radiol 38: 575–581, 1987

39.  Sanchiz F, Millà A, Torner J, et al. Single fraction per day versus two fractions per day versus radiochemotherapy in the treatment of head and neck cancer. Int J Radiat Oncol Biol Phys 19: 1347–1350, 1990.

40.  Wendt TG, Grabenbauer G, Thiel HJ, et al. Simultaneous radio-chemotherapy vs. radiotherapy alone in stage III and IV carcinoma of the head and neck: early results of a randomized study (abstr.). Radiother Oncol 32(Suppl): S145, 1994.

41.  Merlano M, Vitale V, Rosso R, et al. Treatment of advanced squamous-cell carcinoma of the head and neck with alternating chemotherapy and radiotherapy. N Engl J Med 327: 1115–1121, 1992.

42.  Merlano M, Benasso M, Corvò R, et al. Five-year update of a randomized trial of alternating radiotherapy and chemotherapy compared with radiotherapy alone in treatment of unresectable squamous cell carcinoma of the head and neck. J Natl Cancer Inst 88: 583–589, 1996.

43.  Merlano M, Corvò R, Margarino G, et al. Combined chemotherapy and radiation therapy in advanced inoperable squamous cell carcinoma of the head and neck. The final report of a randomized trial. Cancer 67: 915–921, 1991.

44.  SECOG. A randomized trial of combined multidrug chemotherapy and radiotherapy in advanced squamous cell carcinoma of the head and neck. Eur J Surg Oncol 12: 289–295, 1986.

45.  Leyvraz S, Pasche P, Bauer J, et al. Rapidly alternating chemotherapy and hyperfractionated radiotherapy in the management of locally advanced head and neck carcinoma: four-year results of a phase I–II study. J Clin Oncol 12: 1876–1885, 1994.

46.  Crispino S, Colombo A, Ardizzoia A, et al. Larynx preservation with concomitant radiochemotherapy (abstr.). Proc Annu Meet Am Assoc Cancer Res 14: A838, 1995.

C.J. Rosenthal and M. Rotman (Eds.), *Infusion Chemotherapy–Irradiation Interactions*

221

# CHAPTER 21

# Nasopharyngeal carcinoma curability by combined radiation–chemotherapy

K.N. CHOI[1], M. ROTMAN[1], H. AZIZ[1], C. SOHN[1], J. CIRRONE[1],
A. SCHULSINGER[1], D. SCHWARTZ[1], P. CHANDRA[2], T. BRADLEY[2],
A. BRAVERMAN[2] and C.J. ROSENTHAL[2]

*Departments of [1]Radiation Oncology and [2]Medical Oncology, State University of New York, Health Science
Center at Brooklyn, 450 Clarkson Avenue, Brooklyn, NY 11203, USA*

Nasopharyngeal carcinoma spreads through the mucosal linings into adjacent structures. It spreads freely into the nasal cavity anteriorly and to the oropharynx inferiorly. The superior and lateral wall is a muscular tube comprised of the pharyngeal constriction muscles. This is pierced by the Eustachian tubes bilaterally which provides an avenue of spread laterally into the parapharyngeal space and superiorly to the base of skull. In advanced stages, the cancer often destroys the bony walls and base of skull. It also spreads into the base of the brain causing cranial nerve symptoms. Nasopharyngeal cancers develop asymptomatically in cryptic areas and therefore are often not detected until they reach advanced stages. These tumors are generally considered to be surgically unresectable due to their proximity to the base of the skull and cranial nerves in conjunction with widespread lymphatic involvement. Radiation is highly effective in irradiating early stages of nasopharyngeal cancers, but in advanced stages it has difficulty in sterilizing tumor cells embedded in the compact facial bones and base of the skull [1]. Continued efforts have been made to improve the effectiveness of treatment including the use of altered fractionated irradiation and combined chemoradiation. Altered fractionation includes accelerated fractionation. The main strategy of accelerated fractionation is to shorten overall treatment time to decrease the chances of repopulation. Dr. Wang has used a scheme of 1.6 Gy/fraction, twice daily (bid) for a total dose of approximately 70 Gy in 6 weeks. Local control improved from 43 to 71% for T3-T4 lesions compared with once-a-day conventional treatment (70 Gy in 8 weeks with 1.8 Gy/day) [2]. Likewise, 5-year survival improved from 33 to 75% when compared with conventional treatment.

Hyperfractionated regimens have been used to treat advanced head and neck cancers. The most important phenomenon occurring between those fractionations is the repair of sublethal damage [3]. This phenomenon occurs more consistently with later responding tissues compared to early responding tissue. Therefore late responding tissue which is responsible for late radiation damage is spared more by hyperfractionation. This allows the total dose of radiation to be increased by 10–20% which translates into a better local control without an increase in late radiation damage. In an EORTC trial for oropharyngeal cancers $(T_{2,3}, N_{0,1})$, the total dose was increased by 15% from 70 Gy with standard fractions to

80.5 Gy given in a hyperfractionated regimen [4]. The tumor control increased from 40 to 59% with the same rate of late fibrosis (Grades 2 and 3) of 50%, thus the therapeutic ratio was improved.

Nasopharyngeal cancers are highly responsive to chemotherapy, especially to cisplatin based regimens. Various schedules of combined chemo-radiation administration have been used. These include neoadjuvant, concomitant and adjuvant chemotherapy. Unlike other head and neck cancers, most investigators have reported a higher local control and progression free survival with combined chemoradiation compared to radiation alone in nasopharyngeal cancers.

The initial pilot neoadjuvant studies reported higher local control and disease-free survival compared to historical control treated with radiation alone (Table 1) [5–8]. However, there are also negative retrospective studies. Two prospectively randomized neoadjuvant studies are available (Table 2). Chan et al. reported the result of a prospective randomized trial comparing two cycles of neoadjuvant chemotherapy using 5-fluorouracil (5-FU) infusion of 1000 mg/m$^2$ for 3 days and cisplatin bolus 100 mg/m$^2$ followed by radiation (86 Gy) and four cycles of adjuvant chemotherapy of the same regimen [9]. The locoregional failure rate, distant metastatic rate and 2-year disease free survival were not different between the two groups. Recently, the International Nasopharynx Cancer Study Group (INCSG) reported a randomized phase III trial comparing neoadjuvant three cycles of bleomycin, epirubicin and cisplatinum (BEC) followed by radiation to radiation alone (70 Gy) [10]. Three hundred thirty-nine patients with undifferentiated nasopharyngeal carcinoma were randomized. Treatment results were reported with a median followup of 49 months (23–

Table 1

Neoadjuvant chemotherapy and radiation for advanced nasopharyngeal carcinoma (non-randomized study)

| Authors | No. of patients | Chemo Tx (C, cycle) | CR (%) | Rad Tx (Gy) | Post RT CR (%) | L-R failure | DM (%) | DFS (%) | F/U (months) |
|---|---|---|---|---|---|---|---|---|---|
| Al-Kourainy[a] [5] | 8 | CDDP + 5-FU (3C) | 75 (6/8) | 70 | 75 (6/8) | | | 6/8 | 33–57 |
| Dimery[a] [6] | 47 | CDDP + 5-FU (3C) | 21 | 70–72 | 86 | 27 | | 4 years 66 | |
| Tannock[a] [7] | | | | | | | | 3 years | |
| RT 1970–1976 | 140 | 0 | – | 70 | – | 52 | 22 | 34 | 120–204 |
| CT-RT 1981–1983 | 51 | MBC × 2C | 13 | 70 | 82 | 43 | 18 | 34 | 40–72 |
| Teo[a] [8] | | | | | | | | 2 years | |
| RT 1981–1982 | 36 | 0 | – | 61 (2.5, 3.5) | 79* | 30 | 56 | 40 | 60–72 |
| CT-RT 1983 | 13 | VBMF 2C-RT | – | 61 | 0 | 15 | 77 | 13 | 36–48 |
| CT-RT-CT 1984 | 19 | PVMF 2C-RT-2C | – | 61 | 6 | 21 | 42 | 37 | 24–36 |

[a]Acceptable toxicities.
*$P < 0.00003$.

Table 2

Neoadjuvant chemotherapy and radiation for advanced nasopharyngeal carcinoma (prospective randomized studies)

| Authors | No. of patients | Chemo Tx (C, cycle) | CR (%) | Rad Tx (Gy) | Post RT CR (%) | L-R failure | DM (%) | DFS (%) | F/U (months) |
|---|---|---|---|---|---|---|---|---|---|
| Chan [9] | | | | | | | | 2 years | |
| CT-RT-CT | 37 | CDDP + 5-FU 2C-RT-4C | 5 | 66 + 20 | 100 | 16 | 30 | 68 | 47–71 (29) |
| RT | 40 | 0 | – | 66 + 20 | 95 | 15 | 22 | 72 | |
| Cvitkovic[b] [10] | | | | | | | | 3 years | |
| CT-RT | 171 | BEC 3C-RT | 47 | 69 | 55* | | | 47** | 23–70 (49) |
| RT | 168 | 0 | – | 69 | 34 | | | 31 | |

[a]No significant toxicities.
[b]More toxicities with neoadjuvant treatment group. Refusal of treatment (9 versus 5 patients), treatment related death (8 versus 1%, $P < 0.01$).
$*P < 0.01$; $**P < 0.02$.

70 months). There was a significant disease-free survival advantage favoring the neoadjuvant group (47.1 versus 30.5%, $P < 0.02$). Tumor recurrence or progression rate was 34% in the chemoradiation group compared to 55% in the radiation alone group ($P < 0.01$). There was a decrease in the incidence of relapse in both the primary site and distant sites. There was no difference in the overall survival because the number of events needed for analysis has not yet been reached. The therapy induced mortality was higher (8 versus 1%, $P < 0.01$) and the refusal of radiation was also high (9 versus 5 patients) in the neoadjuvant group.

With three cycles of the most effective cisplatin based regimen, neoadjuvant chemotherapy can have a significant impact on disease progression in nasopharyngeal cancer patients. However, treatment related morbidity and mortality increases. There is also the risk of delaying radiation treatment or of patients refusing further treatment after three cycles of chemotherapy.

Concomitant use of chemotherapy and radiation takes advantage of the potential enhancing properties of the chemotherapeutic agents to radiation (Table 3) [5,11,12]. The Radiation Therapy Oncology Group (RTOG) conducted a trial of concomitant cisplatin (100 mg/m$^2$ i.v. bolus) administered every 3 weeks for three courses and radiation (70 Gy delivered with standard fractionation) in patients with locally advanced head and neck cancers [11]. Twenty-seven patients with Stages III or IV (26 Stage IV) nasopharyngeal cancers were included in this study and the treatment results were compared to the 78 patients treated with radiation alone from the RTOG database. The disease-free survival (47 versus 32% at 3 years), overall survival, locoregional failure (30 versus 35%) and the incidence of distant metastases (27 versus 56%) appear to be better in the concomitant chemoradiation group. All patients finished the radiation, but 8 patients (30%) could not complete the entire plan of three courses of cisplatin due to acute toxicities. Four patients (15%) developed major (grade $\geq$ 3) late toxicities.

RTOG, ECOG and SWOG conducted an intergroup phase III study of radiotherapy with or without concomitant cisplatin followed by three courses of 5-FU and cisplatin in patients with Stages III and IV nasopharyngeal cancers [12]. The study was initiated in June 1989

Table 3

Concomitant chemoradiation for advanced nasopharyngeal carcinoma

| Authors | No. of patients | Chemo Tx (C, cycle) | Rad Tx (Gy) | CR (%) | L-R failure (%) | DM (%) | DFS (%) | F/U (months) |
|---|---|---|---|---|---|---|---|---|
| Al-Kourainy [5] | 4 | CDDP + 5FU (3C) | 70 | 100 | | | 75 | 33–57 |
| Al-Sarraf[a] [11]: comparison with radiation data base | | | | | | | | |
| RTOG 81–17 | | | | | | | | 4–63 |
| RT | 78 | CDDP (3C) | 70 | 89 | 35 | 56 | 32 | (34) |
| CT + RT | 27 | 0 | 70 | 81 | 30 | 27 | 47 | |
| Al-Sarraf [12]: prospective randomized study | | | | | | | 2 years | 48 |
| RTOG 88–17, SWOG 88–92, ECOG 2388 | | | | | | | survival | |
| RT | 67 | | 70 | | | | 55* | |
| CT + RT – CT | 71 | CDDP × 3 + RT CDDP + 5FU × 3 | 70 | | | | 80 | |

[a]Acute life threatening hematological complication (7%), late complication >G3 (15%).
*$P > 0.007$.

and closed early in December 1995 because there was a sufficiently great statistically significant advantage observed for patients treated with combined chemoradiotherapy in terms of progression-free and overall survival to meet the criteria for early closure of the study. Although final treatment results are pending in terms of survival, it appears that concomitant chemoradiation regimens do have a major impact on survival. However, longer followup is needed to ascertain the therapeutic benefit gaged on late complications.

Concomitant chemoradiation aims to accomplish synergistic actions between these two modalities. Therefore, more complications are to be expected in the concomitant regimen rather than a sequential regimen.

In an attempt to improve the therapeutic ratio, a strategy using split courses of hyperfractionated radiation and concomitant infusion of cisplatin was initiated in 1983 at the State University of New York Health Science Center at Brooklyn. Twenty-one patients with locally advanced or recurrent cancer of the nasopharynx and paranasal sinus were treated with this regimen. This report includes 10 patients with locally advanced nasopharyngeal cancers with followup of 3–10 years. The characteristics of the 10 patients are listed in Table 4. Nine patients had poorly differentiated squamous cell carcinoma, one had lymphoepithelioma (WHO type 3). One patient had a Stage 3 primary and 9 patients had Stage 4 primary lesions using The American Joint Committee Staging System.

The treatment regimen consisted of three courses of 2 weeks of concomitant continuous infusion cisplatin and twice-a-day irradiation with 1–2 weeks rest between courses (Table 5). The daily irradiation dose was 2.40–2.50 Gy given in two daily 1.2–1.25 Gy fractions using 4–6 h time intervals. The total irradiation dose ranged from 64.8 to 69.4 Gy. Cisplatin was given, via continuous infusion using Hickman catheters or infusa-port with pump on an out-patient basis at doses ranging from 5 to 10 mg/m$^2$ per day. The irradiation treatment was given using parallel opposed portals including the nasopharynx, base of skull, cranial exten-

Table 4

Patient characteristics

| | |
|---|---|
| Total patients | 10 |
| Pathology | |
|    Squamous cell CA | 9 |
|    Lymphoepithelioma (WHO 3) | 1 |
| Stage (AJC) | |
|    III | 1 |
|    IV | 9 |
|       $T_{2,3} N_2$ | 2 |
|       $T_4 N_{1,2,3}$ | 6 |
|       $T_x N_{3B}$ | 1 |

AJC, American Joint Committee.

sion of disease and the upper neck. This was followed by a tumor volume boost treatment using lateral opposed shrinking fields or a three field technique (one anterior and two wedged bilateral ports). The lower neck was treated using a single anterior portal to 5040 cGy with a given dose of a single 180 cGy/fraction when there were no enlarged nodes. The patients were treated on either 4 or 6 MV linear accelerator or a cobalt-60 teletherapy unit. The initial tumor response was complete in 9 patients and partial in 1 patient. The tumor response was evaluated by direct nasopharyngoscopy and complimented by CT and MRI scans. Of the 9 patients who achieved complete response, 7 patients were alive at the time of analysis (36–126 months with a median survival time of 110 months). One patient died at 21 months with marginal recurrence arising in the temporal area. One patient died of lung metastases in 7 months with the primary tumor locally controlled. One patient who had partial response died in 25 months with local disease and metastases to the bones and lung.

The response to treatment was analyzed based on the initial tumor volume and the total dose of irradiation delivered. The tumor size ranged from 3 to 10 cm in average diameter. Two patients failed locally with irradiation doses of 64.8–70.8 Gy.

The acute mucosal and skin reactions were within acceptable limits. The acute skin reactions consisted of mild erythema which became dry hyperpigmented intact skin. The intense erythematous mucosal reaction developed periodically, subsiding during the rest period. Four patients developed petechial mucositis and only 2 patients developed confluent mucositis. Table 6 shows the acute mucosal and hematological reaction. Hematological toxicities were within acceptable ranges. None of the patients developed WBC count less than 2000 or platelet count less than 100 000. In two patients who received cisplatin 10 mg/m$^2$

Table 5

Treatment regimen

| Weeks | 1 | 2 | 3 | 4 | 5 | 6 | 7 | 8 |
|---|---|---|---|---|---|---|---|---|
| Cisplatinum | ___ | ___ | | ___ | ___ | | ___ | ___ |
|   continuous infusion: 5–10 mg/m$^2$/24 h | | | | | | | | |
| Radiation | | | | | | | | |
|   a.m. | ||||| ||||| | | | ||||| ||||| | | | ||||| ||||| | |
|   p.m. | ||||| ||||| | | | ||||| ||||| | | | ||||| ||||| | |
|   120–125 cGy/fraction: 4–6 h between fractions | | | | | | | | |

Table 6

Acute hematological toxicities and mucosal reactions

|                        | Patients      |
| ---------------------- | ------------- |
| Platelet count         |               |
| <100000                | 0             |
| 100000–120000          | 1             |
| >120000                | 9             |
| Leukocyte count        |               |
| <2000                  | 0             |
| 2000                   | 5             |
| >3000                  | 5             |
| Creatinine             |               |
| >1.4                   | 2 (2.0, 1.7)  |
| Mucosal reactions      |               |
| Intense erythema       | 4             |
| Petechial mucositis    | 4             |
| Confluent mucositis    | 2             |

per day, the creatinine level became abnormal (2.0, 1.7). In these two patients, the creatinine slowly returned to normal over a 6-month period.

Late effects on soft tissues were minimal and included mild atrophy or thickening of in-field tissues (RTOG Grade 1 and 2). Severe fibrosis (Grade 3) was not found in any patient. Mild or moderate (Grade 1 or 2) xerostomia developed and lasted for 1 year and then resolved. One patient developed diffuse dental caries requiring multiple tooth extractions without complications. One patient developed otitis media and recovered with antibiotics. Three patients had routine followup hormonal evaluations, including TSH, T3, T4, FSH, LH cortisol level 2–3 years post treatment. All hormonal levels were within normal limits. The eye or optic nerve was included in the treatment ports in all 10 patients. The radiation dose to the eye or optic nerve was calculated using an isodose plan. The optic nerve received 50–69.4 Gy. It is difficult to evaluate these treatments for a long term effect on the optic nerve. However, 4 patients treated with 60–65 Gy to the optic nerve survived 21–110 months without optic nerve damage.

Our treatment scheme exploits the radiopotentiation of cisplatin and the advantages afforded by hyperfractionated irradiation on late responding normal tissues. Instead of increasing the total irradiation dose, as in most hyperfractionated regimens, conventional total doses of 65.0–70.8 Gy were employed with twice-a-day irradiation therapy and concomitant cisplatin infusion. An initial complete response was achieved in 90% of patients despite the advanced and invasive nature of these cases. In followups which ranged from 36 to 126 months, 3 patients failed; 1 patient failed locally, 1 patient failed in the lung with local tumor control and 1 patient failed both locally and in bone. The split courses allowed acceptable acute reactions in spite of concomitant cisplatin infusion. Late complications were minimal probably due to hyperfractionations. The net effect, therefore, of concomitant continuous infusion cisplatin and split-course hyperfractionated irradiation is to increase the therapeutic ratio by improving the response rate without increasing the toxicity. Late complications were so minimal and few as to make it possible to improve the tumor control further by increasing the total irradiation dose. However, an increased survival may not be possible given the propensity for these advanced stage patients to develop distant metastases.

Based on this consideration, further study exploring the potential benefits of post radiation adjuvant chemotherapy is warranted in this high risk group of patients and is being looked at in an RTOG, ECOG, SWOG intergroup study.

## References

1.  Lederman M. Tumors of the upper jaw. J Laryngol 84: 369–401, 1970.
2.  Wang CC. Accelerated hyperfractionation radiation therapy for carcinoma of the nasopharynx. Techniques and results. Cancer 63: 2461–2467, 1989.
3.  Thames HD, Withers RH, Peters LJ, Fletcher GH. Changes in early and late radiation responses with altered dose fractionation: implications for dose-survival relationships. Int J Radiat Oncol Biol Phys 8: 219–226, 1982.
4.  Horiot JC, LeFur R, N'Guyen T, et al. Hyperfractionation versus conventional fractionation in oropharyngeal carcinoma: final analysis of a randomized trial of the EORTC cooperation group of radiotherapy. Radiother Oncol 25: 231–241, 1992.
5.  Al-Kourainy K, Crissman J, Ensley J, et al. Excellent response to cisplatinum-based chemotherapy in patients with recurrent or previously untreated advanced nasopharyngeal carcinoma. Am J Clin Oncol 11: 427–430, 1988.
6.  Dimery IW, Peters LJ, Goepfert H, et al. Effectiveness of combined induction chemotherapy and radiotherapy in advanced nasopharyngeal carcinoma. J Clin Oncol 11: 1919–1928, 1993.
7.  Tannock I, Payne D, Cummings B, et al. Sequential chemotherapy and radiation for nasopharyngeal cancer: absence of long-term benefit despite a high rate of tumor response to chemotherapy. J Clin Oncol 5: 629–634, 1987.
8.  Teo P, Ho JHC, Choy D, et al. Adjuvant chemotherapy to radical radiation therapy in the treatment of advanced nasopharyngeal carcinoma. Int J Radiat Oncol Biol Phys 14: 679–685, 1987.
9.  Chan AT, Teo PML, Leung TWT, et al. A prospective randomized study of chemotherapy adjunctive to definitive radiotherapy in advanced nasopharyngeal carcinoma. Int J Radiat Oncol Biol Phys 33: 569–577, 1995.
10. Cvitkovic E. Preliminary results of a randomized trial comparing neoadjuvant chemotherapy (cisplatin, epirubicin, bleomycin) plus radiotherapy vs radiotherapy alone in Stage IV (>N2M0) undifferentiated nasopharyngeal carcinoma. A positive effect on progression-free survival: International Nasopharynx Cancer Study Group: VUMCA Trial. Int J Radiat Oncol Biol Phys 35: 463–469, 1996.
11. Al-Sarraf M, Pajak TF, Cooper JS, et al. Chemo-radiotherapy in patients with locally advanced nasopharyngeal carcinoma: a Radiation Therapy Oncology Group study. J Clin Oncol 8: 1342–1351, 1990.
12. Al-Sarraf M, LeBlanc M, Gari PGS, et al. Superiority of chemo-radiotherapy (CT-RT) vs radiotherapy (RT) in patients with locally advanced nasopharyngeal cancer. Preliminary results of Intergroup (0099) (SWOG 8892, RTOG 8817, ECOG 2388) Randomized Study. Proc Am Soc Clin Oncol 15: 313, 1996.

C.J. Rosenthal and M. Rotman (Eds.), *Infusion Chemotherapy–Irradiation Interactions*

# CHAPTER 22

# Neo-adjuvant organ-preserving chemotherapy in the management of locally advanced oral cavity and oropharynx cancer: a quantitative evaluation of organ preservation and clinical response

GIOVANNI MANTOVANI[1], VITTORIO GEBBIA[4], ERNESTO PROTO[2], FRANCESCO COSSU[3], ALESSANDRO BIANCHI[2], LUIGI CURRELI[1], MASSIMO GHIANI[1], GIORGIO ASTARA[1], BIANCAROSA LAMPIS[1], DANIELA DESSÌ[1], MARIA CRISTINA SANTONA[1] and ELENA MASSA[1]

[1]*Department of Medical Oncology, Institute of Internal Medicine,* [2]*Department of Surgery, Otolaryngology Branch,* [3]*Department of Radiation Therapy, University of Cagliari, 09124 Cagliari, Italy and* [4]*Chair and Service of Chemotherapy, University of Palermo, 90127 Palermo, Italy*

## 1. Introduction

With the aim of further investigating the effect of neo-adjuvant chemotherapy (NAC) combined with radiation therapy (RT) on organ preservation at head and neck sites different from the larynx, we designed an open, non-randomized, phase II clinical study to assess, as the first endpoint, the feasibility of sparing surgery and of preserving organ/function by using NAC in oral cavity and oropharynx cancer patients, and, as the second endpoint, the clinical response to this treatment approach and its duration. Moreover, an attempt was made to scale the extent of surgery by means of an arbitrary scale assigning different percentages to the different extents of surgical resection. Briefly, the main aim of our study was to avoid or at least substantially reduce the amount of surgery in patients responding to chemotherapy, leaving major surgery as a salvage treatment.

## 2. Patients and methods

### 2.1. Patients

Patients with histologically confirmed, operable, squamous cell carcinoma of the oral cavity and oropharynx were considered eligible for this study. They were also required to have stage III or IV disease without distant metastases according to the staging system of the International Union Against Cancer [1], to have had no previous treatment, to be less than 70 years old, to have a performance status (PS) of 1 or less of the ECOG scale, and to have normal cardiac, hepatic, and renal functions as well as leukocyte counts of >4000/$\mu$l and platelet counts of >100 000/$\mu$l. Patients with both previous or concurrent malignancy were excluded.

Table 1

Organ/function preservation according to the different surgical procedures performed for oral cavity and oropharynx cancer

| Extent of planned surgery before NAC | % Extent of performed surgery after NAC compared to extent of planned surgery before NAC | | | | | |
|---|---|---|---|---|---|---|
| | CRTG | CO | PT | ET | PG | ND/AS |
| CRTG | 0 | 30 | 50 | 80 | 80 | 100 |
| CO | | 0 | 20 | 50 | 50 | 70 |
| PT | | | 0 | 30 | 30 | 50 |
| ET | | | | 0 | 0 | 20 |
| PG | | | | | 0 | 20 |

Arbitrary scale: 100%, organ/function completely preserved; 0%, organ/function completely lost. Abbreviations: NAC, neo-adjuvant chemotherapy; CRTG, composite resection for total glossectomy; CO, commando operation; PT, pull-through; ET, enlarged tonsillectomy; PG, partial glossectomy; ND, neck dissection; AS, avoided surgery.

All patients were initially evaluated by an otolaryngologist and a medical oncologist. Evaluation for resectability was performed at the first visit and only resectable patients were included. A tumor was defined as unresectable if it was fixed to either a bone structure or lymph nodes or if it was too invasive to allow for radical surgical removal. At the same time, the extent of surgery was planned for each patient according to the extent of disease and widespread criteria of well-conducted surgical oncology, assuming that each patient should be submitted to surgical removal of the tumor as first treatment. Moreover, an attempt was made to score the decreasing extent of surgery following NAC by means of an arbitrary scale which is shown in Table 1. A maximum score (100%) was attributed to the patients who completely avoided surgery and a minimum score (0%) was assigned in the case of either no organ preservation or no reduction in the extent of surgical resection performed after NAC compared to that planned before NAC. Initial evaluation included a medical history, clinical examination, upper aerodigestive tract endoscopy, complete blood cell count, complete blood chemistry, urinanalysis, electrocardiogram and chest X-ray. When indicated, computed tomographic (CT) scans of the chest, abdomen, and head and neck regions were obtained. Written informed consent was obtained from each patient prior to treatment, according to the guidelines of the Ethics Committee of the Department of Internal Medicine, University of Cagliari.

## 2.2. Treatment plan

NAC eligible patients were assigned to one of the two different induction chemotherapy regimens according to the time of their accrual. Regimen 1 was the classical Al-Sarraf's: cisplatin (100 mg/m$^2$ i.v. as a 60 min infusion on day 1) with a standard pre- and post-hydration protocol with forced diuresis by 250 cm$^3$ of 18% mannitol plus 5-fluorouracil (5-FU, 1000 mg/m$^2$ per day on days 1–5 as a continuous infusion by peripheral vein), to be repeated every 3 weeks for three cycles. This protocol was effective from February 1991 to February 1993 and was applied to 15 patients (all evaluable).

Regimen 2 was set up by our Institute [2] with the aim of improving the clinical results obtained with Al-Sarraf's regimen by adding vinorelbine, a new semisynthetic *Vinca* alkaloid, which was able to induce a 22% partial response rate in a group of 23 heavily pre-treated patients with recurrent and/or metastatic head and neck squamous cell carcinoma (HNSCC) [3]. It consisted of cisplatin (80 mg/m$^2$ i.v. 60 min infusion on day 1), 5-FU (600 mg/m$^2$ diluted in 500 cm$^3$ of normal saline over 4 h infusion on days 2–5) and vinorel-bine (20 mg/m$^2$ diluted in 250 cm$^3$ of normal saline over 20 min on days 2 and 8). It was effective from March 1993 to April 1995 and was applied to 10 patients (all evaluable).

Three treatment cycles were planned for Regimen 1. Regimen 2 response was first evalu-ated after two cycles of therapy. Treatment duration (number of cycles administered) de-pended on the clinical response obtained. If complete response (CR) was observed after the first two treatment cycles (1st and 2nd cycles), patients were offered radiation therapy as definitive locoregional treatment; if only partial response (PR) was seen, two more cycles (3rd and 4th cycles) were administered. Then, if the tumor continued to shrink, two more cycles (5th and 6th cycles) were employed before definitive locoregional therapy was given. On the other hand, if no further decrease in tumor size was seen after the 4th cycle, patients were submitted to definitive locoregional therapy without any further cycle of chemother-apy. If after the first two cycles (1st and 2nd cycles) "no change" was recorded, two more cycles (3rd and 4th cycles) were administered. In the case of stabilization or progression after the 4th cycle, patients were assigned to locoregional therapy but where only PR was recorded, two more cycles (5th and 6th cycles) were administered. If after the first two cy-cles (1st and 2nd cycles) progression was recorded, where possible, surgery as locoregional therapy or non-cross–resistant chemotherapy were offered.

All patients were again evaluated 3 weeks after the end of the planned chemotherapy by a clinical examination, endoscopy, CT scan and confirmatory biopsy where indicated.

### 2.2.1.  Loco--regional treatment

Patients who achieved a CR were submitted to RT using $^{60}$Co equipment with a planned dose of 65–70 Gy to the involved areas at a 2 Gy fraction per day, 5 fractions per week. Treatment interruptions were allowed for 2 weeks after a dose of 30 Gy when grade III/IV mucositis occurred. Patients achieving a PR $\geq 70\%$ were either not submitted to surgery or submitted to surgery according to the criterion that the extent of organ preservation by sur-gical resection was directly dependent on the clinical response obtained after NAC. Patients achieving a PR $< 70\%$ or a MR were submitted to the surgical resection planned before NAC. Patients in PD underwent surgical resection according to the anatomical tumor exten-sion.

### 2.3.  Toxicity

Toxicity was assessed according to WHO criteria [4].

## 3.  Results

Twenty-five patients with oral cavity and oropharynx cancer (24 males and 1 female, 7 with stage III disease and 18 with stage IV disease) were enrolled from February 1991 to April 1995. All patients were hospitalized in the Department of Medical Oncology, Institute of Internal Medicine, University of Cagliari. The consultant otolaryngologist was always the Vice-Head of the Otolaryngology Branch, Department of Surgery, University of Cagliari.

The consultant Radiation Therapist was the Head, Department of Radiation Therapy, University of Cagliari. The results are updated to February 1996. The 25 patients were all evaluable for response to NAC and 20 of them were evaluable for organ preservation.

### 3.1.  Response to NAC

Patients were evaluable for response if at least two chemotherapy cycles were administered.

All patients were evaluable for response to NAC. A mean of 3.5 cycles per patient (range 2–6) was administered. One patient received only two chemotherapy cycles, 13 patients received three cycles and 5 patients received six cycles. The average dose intensity actually received for each of the drugs included in the two regimens was superior to 75% of the programmed dose intensity.

The CR rate was 26.6% (4/15 patients) and the PR rate was 60% (9/15 patients) with an overall response (OR) rate of 86.6% (13/15 patients) for Regimen 1 (cisplatin + 5-FU); the CR rate was 0% and the PR rate was 80% (8/10 patients) with an OR rate of 80% (8/10 patients) for Regimen 2 (cisplatin + 5-FU + vinorelbine). The mean time to response was 3 months (range 1–8.2).

### 3.2.  Organ/function preservation

The patients evaluable for organ preservation were 20/25. Five patients were not evaluable for the following reasons: 2 refused surgery (1 in PR and 1 in PD), 1 patient in CR decided to undergo the previously planned surgical resection, 1 was unresectable when he required surgery for rapidly progressive disease and 1 patient in PR died after 5 cycles of chemotherapy due to hematologic toxicity.

The patient distribution according to the extent of planned surgery before NAC compared to the surgery performed after NAC is shown in Table 2: it summarizes the extent of organ preservation in 20 evaluable patients.

Five of twenty five (25%) patients completely avoided surgery, 5/20 (25%) patients had a reduced extent of surgical resection, while 10/20 (50%) patients received the previously planned surgical resection. Overall, 10/20 (50%) patients either avoided or achieved a reduction in the previously planned surgical resection attributable to NAC.

Currently (February 1996), 3/5 (60%) patients who did not undergo surgery are alive and have remained continuously disease-free, 1/5 (20%) locally relapsed (time to progression 22.8 months) but could undergo salvage surgery and is currently NED, while 1/5 (20%) died of hematologic toxicity but was relapse-free; 4/5 (80%) patients who achieved partial organ preservation are alive and have remained continuously disease-free, while 1/5 (20%) died of second primary tumor (lung carcinoma) while being NED; 3/10 (30%) patients who received the previously planned surgical resection are alive and disease-free, 1/10 (10%) relapsed but was unresectable and is actually alive with PD, while 5/10 (50%) died of PD (time to progression 16.4, 4.7, 1.9, 5.7, 6.7 months, respectively) and 1/10 (10%) died of another cause (gastrointestinal hemorrhage) but was relapse-free (Table 3).

### 3.3.  Response after all treatment

Twenty-four of twenty-five patients completed all treatment, including loco-regional therapy (1 patient died after the 5th chemotherapy cycle before locoregional treatment): 20/24

Table 2

Patient distribution according to the extent of planned surgery before NAC compared to that performed after NAC

| Extent of planned surgery before NAC | Extent of performed surgery after NAC | No. of patients | Clinical response after NAC | % Organ preservation after surgery (mean) | Time (months) to progression (mean) |
|---|---|---|---|---|---|
| CRTG (4 pts) | CRTG | 3/4 | 2 PR < 70% | 0 | 3.0[a] |
| | | | 1 PD | | 6.7 |
| | | | | | 20.5+ |
| | CO | 1/4 | 1 PR ≥ 70% | 30 | 17.0+ |
| | | | | (7.5) | (13.5+) |
| CO (9 pts) | CO | 3/9 | 2 PR < 70% | 0 | 13.2 |
| | | | | | 16.0+ |
| | | | 1 MR (NC) | | 1.9 |
| | PT | 1/9 | 1 PR ≥ 70% | 20 | 40.5+ |
| | ND | 1/9 | 1 PR ≥ 70% | 70 | 22.5+ |
| | AS | 4/9 | 2 CR | 70 | 12.6[b] |
| | | | | | 8.9+ |
| | | | 2 PR ≥ 70% | | 7.8[c] |
| | | | | | 34.5+ |
| | | | | (41) | (17.5+) |
| PT (4 pts) | PT | 2/4 | 2 PR < 70% | 0 | 4.7 |
| | | | | | 5.7 |
| | PG | 1/4 | 1 PR ≥ 70% | 30 | 22.1+ |
| | AS | 1/4 | 1 CR | 50 | 22.8+ |
| | | | | (20) | (13.8+) |
| ET (3 pts) | ET | 2/3 | 2 PR < 70% | 0 | 16.4 |
| | | | | | 25.1+ |
| | AS | 1/3 | 1 PR ≥ 70% | 20 | 36.5+ |
| | | | | (6.7) | (26.0+) |

NAC, neo-adjuvant chemotherapy; CRTG, composite resection for total glossectomy; CO, commando operation; PT, pull-through; ET, enlarged tonsillectomy; PG, partial glossectomy; ND, neck dissection; AS, avoided surgery
[a]Other cause.
[b]Second primary tumor.
[c]Toxic death (hematologic toxicity).

(83.3%) patients were rendered NED and 1/24 (4.2%) were in objective response (PR), while 3/24 were in PD. The following local modalities were used in the patients rendered NED, after completion of NAC: RT alone in 6/20 (30%) patients, RT plus surgery to the

Table 3

Current status (February 1996) of 20 patients evaluable for organ preservation

| | No. of patients | | |
|---|---|---|---|
| | Alive | Dead | Total |
| Avoided surgery | 4 NED | 1 hematologic toxicity (CR) | 5 |
| Reduced extent of surgical resection | 4 NED | 1 2nd primary tumor (CR) | 5 |
| Underwent previously planned surgery | 3 NED | 5 PD | 10 |
| | 1 PD | 1 another cause (CR) | |

primary tumor site and/or neck dissection in 12/20 (60%) patients, surgery and/or neck dissection alone in 2/20 (10%) patients. The patient in PR underwent RT alone.

## 3.4. Toxicity

Approximately, 20% of patients had grade 3–4 leukopenia and 1 patient died of hematologic toxicity, while anemia was only grade 1–2. Toxicity due to RT was similar to previous experiences in which RT was administered at similar doses without previous chemotherapy: the great majority of patients developed mild to moderate mucositis. Grade 1–2 phlebitis was observed in approximately 50% of patients in both groups and grade 1–2 pain at the tumor site in 30% of patients in the vinorelbine treatment group.

## 4. Conclusions

In the absence of data from randomized controlled trials, our study must be considered as investigational. The ORR of our patients was more than 80% with a CR rate in one chemotherapy group of 26.6%. The OR rates in the literature for primary tumors at all sites of the head and neck have been consistently greater than 80% since the first report on the efficacy of cisplatin and 5-FU by investigators at the Wayne State University [5]. Therefore, the clinical response rate of our series, which included only patients with advanced HNSCC cancer, is consistent with that previously reported in other studies [6–9].

Overall, 10/20 (50%) patients either avoided or achieved a reduction in the previously planned surgical resection attributable to NAC. Moreover, 8/10 (80%) patients who avoided or achieved a reduction in the previously planned surgery are currently alive and NED versus only 3/10 (30%) patients who underwent the previously planned surgery.

As regards the extent of reduced surgery made possible by NAC, the best results were obtained by a group of 9 patients who were planned for commando operation and who had a mean of 41% organ preservation compared to the other three groups (mean 20%, 7.5%, 6.7%) (see Table 2). Our results are quite consistent with those of Pfister et al. [10]. However, it is not the case to stress the better outcome of patients who underwent less surgery (80% actually alive) compared to those who were subjected to the previously planned surgery (30% presently alive) because these differences may be biased due to a positive selection made by NAC, i.e. the patient responders to NAC were those with a better prognosis, irrespective of the subsequent locoregional treatment. In fact, previous studies reported that non-responders to NAC have dismal survival rates [11,12].

In our opinion the two most relevant contributions offered by our study are: (1) to have addressed the question of measuring as precisely as possible the reduction of surgical resection made possible by NAC compared to surgery planned before NAC and (2) to have attempted to avoid or at least substantially reduce the amount of surgery in patients responding to chemotherapy, leaving major surgery as a salvage treatment.

Although the scale provided by us is an arbitrary one, it must be emphasized that it attempts to address the issue of quality of life in cancer patients by a more precise quantification of organ/function sparing surgery, taking into consideration that many patients with oropharynx cancer, if managed surgically, would require total laryngectomy and that the loss of voice has always been considered to have a major impact on the quality of life [13].

*Acknowledgements*

This work was supported by C.N.R., Rome, A.P. "Clinical Applications of Oncological Research", Contract No. 95.00389.PF39. We thank Dr. Roberta Tocco for the preparation of the manuscript.

*References*

1.  International Union Against Cancer. TNM-Classification of Malignant Tumors, 3rd edn. Geneva: UICC, 1978.
2.  Gebbia V, Mantovani G, Agostara B, et al. Treatment of recurrent metastatic squamous cell head and neck carcinoma with a combination of vinorelbine, cisplatin, and 5-fluoruracil: a multicenter phase II trial. Ann Oncol 6: 987–991, 1995.
3.  Gebbia V, Testa A, Valenza R, et al. A pilot study of vinorelbine on a weekly schedule in recurrent and or metastatic squamous cell carcinoma of the head and neck. Eur J Cancer 29A: 1358–1359, 1994.
4.  Miller AB, Hodgstraten B, Staquet M, Winkler A. Reporting results of cancer treatment. Cancer 47: 207–214, 1981.
5.  Al-Kourainy K, Kish J, Ensley J, et al. Achievement of superior survival for histologically negative versus histologically positive clinically complete responders to cisplatin combination in patients with locally advanced head and neck cancer. Cancer 59: 233–238, 1987.
6.  Head and Neck Contracts Program. Adjuvant chemotherapy for advanced head and neck squamous carcinoma: final report. Cancer 60: 301–311, 1987.
7.  Schuller DE, Metch B, Stein DW, et al. Preoperative chemotherapy in advanced resectable head and neck cancer: final report of the Southwest Oncology Group. Laryngoscope 98: 1205–1211, 1988.
8.  The Department of Veterans Affairs Laryngeal Cancer Study Group. Induction chemotherapy plus radiation compared with surgery plus radiation in patients with advanced laryngeal cancer. N Engl J Med 324: 1685–1690, 1991.
9.  Laramore GE, Scott C, Al-Sarraf M, et al. Adjuvant chemotherapy for resectable squamous cell carcinomas of the head and neck: report of Intergroup Study 0034. Int J Radiat Oncol Biol Phys 23: 705–713, 1992.
10. Pfister DG, Harrison LB, Elliot W, et al. Organ-function preservation in advanced oropharynx cancer: results with induction chemotherapy and radiation. J Clin Oncol 13: 671–680, 1995.
11. Ervin TJ, Clark JR, Weichselbaum RR, et al. An analysis of induction and adjuvant chemotherapy in the multidisciplinary management of squamous cell carcinoma of the head and neck. J Clin Oncol 5: 10–20, 1987.
12. Bosl GJ, Strong E, Harrison L, Pfister DG. Chemotherapy and the management of locally advanced squamous cell carcinoma of the head and neck: role in larynx preservation. In: DeVita VT Jr, Hellman S, Rosenberg SA (Eds), Important Advances in Oncology. Philadelphia, PA: Lippincott, pp. 191–203, 1991.
13. Clayman GL, Weber RS, Guillamondegui O, et al. Laryngeal preservation for advanced laryngeal and hypopharyngeal cancers. Arch Otolaryngol Head Neck Surg 121: 219–223, 1995.

C.J. Rosenthal and M. Rotman (Eds.), *Infusion Chemotherapy–Irradiation Interactions*
© 1998 Elsevier Science B.V. All rights reserved

# Combined radiotherapy and intra-arterial chemotherapy for advanced cancer of the oropharynx

LUBOŠ PETRUŽELKA, JAN BETKA, PETR KASÍK, JAN KLOZAR,
HANA HONOVÁ, OLGA PŘIBYLOVÁ, PETR ZATLOUKAL,
LIBOR JUDAS and PETR CECH

*Department of Oncology, Charles University, U nemocnice 2, 128 08 Prague 2, Czech Republic*

## 1. Introduction

The prognosis of patients with advanced cancer of the head and neck is poor with the majority of patients dying from uncontrolled local disease [1]. Because of its propensity to spread locoregionally, the standard treatment of head and neck cancer has historically relied on the locoregional treatment modalities of surgery and radiotherapy. Their success depends upon their ability to excise or sterilize the tumor. The standard treatment with conventional radiotherapy for inoperable patients and those with far advanced unresectable disease has had poor results [2,3]. Primary control and survival might be improved if an appropriate cytotoxic drug could be given concurrently with irradiation to enhance the global effect [4–8]. Concomitant systemic chemotherapy and radiotherapy has resulted in increased disease-free survival and/or survival in several randomized studies [9–13].

The use of intra-arterial therapy as an alternative route to delivery chemotherapy for head and neck cancer is technically more difficult than using systemic intravenous therapy [14]. Intra-arterial chemotherapy would seem to be ideal for the treatment of patients with head and neck cancers because of the accessibility of arterial blood vessels and the frequently localized nature of the malignant disease [15] and was used for more than 30 years for head and neck cancer [16,17]. However, because of catheter-related complications occurring quite frequently, this method was abandoned in many institutions. However, the improvement of intra-arterial infusion technique has renewed interest in regional drug delivery [14]. Complications can be minimized by selecting the right drug delivery system and by judicious use of appropriate chemotherapeutic agents.

This study was designed to evaluate results of intra-arterial chemotherapy and the feasibility of combination with radiotherapy in patients with advanced oropharyngeal carcinoma. We analyzed the following endpoints: survival, freedom from progression time, local control, local and systemic toxicity.

Survival time and time to progression were determined using the Kaplan–Meier method. The log-rank test was used to test for differences between actuarial rates. The Cox proportional hazards model was used to analyze the influence of multiple variables on survival and local control [18]. Variables tested were: age, stage, nodes involvement, radiation dose, duration of chemotherapy, salvage surgery, response and mucosal toxicity. Complications were analyzed using the World Health Organization (WHO) toxicity scoring system [19].

Table 1

| Treatment administration | |
|---|---|
|    Catheterization not achieved | 6 |
|    For technical difficulties | 5 |
|    For blocking the catheter | 1 |
| | |
| Evaluable patients for response | 38 |
|    Intra-arterial chemotherapy only | 1 |
|    Combined chemoradiotherapy | |
|       Sequential | 8 |
|       Concurrent | 29 |

## 2. Patients and methods

Between May 1986 and May 1992, 44 patients were treated with the intention of using in-tra-arterial chemotherapy combined with concurrent radiotherapy. In 6 patients catheteriza-tion was not performed, because of technical difficulties in 5 patients, and for blocking of the catheter in 1 patient. All 38 patients treated with intra-arterial chemotherapy were evalu-able for response and toxicity and were analyzed on "the intention to treat basis". Overall, 29 patients (76%) received the intended chemotherapy and radiation therapy concurrently. Eight patients were treated sequentially. One patient did not receive the planned radiother-apy because of patients non-compliance (Table 1). Patients with previously untreated inop-erable advanced non-metastatic squamous cell carcinoma of the oropharynx were included in the analysis. There were 36 males and 2 females whose ages ranged from 29 to 75 years with a median of 54, 5 with stage III disease and 33 with stage IV (M0). Performance status was from 0 to 2. Patient characteristics and stage distributions are reported in Table 2. The UICC 1979 staging system was used [18]. All patients had normal renal and hepatic func-tions. Eight patients underwent salvage surgery for persistent or recurrent disease.

Standard criteria were used to assess response [19]. Complete response (CR) implies total regression of all evaluable tumor. Response was assessed by at least two observers and in-cluded a repeat clinical and endoscopic examination when applicable. CR was defined as the complete disappearance of clinically detectable disease. Partial response (PR) implied an average reduction of all measurable disease by at least 50% and no appearance of new le-sions. Survival time was assessed from the first day of treatment until death due to any

Table 2

Patient characteristics ($N = 38$)

| | |
|---|---|
| Median age ( range) | 54 (29–75) |
| Sex (m/f) | 36/2 |
| Median PS ( range) | 1 (0–2) |
| Site | Oropharynx |
| Histology | Squamous cell ca |
| Stage III | 5 |
| Stage IV | 33 |
| Period of treatment | 1986–1992 |

cause. Time to disease progression was calculated from the first day of treatment until evidence of local or distant recurrence.

## 2.1. Treatment administration

### 2.1.1. Intra-arterial continuous infusion

Intra-arterial catheter placement was performed after local anesthesia and vertical pre-auricular skin incisions. The catheter was then advanced retrogradely into the external carotid artery until the catheter tip was positioned below the origin of the appropriate branch. The correct position of the catheter was confirmed by the injection of patent blue and radiographically. Re-evaluation of the correct positioning of the catheter was performed routinely every week. The canulation of the opposite external carotid was not used because of combination with radiotherapy.

Our chemotherapy (CT) treatment program consisted of continuous intra-arterial infusion of 10 mg bleomycin (BLM) per day alternating with 10 mg of methotrexate (MTX) per day. A slow continuous infusion (CI) was given by portable external infusion pumps (Pharmacia Deltec CADD-1). Citrovorum Factor (Leucovorinum calcium) was administered the following day after methotrexate. Citrovorum factor was delivered at a dose of 10 mg intramuscularly every 6 h for four doses starting 6 h after methotrexate (Table 3). During the whole period of catheterization, every patient was carefully evaluated daily with a personal interview and physical examination in order to asses general condition, local and drug related toxicities. The local and hematological toxicities were analyzed according to WHO criteria [19]. The intra-arterial chemotherapy was stopped and the catheter was removed in the presence of relevant toxicity associated with patient's noncompliance at any time of the study. The median duration of intra-arterial chemotherapy was 20 days (range 8–36).

### 2.1.2. Radiotherapy (RT)

Patients were treated with cobalt-60 gamma rays. Radiation fields initially encompassed the gross disease covering also the draining lymphatics in the neck. Field reduction occurred at 45 Gy to exclude the spinal cord and to treat only that volume that encompassed the primary tumor and the clinically involved nodes. Total dose (TD) ranged from 48 to 70 Gy (median 60 Gy). During the initial phase daily fraction of 1.5 Gy was given concomitantly with chemotherapy. Later, after chemotherapy was stopped, the daily fraction was increased to 1.8 Gy. The daily dose was 1.8–2.0 Gy/fraction if radiotherapy was given sequentially after chemotherapy (Table 3).

Table 3
Dose schedule

|  | Dose |
|---|---|
| CT | |
| MTX | 10 mg/day |
| BLM | 10 mg/day |
| RT (5 fractions/week) | 60 Gy (48–70) |
| RT + CT | 1.5 Gy/day |
| RT | 1.8 Gy/day |

Table 4

Technique related toxicity

|  | No. (%) |
|---|---|
| Minor local complication | 5 (13.1) |
|   Local extravasation | 2 |
|   Edema | 1 |
|   Fistula | 1 |
|   Bleeding | 1 |
| Neurological complication | 4 (10.5) |
|   Transient weakness | 3 |
|   Transient disorientation | 1 |

## 3.  Results

### 3.1.  Toxicity

#### 3.1.1.  Technique-related toxicity
The technique related toxicity is reported in Table 4. Local complications occurred in 5 patients (13.1%) and central nervous system complications developed in 4 patients (10.5%). These latter consisted of 3 patients with transient motor weakness and 1 with transient disorientation. The five technique-related local toxicities included two cases of local extravasations of the cytostatic agent along the catheter at the site of entry in the cannulated vessel, one case of local edema, one transient bleeding from the tumor and one case of orocutaneous fistula which was spontaneously closed.

#### 3.1.2.  Drug (radiation)-related toxicity
The drug (radiation)-related toxicity is also reported in Table 5. Combined radiotherapy with low dose continuous intra-arterial chemotherapy resulted in a non-significant systemic toxicity. The systemic hematological toxicity observed in 4 patients (10.5%) was moderate and was never greater than grade 2. As expected, the predominant toxicity was locoregional characterized by grade 3 mucositis in 18 (47.3%) patients. Mucositis within the treatment

Table 5

Drug (radiation) related toxicity

|  | No. (%) |
|---|---|
| Local |  |
|   Mucositis grade 3 | 18 (47.3) |
|   Dermatitis grade 2–3 | 3 (7.8) |
| Systemic |  |
|   Hematological grade 2 | 4 (10.5) |
|   Asthenia | 3 |
|   Infection | 1 |
|   Anorexia | 1 |
| Deaths within 2 months following treatment | 2 |

Table 6

Analysis of response to treatment

|  | No. (%) |
| --- | --- |
| Complete response | 6/38 (15.78) |
| Partial response | 21/38 (55.2) |
| Overall response | 27/38 (71) |

volume occurred in all patients, but was most severe in those receiving synchronous chemotherapy. Mucositis grade 3 was observed in 17 of 29 patients (58.6%) treated concurrently. Three patients treated concurrently developed cutaneous toxicities grade 2–3 in limited areas of radiation ports.

Two patients died in the 2 months after treatment due to CNS embolism, and malnutrition and infection, respectively.

## 3.2. Response and survival

At the end of the entire treatment, 6 complete responses (15.8%) and 21 partial responses (55.2%) were obtained. The total response rate was 71% (Table 6). The overall response rate in the subgroup treated concurrently was 72.4% with 5 complete responses and 16 partial responses. The 1-year, 2-year and 3-year survival rate was 60.5, 36.8%, 28.9%, respectively (Table 7) and 65.5, 44.8 and 31%, respectively in the concurrently treated group. Overall survival and freedom from progression time of all patients was calculated by the Kaplan–Meier method and is shown in Figs. 1 and 2. Median time to progression was 11 months and median survival was 17 months.

The impact of prognostic factors on survival and time free from progression was assessed by proportional hazards regression model. Two variables mucosal reaction grade 3 and TNM stage were found to be significant in the prediction of survival and progression free survival (Table 9). The occurrence of grade 3 mucositis during treatment had the lowest $P$ value ($P = 0.0001$, respectively $P = 0.0005$). Survival curves for patients treated with concurrent radiochemotherapy according to the grade of mucosal reactions are shown in Fig. 3 (log-rank test $P = 0.2$). Overall survival for groups treated with concurrent radiochemotherapy according to the response are shown in Fig. 4 ( log-rank test $P = 0.16$).

Thirty-one deaths have occurred. Two patients died in the 2 months after treatment. The first was due to CNS embolism and the second to malnutrition and infection. Twenty-seven (71%) patients died due to local progression, 4 patients died of distant disease progression (10.5%), 2 died of second malignancy and 3 of other medical reasons. Seven patients (18.4%) are alive. Duration of follow-up of surviving patients ranged from 37 to

Table 7

Analysis of survival

|  | No. (%) |
| --- | --- |
| 1 year | 23/38 (60.5) |
| 2 years | 14/38 (36.8) |
| 3 years | 11/38 (28.9) |

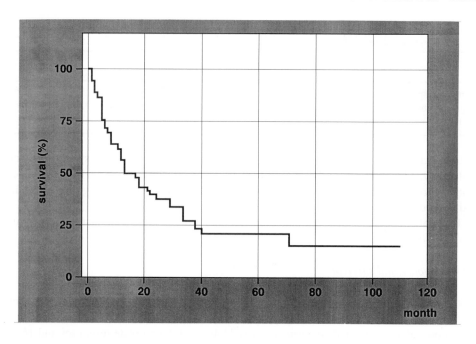

Fig. 1. Overall survival (n = 38).

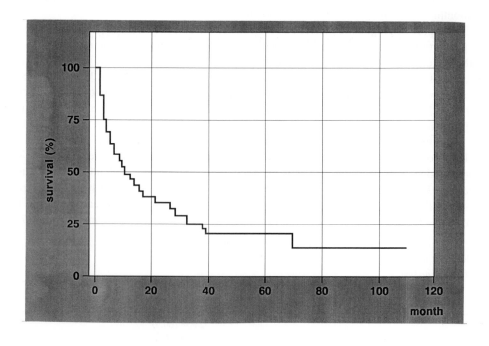

Fig. 2. Overall freedom from progression (n = 38).

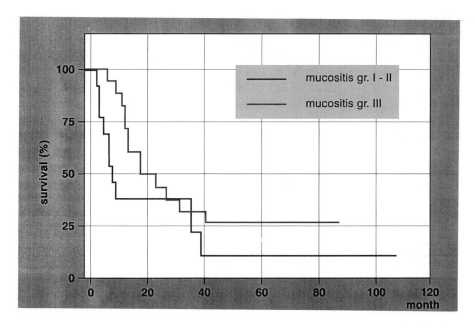

Fig. 3. Overall survival for groups with mucositis (groups I–II and IV).

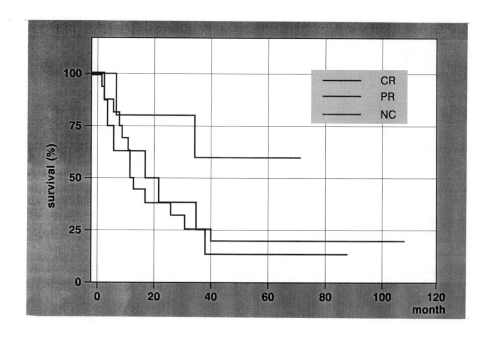

Fig. 4. Overall survival for group treated with concurrent chemotherapy according to response.

Table 8

Long-term survivors (≥36 months)

| Age | Stage | TRT | CT duration (days) | RT (Gy) | Mucositis grade 3 | Survival | Status |
|-----|-------|-----|--------------------|---------|-------------------|----------|--------|
| 74 | IV | CT + RT | 24 | 68 | − | 36 | D |
| 61 | III | CT + RT | 10 | 48 | − | 37 | A |
| 73 | III | CT + RT | 12 | 48 | − | 38 | D |
| 37 | IV | CT + RT | 30 | 56 | + | 40 | D |
| 54 | IV | CT + RT | 27 | 60 | + | 42 | A |
| 47 | IV | CT + RT | 27 | 30 | + | 50 | A |
| 57 | IV | CT + RT | 19 | 62.5 | + | 58 | A |
| 65 | IV | CT + RT | 15 | 70 | − | 69 | D |
| 43 | III | CT + RT | 25 | 60 | + | 72 | A |
| 70 | IV | CT + RT | 12 | 61 | + | 88 | A |
| 57 | II | CT + RT | 23 | 50 | − | 109 | A |

RT, radiotherapy; CT, chemotherapy; D, dead; A, alive.

109 months. All of these were treated with concurrent radiochemotherapy. Six of them are currently disease-free. One patient is surviving with local recurrence developed 72 months after treatment initiation. Eleven patients have survived more than 36 months after treatment (Table 8). All of them were treated with concurrent radiochemotherapy.

## 4. Discussion

Intra-arterial chemotherapy appears to be particularly suited for the management of head and neck cancer, because of the natural tendency of this disease is to recur at the primary site or in regional neck nodes. Distant dissemination occurs late and is a less frequent cause of morbidity and death. The rationale for prolonged arterial infusions is based on several theoretical advantages [21,22]. Achievement of much higher regional drug exposures generally leads to a higher rate of regional toxicities, with a variably lower rate of systemic toxicities [23–26]. There are several elements which are unique to regional intra-arterial chemotherapy as compared to conventional systemic intravenous chemotherapy. The toxicities of intra-arterial chemotherapy are generally different from the usual dose-limiting toxicities of systemic intravenous chemotherapy [27,28]. A major nidus for toxicity is the

Table 9

Cox's proportional hazard regression analysis

| Parameter | Survival | FFP |
|-----------|----------|-----|
| Mucositis (grade 3) | 0.0001 | 0.0005 |
| Stage | 0.004 | 0.042 |
| Response | 0.020 | 0.038 |
| Age (log) | 0.063 | 0.016 |
| Radiation dose (log) | 0.053 | 0.25 |
| CT duration | >0.1 | >0.1 |
| Surgery | >0.1 | >0.1 |

intra-arterial drug delivery system itself. Patients usually require prolonged hospitalization with constant nursing care to keep the catheter in place. The specific patient population in which intra-arterial chemotherapy may have an advantage over systemic drug therapy has yet to be defined. Its indications may be broadened because of progress and advance in the procedures and apparatus used in intra-arterial infusion, such as superselective arterial catheterization [29] and implantable pumps [14]. The concurrent intra-arterial chemotherapy and radiotherapy is associated with high local toxicity and needs intensive medical and nursing supervision, which requires a trained team [30]. Intra-arterial therapy should not be used by physicians who are unwilling to provide the commitment necessary. Experience and dedication are essential ingredients. Controversy still exists because of inappropriate clinical trials failing to directly compare intra-arterial and intravenous drug administration. It appears that the use of concurrent chemoradiotherapy in poor prognosis oropharyngeal cancer can result in occasional remissions of long duration in addition to response rates that are higher than those achieved with conventional radiotherapy. It should be pointed out that the use of the intra-arterial technique could be the reason for prolonged survival in the advanced tumors of the oropharynx.

## 5.  Conclusions

Combined radiotherapy and intra-arterial chemotherapy could produce high antitumor activity in locally advanced oropharyngeal carcinoma. Mucositis was the dose-limiting toxicity in the group of patients treated concurrently. The concurrent intra-arterial chemotherapy and radiotherapy is feasible only with intensive use of supportive care which may contribute significantly to the patient's compliance. The use of this combination outside of clinical trials does not appear justified. Now we plan to optimize our protocol by the use of new generation agents as well as their integration with new radiation fractionation.

## Summary

*Background*: The prognosis of patients with advanced cancer of the head and neck is poor with the majority of patients dying from uncontrolled local disease. The standard treatment for advanced head and neck squamous cell carcinoma has had poor results. The present study was designed to evaluate results of intra-arterial chemotherapy and the feasibility of combination with radiotherapy in patients with advanced oropharyngeal carcinoma. We analyzed the following endpoints: survival, local control and toxicity. *Methods:* Patients with previously untreated inoperable advanced non-metastatic squamous cell carcinoma of the oropharynx were included in the analysis. Between May 1986 and May 1992, 44 patients were treated with intention to use intra-arterial chemotherapy combined with concurrent radiotherapy. In 6 patients catheterization was not performed because of technical difficulties in 5 patients and blocked catheter in 1 patient. All 38 patients treated with intra-arterial chemotherapy were evaluable for response and toxicity. Twenty-nine patients had been treated concurrently with external radiotherapy and 8 sequentially. The treatment protocol consisted of continuous intra-arterial infusion of bleomycin (10 mg/day) alternating with methotrexate (10 mg/day) with leucovorin. The median duration of intra-arterial chemotherapy was 20 days (from 8 to 36). Total dose of radiotherapy ranged from 48 to 70 Gy (median 60 Gy), 5 fractions/week, with a daily dose 1.5 Gy/fraction given concurrently with chemotherapy and 1.8–2.0 Gy given sequentially. Twelve patients underwent salvage surgery for persistent or recurrent disease. *Results:* At the end of the entire treatment, 6 complete responses (15.8%) and 21 partial responses (55.2%) were achieved. The total response rate was 71%. Median survival of all patients was 17 months and the 1-year, 2-year and 3-year survival rates were 60.5, 36.8, and 28.9%, respectively. The most relevant toxicity in the group treated with concurrent chemoradiotherapy was mucositis grade 3 observed in 17 patients. The hematological toxicity observed in 4 patients (10.5%) was only moderate and was never greater than grade 2. Two patients died soon after therapy, one due to CNS embolism, the other from malnutrition and infection. *Conclusion:* Combined radiotherapy and intra-arterial chemotherapy could produce high anti-tumor activity in locally advanced oropharyngeal carcinoma. Mucositis was the dose- limiting toxicity in the group of patients treated concurrently. The concurrent intra-arterial chemotherapy and radiotherapy is feasible only with intensive use of supportive care which may contribute significantly to patient compliance. We now plan to optimize our protocol by the use of new generation agents as well as their integration with new radiation fractionation.

## *References*

1.   Gupta NK, Pointon RCS, Wilkinson PM. A randomized clinical trial to contrast radiotherapy with radiotherapy and methotrexate given synchronously in head and neck cancer. Clin Radiol 38: 575–581, 1987.
2.   Dimery IW, Hong WK. Overview of combined modality therapies for head and neck cancer. J Natl Cancer Inst 85: 95–111, 1993.
3.   Million RR, Cassisi NJ, Clark JR. Cancer of the head and neck. In: DeVita VT, Hellman S, Rosenberg SA (Eds), Cancer Principles and Practices of Oncology, 3rd edn. Philadelphia, PA: Lippincott, pp. 488–590, 1989.
4.   Stupp R, Vokes EE. Fortschritte in der Therapie von Kopf- und Halstumoren. Strahlenther Onkol 171: 140–148, 1995.
5.   Tavorath R, Pfister DG. Chemotherapy for recurrent disease and combined modality therapies for head and neck cancer. Curr Opin Oncol 7: 242–247, 1995.
6.   Vokes EE, Athanasiadis I. Chemotherapy for squamous cell carcinoma of head and neck: the future is now. Ann Oncol 7: 15–29, 1996
7.   Vokes EE, Weichselbaum RR. Chemoradiotherapy for head and neck cancer. Principles Pract Oncol Updates 7: 1–8, 1993.
8.   Vokes EE, Weichselbaum RR. Concomitant chemoradiotherapy: rationale and clinical experience in patients with solid tumors. J Clin Oncol 8: 911–934, 1990.
9.   El-Sayed S, Nelson N. Adjuvant and adjunctive chemotherapy in the management of squamous cell carcinoma of the head and neck region: a meta-analysis of prospective and randomized trials. J Clin Oncol 14: 838–842, 1996.
10.  Vokes EE, Panje WR, Schilsky RL. Hydroxyurea, fluorouracil and concomitant RT in poor prognosis head and neck cancer: phase I–II study. J Clin Oncol 7: 761–768, 1989.
11.  Vokes EE, Haraf DJ, Mick R, et al. Intensified concomitant chemoradiotherapy with and without filgrastim for poor-prognosis head and neck cancer. J Clin Oncol 12: 2351–2359, 1994.
12.  Vokes EE, Kies M, Haraf DJ, et al. Induction chemotherapy followed by concomitant chemoradiotherapy for advanced head and neck cancer: impact on the natural history of the disease. J Clin Oncol 13: 876–873, 1995.
13.  Pinnaro P, Cercato MC, Giannarelli D, et al. A randomized phase II study comparing sequential versus simultaneous chemo-radiotherapy in patients with unresectable locally advanced squamous cell cancer of the head and neck. Ann Oncol 5: 513–519, 1994.
14.  Eckardt A, Kelber, A. Palliative, intraarterial chemotherapy for advanced head and neck cancer using an implantable port system. J Oral Maxillofac Surg 52: 1243–1246, 1994.

15.   Al-Sarraf M. Chemotherapeutic management of head and neck neoplasia. In: Peterson DE, Elias EG, Sonis ST (Eds), Head and Neck Management of the Cancer Patient. Boston, MA: Martinus Nijhoff, pp. 299–311, 1986.

16.   Bierman HR, Shimkin MB, Byron RL, Miller ER. Effects of intra-arterial administration of nitrogen mustard (Abstract). International Cancer Congress, Paris, pp. 186–187, 1950.

17.   Klopp CT, Alford TC, Bateman J. Fractionated intraarterial cancer chemotherapy with methyl bis amine hydrochloride: a preliminary report. Ann Surg 132: 811–832, 1950.

18.   Cox DR. Regression models and life tables. J R Statist Soc 34: 187–220, 1972.

19.   Therasse P (Editor in Chief). A Practical Guide to EORTC Studies. EORTC Data Center, Brussels, 1996.

20.   Hermanek P, Sobin LH (Eds). UICC: TNM Classification of Malignant Tumours, 4th edn. Berlin: Springer, 1987.

21.   Baker SR, Wheeler WH. Long-term intraarterial chemotherapy infusion of ambulatory head and neck cancer patients. Surg Oncol 21: 125–131, 1982.

22.   Baker SR, Forastiere AA, Wheeler R, Medvec B. Intra-arterial chemotherapy for head and neck cancer. Arch Otolaryngol Head Neck Surg 113: 1183–1190, 1987.

23.   Chen H, Gross JF. Intra-arterial infusion of anticancer drugs: Theoretic aspects of drug delivery and review of responses. Cancer Treatment Rep 64: 31–40, 1980.

24.   Collins JM. Pharmacologic rationale for regional drug delivery. J Clin Oncol 2: 498–504, 1984.

25.   Howell SB. Pharmacokinetic principles of regional chemotherapy. In: Aigner KR, Patt YZ, Link KH, Kreidler J (Eds), Regional Cancer Treatment, pp. 1–9, 1988.

26.   Koch U, Herberhold C. Intraarterielle Chemotherapie von Karzinomen im Kopf-halsbereich. Arch Otol Rhin Laryngol 207: 565–567, 1974.

27.   Bilder J. Orální mukositida indukovaná cytostatiky a zářením. Klin Onkol 5: 110–122, 1992.

28.   Mazánek J, Haisová L, Kvapil F. Problematika komplexní protinádorové terapie v orofaciální oblasti. II. Komplikace chemoterapie. Čs Stomat 87: 232–237, 1987.

29.   Šimùnek A, Hlava A, Krajina A. Selective intra-arterial chemotherapy of orofacial carcinomas. Acta Radiol Portuguesa 4: 75–79, 1992.

30.   Petruželka L, Betka J, Kasík P, Judas L. Feasibility and efficacy of combined radiotherapy and intra-arterial chemotherapy for advanced cancer of the oropharynx. Support Care Cancer 4: 241, 1996.

C.J. Rosenthal and M. Rotman (Eds.), *Infusion Chemotherapy–Irradiation Interactions*

# CHAPTER 24

# Neo-adjuvant (primary) organ-preserving chemotherapy in the management of locally advanced laryngeal carcinoma: larynx preservation and clinical response

GIOVANNI MANTOVANI[1], VITTORIO GEBBIA[4], ERNESTO PROTO[2], FRANCESCO COSSU[3], ALESSANDRO BIANCHI[1], LUIGI CURRELI[1], MASSIMO GHIANI[1], ELENA MASSA[1], GIORGIO ASTARA[1], BIANCAROSA LAMPIS[1], DANIELA DESSÌ[1] and MARIA CRISTINA SANTONA[1]

[1]*Department of Medical Oncology, Institute of Internal Medicine,* [2]*Department of Surgery, Otolaryngology Branch,* [3]*Department of Radiation Therapy, University of Cagliari, 09124 Cagliari, Italy and* [4]*Chair and Service of Chemotherapy, University of Palermo, 90127 Palermo, Italy*

## 1. Introduction

The standard treatment for larynx cancer has been surgery whenever possible, usually with larynx removal, followed by irradiation or radiation therapy alone. Despite two decades of investigations, the role of chemotherapy as an adjunct to definitive local treatment of loco-regionally advanced squamous cell carcinoma of the head and neck (HNSCC) is still to be defined. Three approaches of utilizing chemotherapy into the primary management of this disease have been evaluated: (1) neo-adjuvant or induction chemotherapy, (2) adjuvant chemotherapy and (3) concomitant therapy (chemotherapy and local treatment, radiation, given simultaneously). Most randomized clinical trials have aimed at demonstrating the value of these different approaches with regard to two main purposes: (1) improving survival by enhancing locoregional and systemic control and (2) preserving organ function [1].

As the approach combining neo-adjuvant chemotherapy (NAC) with radiation therapy warrants further investigation, we designed an open, non-randomized, phase II clinical study to assess as the first endpoint the feasibility of sparing surgery and of preserving organ/function by using NAC in laryngeal cancer patients, and, as the second endpoint, the clinical response to this treatment approach and its duration. Moreover, an attempt was made to scale the extent of surgery by means of an arbitrary scale assigning different scores to the different extents of surgical resections. Briefly, the main aim of our study was to avoid or at least substantially reduce the amount of surgery in patients responding to chemotherapy, leaving major surgery as a salvage treatment.

## 2. Patients and methods

### 2.1. Patients

Patients with histologically confirmed, resectable, squamous cell carcinoma of the larynx were eligible for this study. They were also required to have stage III or IV disease without distant metastases according to the staging system of the International Union Against Cancer [2], to have had no previous treatment, to be less than 70 years old, to have a performance status (PS) of 1 or less on the ECOG scale, and to have normal cardiac, hepatic, and renal functions as well as leukocyte counts of $> 4000/\mu$l and platelet counts of $>100\ 000/\mu$l. Patients with both previous or concurrent malignancy were excluded.

All patients were initially evaluated by an otolaryngologist and a medical oncologist. Evaluation for resectability was performed at the first visit and only resectable patients were included. A tumor was defined as unresectable if it was fixed to either a bone structure or lymph nodes or if it was too invasive to allow for radical surgical removal. At the same time the extent of surgery was planned for each patient according to the extent of disease and widespread criteria of well-conducted surgical oncology, assuming that each patient should be submitted to surgical removal of the tumor as first treatment. Consequently, the patients were divided into two groups: (A) those requiring total laryngectomy (TL) and (B) those not requiring TL, i.e., patients eligible for conservative surgery. Moreover, an attempt was made to score the decreasing extent of surgery following NAC by means of an arbitrary scale which is shown in Table 1. A maximum score (4) was attributed to the patients who completely avoided surgery when TL was planned for them before NAC and a minimum score (0) was assigned in case of either no organ preservation (TL) or no reduction in the extent of surgical resection performed after NAC compared to that planned before NAC. Initial evaluation included a medical history, clinical examination, upper aerodigestive tract endoscopy, complete blood cell count, complete blood chemistry, urinanalysis, electrocardiogram and chest X-ray. When indicated, computed tomographic (CT) scans of the chest, abdomen, and head and neck regions were obtained. Written informed consent was obtained from each patient prior to treatment, according to the guidelines of the Ethics Committee of the Department of Internal Medicine, University of Cagliari.

## 2.2. Treatment plan

### 2.2.1. Neo-adjuvant chemotherapy

Eligible patients were assigned to one of the two different induction chemotherapy regimens according to the time of their accrual. Regimen 1 was the classical Al-Sarraf's: cisplatin 100 mg/m$^2$ i.v. as a 60 min infusion on day 1 with a standard pre- and post-hydration protocol with forced diuresis by 250 cm$^3$ of 18% mannitol plus 5-fluorouracil (5-FU) 1000 mg/m$^2$ per day on days 1–5 as a continuous infusion by peripheral vein, to be repeated every 3 weeks for three cycles. This protocol was effective from April 1990 to February 1993 and was applied to 20 patients (all evaluable). Regimen 2 was set up by our Institution [3] with the aim of improving the clinical results obtained with Al-Sarraf's regimen, by adding vinorelbine, a new semisynthetic *Vinca* alkaloid, which was able to induce a 22% partial response rate in a group of 23 heavily pretreated patients with recurrent and/or metastatic HNSCC [4]. It consisted of cisplatin 80 mg/m$^2$ i.v. as a 60 min infusion on day 1, 5-FU 600 mg/m$^2$ diluted in 500 cm$^3$ of normal saline over 4 h infusion on days 2–5; and vinorelbine 20 mg/m$^2$ diluted in 250 cm$^3$ of normal saline over 20 min on days 2 and 8. It was effective from March 1993 to February 1995 and was applied to 12 patients (11 evaluable).

Three treatment cycles were planned for Regimen 1. Regimen 2 response was first evaluated after two cycles of therapy. Treatment duration (number of cycles administered) depended on the clinical response obtained. If complete response (CR) was observed after the

Table 1

Arbitrary scale for assessing organ preserving surgery

| Extent of planned surgery before NAC[a] | Extent of performed surgery after NAC[a] | | | | |
|---|---|---|---|---|---|
| | TL | La-STL | MP-STL | H-SGL/ HG | Avoided surgery |
| TL | 0 | 1 | 2 | 3 | 4 |
| La-STL | – | 0 | 1 | 2 | 3 |
| MP-STL | – | – | 0 | 1 | 2 |
| H-SGL/HG | – | – | – | 0 | 1 |

[a]NAC, neo-adjuvant chemotherapy; TL, total laryngectomy; La-STL, sub-total laryngectomy with crico-ioido-aritenoidopexy (according to Labayle); MP-STL, sub-total laryingectomy with crico-ioido-epyglottopexy (according to Mayer-Piquet); H-SGL, horizontal supraglottic laryngectomy (according to Alonso); HG, horizontal glottectomy; Score 0, no organ preservation/No reduction in the extent of surgery; Score 1–4, reduction of different degree in the extent of surgery/avoided surgery.

first two treatment cycles (1st and 2nd cycles), patients were offered definitive locoregional treatment, i.e., surgery and/or radiation therapy; if only partial response (PR) was seen, two more cycles (3rd and 4th cycles) were administered. If then the tumor continued to shrink, two more cycles (5th and 6th cycles) were employed before definitive locoregional therapy was given. On the other hand, if no further decrease in tumor size was seen after the 4th cycle, patients were submitted to definitive locoregional therapy without any further cycle of chemotherapy. If after the first two cycles (1st and 2nd cycles) "no change" was recorded, two more cycles (3rd and 4th cycles) were administered. In the case of stabilization or progression after the 4th cycle, patients were assigned to locoregional therapy but where only PR was recorded, two more cycles (5th and 6th cycles) were administered. If after the first two cycles (1st and 2nd cycles) progression was recorded, where possible, locoregional therapies or non-cross-resistant chemotherapy were offered.

All patients were again evaluated 3 weeks after the end of the planned chemotherapy by a clinical examination, endoscopy, CT scan and confirmatory biopsy where indicated. In particular, several random biopsies were obtained in the area of preexisting primary tumor, when a CR was documented by clinical examination plus endoscopy plus CT scan.

### 2.2.2.  Locoregional treatment

Patients who achieved a CR were submitted to radiation therapy using $^{60}$Co equipment with a planned dose of 65/70 Gy to the involved areas at a 2 Gy fraction per day, 5 fractions per week. Treatment interruptions were allowed for 2 weeks after a dose of 30 Gy when grade III/IV mucositis occurred. Patients with a PR ≥ 70% were submitted to organ-preserving surgery, and those with a PR < 70% were submitted either to radical surgery (TL) or to the same extent of surgical resection as that planned before NAC. To prevent the possible criticism that it is not a sound oncological principle to use smaller surgical excision margins in case of residual disease after radiotherapy or chemotherapy, we assessed the histopathological data of surgical specimens of patient who underwent surgery. However, for primary tumors endowed in specific anatomical sites, radical surgery was performed irrespective of the degree of PR. Patients presenting stable disease were submitted to the same extent of surgery as that initially planned. Patients with disease progression were submitted to locoregional therapy (radical surgery or radiation) or non-cross-resistant chemotherapy.

*2.2.3.  Toxicity*

Toxicity was assessed according to WHO criteria [5].

## 3.  Results

Thirty-two patients (31 males and 1 female, 11 with stage III disease, 21 with stage IV disease) were enrolled from April 1990 to February 1995. All patients were hospitalized in the Department of Medical Oncology, Institute of Internal Medicine, University of Cagliari. The results are updated to September 1995. The 32 patients were all evaluable for response to NAC and 31 were evaluable for organ preservation. One patient was not evaluable for organ preservation as he refused the planned therapy, i.e. surgery, after the 4th chemotherapy cycle.

### 3.1.  Response to neo-adjuvant chemotherapy

All patients were evaluable for response to NAC. There were no substantial differences in the overall response rate (ORR), CR and PR rates, between the two chemotherapy regimens: the ORR was 100% for cisplatin + 5-FU and 92.3% for cisplatin + 5-FU + vinorelbine. A mean of four cycles per patient (range 3–6) was administered. All 32 patients (100%) received at least three cycles and 13/32 (40.6%) received six cycles.

The CR rate was 50% (16/32 patients) and the PR rate was 46.9% (15/32 patients) with an ORR of 96.9%. The mean time to response was 2.5 months (range 1.6–5.1).

### 3.2.  Organ/function preservation

The patient distribution according to the extent of planned surgery before NAC is shown in Table 2. Twenty-three patients required TL (Group A) and 8 patients a conservative laryngectomy (Group B).

The results regarding organ preservation are reported in Table 3. Seven of 23 (30.5%) patients of Group A did not undergo surgery (score 4) and 6/23 (26%) achieved a partial larynx preservation (3/23 score 3, 1/23 score 2, 2/23 score 1), whereas 10/23 (43.5%) received the previously planned TL (score 0).

Table 2

Patient distribution according to the extent of planned surgery before neo-adjuvant chemotherapy

|                               | No. of patients |
| ----------------------------- | --------------- |
| Group A                       |                 |
| Total laryngectomy            | 23              |
|                               |                 |
| Group B                       |                 |
| Conservative laryngectomy     | 8               |
| La-STL                        | 2               |
| MP-STL                        | 1               |
| H-SGL/HG                      | 5               |

Table 3

Extent of organ/function preservation

| Extent of planned surgery before NAC[a] | Extent of performed surgery after NAC | | | | | | | | | | | | | | |
|---|---|---|---|---|---|---|---|---|---|---|---|---|---|---|---|
| | TL | | | La-STL | | | MP-STL | | | H-SGL/HG | | | No surgery | | |
| | P | % | S | P | % | S | P | % | S | P | % | S | P | % | S |
| TL | 10/23 | 43.5 | 0 | 2/23 | 8.7 | 1 | 1/23 | 4.3 | 2 | 3/23 | 13.0 | 3 | 7/23 | 30.5 | 4 |
| La-STL | | | | | | | | | | | | | 2/2 | 100 | 3 |
| MP-STL | | | | | | | | | | | | | 1/1 | 100 | 2 |
| H-SGL/HG | | | | | | | | | | 3/5 | 60.0 | 0 | 2/5 | 40 | 1 |

[a]NAC, neo-adjuvant chemotherapy; P, no. of patients; S, score.

Late salvage laryngectomy for recurrent cancer was required in 2/31 patients (rate 6.5%) after intervals of 18.7 and 47.8 months, respectively.

Five of eight (62.5%) patients of Group B did not undergo surgery: 2 patients were planned for sub-total laryngectomy with crico-ioido-aritenoidopexy, according to Labayle (La-STL), score 3, 1 patient was planned for sub-total laryngectomy with crico-ioido-epyglottopexy, according to Mayer-Piquet (MP-STL), score 2 and 2 patients were planned for horizontal supraglottic laryngectomy, according to Alonso (H-SGL)/horizontal glottectomy (HG), score 1, whereas 3/8 (37.5%) received the previously planned H-SGL/HG surgery (score 0).

Therefore, 12/31 patients (38.7%) completely avoided surgery and 6/31 (19.4%) achieved a reduction in the extent of planned surgical resection: overall, 18/31 patients (58.1%) achieved a reduction in the extent of previously planned surgery attributable to NAC, while 13/31 (41.9%) (10 TL and 3 H-SGL/HG) received the previously planned surgical resection. Thirteen of the 23 patients (56.5%) in Group A (candidates to TL) completely or partially preserved the organ/function, while 5/8 (62.5%) patients of Group B completely preserved the organ. A global score evaluation is reported in Table 4.

Currently, 4/7 (57.1%) patients of Group A who did not undergo surgery are alive and have remained continuously disease-free, 2/7 (28.6%) locally relapsed (time to progression 3.5 and 8.4 months, respectively) and subsequently died of disease progression, while 1/7 (14.3%) died of a second primary tumor (lung adenocarcinoma) but was relapse-free for laryngeal cancer. Five of 6 (83.3%) patients of Group A who achieved a partial larynx preservation are alive and have remained continuously disease-free, while 1/6 (16.7%) relapsed (time to progression 11.7 months) and subsequently died of disease progression. Three of 10

Table 4

Global score assigned to organ/function preservation in 31 patients

| Score | No. of patients | % |
|---|---|---|
| 0 | 13/31 | 41.9 |
| 1 | 4/31 | 12.9 |
| 2 | 2/31 | 6.5 |
| 3 | 5/31 | 16.1 |
| 4 | 7/31 | 22.6 |

(30%) patients who received the previously planned TL are alive and disease-free, while 4/10 (40%) died of disease progression (time to progression 12.7, 11.6, 9.0 and 4.4 months, respectively), 2/10 (20%) died of acute myocardial infarction and 1/10 died of second primary tumor (lung epidermoid carcinoma).

All patients in Group B who completely preserved the organ/function are currently alive: 4/5 (80.0%) have remained continuously disease-free, while 1/5 (20%) locally relapsed (time to progression 18.7 months) but could undergo salvage surgery. One of 3 (33.3%) patients of Group B who received expected conservative surgery is alive and disease-free, 1/3 (33.3%) is currently alive and disease-free (he locally relapsed, time to progression 47.8 months, and had to be subjected to salvage surgery) and 1/3 (33.3%) died of another cause (road accident) while being in CR.

## 3.3. Response after all treatment

After completion of all treatment, including locoregional therapy, 24/32 (75%) patients were rendered NED and 7/32 were in objective response (PR). The following local modalities were used in these patients after completion of NAC: RT alone in 14/24 (58.3%) patients, RT plus surgery to the primary tumor site and/or neck dissection in 1/24 patients (4.2%), surgery and/or neck dissection alone in 9/24 (37.5%) patients. Only one patient out of all (10) submitted to surgical resection had positive surgical excision margins.

## 3.4. Toxicity

The two chemotherapy regimens had different toxicity only for Grade 3–4 anemia and thrombocytopenia and for Grade 1–2 pain at the tumor site, which were higher in the cisplatin + 5-FU + vinorelbine group. Overall, NAC-associated toxicity was similar for the two regimens. Approximately 10–15% of the patients had grade 3–4 hematologic or gastrointestinal (nausea and vomiting) toxicity. No chemotherapy-related death was observed. Toxicity due to RT was similar to previous experiences in which RT was administered at similar doses without previous chemotherapy; the great majority of patients developed mild to moderate mucositis.

## 4. Conclusions

Our study was designed and set up as a "pilot" non-randomized, being single-center with no large patients accrual and this may be its main limitation; nevertheless, we believe that the number of patients included is adequate for this type of study and the conclusions to the addressed endpoints are significant. A second possible limitation would be the two different chemotherapy regimens used in our study in two different periods of time, but this was overcome by showing that, as stated above in the Section 3, there were no significant differences in response rates between the two regimens.

Approximately 60% of patients achieved a substantial reduction in the extent of previously planned surgery thus preserving organ/function. Furthermore, 3 patients, although subjected to the previously planned conservative surgery, that is H-SGL/HG, preserved function; overall, 21/31 (67.7%) patients preserved function and only 10/31 (32.3%) patients lost function. Our results are consistent with the findings of the studies reported above.

The assessment of treatment outcome of our patients by the Performance Status Scale for Head and Neck Cancer Patients confirmed that anatomical organ preservation was paralleled by a very successful function preservation.

In our opinion the two most relevant contributions offered by our study are: (1) to have addressed the question of measuring as precisely as possible the reduction of surgical resection made possible by NAC compared to surgery planned before NAC and this not only for TL but for all extents of surgical treatment and (2) to have attempted to avoid or at least substantially reduce the amount of surgery in patients responding to chemotherapy, leaving major surgery as a salvage treatment.

Although the scale provided by us is an arbitrary one, it must be emphasized that our goal was to address the issue of quality of life in cancer patients by a more precise quantification of organ/function sparing surgery, taking into consideration that the loss of the larynx, i.e., voice, has always been considered to have a major impact on the quality of life and that the long-standing interest in voice preservation had a major role in the development of larynx-preserving surgery [6].

## Acknowledgements

This work was supported by C.N.R., Rome, A.P. "Clinical Applications of Oncological Research", Contract No. 95.00389.PF39. We thank Dr. Roberta Tocco for the preparation of the manuscript.

## References

1.  Glisson BS, Ki Hong E. Primary chemotherapy of advanced head and neck cancer: where do we go from here? J Natl Cancer Inst 88: 567–568, 1996.
2.  Hermanek P, Sobin LH (Eds). International Union Against Cancer: TNM Classification of Malignant Tumours, 4th edn., 2nd rev. Berlin: Springer, 1992.
3.  Gebbia V, Mantovani G, Agostara B, et al. Treatment of recurrent and/or metastatic squamous cell head and neck carcinoma with a combination of vinorelbine, cisplatin, and 5-fluoruracil: a multicenter phase II trial. Ann Oncol 6: 987–991, 1995.
4.  Gebbia V, Testa A, Valenza R, et al. A pilot study of vinorelbine on a weekly schedule in recurrent and or metastatic squamous cell carcinoma of the head and neck. Eur J Cancer 29A: 1358–1359, 1994.
5.  Miller AB, Hodgstraten B, Staquet M, Winkler A. Reporting results of cancer treatment. Cancer 47: 207–214, 1981.
6.  Clayman GL, Weber RS, Guillamondegui O, et al. Laryngeal preservation for advanced laryngeal and hypopharyngeal cancers. Arch Otolaryngol Head Neck Surg 121: 219–223, 1995.

C.J. Rosenthal and M. Rotman (Eds.), *Infusion Chemotherapy–Irradiation Interactions*
1998 Elsevier Science B.V.

# CHAPTER 25

# In-field locally relapsed head and neck tumors treated with re-irradiation enhanced by simultaneous low-dose cisplatin

FEDERICO LONARDI, GIOVANNI PAVANATO, VITTORIO D. FERRARI,
GIORGIO BONCIARELLI and ANTONIO JIRILLO

*Dipartimento di Terapie Oncologiche Integrate, ULSS 21, 37045 Legnago (VR), Italy*

## 1. Introduction and aims

Platin compounds have been frequently associated with radiation therapy (RT) as agents being able to potentiate the radiation induced damage, i.e., as "sensitizers". Basically, mechanisms of interaction between platin compounds and radiation include reduction/inhibition of sublethal damage repair and radiosensitization of hypoxic/oxic cells, although some aspects of the modulation are not completely known. The sensitizing effect of platin compounds, with particular reference to cisplatin (CP), has been reported in a large variety of both in vitro and in vivo laboratory studies which have given stronger support to the rationale of combination, focusing on the importance of the timing factor. CP fully enhances cytotoxicity when given concurrently or in close temporal relationship with radiation [1–4]. Administering CP shortly before each RT fraction is considered to produce the greatest cell-kill effect. These experimental findings have been translated in some phase II–III trials which demonstrated the feasibility and efficacy of the combination in the first line treatment of advanced solid neoplasms, especially head and neck and non-small-cell lung cancer [5–10]. The potentiation of radiation by CP, however, may be also considered in the treatment of seriously affected advanced cancer patients with mid-term life expectancy to obtain good long-lasting symptom relief without producing relevant toxicity, thus improving the quality of residual life. In particular, the combination of CP and RT is worth considering when symptomatic in-field RT failures are to be treated after previous heavy therapies [11,12].

Head and neck tumors locoregionally relapsed after first line chemotherapy and/or RT are often hardly manageable, as they are usually not suitable for more radical treatment. Patients often present with poor performance status (PS), are heavily symptomatic and their compliance to further aggressive therapy is generally low. We chose to combine radiation with low-dose cisplatin for the re-treatment of symptomatic in-field recurrences in head and neck cancer patients in order to evaluate the feasibility, efficacy and tolerance in such critical patients, who should have palliation as the main therapeutic goal.

## 2. Patients and methods

Thirteen consecutive unselected male patients, median age 58 (range 47–75), all previously treated from 1990 to 1995 with adjuvant or curative RT (7/13 also with single agent or combination chemotherapy), suffering from in-field recurrence of head and neck carcinomas, entered a chemo-radiation therapeutic program with palliative intent. All patients entered re-treatment after a median interval of 14 months (range 5–72) from previous RT, with median PS 2 (range 1–3, ECOG) and symptomatic disease (pain, dysphagia). Owing to the previous heavy therapy and the poor conditions, they were deemed unfit for further aggressive approaches. Treatment consisted of re-irradiation enhanced by simultaneous low-dose CP at 5 mg/m² bolus without hydration, administered daily 30–60 min before each RT fraction. The total amount of CP varied from 40 to 100 mg/m² (median 65 mg/m²), depending on the number of RT fractions given.

As the spinal chord had to be spared and previous doses of radiation were high in most cases, the residual amount of RT still disposable was quite limited. It was determined through NSD/TDF and $\alpha/\beta$ calculations and delivered with standard fractionation (180–200 cGy per daily fraction) using cobalt-60 and 6-MV LinAc units. A median of 2520 cGy (range 1600–3600 cGy) could be given in 13 (8–20) daily fractions. Most treatments (10/13) were performed on an outpatient basis. Patients' features are reported in Table 1.

## 3. Results

The evaluation of objective and subjective responses was performed at the end of treatment, 2 months later and 2–3 months thereafter. Eleven of thirteen patients were evaluable according to WHO criteria: 4/13 patients had PR, 4/13 had SD and 3/13 PD. Two patients had SD at the end of re-RT, but did not present for late evaluation of response due to early death. Response duration was 4, 4, 4+ and 17 months in PR patients; 4, 4, 4, 15 months in SD patients. All patients presenting either PR or SD experienced good remission (≥50%) of symptoms (evaluation was made through the Visual Analogic Scale). One patient had a brief pain recovery despite PD. Two patients with PR and two with SD had been treated with cisplatin-based combination chemotherapy before undergoing re-treatment.

Table 1

Characteristics of patients

| Patient | Age | Site of primary tumor | Previous radiation therapy (cGy) | Site of recurrence | Previous chemotherapy |
|---|---|---|---|---|---|
| 01 | 55 | Oropharynx | 7000 | Local | No |
| 02 | 60 | Tonsil | 6000 | Local | Yes |
| 03 | 54 | Larynx | 5400 | Neck | Yes |
| 04 | 48 | Larynx | 5000 | Neck | Yes |
| 05 | 67 | Larynx | 6000 | Local | Yes |
| 06 | 75 | Cheek mucosa | 5040 | Local | No |
| 07 | 58 | Larynx | 6000 | Neck | Yes |
| 08 | 63 | Oropharynx | 4400 | Local/neck | No |
| 09 | 49 | Hypopharynx | 6150 | Local | No |
| 10 | 47 | Retrom. trigone | 6775 | Local/neck | No |
| 11 | 58 | Tonsil | 7000 | Local/neck | Yes |
| 12 | 66 | Tongue | 5400 | Local | Yes |
| 13 | 65 | Retrom. trigone | 5400 | Local | No |

Table 2

Re-treatment and results

| Patient | Time to re-irradiation[a] | Re-RT/Fr.[b] | CP[b] | Response (WHO) | Response duration (months) |
|---|---|---|---|---|---|
| 01 | 18 | 1980/11 | 5/55 | SD | 4 |
| 02 | 13 | 1800/10 | 5/50 | n.e. | n.e. |
| 03 | 09 | 3600/20 | 5/100 | PR | 4 |
| 04 | 09 | 2600/13 | 5/65 | PR | 4 |
| 05 | 40 | 3000/15 | 5/75 | PD | – |
| 06 | 05 | 1980/11 | 5/55 | PD | – |
| 07 | 24 | 2400/12 | 5/60 | SD | 4 |
| 08 | 10 | 3000/15 | 5/75 | n.e. | n.e. |
| 09 | 72 | 3060/17 | 5/85 | PR | 17 |
| 10 | 14 | 1600/08 | 5/40 | SD | 4 |
| 11 | 33 | 2520/14 | 5/70 | SD | 15 |
| 12 | 17 | 2520/14 | 5/70 | PD | – |
| 13 | 10 | 2160/12 | 5/60 | PR | 4 |

[a]From the end of pervious RT.
[b]Re-RT/Fr, re-irradiation dose (cGy)/number of fractions; CP, cisplatin daily dose/total amount administered $(mg/m^2)$; n.e., not evaluable.

All patients were monitored weekly with blood count, BUN and creatinine, during treatment and 1 week later. Neither hematologic toxicity nor renal function impairment emerged. As to non-hematologic toxicity, slight nausea occurred in 5 patients at the very beginning of CP administrations, but did not require baseline anti-emetic therapy. Mucositis was present in 9/13 patients, higher in those who underwent chemotherapy, but it never exceeded grade II. Local examination did not reveal significant early RT-related sequelae.

The results are reported in Table 2.

## 4. Conclusions

Most patients with locoregionally advanced head and neck cancer recur despite heavy surgical–chemoradiation intensive therapeutic programs. More frequently, the site of failure is the same head and neck region. Out-of-trial patient populations scarcely benefit from "salvage" therapies due to low compliance, poor PS, resistant disease, etc. Chemotherapy for recurrent cancer does not offer responses better than 30% and survival does not normally exceed 4–6 months. Therefore, the main goal of re-treatment in unselected patients is not to improve survival, but to offer a good chance of palliation in these otherwise untreatable patients, without worsening the quality of residual life. Our data, although very limited, match similar reports from other groups [11–14] and are consistent with our aim, supporting the feasibility, efficacy, low toxicity and good tolerance of this combined re-treatment approach. In our opinion concurrent CP-RT deserves consideration in the palliation of recurrent symptomatic head and neck cancer patients when more aggressive therapeutic choices are not allowed. The encouraging response rate and duration we observed led us to extend this combined schedule to more advanced solid tumor in-field failures, using infusional CP via central venous access devices and portable pumps.

## Summary

*Background.* In-field locally relapsed head and neck (H&N) tumors are often hardly manageable, due to previous heavy treatments, poor patient conditions and low compliance. Reirradiation (reRT) can be combined with cisplatin (CP) to allow cell-kill enhancement with better preservation of surrounding tissue, thus offering good chance of palliation. *Methods.* Thirteen consecutive male patients (all previously treated with chemo-radiotherapy), suffering from relapsed symptomatic H&N tumors, underwent reRT plus simultaneous daily low-dose CP (5 mg/m²) as "sensitizer". CP amount ranged from 40 to 100 mg/m² (median 65) and total dose of RT 16–36 Gy (median 25.20). *Results.* According to WHO criteria, 4/13 patients had PR, 4/13 had SD and 3/13 PD. Two patients were not evaluable. Median response duration was 4–17 months in PR patients and 4–15 months in SD patients. All responding (PR + SD) patients had good symptom relief and there was no significant early toxicity, either from CP or RT. *Conclusions.* ReRT plus low-dose CP is feasible, low toxic and deserves consideration in patients with H&N recurrences not suitable for more aggressive treatments.

## References

1.  Steel GG. The search for therapeutic gain in the combination of radiotherapy and chemotherapy. Radiother Oncol 11: 31–53, 1988.
2.  Coughlin CT, Richmond RC. Biologic and clinical developments of cisplatin combined with radiation: concepts, utility, projections for new trials and the emergence of carboplatin. Semin Oncol 16(Suppl 6): 31–43, 1989.
3.  Schwachofer JHM, Crooijmans RPMA, Hoogenhout J, et al. Effectiveness in inhibition of recovery of cell survival by cisplatin and carboplatin: influence of treatment sequence. Int J Radiat Oncol Biol Phys 20: 1235–1241, 1991.
4.  Baterlink H. Does timing have an impact on the combination of radiotherapy and chemotherapy? Proc 4th Rome Int Symp Chemotherapy and Radiotherapy: an Integrated Approach. Rome, 1996.
5.  Schaake-Koning C, Van Den Bogaert W, Dalesio O, et al. Effects of concomitant cisplatin and radiotherapy on inoperable non-small-cell lung cancer. N Engl J Med 326: 524–530, 1992.
6.  Aisner J, Jacobs M, Sinabaldi V, et al. Chemoradiotherapy for the treatment of regionally advanced head and neck tumors. Semin Oncol 21(Suppl 2) 35–44, 1994.
7.  Vokes EE, Weichselbaum RR, Lippman SM, et al. Head and neck cancer. N Engl J Med 328: 184–194, 1993.
8.  Sweeney PJ, Haraf DJ, Vokes EE, et al. Radiation therapy in head and neck cancer: indications and limitations. Semin Oncol 21: 296–303, 1994.
9.  Vokes EE, Weichselbaum RR. Concomitant chemoradiotherapy: rationale and clinical experience in patients with solid tumors. J Clin Oncol 8: 911–934, 1990.
10. Marcial VA, Pajak TF, Mohiuddin M, et al. Concomitant cisplatin chemotherapy and radiotherapy in advanced mucosal squamous cell carcinoma of the head and neck. Long term results of the Radiation Therapy Oncology Group Study 81–17. Cancer 66: 1861–1868, 1990.
11. Brando V, Airoldi M, Orecchia R, et al. Re-irradiation (RI) and chemotherapy (CT) in locally recurrent (LR) head and neck cancer (HNC). Proc Am Soc Clin Oncol 11: 804, 1992.
12. Uhlmann D, Monyak D, Lee C, et al. Simultaneous chemotherapy and radiation therapy (RT) for recurrent squamous cell carcinoma (SSC) of the head & neck. Proc Am Soc Clin Oncol 11: 803, 1992.
13. Weichselbaum RR, Haraf DJ, Vokes E. Concurrent chemoradiotherapy for locally advanced recurrent head and neck cancer (HNC). Proc 4th Int Symp Chemotherapy and Radiotherapy: an Integrated Approach. Rome, 1996.
14. Ciabattoni A, Mantini G, Trodella L, et al. Radio-chemotherapy combination for palliative treatment: the experience of a radio-chemotherapy day-hospital. Proc 4th Int Symp Chemotherapy and Radiotherapy: an Integrated Approach. Rome, 1996.

C.J. Rosenthal and M. Rotman (Eds.), *Infusion Chemotherapy–Irradiation Interactions*
© 1998 Elsevier Science B.V. All rights reserved

# Non-resectable non-small-cell lung carcinoma: continuous infusion of cisplatin and concurrent radiotherapy plus adjuvant surgery

AMEDEO V. BEDINI[1], LUCA TAVECCHIO[1], ALBERTO GRAMAGLIA[2],
SERGIO VILLA[2], FRANCO MILANI[2], MAURO PALAZZI[2]
and GIANNI RAVASI[1]

[1]*Thoracic Surgery Department and* [2]*Radiotherapy Department, Istituto Nazionale Tumori, Via G. Venezian 1, 20133 Milano, Italy*

## 1. Introduction

High-dose radiation therapy (RT) is currently used in clinical practice for the treatment of locally advanced, inoperable non-small-cell lung carcinoma (NSCLC). However, 95% or more of the patients die without achieving long-term survival, locoregional failure being the main cause of death [1]. Concurrent cisplatin (CDDP) delivery has been introduced into RT schedules to improve the locoregional control by virtue of its radioenhancement properties. We have been investigating the concurrent administration of CDDP by continuous infusion since 1988 [2]. In this chapter we report the results of our second phase II study on this topic, involving patients with non-resectable stage III NSCLC in whom adjuvant surgery was systematically evaluated.

## 2. Patients and methods

Patients were eligible for the study if they had non-resectable stage III NSCLC [3]. Entry criteria included a pathological diagnosis, absence of distant metastases, functional operability, age less than 75 years, ability to be treated in the outpatient setting, normal blood cell counts and renal function, and informed consent. Criteria of non-resectability were T4 stage and/or N2 spread with presence of at least one mediastinal node ≥3 cm in diameter and/or involvement of three or more nodal stations, classified according to the criteria of the American Thoracic Society [4]. Nodes were considered positive when they had a diameter ≥1.5 cm on CT or MRI. Physical examination, chest X-rays, bronchoscopy, and computed studies of the brain, chest and upper abdomen were the routine staging procedures. A non-invasive diagnosis of a T4 stage was admitted in the case of vocal cord paralysis, compression of the trachea at bronchoscopy, or vertebral or great vessel involvement observed in computed studies. Pathological confirmation of clinical involvement of mediastinal nodes was mandatory except in those patients having a nodal diameter ≥4 cm, vocal cord paralysis, or a T4 primary tumor. A bone scan was performed only when skeletal pain and/or tenderness, alkaline phosphatase exceeding 108 IU/dl, or hypercalcemia were present. Patients with superior vena cava syndrome, malignant pleural effusion, N3 involvement, previous RT and/or response to previous chemotherapy were excluded.

Treatment consisted of RT and concurrent continuous infusion of CDDP. A continuous radiation course was planned. The projected standard total dose was 50 Gy, with daily doses of 2 Gy given 5 days a week. Higher total doses were admitted, but not exceeding 60 Gy. Radiotherapy was delivered by means of a 6 MV or 15 MV linear accelerator. Target volumes were localized with a standard simulation procedure on the basis of the available computed studies of the chest. The gross tumor volume (GTV) with 2 cm wide margins and the node-bearing areas judged to be at high risk of subclinical malignant spread were the planning target volume of the first phase of treatment (PTV 1). The node-bearing areas at risk were the homolateral hilum, the mediastinum with the lower margin ranging from 3 cm distal to the tracheal carina down to the diaphragm, according to the location of the primary tumor and the extent of clinical nodal involvement, the contralateral hilum in selected cases of extensive mediastinal involvement, both supraclavicular fossae in case of an upper lobe primary and/or involvement of upper mediastinal nodes. The dose given in PTV 1 was 40 Gy in 4 weeks (no inhomogeneity correction). Almost all treatments were delivered by means of 2 anterior and posterior opposite individually shielded portals, but in some instances 3 or 4 portals were required. Any portions of the spinal cord were specifically excluded in the second treatment phase (PTV 2), and GTV was treated with 1–2 cm margins. The dose of PTV 2 ranged from 10 to 20 Gy in 1–2 weeks, respectively, given with parallel opposite oblique or lateral fields. The total dose to any portion of the spinal cord was estimated not to exceed 45 Gy. Continuous infusion of CDDP was started each week of RT before the first weekly RT fraction and suspended after the last, or 96–100 h later. The daily dose was 4 mg/m$^2$ and the total projected dose for a 5-week course was 80 mg/m$^2$. CDDP infusion was delivered by a tunnelled central catheter and a portable pump. A daily oral fluid intake of 1.5–2 l was prescribed to patients during CDDP delivery. Treatment was given on a full outpatient basis.

Acute toxicities were defined as those occurring within 3 months from the start of treatment. Hematologic, renal and gastrointestinal toxicities were graded according to the World Health Organization criteria [5]. Other toxicities were classified as follows: mild dysphagia requiring soft diet without any need for narcotic analgesics was scored as acute esophageal radiation toxicity grade 1, and moderate dysphagia requiring purée or liquid diet as grade 2. Mild symptoms or dry cough or dyspnea on exertion were designated as acute lung radiation morbidity grade 1; persistent cough requiring antitussive agents, dyspnea with minimal effort but not at rest as grade 2. Severe cough, dyspnea at rest, clinical or radiologic evidence of acute pneumonitis, need for intermittent $O_2$ or steroids were assessed as grade 3 toxicity. Vascular toxicity was graded as follows: peripheral thrombophlebitis with an Eastern Cooperative Oncology Group (ECOG) performance status <3 [6] not requiring catheter removal, was graded 1. Peripheral thrombophlebitis with an ECOG performance status 3, was graded 2. Any thrombosis proximal to the catheter access but not affecting the vena cava, was assessed as grade 3 toxicity. Catheter removal was performed for vascular toxicities >1. Therapy was suspended until recovery in case of any other grade 3 toxicity. Patients were judged compliant with treatment if they received a minimum of 48 Gy and a total CDDP dose of at least 64 mg/m$^2$, corresponding to four full-time weekly infusions.

Brain, chest and upper abdomen computed studies were obtained 6 weeks after treatment completion for response assessment according to the ECOG criteria [6]. Patients without distant metastases and locoregional progression were subsequently submitted to broncho-

scopy and reassessment of the operative risk. They were then operated, unless unequivoca-
ble technical non-resectability was presumed. No further treatment was prescribed.

Patients were controlled quarterly in the first 2 years of follow-up, and every 6 months
thereafter. Observed and progression-free survival curves were computed according to the
life-table method at every 1-week interval, taking the start of treatment as time zero. Deaths
not due to cancer were computed as failures in progression-free survival curves.

## 3. Results

Eighty patients entered the study from January 1990 to September 1993. Their characteristics are shown in Table 1. Violations of the entry criteria were assessed in 5 cases on review
of the clinical records. Histology was not available in 1 patient coming from another institution who had been pretreated with chemotherapy. Pathological confirmation of mediastinal
nodes $>1.5 < 4$ cm in diameter was not obtained in one patient with $T < 4$. Three T4 N0
tumors were not submitted to an invasive diagnosis although this was requested by the entry
criteria.

Five patients interrupted treatment because of early distant progression (1 case), toxicity
(2 cases), or deviation from protocol rules (2 cases). The remaining 75 patients received the
initially provided dose of RT but 5 of them received a cumulative CDDP dose of less than
64 mg/m$^2$ due to catheter removal (3 cases), toxicity (1 case), or deviation from protocol
rules (1 case). Seventy patients (87.5%) were fully compliant with the treatment schedule.
All patients were evaluable for toxicity, the features of which are shown in Table 2. The
locoregional clinical response frequencies are shown in Table 3. Thirty-eight patients did
not undergo surgery; this was due to distant metastases in 14 cases, persistent unresectability
in 13, and a prohibitive or high surgical risk in 10. One patient refused operation. Of the 42
patients submitted to surgery, 6 had achieved a clinical complete response, 30 a partial response, and 5 stabilization of disease. The locoregional response was assessed as non-
evaluable in the remaining patient. An exploratory thoracotomy because of persistent unre-

Table 1

Demographic data

| | |
|---|---|
| Male/female ratio | 75/5 |
| Mean age (range) | 55 (38–74) |
| Performance status | |
|    0 | 35 |
|    1 | 43 |
|    2 | 2 |
| Presence of symptoms | 75 |
| Stage | |
|    T < 4   N2   M0 | 32 |
|    T4   N < 2   M0 | 28 |
|    T4   N2   M0 | 20 |
| Histology | |
|    Squamous | 41 |
|    Adenocarcinoma | 28 |
|    Other or undetermined NSCLC | 11 |
| Pretreatment (chemotherapy) | 3 |

Table 2

Percent frequency of toxicity

| | Grade | | | |
|---|---|---|---|---|
| | 1 | 2 | 3 | Total |
| Leukopenia | 7.5 | 5 | – | 12.5 |
| Nephrotoxicity | 5 | – | – | 5 |
| Nausea/vomiting | 21.2 | 10 | 1.2 | 32.5 |
| Esophagitis | 43.7 | 18.7 | – | 62.5 |
| Lung toxicity | 8.7 | 2.5 | 2.5 | 13.7 |
| Vascular toxicity | 1.2 | 2.5 | 1.2 | 5 |

sectable disease was performed in 5 cases. Four sublobar resections, 18 lobectomies or bilobectomies (one with a bronchoplastic procedure and 4 with chest wall resections), 4 left and 7 right pneumonectomies were performed. Extensive biopsies showing no viable tumor were done in 4 cases in whom a right pneumonectomy had to be performed. Resection was feasible in these 4 cases, but judged at excessive risk (see below). Intraoperative staging was very difficult due to fibrosis, and the maneuvers required very high skill and care. There were 7 postoperative deaths. One occurred after an exploratory thoracotomy due to an acute hypertensive contralateral pneumothorax, one after a lobectomy plus chest wall resection due to a pulmonary embolism. Five deaths occurred following a right pneumonectomy for bronchial stump fistula (2 cases), empyema without fistula (1 case), pulmonary embolism (1 case), and adult respiratory distress syndrome (1 case). No viable tumor was found in the specimens of 3 of the 5 patients who died after a right pneumonectomy.

Nineteen of the patients submitted to surgery were assessed as having no viable residual tumor tissue, 11 microresidual foci of carcinoma, the remaining 12 as having gross residual tumor; this was radically resected in 4 cases, resected with macroscopic radicality although with unradical margins at microscopic evaluation in 3, and only explored in 5. Forty-one patients began their follow-up observation without clinical evidence of disease, 30 of them radically resected with tumor-free margins.

Overall, 66 patients had suffered a failure by the time of follow-up closure, November 30, 1996, in all cases but 1 within 4 years of time zero. Distant metastases as the only mo-

Table 3

Frequency of clinical responses

| Locoregional response | Distant metastases | | |
|---|---|---|---|
| | No | Yes | Total |
| CR | 10 | 0 | 10 |
| PR | 42 | 6 | 48 |
| SD | 11 | 2 | 13 |
| NE | 2 | 5 | 7 |
| PRO | 1 | 1 | 2 |
| Total | 66 | 14 | 80 |

CR, complete response; PR, partial response; SD, stable disease; NE, non-evaluable; PRO, progression.

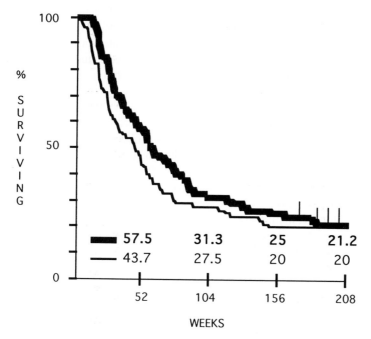

Fig. 1. Progression-free and observed (bold line) survival curves. Vertical marks indicate censored patients.

dality of first failure occurred in 23 patients, locoregional progression in 19, and a combination of the two in 5. The site of first failure remained undetermined in 3 cases. One patient had a new primary. Failures not due to cancer had surgery as the main cause (7 cases). Acute massive hemoptysis killed 3 unresected patients without clinical evidence of disease at 26, 56 and 77 weeks. Two patients died of myocardial infarction, and one of pulmonary edema. One patient died of acute massive bleeding due to a gastric peptic ulcer. One patient who was excluded from surgery at our institution for high risk, was submitted to a left pneumonectomy at another hospital but died in the postoperative period due to respiratory insufficiency. The overall progression-free and observed survival curves are shown in Fig. 1. The median time to progression was 47 weeks. The median observed survival was 59 weeks. Histology did not show any appreciable impact on prognosis. The main features of the 14 currently surviving and disease-free patients consist of a previous resection (11 cases) and achievement of a pathological complete response (7 cases). Two survivors had violated the entry criteria. Observation of the 30 radically resected patients revealed 19 failures at the date of follow-up closure. Distant progression was detected in 6 cases, locoregional relapse in 3, and combined progression in 2. There were 5 deaths due to surgery, 2 due to myocardial infarction, and 1 due to pulmonary edema. The 4-year observed survival rate was 46.2% in this subset of patients.

## 4. Conclusions

The radioenhancement effects of CDDP have stimulated several clinical studies on the treatment of NSCLC, some of them utilizing low doses of CDDP [2,7–13]. The EORTC group [11] randomized 331 patients to receive 55 Gy in a 20-fraction, 6-week split-course of RT, or the same plus CDDP given in a weekly bolus dose of 30 mg/m$^2$ delivered on day 1 of each treatment week, or the same weekly dose fractionated in five administrations of 6 mg/m$^2$, given on each day of RT just before each fraction. This study is of particular interest since it assessed not only the impact of CDDP administration, but also the dose fractionation of this drug, whose delivery at repeated low doses significantly improved the outcome due to a better locoregional control. An overall positive trend in favor of combined therapies was seen.

Extreme hyperfractionation of the CDDP dose, as is obtained with continuous infusion, should allow further improvement both of the radioenhancement effect and the therapeutic index [14–17]. Our group has been investigating this field in the clinical setting since 1988 [2]. Our first phase II trial on 38 patients consisted of 50 Gy in a 7-week split-course of 25 fractions given in 5 weeks plus concurrent weekly CDDP doses of 30 mg/m$^2$ given as a 120-h infusion [12]. Due to its main features, this schedule could be roughly considered as the 4th arm of the aforementioned EORTC study. We gave a split-course of radiation treatment which is far from an optimal schedule, to limit the dose intensity of CDDP and the related toxicity, and to allow therapy to be administered in a full outpatient basis. A high rate (80%) of locoregional objective responses was observed. Surgery was introduced as adjuvant treatment in half of the patients. A pathological complete response was observed in one case. Toxicities were mild to moderate, in contrast to the non-negligible toxicities observed in the EORTC study. These results induced us to optimize the design of the RT schedule by adopting a continuous-course. Moreover, our own observations allowed us [2] to lower the dose of CDDP. These choices form the basis of the design of the study object of the present chapter.

The adopted schedule of treatment was well manageable in the outpatient setting, and the overall frequency of grade 3 acute toxicity was low, namely 5%. The most relevant adverse reaction, esophagitis, was due to RT. A reliable analysis of late toxicities was not feasible; about 70% of the patients dropped out for evaluation due to resection or short-term death, within 1 year of time zero. However, we did not observe any case of late toxicity at sites other than the lung. We did not see any cases of severe symptomatic fibrosis or pneumonitis, or respiratory insufficiency, although some patients required temporary delivery of low-dose steroids. Most of the patients had chest films showing faint or moderate shadowing without distortion of anatomy in the follow-up period. Three unresected patients died due to acute massive hemoptysis in the follow-up period, with no evidence of persistent disease at a recent restaging. We were not able to assess if these cases of bronchovascular fistulas were due to late effects of treatment.

Surgery was feasible following a chemoradiotherapy schedule in which the radiation treatment had features of a radical treatment in terms of doses, fractionation and portals. To our knowledge no other experiences have been reported in this field. Surgery allowed us to verify that the clinical post-treatment staging has poor predictability, underestimating the true extent of response. Moreover, surgery rendered roughly one-fifth of the initial 80 patients disease-free, and established itself as a significant feature in long-term survivors. However, it can "a posteriori" be considered as an overtreatment in slightly less than one-half of the operated patients in view of their achievement of a true complete response with radiochemotherapy only, and in a further one-fifth submitted to non-radical surgery. The right pneumonectomies weighed heavily upon the surgical mortality and formed an unacceptable risk. This observation prompted us to avoid resection if a right pneumonectomy was needed, when extensive intraoperative biopsies did not prove persistence of disease. New means of predictive post-treatment restaging are needed.

This treatment showed a surgically proven high activity. No viable tumor was detected in the specimens of 15 resected patients (18.75%), or in those of a further 4 (5%) submitted to extensive intraoperative biopsies at all disease sites diagnosed by pretreatment staging. We did not find any other experiences with preoperative RT ± chemotherapy reporting such a high rate of pathological complete responses in the literature. We believe that this is a strong argument in favor of the radioenhancement effects of CDDP given concurrently in continuous infusion. A clinical study on the pharmacokinetics of CDDP delivered according to this schedule was subsequently undertaken by our group. It was pointed out that the plasma concentrations of the ultrafilterable platinum were in the order of magnitude of those required for achieving radioenhancement effects in vitro. These data are currently under consideration for publication.

One further argument supporting the effectiveness of this treatment schedule comes from the observation of a low rate of locoregional progression as the first modality of failure. In fact the overall rate of patients developing locoregional failure, alone or combined with distant progression, was 30%. This result can be explained by the efficacy of the chemoradiotherapy in itself and by the application of adjuvant resection in about one-half of the patients.

In conclusion, radical RT can be safely combined with concurrent low-dose continuous infusion of CDDP, resulting in a low-toxicity treatment of high activity. Surgery can improve the rate of complete responses, but its role needs refinement. This treatment is worthy of a phase III study.

## Summary

The current treatment of locally advanced non-small-cell lung carcinoma is radical radiotherapy. However, only 5% or less of the patients achieve long-term survival, locoregional failure being the main cause of death. Radiotherapy and infusional cisplatin as a radioenhancer to improve the locoregional control, were delivered to 80 stage III patients in a phase II study, in which surgery was used as adjuvant treatment. A total of 50 Gy were administered (daily doses of 2 Gy, given 5 days a week). Continuous infusion of cisplatin (daily dose 4 mg/m$^2$) was started before each first weekly radiotherapy fraction and suspended after the last. The rate of grade 3 toxicities was 5%. The locoregional response rate was 72.5%. Five exploratory thoracotomies, 7 right pneumonectomies, and 26 other operations were performed. There were 7 postoperative deaths (5 after a right pneumonectomy). Nineteen operated patients were assessed as having no viable tumor. The median disease-free and observed survival were 47 and 59.5 weeks. Locoregional failure occurred in 24 patients. The 4-year survival was 21.1%. Radical radiotherapy combined with cisplatin in continuous infusion was a low-toxicity treatment of high activity. Adjuvant surgery was feasible, but the risk of the right pneumonectomy was unacceptable. The rate of locoregional progression was low, probability due to the efficacy of the chemoradiotherapy in itself and the application of an adjuvant resection in half the patients. However, the role of surgery needs refinement. This treatment is worthy of a phase III study.

# References

1. Saunders MI, Bennet MH, Dische S, et al. Primary tumor control after radiotherapy for carcinoma of the bronchus. Int J Radiat Oncol Biol Phys 10: 499–501, 1984.
2. Bedini AV, Tavecchio L, Milani F, et al. Prolonged venous infusion of cisplatin and concurrent radiation therapy for lung carcinoma. A feasibility study. Cancer 67: 357–362, 1991.
3. Mountain CF. A new international staging system for lung cancer. Chest 89(Suppl): 225–232, 1986.
4. Tisi GM, Friedman PJ, Peters RM, et al. Clinical staging of primary lung cancer. Am Rev Respir Dis 127: 659–669, 1983.
5. Miller AB, Hoogstraten B, Staquet M, Winkler A. Reporting results of cancer treatment. Cancer 47: 207–214, 1981.
6. Oken MM, Creech RH, Tormey DC, et al. Toxicity and response criteria of the Eastern Cooperative Oncology Group. Am J Clin Oncol 5: 649–655, 1982.
7. Van Harskamp G, Boven E, Vermorken JB, et al. Phase II trial of combined radiotherapy and daily low-dose cisplatin for inoperable, locally advanced non-small cell lung cancer (NSCLC). Int J Radiat Oncol Biol Phys 13: 1735–1738, 1987.
8. Soresi E, Clerici M, Grilli R, et al. A randomized trial comparing radiation therapy vs radiation therapy plus cis-dichlorodiammine platinum (II) in the treatment of locally advanced non-small cell lung cancer. Semin Oncol 6(Suppl 7): 20–25, 1988.
9. Ellerbroek N, Fossella FV, Rich TA, et al. Low-dose continuous infusion cisplatin combined with external beam irradiation for advanced colorectal adenocarcinoma and unresectable non-small cell lung carcinoma. Int J Radiat Oncol Biol Phys 20: 351–355, 1991.
10. Trovò MG, Minatel E, Franchin G, et al. Radiotherapy versus radiotherapy enhanced by cisplatin in stage III non-small cell lung cancer. Int J Radiat Oncol Biol Phys 24: 11–15, 1992.
11. Schaake-Koning C, van den Bogaert W, Dalesio O, et al. Effects of concomitant Cisplatin and radiotherapy on inoperable non-small-cell lung cancer. N Engl J Med 236: 524–530, 1992.
12. Bedini AV, Tavecchio L, Milani F, et al. Non-resectable stage IIIa-b lung carcinoma: a phase II study on continuous infusion of cisplatin and concurrent radiotherapy (plus adjuvant surgery). Lung Cancer 10: 73–84, 1993.
13. Blanke R, Ansari R, Mantravadi R, et al. Phase III trial of thoracic irradiation with or without cisplatin for locally advanced unresectable non-small cell lung cancer: a Hoosier Oncology Group protocol. J Clin Oncol 13: 1425–1429, 1995.
14. Lokich JJ. Phase I study of cis-diamminnedichloroplatinum (II) administered as a constant 5-day infusion. Cancer Treatment Rep 64: 905–908, 1980.
15. Patton TF, Himmelstein KJ, Belt R, et al. Plasma levels and urinary excretion of filterable platinum species following bolus injections and iv infusion of cis-dichlorodiamminoplatinum (II). Cancer Treatment Rep 62: 1359–1362, 1978.
16. Reece PA, Stafford I, Abbott RL, et al. Two- versus 24-hour infusion of cisplatin: pharmacokinetic considerations. J Clin Oncol 7: 270–275, 1989.
17. Vermorken JB, van der Vijgh WJF, Klein I, et al. Pharmacokinetics of free and total platinum species after rapid and prolonged infusions of cisplatin. Clin Pharmacol Ther 39: 136–144, 1986.

C.J. Rosenthal and M. Rotman (Eds.), *Infusion Chemotherapy–Irradiation Interactions*
269

# CHAPTER 27

# Chemoradiation for gynecological cancers

## MADHU J. JOHN

*University of California, San Francisco, Radiation Oncology Services, Kaweah Delta Cancer Care Center, Visalia, CA and The Cancer Center at Saint Agnes, Fresno, CA, USA*

## 1. Introduction

The efficacy of chemoradiation in improving cure rates and its use in organ preservation in several solid tumors in humans has not been duplicated yet in gynecological cancers. There are several reasons for this. In cervical cancer, the cure rates with conventional radiotherapy (RT) or surgery are excellent, particularly with early stage disease which comprises the vast majority diagnosed in this country. The innumerable "promising" chemoradiation studies involve a heterogeneous population including early stage patients with "poor prognostic features" in whom the impact of chemoradiation would be difficult to prove since they already have higher cure rates. In ovarian cancers and papillary endometrial cancers, chemoradiation in concurrent mode has simply not been attempted in light of the whole abdominal RT fields required or the relative inefficacy of drugs available for these cancers. Finally, cancers of the vagina, vulva, advanced cancer of the cervix and papillary endometrial cancers are infrequent to the point that large phase III protocols are just not practical in this country.

Yet the basic rationale for chemoradiation in general holds true for several gynecological cancers. The cure rates for Stage III and IVA ovarian cancer, traditionally treated with surgery and chemotherapy in this country, has not essentially changed in the last 20 years. Locally advanced cervical cancer conventionally treated with RT alone has had stagnant cure rates since the advent of megavoltage RT 40 years ago. The culture of our times has persuaded all of us to address quality of life issues and its corollaries of organ and function preservation. Thus, we seek alternatives to the radical surgeries used in the treatment of the vagina and vulva. And then we have the population of elderly patients with co-morbid conditions that preclude definitive surgery as a treatment option. It is incumbent on us to find alternate means to treat these medically challenged patients effectively and chemoradiation might be one such option to allow them a decent chance for cure.

## 2. Cervical cancer

### 2.1. Current standard management

The standard combination of external beam RT and intracavitary brachytherapy (BT) was established about 4 decades ago for locally advanced cervical cancers (ACC). Despite investigations exploring a multitude of adjuvant treatment options to RT, none have shown conclusively to be superior to the standard combination of RT + BT. Several reasons can be cited for this apparent lack of improvement in cure rates: (1) The universally accepted FIGO staging system is a clinical one that does not incorporate variables as important as tumor bulk and lymph node involvement. Thus a wide variation in study populations may subvert comparative studies – even randomized ones. (2) In studies of ACC, patients with Stage IIB with cure rates of 60–75% are lumped together with patients with more advanced stages of III and IVA (cure rates of 0–50%) particularly in developed countries where the latter group is a relatively rare population. Even Stage IIB patients are a heterogeneous group with a wide range of prognostic factors including unilateral versus bilateral parametrial involvement shown by multivariate analysis to be a highly significant variable [1]. (3) Even though local tumor control is the principal focus of most of these studies, it is apparent that especially in Stage III and IVA the incidence of distant metastases alone or in conjunction with local failure is a prominent feature of disease recurrence.

## 2.2. Rationale for chemoradiation

The reasons for the continued investigation of combining RT and chemotherapy in ACC are as follows: (1) Despite an apparent improvement (50% at 5 years) in cure rates in a few small multi-institutional studies, and in major treatment centers, larger multi-institutional and multi-national studies show cure rates between 0–30% for Stage III and IVA cervical cancer (Table 1) [1–6]. (2) Chemotherapy appears to be the most facile and available modality in developing countries where this cancer reaches endemic or epidemic proportions. (3) A fairly large number of newer systemic agents with activity against cervical cancer are now available but have not yet been tested in chemoradiation protocols to any significant degree (paclitaxel, interferon, ifosfamide). (4) The theoretical and practical importance of addressing latent systemic disease cannot be addressed by modalities that focus on increasing local control (hyperthermia, neutron beam RT, radiosensitizers). (5) Sub-populations of patients with clinically early disease have been established to have poor outcomes with standard treatment (very bulky Stage I or II cervical cancer, Stage IIB patients with bilateral parametrial disease). (6) The sheer number of "promising" phase II chemoradiation studies inspite of wide variations in RT and chemotherapy dose, suggest that the definition of optimal intensity and quality of chemoradiation regimens should be the central aim of future protocols.

Table 1

Selected series depicting actuarial rates for Stage III and IVA cervical cancer treated by radiotherapy alone

| Series | No. of patients | 5 year survival (%) | Major toxicity (%) |
|---|---|---|---|
| 1. Medical Research Council, UK [2] | 148 | 23 | 4 |
| 2. Patterns of Care, USA [1,3] | 259 | 24[a,b] | 14 |
| 3. Duke University [4] | 203[b] | 33[b] | 5 |
| 4. Mallinckrodt Institute of Radiology [5] | 313 | 30 | 10–14 |
| 5. Kottmeier (World Average) [6] | >500 | 28 | NS |

NS, not stated.
[a]Four-year overall survival.
[b]Stage III only.

## 2.3.  Chemoradiation for ACC

Aside from tumor volume or bulk, which is considered in all quarters to be the single most important prognostic variable, a large number of factors have been independently associated with poor outcome. These include histological features of adenocarcinoma, poorly differentiated squamous cancers, small cell cancer, lymphovascular and perineural invasion and endometrial extension, host factors such as anemia, poor performance status, anatomical constraints that preclude adequate brachytherapy and the so-called yWACC syndrome (the younger woman with aggressive cervical cancer). Only some of these factors have been shown unequivocally to be poor prognostic factors and they relate variably to overall response to treatment, specific response to RT, a high local recurrence rate or distant metastatic rate. Stage IIB disease represents a wide range of tumors, some with minimal volume, few of the above poor prognostic features and a high cure rate of 60–75% and others with greater tumor volumes and more of the above poor prognostic features and a cure rate of 40–60%. Since most studies do not stratify their Stage IIB patients according to these variables, we deal here with studies relating to Stage III and IVA disease alone. In these patients the stagnant cure rates over four decades makes modest improvements in outcome worthwhile.

The chemoradiation experience with Stage III and IVA cervical cancers can be categorized into neoadjuvant and concurrent groups. A large number of reports have published their experience with the use of various combinations of drugs followed by definitive RT. While these combinations have achieved complete response rates and the overall response rates of 0–50% and 10–100%, respectively, none have resulted in superior eventual outcome compared to RT alone. Indeed, several randomized prospective studies comparing RT alone versus sequential chemotherapy followed by RT have not shown any significant improvement in disease-free and actuarial survival [7–11], very much like the experience with head and neck cancers. One of the largest trials, reported by Tattersall et al., showed a significantly improved local control and survival with standard RT compared to neoadjuvant epirubicin and cisplatin followed by standard RT [9].

The experience with concurrent chemotherapy and RT and be categorized into four groups:

1.  *The Hydrea Trials*: The concurrent use of hydroxyurea and RT introduced by Hreshchyshyn was investigated subsequently in several randomized studies by Piver et al and by the Gynecology Oncology Group (GOG) [12–14]. Some of these studies used subgroup analysis and did not present outcomes related to randomization. Nevertheless, the GOG has accepted the hydroxyurea + RT combination as the standard treatment for ACC against which other regimens are tested. In any case, none of these trials ever showed chemoradiation with hydroxyurea to be superior to RT alone in Stage III and IVA patients.

2.  *Radiation Therapy Oncology Group (RTOG) studies*: The RTOG combined with the Northern California Oncology Group initially presented the results of treating 38 patients (27 patients with Stage III) with a combination of 5-fluorouracil (5-FU) + mitomycin C and 5-FU + cisplatin concurrently with pelvic RT and BT [15]. A 2-year survival rate of 63% was noted in this group with a 11% incidence of grade 3 non-hematalogic toxicity. An additional 60 patients with similar disease were treated with minor adjustments of RT and chemotherapy in a second phase II trial. The mature 5-year actuarial survival for Stage III and IVA patients in this group was 39% [16]. The

RTOG has recently completed accrual to a randomized study comparing patients treated for ACC by concurrent 5-FU + cisplatin and RT versus patients treated with pelvic and para-aortic RT only.

3.  *The Princess Margaret Series*: Thomas et al. reported on a series of patients with cervical cancer treated with concurrent 5-FU and RT with and without mitomycin C [17]. The 3-year survival for 99 patients with Stage III and IV disease was 42%. A significantly increased incidence of bowel toxicity found an multivariable analysis to be attributable to mitomycin C alone, although a variety of RT doses, fractions and field sizes were used.

4.  *Miscellaneous Concurrent Chemoradiation Trials*: The vast majority of concurrent chemoradiation trials for ACC have used the combinations of 5-FU and mitomycin C or 5-FU and cisplatin with RT based on the successful experience with anal and esophageal cancers using the same combinations. These are generally single institution studies reporting early results and concluding that more follow-up data are required and that prospective studies should be conducted [18]. At this writing, no prospective randomized trial comparing standard RT versus RT with concurrent 5-FU + cisplatin/ mitomycin C have been reported in direct contrast to the large number of trials conducted with sequential chemoradiation.

## 2.4. Discussion

Table 1 shows the survival rate for Stages III and IVA cervical cancer treated by RT alone from larger published studies. The Patterns of Care statistics relate to 163 institutions throughout the United States and reflects the "true situation" in this country rather than single large institution results. There is no reason to believe that cure rates for advanced cervical cancer have improved in recent years. In fact, according to the National Cancer Institute's Surveillance, Epidemiology, and End Results (SEER) program, the overall 5-year survival rate for cervical cancers has remained unchanged from 1974 (when the original Patterns of Care study was undertaken) to 1992 [19]. Moreover, it continues to be the most common female cancer and the most common cancer-related cause of death (male or female) in many developing countries [20].

Table 2 depicts a selection of studies combining various chemotherapies concurrently with RT in Stages III and IVA cervical cancers [13,16,17,21–23]. Large studies, let alone randomized ones, are hard to come by. Large randomized studies have only studied sequential chemoradiation and these have uniformly shown no advantage compared to RT alone [18]. The studies depicted in Table 2 show a wide range of responses and 3–5-year survival data, but major toxicity to be on par with the experience of RT alone. The RTOG multi-institutional study combining 5-FU + mitomycin C + cisplatin with RT doses in the lower range of accepted standards, yielded a low incidence of major complications and perhaps a modest increase in 5-year survival over RT alone in historical cohorts [16].

So where do we go from here? It is true that the "gold standard" of treatment of ACC remains a combination of external RT and BT. It is also true that the large number of tantalizing Phase II studies using a concurrent combination of chemotherapy and irradiation makes chemoradiation the most likely modality to become the new standard for ACC. There are reasons for optimism. Newer drugs which are active against cervical cancer and are known to have radio-additive effects are now available. Paclitaxel, ifosfamide and interferons have shown significant activity against cervical cancer both in in vitro and in vivo

Table 2

Selected series depicting actuarial survival rates for Stages III and IVA cervical cancers treated by concurrent chemoradiation

| Series | No. of patients | Drugs | 5 year survival (%) | Major toxicity (%) |
|---|---|---|---|---|
| 1. RTOG 85–15 [16] | 30 | MPF | 39 | 5 |
| 2. Princess Margaret [17] | 99 | F ± M | 42[a] | 7–22 |
| 3. Heaton et al. [21] | 29 | FP | 65[b] | 4 |
| 4. Ludgate et al. [22] | 38 | FM | 71[c] | 5 |
| 5. Fields et al. [23] | 28 | P | 60[d] | NS |
| 6. GOG [13] | 53 | H | 47 | 8 |

M, mitomycin C; P, cisplatin; F, 5-fluorouracil; H, hydroxyurea. NS, not stated.
[a]Three-year survival.
[b]Median follow up 29 months.
[c]Median follow up 20 months.
[d]Median follow up 65 months.

studies [24–26]. They are currently being tested in Phase I and II trials in combination with RT by major cooperative groups. The combinations of "old and "new" drugs have been shown to have excellent response rates superior to their individual activity in ACC [26]. For example, the combination of ifosfamide and cisplatin yielded a 62% response rate in patients with advanced and metastatic cervical cancer [27]. The combination of etoposide, ifosfamide/mesna and cisplatin have shown a 57% complete response rate sustained for 7 to 24 months in advanced and metastatic cervical cancer [28].

With current resources, one way to proceed would be to test several combinations of effective chemotherapy combinations (which are also radio-additive) in a chemoradiation course in patients with Stage III and IVA cervical cancers. For example, the combinations of 5-FU + cisplatin, cisplatin + taxol, 5-FU + mitomycin C or etoposide + ifosfamide/mesna + cisplatin, could be distributed through a course of external RT and BT. The advantages of such combinations over the use of a single combination, say 5-FU + cisplatin repeatedly through irradiation, are the potential for preventing the development of resistant phenotypes, for a broad range of cell kill in a heterogeneous tumor and for preventing overlapping toxicities that might otherwise prolong treatment time.

If such a chemoradiation combination is found to be feasible, effective and with acceptable toxicity, one could then move on to a randomized prospective trial comparing RT alone versus the chemoradiation regimen described above. This study should include Stage III and IVA patients only and avoid the considerable inhomogeneities found in Stage IIB patients. The study should be conducted in collaboration with centers of excellence in countries where ACC is endemic, such as in South America and Asia. This would ensure that a large numbers of patients can be accrued into the protocol and modest survival improvements of 5–10 % over standard treatment would be more easily evident. Finally, if a difference is indeed shown by this randomized trial in favor of chemoradiation, one could then proceed to use the combination in other patient groups, such as Stage IIB patients with bilateral parametrial involvement, "bulky" Stage IB patients, patients with endometrial extension of cervical cancer and patients with the yWACC syndrome.

## 3.  Cancer of the vulva

### 3.1.  Current standard management

The traditional treatment of vulvar carcinoma has been radical vulvectomy and bilateral inguinal node dissection [29,30]. Over the last 2 decades attempts have been made to use treatment methods that reduce morbidity, sexual dysfunction and urinary incontinence. FIGO Stage I patients now frequently undergo limited resection with wide local excision or modified radical vulvectomy with lymph node dissections instead of radical vulvectomy. For Stage II disease, as well, the standard treatment of radical vulvectomy and inguinal node dissection has been replaced by modified vulvectomy with a negative pathological margin. For Stage III disease, radical vulvectomy and postoperative inguinal mode irradiation is the treatment of choice where as pelvic exenteration is the standard treatment for Stage IVA and recurrent cancer patients.

The cure rates achieved by radical surgery for Stage I and II are 70 and 49%, respectively, whereas for Stages III and IV vulvar cancer the cure rate is 30% and 8%, respectively [6]. With recent improvements in surgical techniques and perhaps due to earlier diagnosis and patient awareness, these cure rates may have increased in all stages [19,29].

### 3.2.  Rationale for chemoradiation

Vulvar cancers occur most frequently in women in the 7th decade of life. These women are frequently afflicted by medical conditions that preclude a definitive surgical approach. Secondly, the morbidity of radical vulvectomy and/or inguinal node dissection can be considerable. Side-effects include wound dehiscence, lymphedema, urinary stress incontinence and psychosexual sequelae [30,31]. Patterns of failure following radical surgery are difficult to ascertain considering the variation in patient population and treatment methods. Nevertheless, an overall 20% local recurrence rate and a 25% rate of pelvic and distant metastases have been described [32].

The impressive results of chemoradiation in other solid tumors such as the anal cancer and esophagus have given impetus to a number of investigators to attempt combined modality in lieu of radical surgery or pre-operatively to minimize the extent of surgery in vulvar cancer [33–43]. Several of these studies suggest that chemoradiation would provide equal or better local control compared to historic cohorts.

Thus, the rationale for the use of chemoradiation in advanced vulvar cancers is to provide an alternative to radical surgery for Stage I and II patients who are medically inoperable or those who fail locally after surgery. In addition, it may provide an alternative to radical surgery with reduced sequelae but without reduction in cure rates achievable by surgery. It also appears to have the potential to increase local control and survival in patients with more advanced Stage III and IVA disease.

### 3.3.  Chemoradiation experience

Most of the studies employing chemoradiation in vulvar cancer have used the concurrent approach. Two studies employing neoadjuvant chemotherapy and chemoradiation are of interest. First, an Italian study described 21 patients with Stage IVA vulvar cancer treated with cisplatin, bleomycin and methotrexate prior to surgery [44]. The 3-year survival rate

Table 3

Selected series of patients with vulvar carcinoma treated with chemoradiation

| Author | No. of patients | Drugs | RT dose (Gy) | DFS% | Followup median (months) | Severe toxicity (%) (grades 4 + 5) |
|---|---|---|---|---|---|---|
| Thomas [36] | 24 | FM | 51 | 54 | 20 | 22 versus 7 ± mitomycin C |
| Berek [39] | 12 | FP | 44–54 | 84[a] | 37 | 0 |
| Russell [40] | 25 | FPM | 54 | 56 | 24 | Less severe than anticipated |
| Koh [41] | 20 | FPM | 54 | 49 (5 years) | NS | 5 |

F, 5-fluorouracil; M, mitomycin C; P, cisplatin. NS, not stated.
[a]Two patients salvaged by surgery.

was 24%. Almost 50% of patients failed locally, persuading the investigators to add RT in their next trial.

Yet another Italian trial described prospectively treating 58 patients with 54 Gy RT delivered in split course fashion combined with 5-FU and mitomycin C followed by limited surgery including wide local excision and inguinal lymphadenectomy. The severe toxicity rate was 10% and there were 3 early deaths. The actuarial 2-year survival rate was 36% [43].

Table 3 describes selected reports of concurrent chemoradiation in vulvar cancers [36, 39–41]. In general, most patients included in these series had Stage III or IV disease or were considered medically inoperable. As in cervical cancer, most series employed 5-FU and mitomycin C or 5-FU and cisplatin. The RT dose ranged from 44 to 54 Gy. Aside from the experience of Thomas et al. who described a 22% incidence of severe bowel toxicity attributable to mitomycin C, severe toxicity rate was acceptable.

### 3.4. Summary

A large number of single institution pilot studies have described the feasibility and efficacy of concurrent chemoradiation in vulvar cancers. With increasing attention to quality of life issues, such as organ preservation and psychosexual aspects, chemoradiation is being increasingly used as definitive treatment or as a prelude to limited surgery. A current prospective Phase II RTOG study will evaluate the feasibility of definitive chemoradiation in patients with clinically negative groin nodes and the value and feasibility of chemoradiation given post-operatively to patients with positive groin nodes who have undergone superficial groin node dissection.

## 4. Cancer of the ovary

### 4.1. Background

Ovarian cancer is the leading cause of death from a gynecological malignancy in the United States. It is generally treated by surgical extirpation followed by combination chemotherapy or abdomino-pelvic irradiation. The 5–10-year cure rates for early stage patients varies from 60 to 80%; for patients with advanced disease the cure rates range from 10 to 30% [45]. Overall, the 5-year survival rates are between 10 and 35% because most patients present with advanced (Stage III and IV) disease. These figures have remained essentially unchanged for over 20 years inspite of improvements in surgical technique and in the delivery of radiotherapy and chemotherapy.

There are several variables that are responsible for these poor cure rates. The volume of residual disease following cytoreductive surgery is the most powerful predictor of treatment success or failure. Other less important variables included tumor grade, stage, patient age, and histological type [46]. A meta-analysis of 9 reports on Stage III ovarian cancers shows that when no gross residual tumor was present after surgery, the cure rate was about 65%; in patients with smaller residual tumors (<2 cm), the survival rates were about 35% and with larger residual tumors (>2 cm), the cure rate was 18%. In Stages III and IV patients, optimal tumor resection to <2 cm is possible only in about 30% of patients [47]. Even in patients achieving an apparent complete remission following cisplatin-based chemotherapy, about 60% are found to have residual disease at second-look laparotomy [48].

Most protocols for ovarian cancer consist of initial debulking surgery followed by cisplatin-based chemotherapy followed by a second surgical effort and culminating in a course of whole abdominal RT. In fact, the National Comprehensive Cancer Network (NCCN) in its publication of guidelines for the treatment of ovarian cancer recommended the above schema in general [49]. However, the emphasis was on paclitaxel–cisplatin combination both for initial chemotherapy, as well as following second-look surgery. Despite the fact that paclitaxel–cisplatin combinations may be superior to previously used cisplatin-based chemotherapy, it appears unlikely to impact long term survival significantly in patients with Stage III and IV ovarian cancers.

## 4.2. Chemoradiation experience

Early experience with chemoradiation was obtained when whole abdominal radiotherapy (WAR) was used as "salvage" therapy for patients who failed cisplatin-based chemotherapy. A moving-strip technique was used with relatively large fractions of RT resulting in severe marrow toxicity, radiation enteritis, and often early discontinuation of radiotherapy [50]. This RT delivery was changed to an open-field technique with low doses per fraction. Kong et al reported on 21 patients treated with an open-field technique and hyperfractionation with 100 cGy twice daily, 6 h apart to a total of 3000 cGy and a 1500 cGy pelvic boost. Treatment was well tolerated with one patient unable to complete the prescribed dose [51].

Inspite of establishing a safe method of RT delivery, the results in terms of disease eradication were essentially unchanged. Fuks noted in a meta-analysis of 23 studies, that if tumor residual of >1 cm was present at second surgery, additional RT was quite useless – just as intraperitoneal chemotherapy or second-line chemotherapy would be [45]. The reasons for these disappointing results are felt to be probably due to the prolonged delivery of chemotherapy and the development of multi-drug cross resistance and cross resistance between cisplatin and radiotherapy. The development of cross resistance between drugs and radiation was confirmed by subsequent in vitro studies [52, 53].

Table 4

Chemoradiation strategies for ovarian cancer

| | | | | |
|---|---|---|---|---|
| A. Chemotherapy (short, intensive 1–2 cycles, cytokines) | → | Surgery | → | Chemoradiation (concurrent, reduced RT and CT doses, radioprotectors, intense hematological support) |
| B. Surgery | → | Chemoradiation | → | Maintenance chemotherapy (alternating non-cross resistant drugs) |

## 4.3.  Suggested chemoradiation strategies

Based on the experience to date and some of the lessons learned in the treatment of other solid tumors, a few basic tenets can be drawn for future chemoradiation protocols. Two potential strategies are outlined in Table 4.

With regard to radiotherapy, the use of hyperfractions with low dose per fraction and the technique of open fields is mandatory. Regarding chemotherapy it would be best to use two or more effective combinations in alternating fashion, e.g. one paclitaxel-based chemotherapy regimen with another platinum-based combination. If chemotherapy is used sequentially than it should be dose intensive but with only 1 or 2 cycles immediately prior to surgery.

Preferably WAR should be used simultaneously with chemotherapy. This may entail the use of even lower individual RT fractions, lower total abdominal and pelvic dose, lower doses of chemotherapy and hematological support with prophylactic use of cytokines if necessary.

## 5.  Conclusions

Chemoradiation in the treatment of locally advanced gynecological cancers serves a three-fold purpose: to increase cure rates compared to surgery or radiotherapy alone; to allow for anatomic and function preservation; and to offer a reasonable chance for cure to those women whose general condition does not allow for extensive surgical treatment.

Locally advanced cancer of the cervix is best treated with radical radiotherapy but cure rates have remained static for several decades. A host of phase II studies employing various combinations of drugs and concurrent RT have yielded compelling but inconclusive results. The availability of newer effective drugs makes it likely that this avenue of investigation will be pursued further, at least in the near future.

For cancers of the vulva the primary reason to use chemoradiation is to avoid the considerable morbidity that is associated with the standard treatment of radical vulvectomy. Inspite of its low incidence, multiple small reports on the feasibility and efficacy of chemoradiation in vulvar cancer have appeared in the literature. It appears likely that chemoradiation alone or with limited surgery will become the new standard of therapy for locally advanced vulvar cancer in the near future.

The management of ovarian cancer remains an enigma. The use of post-operative chemotherapy or whole abdominal RT has not yielded any improvement in survival in the last two decades due to several reasons. The incorporation of the radio-additive drug, paclitaxel, into treatment protocols for this disease holds some promise. Yet for Stages III and IV ovarian cancer, the prospects appear dismal unless a drastic re-thinking in strategy is made.

## References

1. Lanciano RM, Won M, Hanks GE. A reappraisal of the International Federation of Gynecology and Obstetrics staging system for cervical cancer. A study of Patterns of Care. Cancer 69: 482–487, 1992.
2. Watson ER, Halnan KE, Dische S, et al. Hyperbaric oxygen and radiotherapy: a Medical Research Council trial in carcinoma of the cervix. Br J Radiol 51: 879–887, 1978.
3. Hanks GE, Herring DF, Kramer S. Patterns of care outcome studies - results of the national practice in cancer of the cervix. Cancer 51: 959–967, 1983.
4. Montana GS, Fowler WC, Varia MA, et al. Carcinoma of the cervix. Results of radiation therapy. Cancer 57: 148–154, 1986.
5. Perez CA. Uterine cervix. In: Perez CA, Brady LW (Eds), Principles and Practice of Radiation Oncology, 2nd edn. Philadelphia, PA: Lippincott, pp. 1143–1202, 1992.
6. Kottmeier HL, Kolstad P, McGarrity KA, et al. (Eds). Annual Report on the Results of Treatment in Gynecological Cancer, Vol 18. Stockholm: International Federation of Obstetrics and Gynecology, 1982.
7. Chauvergne J, Rohart J, Heron JF, et al. Randomized phase III trial of neoadjuvant chemotherapy (CT) + radiotherapy (RT) vs. RT in Stage IIB, III carcinoma of the cervix (CACX): a comparative study of French Oncology Centers. Proc Am Soc Clin Oncol 7: 136, 1988.
8. Souhami L, Gil RA, Allan SE, et al. A randomized trial of chemotherapy followed by pelvic radiation therapy in Stage IIIB carcinoma of the cervix. J Clin Oncol 9: 970–977, 1991.
9. Tattersall M H, Lorvidhaya V, Vootiprux V, et al. Randomized trial of epirubicin and cisplatin chemotherapy followed by pelvic radiation in locally advanced cervical cancer. Cervical Cancer Study Group of the Asian Oceanian Clinical Oncology Association. J Clin Oncol 13: 444–451, 1995.
10. Sundfor K, Trope CG, Hogberg T, et al. Radiotherapy and neoadjuvant chemotherapy for cervical carcinoma. Cancer 77: 2371–2378, 1996.
11. Leborgne F, Leborgne JH, Doldan R, et al. Induction chemotherapy and radiotherapy of advanced cancer of the cervix: a pilot study and phase III randomized trial. Int J Radiat Oncol Biol Phys 37: 343–350, 1997.
12. Hreschyshyn MM. Hydroxurea with irradiation for cervical carcinoma - a preliminary report. Cancer Chemother Rep 52: 601, 1968.
13. Piver MS, Barlow JJ, Vongtama V, Webster J. Hydroxyurea and radiation therapy in advanced cervical cancer. Am J Obstet Gynecol 120: 969, 1974.
14. Stehman FB, Bundy BN, Thomas G, et al. Hydroxyurea versus misonidazole with radiation in cervical carcinoma: long-term follow-up of a Gynecology Oncology Group trial. J Clin Oncol 11: 1523–1528, 1993.
15. John M, Flam M, Sikic B, et al. Preliminary results of concurrent radiotherapy and chemotherapy in advanced cervical carcinoma: a phase I-II prospective intergroup NCOG and RTOG study. Gynecol Oncol 37: 1–5, 1990.
16. John M, Flam M, Caplan R, et al. Final results of a phase II chemoradiation protocol for locally advanced cervical cancer: RTOG 85–15. Gynecol Oncol 61: 221–226, 1996.
17. Thomas G, Dembo A, Fyles A, et al. Concurrent chemoradiation in advanced cervical cancer. Gynecol Oncol 27: 446, 1990.
18. John M, Flam M. Gynecologic system. In: John M, Flam M, Legha S, Phillips T (Eds), Chemoradiation: an Integrated Approach to Cancer Treatment. Philadelphia, PA: Lea and Febiger, pp. 374–383, 1993.
19. Kosary CL, Ries LA, Miller BA, et al. (Eds). SEER Cancer Statistics Review 1973–1992: Tables and Graphs. National Cancer Institute, NIH Publication No. 96: 2789, Bethesda, MD, 1995.
20. Herrero R. Epidemiology of cervical cancer. Monogr Natl Cancer Inst 21: 1–6, 1996.
21. Heaton D, Yordan E, Reddy S, et al. Treatment of 29 patients with bulky squamous cell carcinoma of the cervix with simultaneous cisplatin, 5-fluorouracil and split-course hyperfractionated radiation therapy. Gynecol Oncol 38: 323–327, 1990.
22. Ludgate S, Crandon A, Hudson C, et al. Synchronous 5-fluorouracil, mitomycin C and radiation therapy in the treatment of locally advanced carcinoma of the cervix. Int J Radiat Biol Phys 15: 893–899, 1988.

23.   Fields AL, Anderson, PS, Goldberg, GL, et al. Mature results of a phase II trial of concomitant cis-platin/pelvic radiotherapy for locally advanced squamous cell carcinoma of the cervix. Gynecol Oncol 61: 416–422, 1986.

24.   Lippman SM, Kavanagh JJ, Paredes-Espinoza M, et al. 13-cis-Retinoic acid plus interferon alpha-2a: Highly active systemic therapy for squamous cell carcinoma of the cervix. J Natl Cancer Inst 84: 241–245, 1992.

25.   Angioli R, Sevin B, Perras JP, et al. Rationale of combining radiation and interferon for the treatment of cervical cancer. Oncology 49: 445–449, 1992.

26.   Thigpen T, Vance R, Khansur T, Malamud F. The role of paclitaxel in the management of patients with carcinoma of the cervix. Semin Oncol 24: S2-41–S2-46, 1997.

27.   Cervellino JC, Araujo CE, Sanchez O, et al. Cisplatin and ifosfamide in patients with advanced squamous cell carcinoma of the uterine cervix. Acta Oncol 34: 257–259, 1995.

28.   Kredentser DC. Etoposide (VP-16), Ifosfamide/Mesna and cisplatin chemotherapy for advanced and recurrent carcinoma of the cervix. Gynecol Oncol 40: 145–148, 1991.

29.   Hoskins WJ, Perez CA, Young RC. Gynecologic tumors. In: DeVita VT Jr, Hellman S, Rosenberg SA (Eds). Cancer: Principles and Practice of Oncology, 4th edn. Philadelphia, PA: Lippincott, pp. 1152–1225, 1993.

30.   Di Saia PJ, Creasman WT. Clinical Gynecologic Oncology, 4th edn. St Louis, MO: Mosby, pp. 238–272, 1993.

31.   Anderson HL, Hacker WP. Psychosexual adjustment after vulvar surgery. Obstet Gynecol 62: 457–462, 1983.

32.   Corn BW, Lanciano RM. Combined modality treatment for carcinomas of the uterine cervix and vulva. Curr Opin Oncol 6: 524–530, 1994.

33.   Kalra JK, Grossman AM, Krumholz BA, et al. Preoperative chemoradiotherapy for carcinoma of the vulva. Gynecol Oncol 12: 256, 1981.

34.   Levin W, Goldberg G, Altaras M, et al. The use of concomitant chemotherapy and radiotherapy prior to surgery in advanced stage carcinoma of the vulva. Gynecol Oncol 25: 20, 1986.

35.   Evans LS, Kersh CR, Constable WC, et al. Concomitant 5-fluorouracil, mitomycin C, and radiotherapy for advanced gynecologic malignancies. Int J Radiat Oncol Biol Phys 15: 901, 1988.

36.   Thomas G, Dembo A, DePetrillo A, et al. Concurrent radiation and chemotherapy in vulvar carcinoma. Gynecol Oncol 34: 263, 1989.

37.   Carson LF, Twiggs LB, Adcock LL, et al. Multimodality therapy for advanced and recurrent vulvar squamous cell carcinoma. J Reprod Med 35: 1029, 1990.

38.   Roberts WS, Hoffman MS, Kavanagh JJ, et al. Further experience with radiation therapy and concomitant intravenous chemotherapy in advanced carcinoma of the lower female genital tract. Gynecol Oncol 43: 233, 1991.

39.   Berek JS, Heaps JM, Fu YS, et al. Concurrent cisplatin and 5-fluorouracil chemotherapy and radiation therapy for advanced-stage squamous carcinoma of the vulva. Gynecol Oncol 42: 197, 1991.

40.   Russell AH, Mesic JB, Scudder SA, et al. Synchronous radiation and cytotoxic chemotherapy for locally advanced or recurrent squamous cancer of the vulva. Gynecol Oncol 47: 14, 1992.

41.   Koh WJ, Wallace JH III, Greer BE. Combined radiotherapy and chemotherapy in the management of local-regionally advanced vulvar cancer. Int J Rad Oncol Biol Phys 26: 809, 1993.

42.   Wahlen SA, Slater JD, Wagner RJ, et al. Concurrent radiation therapy and chemotherapy in the treatment of primary squamous cell carcinoma of the vulva. Cancer 75: 2289–2294, 1995.

43.   Landoni F, Maneo A, Zanetta G, et al. Concurrent preoperative chemotherapy with 5-fluorouracil and mitomycin C and radiotherapy (FUMIR) followed by limited surgery in locally advanced and recurrent vulvar carcinoma. Gynecol Oncol 61: 321–327, 1996.

44.   Benedetti-Panici P, Greegi S, Scambia G, et al. Cisplatin (P), bleomycin (B) and methotrexate (M) preoperative chemotherapy in locally advanced vulvar carcinoma. Gynecol Oncol 50: 49–53, 1993.

45.   Fuks Z. Ovarian cancer. In: Horwich A (Ed), Combined Radiotherapy and Chemotherapy in Clinical Oncology. London: Edward Arnold, pp. 165–182, 1992.

46.   Dembo AJ, Bush RS. Choice of post-operative therapy based on prognostic factors. Int J Radiat Biol Phys 8: 893–899, 1982.

47.   Beilinson JL, Lee KR, Jarell MA, McClure M. Management of epithelial ovarian neoplasms using platinum based regimen. A 10 year experience. Gynecol Oncol 37: 66–73, 1990.

48.    Fuks Z. Questioning current policies for the curative management of ovarian carcinoma. Israel J Med Science 24: 572–579, 1988.
49.    NCCN Ovarian Cancer Practice Guidelines. Oncology 10: S293–310, 1996.
50.    Peters WA, Blaski JC, Bagley CM, et al. Salvage therapy with whole abdominal irradiation in patients with advanced carcinoma of the ovary previously treated by combination chemotherapy. Cancer 58: 880–882, 1986.
51.    Kong JS, Peters LJ, Wharton, JT, et al. Hyperfractionated split course whole abdominal radiotherapy for ovarian carcinoma: tolerance and toxicity. Int J Radiat Oncol Biol Phys 14: 1–7, 1988.
52.    Louie KG, Behrens BC, Kinsella, TJ, et al. Radiation survival parameters of antineoplastic drug-sensitive and resistant human ovarian cancer cell lines and their modification by buthionine sulphoximine. Cancer Res 45: 2110–2115, 1985.
53.    Rotmesch J, Schwartz JL, Atcher RW, et al. The inherent cellular radiosensitivity of epithelial ovarian carcinoma. Gynecol Oncol 35: 282–285, 1989.

C.J. Rosenthal and M. Rotman (Eds.), *Infusion Chemotherapy–Irradiation Interactions*

# CHAPTER 28

# Multimodality treatment for adult advanced soft tissue sarcomas: results of combined radio-chemotherapy

RAFFAELLA PALUMBO[1,2], FAUSTO BADELLINO[1,3],
GIUSEPPE CANAVESE[1,3] and SALVATORE TOMA[1,2]

[1]*National Institute for Cancer Research, Largo Rosanna Benzi, n. 10, 16132 Genova, Italy,* [2]*Department of Experimental and Clinical Oncology, University of Genova, Genova, Italy and* [3]*Division of Surgical Oncology, National Institute for Cancer Research, Genova, Italy*

## 1. Introduction

The optimal treatment of advanced soft tissue sarcomas (STS) remains a challenge for the multidisciplinary approach in modern oncology, in view of both adequate local control and prevention of distant metastases. In fact, primary tumors are often large and invade the locomotor system, while blood-borne distant metastases are present at the time of diagnosis in most cases. Surgery, when feasible, remains essential as first line treatment of STS, but anatomic location and/or local invasiveness often prevent radical resection. In addition, patients with high-grade, large tumors and recurrent local disease are at high risk for developing distant metastases; despite optimal local control, 40–60% of patients with STS die within 5 years, due to metastatic disease, predominantly in the lung and liver. At the present time, the advanced and/or metastatic stage of disease does not allow an option for curative treatment, the intention of systemic chemotherapy (CT) or potentially adequate radiotherapy (RT) being only palliative.

During the past two decades, multimodality approaches in advanced STS have been extended. Chiefly, limb-sparing protocols have progressed, becoming the treatment of choice for most STS of the extremities, which represent about 60% of all STS, while new treatment modalities (e.g., isolated limb perfusion and intraarterial CT) have entered clinical trials. Combined schedules have taken several forms: CT alone, RT alone, or a combination of the two. In the following review theoretical hypothesis and clinical evidences underlying the development of integrated strategies in STS are reported, in order to give a focus on the actual role of combined radio-chemotherapy treatment in advanced and/or metastatic disease.

## 2. Preoperative and postoperative radiotherapy

The routine use of radiation therapy (RT) in treatment of STS is relatively recent, being essentially used in an adjuvant setting. Adjuvant RT after limb-sparing surgery has largely improved local control [1–8], but treatment-related toxicity remains a major problem. In 1982 a first randomized trial compared conservative limb-sparing surgery and RT with amputation, showing no effect of local failure (15% in the conservative arm) on overall survival [3]. A comparable survival time for advanced sarcoma patients treated with limb preservation versus amputation has been further demonstrated from retrospective studies and randomized trials [5–10]. These results suggested that no clear relationship exists between local control and distant recurrence. This issue remains controversial, most explicitly so in low-grade STS [11–13].

Preoperative RT alone has also been used in STS; with regimens generally involving 50–60 Gy delivered over 5–6 weeks, a 5-year local control rate of 86% has been reported, being very much lower in larger tumors [14–16]. A more recent report from Massachusetts General Hospital (Boston, MA) on 132 consecutive patients with unresectable extremity STS treated with preoperative RT followed by surgery showed no importance of the surgical margins on the local control rate (97% and 82%, respectively, for 104 tumors with negative margins and 28 tumors with positive margins). In this study, one of the major problems resulted that of increased morbidity due to difficult wound healing [17].

## 3. Preoperative and postoperative chemotherapy

The strategy of systemic CT has been integrated in the multidisciplinary approach of advanced STS either before (neoadjuvant) or after (adjuvant) locally curative treatment, mainly in order to eradicate distant micrometastases thought to be present at the time of diagnosis. Studies of preoperative CT without RT are few, but generally disappointing, with poor local control and limb salvage rates. Some benefit has been suggested in patients with bulky STS, because formerly inoperable cases were rendered operable [18–21]. Only 40% response rate has been achieved with doxorubicin-based preoperative CT, and local recurrence rates up to 34% have been reported when the regimen was combined with conservative surgery [20]. Preoperative CT alone appears to offer the unique advantage of determination of in vivo sensitivity to chemotherapeutic agents; patients responding to neoadjuvant CT have longer survival times than do those who do not respond, but a satisfactory limb-salvage rate cannot be achieved [19,20].

As far as adjuvant CT in STS is concerned, the available results are clearly controversial. Even if two recent meta-analysis suggested that some patients may benefit from postoperative CT [22–23], most of the 15 published randomized trials are too small or take too much time because of slow accrual. On the whole, these studies failed to demonstrate a significant impact of CT on overall survival, while showing an advantage in terms of disease-free survival or decreased local recurrence rate [24]. A maximal combined approach in patients with unfavorable sarcomas has recently been reported, which combined an intensive pre- and postoperative chemotherapeutic regimen with surgery and RT; the results are not different from those of historical controls [25]. At present, adjuvant CT should be recommended only in the setting of a clinical controlled trial.

## 4. Combined radio-chemotherapy

The approach of combined CT with RT in a preoperative setting was pioneered by the group at the University of California. In two consecutive trials, Eilber and co-workers combined preoperative intraarterial doxorubicin (30 mg/day for 3 consecutive days) with 35 Gy in

350 cGy fractions over 10 days in patients with sarcoma of the extremity. In their early experience, a total of 77 patients with high-grade, advanced extremity STS were treated, 96% of whom were able to have limb-salvage surgery (74/77). Local recurrences were observed in 4% of patients, and overall survival rate was 76% at a median follow-up of 32 months [26]. However, a high treatment-related complication rate was detected (35% of cases, 17% of whom required further surgical procedures). Thus, following RT dosages were decreased to 17.5 Gy and ultimately modified in 8 fractions of 28 cGy; in the additional 105 patients treated, local recurrence occurred in 8% of patients, and the amputative surgery rate was reduced to 2.8% [27].

Similar experiences, with minor variations in dosing and RT schedules, have also been published, with relatively short follow-ups [28–31]. In general, it appeared that the use of larger fractions of RT, in association with CT, improved local control, but was associated with increased normal tissue toxicity.

To date, controversies remain regarding some major issues in similar combined approaches in the advanced stage of disease, such as the appropriate fraction size and the timing of RT in relation to surgery. The report of Levine et al. is unique regarding the timing of RT relative to surgical resection [32]. This study evaluated a 10-day preoperative regimen of intraarterial doxorubicin (10 mg/m$^2$ per day) with concomitant RT (25 Gy in 10 daily fractions over 2 weeks); adjuvant RT was administered in all patients whose margins were considered "close", using 180 cGy fractions, 5 days per week. The low rate of reported local recurrences (4%) in the whole group support a role for such a "sandwich" approach; on the other hand, the 25% local failure in patients only given preoperative RT suggested that the dose of 2.500 cGy, administered with concomitant intraarterial doxorubicin, was inadequate therapy to an optimal local control. In addition, complications related to the intraarterial infusion were significant, occurring in 26% of patients, 7% of whom required additional surgery.

The benefit of intraarterial CT has been questioned [33]. Two randomized trials, one in STS and the other in osteosarcoma, failed to demonstrate a significant advantage for regional compared with systemic CT, in regard to limb salvage, local recurrences, and complications [34,35]. Therefore, we agree with Levine et al. that the role of intraarterial infusions as a part of multimodality treatment needs to be reconsidered [32].

## 5.  Concomitant chemo-radiotherapy

With the aim of a better therapeutic ratio, different concentrations and scheduling of drugs acting as radiosensitizers have been tested in advanced solid tumors; effective improvement in objective responses and survival have been obtained in relatively limited clinical experiences, such as advanced cancer of the head and neck, anus, esophagus, hepatic metastases of gastrointestinal and gynecologic tumors [36].

The rational of concomitant chemo-radiotherapy is based on spatial cooperation and synergistic effect between CT and RT, when used together. The aim is to improve both local control, enhancing RT activity, and distant subclinical metastases eradication, by early CT administration [37].

The concurrent use of anthracyclines and RT seemed to provide more than simply additive effects in different malignant tumors [38], suggesting synergistic activity between the two agents. A radiosensitivizing effect of doxorubicin, certainly the most active drug in advanced STS, has been shown by early experimental data on both animal and human cancer cells [39,40]. The mechanism of the radiosensitizing effect of doxorubicin is still a subject of speculation. Possible interactions concern an inhibition of mitochondrial respiration, as well as an improved oxygenation and radiosensitivity of the tumoral hypoxic cells [41]; an inhibition of enzymatic repair following RT has also been reported [42].

Despite the synergism between doxorubicin and RT in experimental systems, there have been only a few clinical trials of this combination.

The first clinical evidence of antitumor activity of such a regimen was obtained on patients with unresectable gynecologic cancers by Watring et al. in the early 1970s. The adopted schedule consisted of 6-weekly treatments of 13 mg/m$^2$ of intravenous doxorubicin followed by 200 cGy/day of supervoltage RT for 5 days. Four of the 5 treated patients responded to treatment, with moderate hematological toxicity [43]. A following controlled study tested the activity of doxorubicin alone versus doxorubicin–RT combination on 33 patients with advanced, inoperable esophageal cancer [44]. A significantly higher OR rate was observed in the combined treatment group (60% versus 33% of the group receiving the anthracycline alone). A longer response duration was also reported (8.6 months compared to 3.2 months, respectively).

As far as STS is concerned, a first experience was reported by Sordillo et al. in 1982; a series of 53 patients with advanced solid tumors was treated with five weekly injections of low-dose doxorubicin (total 60 mg/m$^2$), each followed in 90 min by RT (total dose of 2900 cGy over a 5-week period). In this preliminary report, the combined treatment gave best results in the group of patients with advanced and/or metastatic STS, producing an OR of 62% (18/29), with nearly absent toxicity [45]. An important observation was the lack of response to the low doses of doxorubicin in tumors located outside of the RT field, as well as the low response rate in patients given RT alone to other lesions, before or after the combined treatment. These data indicated the necessity of combining the two agents to achieve a significant response. A few years later, Turner et al. described an excellent response achieved in a patient with extensive, unresectable sarcoma of a lower limb, after six cycles of doxorubicin by continuous infusion and RT combination; the response obtained was maintained at a follow-up evaluation more than 7 years later [46].

The first important clinical experience with concomitant chemo-radiotherapy was in the late 1980s by Rosenthal and Rotman, who in a pilot study on patients with advanced solid tumors studied the kinetics of doxorubicin given by means of continuous infusion over 5 consecutive days [47]. A steady level of doxorubicin at 60 ng/ml for 100 h was obtained after administration of 60 mg/m$^2$ of the drug over 120 h, while a decline to 50% of the dose after giving the same dosage as an intravenous bolus was observed. Further, doxorubicin administered by continuous intravenous infusion for up to 96 h at a dose of 20 mg/m$^2$ had been previously found to have significantly less cardiotoxic effects [48].

Based on these data, the authors postulated that concomitant administration of low dose doxorubicin in continuous infusion with daily pulses of RT could improve the therapeutic index of these two modalities of treatment. Thus a doxorubicin dose of 12 mg/m$^2$ per day was chosen combined with concurrent RT (150 or 200 cGy/day daily session for trunk or extremity lesions, respectively) for 5 consecutive days, every 3 weeks. The treatment was feasible and active, producing an objective response rate (OR) of 73% on a small series of 11 patients with advanced or recurrent STS (4 complete and 4 partial responses). In addition, half of the hepatoma patients (2/4) who entered the study obtained a partial remission. The most significant results of this study were the lack of cardiac toxicity of doxorubicin protracted infusion, concomitantly with RT, and its radiation-enhancing effect in such a high percentage of sarcoma patients [49]. Remarkable was the fact that complete and partial responses were obtained with RT dosages ranging from 1500 to 3000 cGy, which are much lower than those usually used to produce similar results with RT alone; in addition, two of the responder patients had been previously irradiated on the same lesions.

The interesting therapeutic ratio obtained by Rosenthal and Rotman prompted us to further investigate the potential activity of a similar approach in patients affected with advanced STS.

The first step of our investigation was to verify the feasibility and activity of such a combined regimen in sarcoma patients. From 1988 to 1990, 17 patients with locally advanced and/or metastatic STS entered a phase II study. We adopted the treatment schedule previously described [47]. Doxorubicin was administered through portable infusion pumps (Multiday Infusor, 0.5 ml/h, Baxter Healthcare Corp., USA; CADD-1, 5100HFX, Pharmacia Deltec, St. Paul, MN, USA) connected to a central venous catheter (port-a-cath). Radiotherapy was given for 5 consecutive days, at a dose of 150 or 200 cGy/day, for trunk or extremity lesions, respectively, concomitantly with doxorubicin infusion. Cycles were repeated every 3 weeks. Treatment was given on an outpatient basis. An overall response rate of 46% was obtained on the 15 evaluable patients, with 1 complete and 6 partial responses, that reached 54% in the non-pretreated group and 75% in patients with better performance status (0–1 according to ECOG criteria). Toxicity was very low, and treatment well tolerated [50].

In the light of these results, we extended our study to evaluate the effectiveness of the tested regimen on a larger number of patients; concomitantly, an analysis of potential prognostic factors predictive of clinical response and survival was carried out. In 1994, we reported an OR rate of 53% on the enlarged series of 30 patients, with 2 complete and 14 partial remissions. Again, the pretreated patients (6 with CT and 4 with RT) had the lower percentage of ORs (33% versus 58% of the non-pretreated group). In addition, we confirmed that patients with better performance status showed a better response to treatment, compared to those with performance status $\geq 2$ (65% versus 14%). In all evaluable patients, the median survival time was 34 weeks (range 4–129), being 44 weeks in responders versus 24 weeks in non-responders; the pretreated group showed a median overall survival of 26 weeks. Neither treatment delay nor dose reduction was required due to side effects. Dose-limiting toxicity was acceptable, even in pretreated patients, and no sign of therapy-related hepatic or renal toxicity was observed. Especially, cardiotoxicity was nearly absent; only 2 patients, 1 of which was pretreated with anthracyclines, experienced temporary and reversible tachycardia [51].

This study confirmed our preliminary data on the effectiveness of a concomitant chemo-radiotherapy treatment, showing the possibility of achieving a good response rate (over 50%) in locally advanced and/or metastatic STS, with low overall toxicity. Thus, the chance of using both doxorubicin and RT at low doses seemed to be effective in improving the therapeutic index and raising the number of eligible patients.

Finally, in these last 3 years, our further investigation was focused on the possibility of a dose intensification of such a regimen, in an attempt to improve the OR rate and allow the possibility of further adequate surgery. In view of this end-point, we tested two possibilities: (1) to reduce the interval between two consecutive courses of treatment (every 2 weeks versus every 3 weeks in the previous experience), adding the use of granulocyte colony-stimulating factors ($200 \mu g/m^2$ per day, subcutaneously, from day 6 to day 10 of each cycle); (2) to associate other antineoplastic agents (e.g., intravenous ifosfamide or dacarbazine).

Table 1

Results of concomitant continuous infusion doxorubicin and radiotherapy in advanced soft tissue sarcomas

| Author | Year | Evaluable patients | Treatment | | Response | | | | | Response duration (weeks) | |
|---|---|---|---|---|---|---|---|---|---|---|---|
| | | | Doxorubicin | RT | CR | PR | MR | SD | OR (%) | Median | Range |
| Sordillo et al. [45] | 1982 | 29 | 20 mg/m²/day i.v.[a] weekly injection Over 5 weeks | 580 cGy weekly session[b] Over 5 weeks | 6 | 12 | 3 | 8 | 18/29 (62) | 22 | 1–52 |
| Turner et al. [46] | 1986 | 1 | 12 mg/m² per day c.i. days 1–5 Over 6 cycles | 5400 cGy days 1–5 Over 6 cycles | 1 | – | – | – | 1/1 (100) | 7 years | – |
| Rosenthal and Rotman [47] | 1988 | 9 | 12 mg/m²/day c.i. days 1–5 Every 3 weeks | 150 or 200 cGy/day[c] days 1–5 Every 3 weeks | 4 | 3 | – | 2 | 7/9 (78) | 38 | 18–204 |
| Rosenthal and Rotman [49] | 1991 | 11[d] | 12 mg/m² per day c.i. days 1–5 Every 3 weeks | 150 or 200 cGy/day[c] days 1–5 Every 3 weeks | 4 | 4 | – | 3 | 8/11 (73) | 41 | 18–204 |
| Toma et al. [50] | 1991 | 15 | 12 mg/m² per day c.i. days 1–5 Every 3 weeks | 150 or 200 cGy/day[c] days 1–5 Every 3 weeks | 1 | 6 | 6 | 2 | 7/15 (47) | 28 | 5–86 |
| Toma et al. [51] | 1994 | 30 | 12 mg/m² per day c.i. days 1–5 Every 2–3 weeks[e] | 150 or 200 cGy/day[c] days 1–5 Every 2–3 weeks | 2 | 14 | 6 | 8 | 16/30 (53) | 30 | 5–129 |
| Palumbo et al. [52] | 1996 | 35[d] | 12 mg/m² per day c.i. days 1–5 Every 2–3 weeks[e] | 150 or 200 cGy/day[c] days 1–5 Every 2–3 weeks | 3 | 17 | 8 | 11 | 20/35 (57) | 37 | 5–261 |

RT, radiotherapy; Doxo, doxorubicin; CR, complete response; PR, partial response; MR, minor response; SD, stable disease; i.v., intravenously; c.i., continuous infusion. [a]Total dose of 60 mg/m². [b]90 min after each dose of Doxo, total dose of 2900 cGy. [c]For trunk or extremity lesions, respectively. [d]The previous series is included. [e]With granulocyte colony-stimulating factor support, 200 $\mu$g/m² per day subcutaneously, from days 6 to 10.

In a recent update of our experience on 35 patients [52], we confirmed the activity of the tested regimen, reporting an OR rate of 57% (20/35, with 3 complete and 17 partial remissions). The ORs were obtained with median doxorubicin dose of 180 mg/m$^2$ (range 120–360) and median RT dose of 3000 cGy (range 2000–6000). An accelerated CT/RT schedule with granulocyte colony-stimulating factor support did not increase overall toxicity. After 2–3 cycles of treatment, 13 responder patients underwent surgery, which was radical in all but one case. At a median follow-up of 36 months (range 15–96), the median survival time was 12 months in the whole group of patients (range 2–61) and 22.2 months in the 19 responders (range 4.6–61), reaching 38 months in patients who underwent radical surgery. We would underline that in no case did the preoperative regimen compromise further adequate surgery.

In the extended prognostic factors analysis, the achievement of an objective response was found to have an impact on median overall survival. A suggestion emerged that a regimen dose intensification might allow a better probability of clinical response (82% ORs in the 2-week schedule versus 69% in the 3-week schedule). Clearly, due to the small series studied, no definitive conclusion can be drawn.

On the contrary, no evident improvement in treatment response was observed in the small series in which CT/RT regimen was combined with intravenous ifosfamide (1.2 g/m$^2$ per day, for 5 consecutive days) or dacarbazine (200 mg/m$^2$ per day, over 5 consecutive days), while increased overall toxicity occurred.

In conclusion, our experience shows that concomitant CT/RT regimen is active and well tolerated in STS, also in advanced/metastatic and pretreated disease. The extended follow-up data confirm our preliminary observations: OR rate of 46% in the preliminary trial, 53% in the extended study, and 57% in the updated series. Overall, previous data and our own experience (Table 1) suggest that a similar combined approach produces a percentage of ORs ranging from 47% to 78%, which seems to be better than that obtained with more aggressive polychemotherapeutic schedules; in advanced/metastatic disease, anthracycline-based regimens produce OR rates ranging from 22% to 42%, with significant overall toxicity [53–58]. Specifically, in our investigation, the possibility of a radical surgical approach after the combined schedule emerged as a significant issue.

Two important aspects need to be additionally underlined: the feasibility of a similar treatment in an outpatient regimen, with no required hospitalization due to toxicity, which suggests a satisfactory cost/benefit ratio; good patient compliance to the adopted system of CT delivery by portable infusion pumps, which focuses on the quality of life issue.

In our opinion, concomitant chemo-radiotherapy regimen appears to be a useful approach in sarcoma patients, in both primary tumors, when adequate surgery is the major goal, and advanced/metastatic disease, in which systemic CT or potentially therapeutic RT remain palliative in intent.

The usefulness of this chemo-radiotherapy approach in less advanced stages of disease (neo-adjuvant setting) deserves further investigation; its actual role in multimodality strategies for STS needs to be verified through randomized controlled trials.

*Summary*

*Background:* The optimal treatment of advanced soft tissue sarcomas (STS) remains a challenge for the multidisciplinary approach in modern oncology, in view of both adequate local control and prevention of distant metastases. During the past two decades, multimodality approaches in advanced and/or metastatic STS have been extended. Combined schedules have taken several forms: chemotherapy (CT) alone, radiotherapy (RT) alone, or a combination of the two. *Methods:* The theoretical hypothesis and available clinical evidences underlying the development of integrated strategies in STS are reviewed; our own experiences, specifically focused on the actual role of combined CT-RT in advanced disease, are also presented. *Results:* Considered in the whole, previous data and our own experience suggest that concomitant CT-RT regimen is well tolerated and active in STS, also in advanced/metastatic and pretreated disease. The observed percentage of objective responses, ranging from 47% to 78%, seems to be better than that obtained with more aggressive polychemotherapeutic schedules. Specifically, in our investigation, the possibility of a radical surgical approach following the combined treatment emerged as a significant issue. *Conclusions:* Concomitant CT-RT regimen appears to be a useful approach in sarcoma patients, in both primary tumours, when adequate surgery is the major goal, and advanced/metastatic disease, in which systemic CT or potentially therapeutic RT remain palliative in intent. The usefulness of such an approach in less advanced stages of disease (neo-adjuvant setting) deserves further investigation; its actual role in multimodality strategy for STS needs to be verified through controlled clinical trials.

## References

1.  Eilber FR, Mirra JJ, Grant TT, et al. Is amputation necessary for sarcomas? A seven-year experience with limb-salvage. Ann Surg 192: 431–438, 1980.
2.  Lindberg RD, Martin RG, Romsdahl MM, et al. Conservative surgery and postoperative radiotherapy in 300 adults with soft tissue sarcomas. Cancer 47: 2391–2397, 1981.
3.  Rosenberg SA, Tepper J, Glatstein E, et al. The treatment of soft tissue sarcomas of the extremities: prospective evaluation of limb-sparing surgery plus radiation therapy compared with amputation and the role of adjuvant chemotherapy. Ann Surg 196: 305–315, 1982.
4.  Karakousis CP, Emrich LJ, Rao U, et al. Feasibility of limb-salvage and survival in soft tissue sarcomas. Cancer 56: 484–491, 1986.
5.  Suit HD. In: Pinedo HM, Verweij J (Eds), Treatment of Soft Tissue Sarcoma. Dordrecht: Kluwer, pp. 65–74, 1989.
6.  Williard WC, Hajdu SI, Casper ES, Brennan MF. Comparison of amputation with limb-sparing operations for adult soft tissue sarcoma of the extremity. Ann Surg 215: 269–275, 1992.
7.  Harrison LB, Franzese F, Gaynor JJ, Brennann MF. Long-term results of a prospective randomized trial of adjuvant brachytherapy in the management of completely resected soft tissue sarcomas of the extremities and superficial trunk. Int J Radiat Oncol Biol Phys 27: 259–265, 1993.
8.  Pisters PWT, Harrison LB, Woodruff JM, et al. A prospective randomized trial of adjuvant brachytherapy in the management of soft tissue sarcomas of the extremities and superficial trunk. J Clin Oncol 12: 1150–1155, 1994.
9.  Keus RB, Rutgers EJTh, Ho Gortzak E, et al. Limb-sparing therapy of extremity soft tissue sarcomas: treatment outcome and long-term functional results. Eur J Cancer 30A: 1459–1463, 1994.
10. Dinges S, Budach V, Feldmann HJ, et al. Local recurrences of soft tissue sarcomas in adults: a retrospective analysis of prognostic factors in 102 cases after surgery and radiation therapy. Eur J Cancer 30A: 1636–1642, 1994.
11. Pisters PWT, Harrison LB, Leung DH, et al. Long term results of a prospective randomized trial evaluating the role of adjuvant brachytherapy in soft tissue sarcoma. J Clin Oncol 14: 859–868, 1996.
12. Heslin MJ, Woodruff J, Brennann MF. Prognostic significance of a positive microscopic margin in high-risk extremity sarcoma: implications for management. J Clin Oncol 14: 473–478, 1996.
13. Brennan MF. The enigma of local recurrence. Ann Surg Oncol 4: 1–12, 1997.

14.  Suit HD, Proppe KH, Mankin HJ, Woods WC. Preoperative radiation therapy for sarcoma of the soft tissue. Cancer 47: 2269–2274, 1981.

15.  Suit HD, Mankin HJ, Wood WC, Proppe KH. Preoperative, intraoperative and postoperative radiation in the treatment of primary soft tissue sarcoma. Cancer 55: 2659–2667, 1985.

16.  Tepper JE, Suit HD. Radiation therapy for soft tissue sarcomas. Cancer 55: 2273–2277, 1985.

17.  Sadosky C, Suit HD, Rosenberg A, et al. Preoperative radiation, surgical margins, and local control of extremities sarcomas of soft tissue. J Surg Oncol 5: 223–230, 1993.

18.  Lokich JJ. Preoperative chemotherapy in soft tissue sarcoma. Surg Gynecol Obstet 148: 512–516, 1979.

19.  Rouesse JG, Friedman S, Sevin DM, et al. Preoperative induction chemotherapy in the treatment of locally advanced soft tissue sarcomas. Cancer 60: 296–300, 1987.

20.  Pezzi CM, Pollock RE, Evans HL, et al. Preoperative chemotherapy for soft-tissue sarcomas of the extremities. Ann Surg 211: 476–481, 1990.

21.  Casali P, Pastorino U, Santoro A, et al. Epirubicin, ifosfamide, and dacarbazine (EID) combined with surgery in advanced soft tissue sarcomas (abstr.). Proc Am Soc Clin Oncol 10: 353, 1991.

22.  Zalupski MM, Ryan JR, Hussein ME, et al. Defining the role of adjuvant chemotherapy for patients with soft tissue sarcoma of the extremities. In: Salmon SE (Ed), Adjuvant Therapy of Cancer VII. Philadelphia, PA: JB Lippincott, pp. 385–392, 1993.

23.  Tierny JF, Mosseri V, Stewart LA, et al. Adjuvant chemotherapy for soft tissue sarcoma: review and meta-analysis of the published results of randomized clinical trials. Br J Cancer 72: 469–475, 1995.

24.  Gortzak E, van Coevorden F. Soft tissue sarcoma – messages from completed randomized trials. Eur J Surg Oncol 21: 469–477, 1995.

25.  Casper ES, Gaynor JJ, Harrison LB, et al. Preoperative and postoperative adjuvant chemotherapy for adults with high grade soft tissue sarcoma. Cancer 73: 1644–1651, 1994.

26.  Eilber FR, Morton DL, Eckardt J, et al. Limb salvage for skeletal and soft tissue sarcoma. Cancer 53: 2579–2584, 1984.

27.  Eilber FR, Giuliano AE, Huth J, et al. Limb salvage for high-grade soft tissue sarcomas of the extremity: experience at the University of California, Los Angeles. Cancer Treatment Symp 3: 49–57, 1985.

28.  Denton JW, Dunham WK, Slater M, et al. Preoperative regional chemotherapy and rapid-fraction irradiation for sarcomas of the soft tissue and bone. Surg Gynecol Obstet 158: 545–551, 1984.

29.  Goodnight JE, Bargar WL, Voegell T, Blaisdell FW. Limb-sparing surgery for extremity sarcomas after preoperative intraarterial doxorubicin and radiation therapy. Am J Surg 150: 109–113, 1985.

30.  Temple WJ, Russell JA, Arthur K, et al. Neoadjuvant treatment in conservative surgery of peripheral sarcomas. Can J Surg 32: 361–365, 1989.

31.  Wanebo H, Temple WJ, Popp MB, et al. Combination regional therapy for extremity sarcoma. Arch Surg 125: 355–359, 1990.

32.  Levine EA, Trippon M, Das Gupta TK. Preoperative multimodality treatment for soft tissue sarcomas. Cancer 71: 3685–3689, 1993.

33.  Bramwell VHC. Intraarterial chemotherapy of soft-tissue sarcomas. Semin Surg Oncol 4: 66–72, 1988.

34.  Eilber FR, Giuliano JF, Huth JF, et al. Intravenous (IV) vs intraarterial (IA) Adriamycin, 2800r radiation and surgical excision for extremity soft tissue sarcomas: a randomized prospective trial. Proc Am Soc Clin Oncol 9: 309, 1990.

35.  Winkler K, Bielack S, Delling G, et al. Effect of intraarterial versus intravenous cisplatin, in addition to systemic doxorubicin, high-dose methotrexate, and ifosfamide, on histologic tumor response in osteosarcoma. Cancer 66: 1703–1710, 1990.

36.  Rotman MZ. Chemoirradiation: a new initiative in cancer treatment. Radiology 184: 319–327, 1992.

37.  Vokes EE, Weihselbaum RR. Concomitant chemoradiotherapy: rationale and clinical experience in patients with solid tumors. J Clin Oncol 8: 911–934, 1990.

38.  Phillips TL, Fu K. Quantification of combined radiation therapy and chemotherapy effects on critical normal tissues. Cancer 37: 1186–1200, 1976.

39.  Byfield JE, Lee YC, Tu L. Molecular interactions between Adriamycin and x-ray damage in mammalian tumor cells. Int J Cancer 19: 186–193, 1977.

40.  Kimler BF, Loeper DB. The effect of Adriamycin and radiation on G cell survival. Int J Radiat Oncol Biol Phys 3: 1297–1300, 1979.

41.  Durand RE. Adriamycin: a possible indirect radiosensitizer of hypoxic tumor cells. Radiology 119: 217–222, 1976.

42. Byfield JE, Lynch M, Kulhaman F, et al. Cellular effects of combined Adriamycin and X irradiation in human tumor cells. Int J Cancer 19: 194–201, 1977.

43. Watring WG, Byfield JE, Lagasse LD, et al. Combination of adriamycin and radiation therapy in gynecologic cancers. Gynecol Oncol 2: 518–526, 1974.

44. Kolaric K, Maricic Z, Roth A, Dujmovic I. Adriamycin alone and in combination with radiotherapy in the treatment of inoperable esophageal cancer. Tumori 63: 485–491, 1977.

45. Sordillo PP, Magill GB, Schauer PK, et al. Preliminary trial of combination therapy with adriamycin and radiation in sarcomas and other malignant tumors. J Surg Oncol 21: 23–26, 1982.

46. Turner S, Shetty R, Gandhi H, et al. Combination of radiation with concomitant continuous Adriamycin infusion in a patient with partially excised pleomorphic soft tissue sarcoma of the lower extremity. In: Rosenthal CJ, Rotman M (Eds), Clinical Applications of Continuous Infusion Chemotherapy and Concomitant Radiation Therapy. New York: Plenum, 1986.

47. Rosenthal CJ, Rotman M. Pilot study of interaction of radiation therapy with doxorubicin by continuous infusion. Natl Cancer Inst Monogr 6: 285–290, 1988.

48. Legha S, Benjamin R, Mackay B, et al. Reduction of cardiotoxicity by prolonged continuous intravenous infusion. Ann Intern Med 96: 133–138, 1982.

49. Rosenthal CJ, Rotman M. Concomitant continuous infusion Adriamycin and radiation: evidence of synergistic effect in soft tissue sarcomas. In: Rotman M, Rosenthal CJ (Eds), Concomitant Continuous Infusion Chemotherapy and Radiation. Heidelberg: Springer-Verlag, pp. 271–280, 1991.

50. Toma S, Palumbo R, Sogno G, et al. Concomitant radiation-doxorubicin administration in locally advanced and/or metastatic soft tissue sarcomas: preliminary results. Anticancer Res 11: 2085–2090, 1991.

51. Toma S, Palumbo R, Grimaldi A, et al. Concomitant radiation-Doxorubicin administration in locally advanced and/or metastatic soft tissue sarcomas. In: Banzet P, Holland JF, Khayat D, Weil M (Eds), Cancer Treatment. An Update. Paris: Springer-Verlag, pp. 581–583, 1994.

52. Palumbo R, Grimaldi A, Canavese G, et al. Concomitant radio-chemotherapy at low doses in locally advanced and/or metastatic soft tissue sarcomas (STS): long-term followup. Ann Oncol 7: 117 (abstr 562P), 1996.

53. Borden EC, Amato DA, Rosenbaum C, et al. Randomized comparison of three Adriamycin regimens for metastatic soft tissue sarcomas. J Clin Oncol 5: 840–850, 1987.

54. Toma S, Palumbo R, Sogno G, et al. Doxorubicin (or epidoxorubicin) combined with ifosfamide in the treatment of adult advanced soft tissue sarcomas. Ann Oncol 3: 119–123, 1993.

55. Edmonson JH, Ryan LM, Blum RH, et al. Randomized comparison of doxorubicin alone versus ifosfamide plus doxorubicin or mitomycin, doxorubicin, and cisplatin against advanced soft tissue sarcomas. J Clin Oncol 11: 1269–1275, 1993.

56. Antman K, Crowley J, Balcerzak SP, et al. An intergroup phase III randomized study of doxorubicin and dacarbazine with or without ifosfamide and mesna in advanced soft tissue sarcomas. J Clin Oncol 11: 1276–1285, 1993.

57. Schutte J, Mouridsen HT, Steward W, et al. Ifosfamide plus doxorubicin in previously untreated patients with advanced soft tissue sarcoma. Eur J Cancer 26: 558–561, 1990.

58. Santoro A, Tursz T, Mouridsen H, et al. Doxorubicin versus CYVADIC versus Doxorubicin plus ifosfamide in first-line treatment of advanced soft tissue sarcomas: a randomized study of the European Organization for Research and Treatment of Cancer Soft Tissue and Bone Sarcoma Group. J Clin Oncol 13: 1537–1545, 1995.

# SECTION III

## FUTURE DIRECTIONS:
## MOLECULAR BIOLOGY ADVANCES – POTENTIAL CLINICAL
## APPLICATIONS TO CHEMO–RADIATION

- – Apoptosis Enhancement
- – Antiangiogenic Therapy
- – Gene Therapy
- – Suppressor Gene Repair

*"There are no such things as incurables; there are only things for which man has not found a cure."*

Bernard M. Baruch

C.J. Rosenthal and M. Rotman (Eds.), *Infusion Chemotherapy–Irradiation Interactions*
© 1998 Elsevier Science B.V. All rights reserved

# CHAPTER 29

# Apoptosis as a target for chemotherapeutic drug development

RUTH W. CRAIG and ALAN EASTMAN

*Department of Pharmacology and Toxicology, Dartmouth Medical School, Hanover, NH 03755-3835, USA*

## 1. Introduction

The phenomenon of cell death by apoptosis was meticulously documented more than 25 years ago by Wyllie et al. [1]. The term apoptosis derives from a Greek word used to describe "the dropping off or falling off, as petals from a flower or leaves from a tree". Apoptotic cell death can be contrasted to necrotic cell death; necrotic cell death is characterized by cell swelling followed by lysis of the cell membrane, and often occurs in response to external cell injury. On the other hand, apoptotic cell death is characterized by cell shrinkage and the degradation of internal cell components (e.g., by proteases and DNases), which occur prior to lysis of the cell membrane. Hallmarks of apoptosis include cell membrane blebbing, nuclear condensation/fragmentation, and DNA digestion into oligonucleosome-length fragments. Once initiated, the changes that typify apoptotic cell death proceed in a predetermined, stereotypic fashion, which is thought to be mediated through an internally coded molecular program. It is for this reason that apoptotic cell death has been referred to as an "internal cell suicide". Another prominent difference between apoptosis and necrosis is that necrosis generally elicits an inflammatory response, while little inflammation is seen in the case of apoptosis. This is because inflammatory stimuli are not released in apoptosis, since the cell degradation is contained within an intact cell membrane. In addition, in the intact animal, cells undergoing apoptosis can be engulfed by either neighboring cells or phagocytes, completely avoiding the release of cell contents. Because of the lack of inflammation and because apoptosis can occur rapidly (cells may be disposed of nearly completely within an hour or less), the only alteration seen in tissues undergoing rapid apoptosis may be a minute fraction of dying cells [2]. It is largely for this reason that the critical importance of apoptosis in many physiologic as well as pathologic processes has only been recognized relatively recently. Now that its importance has been recognized, research on this unique mode of cell death is moving forward at an explosive pace.

Apoptotic cell death can occur as part of the normal development of the organism, an example being the loss of the webs between the digits. Such instances of developmentally regulated apoptosis have been referred to as "programmed cell death". Another example of naturally occurring apoptosis is seen in the immune system, where large numbers of cells are generated but only a small fraction of these are useful and are retained, while the remainder undergo apoptosis [3]. Apoptosis also occurs in response to DNA damage, where activation of the internal apoptotic suicide program serves to prevent the propagation of potentially mutagenic or carcinogenic lesions [4–6]. A wide variety of chemotherapeutic drugs also cause cell death by apoptosis. While many of these drugs act on DNA (e.g., cisplatin) [7], even drugs that act at non-nuclear targets cause cell death by apoptosis (e.g., drugs that act on microtubules such as vinblastine and paclitaxel) [8–11]. Thus, a wide variety of currently used chemotherapeutic drugs are efficacious because they activate the normal apoptotic program in cancer cells [12,13]. When tumors exhibit resistance to therapy, it is frequently due to alterations in components of the apoptotic machinery, such as alterations in p53 or a BCL2 family member, that result in a diminished ability to activate apoptosis [14].

The genes and gene products that orchestrate the apoptotic program are beginning to be elucidated. These include genes in three general categories, (i) gene products involved in the initiation and transmission of signals for survival or death, (ii) gene products involved in regulating the cell death decision based on the signals received, and (iii) gene products involved in carrying out the cell death program. A schematic demonstrating the proposed relationship between these various types of gene products is shown in Fig. 1. The most downstream components in this scheme, the cell death effectors, include enzymes that degrade key cell components; these are primarily proteases of the caspase or interleukin-1$\beta$ converting enzyme (ICE) family. Upstream of these death effectors are the cell death regulators, the principal regulators characterized to date being members of the BCL2 family. Further upstream are a wide variety of signaling molecules, which may influence both the cell death regulators and the cell death effectors. Each of these categories of molecules contains potential targets for chemotherapeutic agents, as discussed in turn below. The cell death ef-

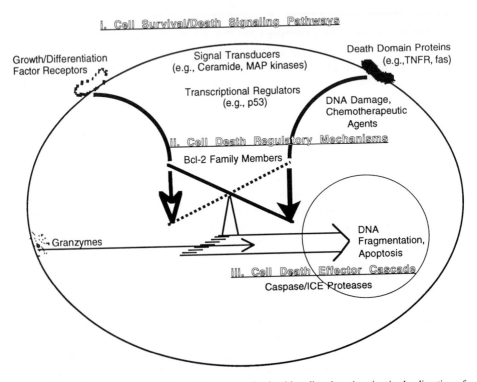

Fig. 1. The balance between cell survival and death can swing in either direction. A swing in the direction of cell death is represented as a clockwise swing (filled arrow on solid line). A swing in the direction of cell viability is represented as a counterclockwise swing (open arrow on dotted line).

fector portion of the pathway is covered first, as it represents conceptually the simplest phase of the apoptotic program.

## 2.   Cell death effectors: the caspase/ICE protease cascade

The role of the caspase/ICE protease family in apoptosis was discovered through the pioneering work of Horvitz et al. [15]. These investigators were interested in genes involved in programmed cell death in the nematode *Caenorhabditis elegans*, where the precise developmental timing of the death of individual cells has been well characterized. One of the genes involved, the *Caenorhabditis elegans* death gene 3 (ced3), proved to be a member of a unique family of cysteine proteases, the ICE family. The distinguishing characteristic of proteases in this family is that they carry out proteolytic cleavage immediately downstream of an aspartic acid (Asp) residue. The founding member of this family, ICE itself (now called caspase I for <u>c</u>ysteine <u>asp</u>artic acid <u>p</u>rotease I) [16] had previously been identified as the protease that activates interleukin-1$\beta$ through cleavages at Asp residues [17]. A growing number of additional members of this family have since been identified [18], one example being a protease termed CPP32 (also called caspase 3) [19,20]. Most of the caspases are themselves activated by proteolytic cleavages at Asp residues, in addition to causing such Asp cleavages in other proteins. Because of this, various members of the caspase family can activate other more downstream members, resulting in amplifying cascades of proteolyic cleavages [21]. A recent exciting development in this field is the discovery of the FLICE protease [22], which may be an "initiator" protease in the sense that it may lie at the beginning of one such cascade and may be subject to triggering through cell surface molecules such as the tumor necrosis factor receptor (TNFR) or the fas antigen. These death domain-containing proteins and their associated signaling molecules are reviewed by Cleveland and Ihle [23].

While the cleavage of interleukin-1$\beta$ itself probably does not have a role in apoptosis, a host of other substrates for these enzymes have been identified and these may more directly relate to apoptosis. Some of the known substrates include poly-ADP ribose polymerase (PARP) and lamins [24,25], although it is not known whether these or other as-yet unidentified substrates are critical for apoptosis. Proteolytic cleavage of lamin, for example, might be expected to compromise the structural integrity of the nucleus, contributing to the nuclear condensation seen during apoptosis. Activation of the caspase cascade is also associated with the activation of endonucleases. The latter carry out the DNA degradation that occurs in apoptosis, although exactly which nuclease(s) are involved and how they are activated remains in question [26–28].

Blockade of the caspase cascade results in inhibition of apoptosis [19,29]. Different caspases exhibit differences in the specificity of the site at which they cleave, principally differences in the three amino acid residues upstream of the conserved Asp. Based on this fact, inhibitors have been developed that differentially target different caspases. Thus, ICE can be inhibited by a small peptide derivative containing the four amino acid residues Tyr-Val-Ala-Asp (YVAD), while CPP32 can be inhibited a derivative containing the residues Asp-Val-Glu-Asp (DVED) [19]. Another similar small peptide (zVAD-FMK) appears to inhibit many caspase family members.

While the above peptide derivatives can inhibit apoptosis in cultured cell systems very effectively [29], it would be premature to assert that these, or other caspase inhibitors that might be developed, will be useful drugs. However, drugs capable of exerting antiapoptotic effects through inhibition of caspases may prove to have utility in the treatment of diseases involving inappropriately high levels of cell death. Examples might include neural degenerative disorders or myelodysplastic syndrome, the latter having recently been found to involve extensive cell death by apoptosis [30]. It would also be premature to attempt to predict whether such drugs could be made selective enough to affect cell death in the desired cells without causing other undesired side effects. On one hand, there appears to be considerable redundancy in the caspase system and disruption of a particular one of these proteases can have restricted effects on cell death [31–33]; this might suggest that broad specificity would be required for an effective inhibitor, which would in turn suggest an increased likelihood of side effects. However, the complexity of the web of proteases appears instead to present opportunities for selectivity. Thus, loss of a specific protease can effectively inhibit cell death stimulated by certain agents but not by others (e.g., targeted disruption of the ICE gene results in loss of the apoptotic response to stimulation of the fas antigen but not irradiation) [32]. In addition, loss of different proteases results in differential effects (e.g., targeted disruption of CPP32 results in prominent effects on apoptosis in the developing brain and early death of the organism, while targeted disruption of ICE does not result in a prominent developmental effect) [32,34]. Recent results indicate that inhibitors of CPP32 can inhibit death in neuronal cells, although factors beyond the inhibition of this specific protease may be involved [35]. Whether this type of inhibitor could be applied for human therapy is an open question. Overall, the caspase/ICE protease cascade represents a completely novel potential drug target; caspase inhibitors are extremely efficacious in model systems and it remains to be learned whether this approach can be exploited for therapeutic benefit.

## 3. Cell death regulators: the BCL2 family

Cell death can also be manipulated upstream of the caspase/ICE protease cascade [29,36, 37], at the level of the cell death regulators. These death regulators, principally members of the BCL2 gene family, can be visualized as functioning as a balance. On the one hand, this balance can swing towards death (represented as a clockwise swing in Fig. 1, filled arrow on solid line). Alternatively, the balance can swing towards viability (represented as a counterclockwise swing in Fig. 1, open arrow on dotted line).

The BCL2 family of cell death regulators contains an ever-increasing number of members [38–41], some of which promote cell death (e.g., BAX) [42] and others of which promote cell viability (e.g., BCL2, BCLX, MCL1) [43–47]. The mechanisms through which this family influences the caspase cascade and cell death are poorly understood. The various members of this family are the subject of intense current research [48–53], since an understanding of their mechanisms of action might have profound implications for the treatment, not only of diseases where cell death is accelerated, but also of diseases where cell death is inhibited. The most prominent example of the latter type of disease is cancer, where a more direct means of activating the death pathway (or inactivating inhibitors of this pathway) would represent a potentially very valuable therapeutic approach. Other diseases might include autoimmune disorders, which are thought to result from the persistence of lymphocyte clones that would normally have been eliminated. Inhibition of BCL2 expression (e.g., with antisense oligonucleotides) [54] is effective in causing death in cultured cancer cells. One reason that an analogous approach might prove to be clinically useful is that the BCL2 gene products complement the actions of proliferation-stimulating oncogenes such as MYC [46]. For example, only a fraction of BCL2 transgenic mice develop tumors and these tumors occur only after a long latency [55]; however, when BCL2 transgenic mice are crossed with mice that overexpress MYC, tumor development is synergistically accelerated [38]. When the MYC gene is expressed in the absence of BCL2, on the other hand, it can actually cause cell death [56,57]. Therefore, inhibition of the viability-promoting effects of genes such as BCL2 has the potential to cause rapid cell death in tumors that simultaneously overexpress proliferation-stimulating genes such as MYC and probably other oncogenes.

While the mechanism of action of the BCL2 family members is only beginning to be elucidated, several important properties of this family have been established. Much of what is known about the family is based on the ground-breaking work of Korsmeyer and colleagues, who first demonstrated that BCL2 inhibits apoptosis through an interaction with BAX [41,42]. This work has led to the hypothesis that the relative amount of BCL2 versus BAX determines cell viability; high levels of BAX relative to BCL2 are thought to promote BAX:BAX homodimerization and cell death, while high levels of BCL2 relative to BAX promote BCL2:BAX heterodimerization and cell viability. Although drugs capable of interfering with these interactions have not yet been described, such drugs could have tremendous therapeutic potential. For example, drugs might be designed that prevent BCL2:BAX heterodimerization (or BCLX:BAX or MCL1:BAX heterodimerization), thus freeing BAX for homodimerization and causing apoptosis. This strategy is similar to that used by the endogenous regulator BAD, another member of the BCL2 family, which can bind to BCLX and free BAX for homodimerization, promoting cell death [58] (discussed further below).

The structure of a viability promoting member of the BCL2 family, BCLX, has recently been solved [59]. Interestingly, the structure consists largely of alpha helices and is reminiscent of that of the pore-forming domains of bacterial toxins, which are capable of inserting into membranes to form pores or channels. Correspondingly, BCLX has recently been found to have ion channel activity in synthetic lipid membranes [60]. In a finding that may be related, BCL2 appears to prevent the increase in mitochondrial permeability that occurs during apoptosis [61,62], in keeping with the fact that BCL2 family members are localized in internal cell membranes such as the mitochondrial outer membrane [44,63–66]. Overall, a confluence of clues from different systems is beginning to suggest that BCL2 family members may act to affect the permeability of internal cell membranes. In fact, very recent findings also suggest that a novel apoptotic protease contained within the mitochondrial intermembrane space is released in response to apoptotic stimuli, release being inhibited by BCL2 [62]. Cytochrome *c*, which is also localized in the intermembrane space, is similarly released during apoptosis and its release is inhibited by BCL2 [49,67,68]. Although highly speculative, it is possible then that death promoting gene products such as BAX might promote the apoptosis-associated increase in mitochondrial permeability, which is reversed when BAX is complexed with BCL2 (or BCLX, MCL1, etc.). If this is a valid model, it might then be possible, in addition to interfering with the interaction between BCL2 family members, to directly target their pore/permeability functions.

As with the caspase inhibitors, research on the possibility of targeting BCL2 family members for therapeutic benefit is in its infancy. The different BCL2 family members exhibit considerable tissue- and differentiation stage-specificity of expression [39,69–72]. Nonetheless, one can anticipate the potential for problems of selectivity, since there are many complex interactions between different family members (e.g., BAX interacts with

BCL2, BCLX and MCL1) [41] and it is not clear whether one of these interactions could be inhibited to the exclusion of others. However, the structural basis for the interactions is beginning to be determined [73] and differences between the interactions are already beginning to be uncovered, such as the finding that BAD binds more tightly to BCLX than BCL2 [58]. In spite of potential problems, there is good reason to hope that further exploration of the BCL2 family as a potential therapeutic target will bear fruit. One reason is that drugs that target the gene products involved in cell death would invoke a mechanism different from that utilized by most chemotherapeutic agents, which generally inhibit proliferation. Such anti-viability drugs might then be useful in combination with traditional agents, where the different modes of action might yield additive or synergistic effects and possibly non-overlapping toxicities. Such drugs might also be useful for chronic phase or indolent cancers, for which little is presently available in terms of therapy. An example of such a cancer is follicular lymphoma with the t(14;18) chromosome translocation, where BCL2 was first discovered [74,75]. This lymphoma can remain at a non-aggressive indolent stage for an extended period of years before converting to an overt life-threatening malignant disease.

## 4. Pathways involved in initiating and transmitting signals for cell survival or death

Just as the BCL2 family can regulate the downstream caspase cascade, BCL2 family members can in turn be regulated by upstream pathways involved in the initiation and transmission of signals for cell viability or death. For example, many cell surface receptors involved in the stimulation of cell growth and differentiation also promote cell survival (Fig. 1). Other signaling pathways promote cell death, such as those initiated through death domain containing proteins such as the TNF receptor or the fas antigen [23]. This can be envisioned as a tilting of the balance in the clockwise direction, to allow the caspase effector cascade to proceed.

Although these signaling pathways are incompletely understood at present and probably involve a host of mechanisms, their effects appear in some cases to be mediated through effects on members of the BCL2 family. For example, BCL2 and BAD are subject to post-translational regulation by phosphorylation [8–10,76–78]. In the case of BAD, phosphorylation is promoted by interleukin-3, a growth factor required for cell survival. This phosphorylation prevents BAD from binding to and inhibiting the effects of BCLX, resulting in enhanced viability [78,79]. It is not known which enzymes mediate the phosphorylation of either BCL2 or BAD, although PKC and the raf protocogene might be involved [8,76, 77].

Some of the mediators in these cell survival/death signaling pathways are beginning to be identified. For example, the lipid mediator ceramide is known to promote cell death, although the mechanism of this effect is not known [80,81]. The MAP kinase family of proline-directed serine/threonine kinases also appears capable of having profound effects on cell viability. Thus, in neuronal PC12 cells, the balance between activation of two different branches of the MAP kinase family [the extracellular signal regulated kinases (ERKs) versus c-jun N-terminal kinase (JNK)] appears to determine whether cells live or die [82]. Inhibition of ERKs (by transfection with dominant-negative expression constructs) promotes death, while inhibition of JNK promotes viability. A chemical inhibitor exhibiting exquisite selectivity for the former as compared to the latter has already been identified [83].

Activation of cell signaling pathways frequently leads to effects on transcriptional regulators, which can then alter gene expression [84,85]. p53 is a well studied example of a gene product that is upregulated in response to cell death stimuli (e.g., DNA damage) [86] and can promote cell death by apoptosis [4]. p53 is mutated in a wide variety of tumor types, and presumably contributes to the cancer phenotype by allowing damaged cells to remain viable. Replacement of normal p53 function, if this were possible, might then have therapeutic value in many of the tumors that exhibit alterations in p53. Since recent data suggest that p53 may act through activation of BAX [53,87,88], one could consider the possibility of developing a therapy based on triggering BAX expression by an alternate means, bypassing the requirement for p53.

Finally, some cell death signaling pathways appear to circumvent the BCL2 cell death regulatory mechanisms, allowing for a more direct triggering of the caspase cascade. An example of this is cell death induced by cytotoxic T cells, which release proteolytic granzymes into the target cell [89]. Therapeutic exploitation of such a powerful mechanism has the potential of eliciting widespread cell death and thus undesirable side effects. However, if agents utilizing analogous mechanisms of action could be developed to specifically target tumor cells, they might be highly efficacious.

## 5. Conclusions

The process of cell death by apoptosis can be considered to proceed in three phases, being initiated through cell death signaling pathways, being regulated by members of the BCL2 family, and being carried out by the caspase/ICE protease cascade. The decision as to whether a cell lives or dies can be influenced at points within each of these phases. Each of these phases thus presents the potential for developing novel means for therapeutic intervention in diseases involving inappropriately low or inappropriately high rates of cell death.

## Summary

The gene products that control apoptotic cell death can be grouped into three general categories. These are (i) gene products involved in initiating or transmitting signals for cell survival or death, (ii) gene products involved in regulating the cell death decision based on the signals received, and (iii) gene products involved in carrying out the cell death program. The major genes in the latter category, the "cell death effectors", are proteases of the caspase (interleukin-1$\beta$ converting enzyme) family. Upstream of these proteases are the cell death regulators, principally members of the BCL2 family, which can either promote or inhibit the death effector pathway. Further upstream lie a wide array of cell death initiating/signaling pathways, which can modulate both the death regulators and the death effectors. Each of these categories of gene products represents a potentially valuable target for chemotherapeutic drug development.

## Acknowledgments

Ruth Craig is supported by grant #CA57359 from the National Cancer Institute.

# References

1.  Wyllie AH, Kerr JFR, Currie AR. Cell death: the significance of apoptosis. Int Rev Cytol 68: 251–305, 1980.
2.  Wyllie AH. Apoptosis. Br J Cancer 67: 205–208, 1993.
3.  McCarthy NJ, Smith CA, Williams GT. Apoptosis in the development of the immune system: growth factors, clonal selection and bcl-2. Cancer Metast Rev 11: 157–178, 1992.
4.  Kastan MB, Canman CE, Leonard CJ. p53, cell cycle control and apoptosis: implications for cancer. Cancer Metast Rev 14: 3–15, 1995.
5.  Kuerbitz SJ, Plunkett BS, Walsh WV, Kastan MB. Wild-type p53 is a cell cycle checkpoint determinant following irradiation. Proc Natl Acad Sci USA 89: 7491–7495, 1992.
6.  Lane DP. p53, guardian of the genome. Nature 358: 15–16, 1992.
7.  Demarcq C, Bunch RT, Creswell D, Eastman A. The role of cell cycle progression in cisplatin-induced apoptosis in Chinese hamster ovary cells. Cell Growth Differ 5: 983–993, 1994.
8.  Blagosklonny MV, Giannakakou WS, El-Deiry SE, et al. Raf-1/bcl-2 phosphorylation: a step from microtubule damage to cell death. Cancer Res 57: 130–135, 1997.
9.  Haldar S, Chintapalli J, Croce CM. Taxol induces bcl-2 phosphorylation and death of prostate cancer cells. Cancer Res 56: 1253–1255, 1996.
10. Haldar S, Basu A, Croce CM. Bcl2 is the guardian of microtubule integrity. Cancer Res 57: 229–233, 1997.
11. Martin SJ, Cotter TG. Specific loss of microtubules in HL-60 cells leads to programmed cell death (apoptosis). Biochem Soc Trans 18: 299, 1989.
12. Kaufmann SH. Induction of endonucleolytic DNA cleavage in human acute myelogenous leukemia cells by etopside, camptothecin, and other cytotoxic anticancer drugs: a cautionary note. Cancer Res 49: 5870–5878, 1989.
13. Lowe SW, Ruley HE, Jacks T, Housman D. p53-dependent apoptosis modulates the cytotoxicity of anticancer agents. Cell 74: 957–967, 1993.
14. Datta R, Manome Y, Taneja N, et al. Overexpression of Bcl-$X_L$ by cytotoxic drug exposure confers resistance to ionizing radiation-induced internucleosomal DNA fragmentation. Cell Growth Differ 6: 363–370, 1995.
15. Yuan J, Shaham S, Ledoux S, et al. The C. elegans cell death gene ced-3 encodes a protein similar to mammalian interleukin-1 beta-converting enzyme. Cell 75: 641–652, 1993.
16. Alnemri ES, Livingston DJ, Nicholson DW, et al. Human ICE/CED-3 protease nomenclature. Cell 87: 171, 1996.
17. Cerretti DP, Kozlosky CJ, Mosley B, et al. Molecular cloning of the interleukin-1 beta converting enzyme. Science 256: 97–100, 1992.
18. Martin SJ, Green DR. Protease activation during apoptosis: death by a thousand cuts? Cell 82: 349–352, 1995.
19. Nicholson DW, Ali A, Thornberry NA, et al. Identification and inhibition of the ICE/CED-3 protease necessary for mammalian apoptosis. Nature 376: 37–43, 1995.
20. Schlegel J, Peters I, Orrenius S, et al. CPP32/Apopain is a key interleukin 1beta converting enzyme-like protease involved in fas-mediated apoptosis. J Biol Chem 271: 1841–1844, 1996.
21. Enari M, Talanian RV, Wong WW, Nagata S. Sequential activation of ICE-like and CPP32-like proteases during Fas-mediated apoptosis. Nature 380: 723–726, 1996.
22. Muzio M, Chinnaiyan AM, Kischkel FC, et al. FLICE, a novel FADD-homologous ICE/CED-3-like protease, is recruited to the CD95 (Fas/Apo-1) death-inducing signaling complex. Cell 85: 817–817, 1996.
23. Cleveland JL, Ihle JN. Contenders in FasL/TNF Death Signaling. Cell 81: 1–20, 1995.
24. Lazebnik YA, Kaufmann SH, Desnoyers S, et al. Cleavage of poly(ADP-ribose) polymerase by a proteinase with properties like ICE. Nature 371: 346–347, 1994.
25. Orth K, Chinnaiyan AM, Garg M, et al. The CED-3/ICE-like protease Mch2 is activated during apoptosis and cleaves the death substrate lamin A. J Biol Chem 271: 16443–16446, 1996.
26. Eastman A. Deoxyribonuclease II in apoptosis and the significance of intracellular acidification. Cell Death Differ 1: 7–10, 1994.
27. Hughes FM, Cidlowski JA. Apoptotic DNA degradation: evidence for novel enzymes. Cell Death Differ 1: 11–18, 1994.

28. Peitsch MC, Polzar B, Tschopp J, Mannherz HG. About the involvement of deoxyribonuclease I in apoptosis. Cell Death Differ 1: 1–6, 1994.

29. Armstrong RC, Aja T, Xiang J, et al. Fas-induced activation of the cell death-related protease CPP32 Is inhibited by Bcl-2 and by ICE family protease inhibitors. J Biol Chem 271: 16850–16855, 1996.

30. Raza A, Gezer S, Mundle S, et al. Apoptosis in bone marrow biopsy samples involving stromal and hematopoietic cells in 50 patients with myelodysplastic syndromes. Blood 1: 268–276, 1995.

31. Enari M, Hug H, Nagata S. Involvement of an ICE-like protease in Fas-mediated apoptosis. Nature 375: 78–81, 1995.

32. Kuida K, Lippke JA, Ku G, et al. Altered cytokine export and apoptosis in mice deficient in interleukin-1 beta converting enzyme. Science 267: 2000–2003, 1995.

33. Los M, Van de Craen M, Penning LC, et al. Requirement of an ICE/CED-3 protease for Fas/APO-1-mediated apoptosis. Nature 375: 81–83, 1995.

34. Kuida K, Zheng TS, Na S, et al. Decreased apoptosis in the brain and premature lethality in CPP32-deficient mice. Nature 384: 368–372, 1996.

35. Stefanis L, Park DS, Yan CY, et al. Induction of CPP32-like activity in PC12 cells by withdrawal of trophic support. Dissociation from apoptosis. J Biol Chem 271: 30663–30671, 1996.

36. Chinnaiyan AM, Orth K, O'Rourke K, et al. Molecular ordering of the cell death pathway: Bcl-2 and Bcl-$X_L$ function upstream of the CED-3-like apoptotic proteases. J Biol Chem 271: 4573–4576, 1996.

37. Srinivasan A, Foster LM, Testa MP, et al. Bcl-2 expression in neural cells blocks activation of ICE/CED-3 family proteases during apoptosis. J Neurosci 16: 5654–5660, 1996.

38. Cory S, Strasser A, Jacks T, et al Enhanced cell survival and tumorigenesis. Cold Spring Harbor Symp Quant Biol LIX: 365–375, 1994.

39. Cory S. Regulation of lymphocyte survival by the bcl-2 gene family. Ann Rev Immunol 13: 513–543, 1995.

40. Craig RW. The bcl-2 gene family. Semin Cancer Biol 6: 35–43, 1995.

41. Yang E, Korsmeyer SJ. Molecular thanatopsis: a discourse on the BCL2 family and cell death. Blood 88: 386–401, 1996.

42. Oltvai ZN, Milliman CL, Korsmeyer SJ. Bcl-2 heterodimerizes in vivo with a conserved homolog, bax, that accelerates programmed cell death. Cell 74: 609–619, 1993.

43. Boise LH, Gonzalez-Garcia M, Postema CE, et al. bcl-x, a bcl-2-related gene that functions as a dominant regulator of apoptotic cell death. Cell 74: 597–608, 1993.

44. Hockenbery D, Nunez G, Milliman C, et al. Bcl-2 is an inner mitochondrial membrane protein that blocks programmed cell death. Nature 348: 34–336, 1990.

45. Kozopas KM, Yang T, Buchan HL, et al. MCL1, a gene expressed in programmed myeloid cell differentiation, has sequence similarity to BCL2. Proc Natl Acad Sci USA 90: 3516–20, 1993.

46. Vaux DL, Cory S, Adams JM. Bcl-2 gene promotes hemopoietic cell survival and cooperates with c-myc to immortalize pre-B cells. Nature 335: 440–442, 1988.

47. Zhou P, Qian L, Kozopas, K, Craig RW. MCL-1, a BCL-2 family member, delays hematopoietic cell death under a variety of apoptosis-inducing conditions. Blood 89: 630–643, 1997.

48. Chinnaiyan AM, O'Rourke K, Dixit VM. Interaction of CED-4 with CED-3 and CED-9: a molecular framework for cell death. Science 275: 1122–1126, 1997.

49. Kluck RM, Bossy-Wetzel E, Newmeyer DD. The release of cytochrome c from mitochondria: a primary site for Bcl-2 regulation of apoptosis. Science 75: 1132–1136, 1997.

50. Rampino N, Yamamoto H, Ionov Y, et al. Somatic frameshift mutations in the BAX gene in colon cancers of the microsatellite mutator phenotype. Science 275: 967–969, 1997.

51. Spector MS, Desnoyers S, Hoeppner DJ, Hengartner MO. Interaction between the C. elegans cell-death regulators CED-9 and CED-4. Nature 385: 653–656, 1997.

52. Wu D, Len HD, Nunez G. Interaction and regulation of subcellular localization of CED-4 by CED-9. Science 275: 1126–1129, 1997.

53. Yin C, Knudson CM, Korsmeyer SJ, Van Dyke T. Bax suppresses tumorigenesis and stimulates apoptosis in vivo. Nature 385: 637–640, 1997.

54. Kitada S, Miyashita T, Tanake S, Reed JC. Investigations of antisense oligonucleotides targeted against bcl-2 RNAs. Antisense Res Dev 3: 157–169, 1993.

55. McDonnell TJ, Korsmeyer SJ. Progression from lymphoid hyperplasia to high-grade malignant lymphoma in mice transgenic for the t(14; 18). Nature 349: 254–256, 1991.

56.  Bissonnette RP, Echeverri F, Mahboubi A, Green DR. Apoptotic cell death induced by c-myc is inhibited by bcl-2. Nature 359: 552–554, 1992.

57.  Evan GI, Wyllie AH, Gilbert CS, et al. Induction of apoptosis in fibroblasts by c-myc protein. Cell 69: 119–128, 1992.

58.  Yang E, Zha J, Jockel J, et al. Bad, a heterodimeric partner for bcl-$x_L$ and bcl-2 displaces bax and promotes cell death. Cell 80: 285–291, 1995.

59.  Muchmore SW, Sattler M, Liang H, et al. X-ray and NMR structure of human Bcl-$x_L$, an inhibitor of programmed cell death. Nature 381: 335–341, 1996.

60.  Minn AJ, Velez P, Schendel SL, et al. Bcl-x(L) forms an ion channel in synthetic lipid membranes. Nature 23: 353–357, 1997.

61.  Zamzami N, Marchetti P, Castedo M, et al. Sequential reduction of mitochondrial transmembrane potential and generation of reactive oxygen species in early programmed cell death. J Exp Med 182: 367–77, 1995.

62.  Susin SA, Zamzami N, Castedo M, et al. Bcl-2 inhibits the mitochondrial release of an apoptogenic protease. J Exp Med 184: 1331–1341, 1996.

63.  de Jong D, Prins FA, Mason DY, et al. Subcellular localization of the bcl-2 protein in malignant and normal lymphoid cells. Cancer Res 54: 256–260, 1994.

64.  Monaghan P, Robertson D, Andrew T, et al. Ultrastructural localization of BCL-2 protein. J Histochem Cytochem 40: 1819–1825, 1992.

65.  Nakai M, Takeda A, Cleary ML, Endo T. The bcl-2 protein is inserted into the outer membrane but not into the inner membrane of rat liver mitochondria in vitro. Biochem Biophys Res Commun 196: 233–239, 1993.

66.  Yang T, Kozopas K, Craig RW. The intracellular distribution and pattern of expression of MCL-1 overlap with, but are not identical to, those of BCL-2. J Cell Biol 128: 1173–1184, 1995.

67.  Liu X, Kim CN, Yang J, et al. Induction of apoptotic program in cell-free extracts: requirement for dATP and cytochrome c. Cell 86: 147–157, 1996.

68.  Yang J, Liu X, Wang X. Prevention of apoptosis by Bcl-2: release of cytochrome c from mitochondria blocked. Science 275: 1129–1132, 1997.

69.  Krajewski S, Tanaka S, Takayama S, et al. Investigation of the subcellular distribution of the bcl-2 oncoprotein: residence in the nuclear envelope, endoplasmic reticulum, and outer mitochondrial membranes. Cancer Res 53: 4701–4714, 1993.

70.  Krajewski S, Krajewska M, Shabaik A, et al. Immunohistochemical analysis of in vivo patterns of Bcl-x expression. Cancer Res 54: 5501–5507, 1994.

71.  Krajewski S, Bodrug S, Krajewska M, et al. Immunohistochemical analysis of Mcl-1 protein in human tissues: differential regulation of Mcl-1 and Bcl-2 protein production suggests a unique role for Mcl-1 in control of programmed cell death. Am J Pathol 146: 1309–1319, 1995.

72.  Moore NC, Anderson G, Williams GT, et al. Developmental regulation of bcl-2 expression in the thymus. Immunology 81: 115–119, 1994.

73.  Sattler M, Liang H, Nettesheim D, et al. Structure of BCLX-BAK peptide complex: recognition between regulators of apoptosis. Science 275: 983–986, 1997.

74.  Tsujimoto Y, Croce CM. Analysis of the structure, transcripts, and protein products of bcl, the gene involved in human follicular lymphoma. Proc Natl Acad Sci USA 83: 5214–5218, 1986.

75.  Cleary ML, Smith SD, Sklar J. Cloning and structural analysis of cDNA for bcl-2 and a hybrid bcl-2/immunoglobulin transcript resulting from the t(14;18) translocation. Cell 47: 19–28, 1986.

76.  May WS, Tyler PG, Ito T, et al. Interleukin-3 and bryostatin-1 mediate hyperphosphorylation of BCL2 alpha in association with suppression of apoptosis. J Biol Chem 269: 26865–26870, 1994.

77.  Wang HG, Rapp UR, Reed JC. Bcl-2 targets the protein kinase Raf-1 to mitochondria. Cell 87: 629–38, 1996.

78.  Zha J, Harada H, Yang E, et al. Serine phosphorylation of death agonist BAD in response to survival factor results in binding to 14–3–3 not BCL-X(L). Cell 87: 619–28, 1996.

79.  Gajewski TF, Thompson CB. Apoptosis meets signal transduction: elimination of a BAD influence. Cell 87: 589–592, 1996.

80.  Hannan YA, Obeid LM. Ceramide: an intracellular signal for apoptosis. Trends Biol Sci 20: 73–77, 1995.

81.  Santana P, Pena LA, Haimovitz-Friedman A, et al. Acid sphingomyelinases-deficient human lymphoblasts and mice are defective in radiation-induced apoptosis. Cell 86: 189–199, 1996.

82.  Xia Z, Dickens M, Raingeaud J, et al. Opposing effects of ERK and JNK-p38 MAP kinases on apoptosis. Science 267: 1326–1331, 1995.

83.   Alessi DR, Cuenda A, Cohen P, et al. PD 098059 is a specific inhibitor of the activation of mitogen-activated protein kinase kinase in vitro and in vivo. J Biol Chem 270: 27489–27494, 1995.

84.   Karin M. Signal transduction from the cell surface to the nucleus through the phosphorylation of transcription factors. Curr Opin Cell Biol 6: 415–24, 1994.

85.   Treisman R. Ternary complex factors: growth factor regulated transcriptional activators. Curr Opin Genet Dev 4: 96–101, 1994.

86.   Kastan MB, Onyekwere O, Sidransky D, et al. Participation of p53 protein in the cellular response to DNA damage. Cancer Res 51, 6304–11, 1991.

87.   Miyashita T, Krajewski S, Krajewska M, et al. Tumor suppressor p53 is a regulator of bcl-2 and bax gene expression in vitro and in vivo. Oncogene 9: 1799–1805, 1994.

88.   Zhan Q, Fan S, Bae I, et al. Induction of *BAX* by genotoxic stress in human cells correlates with normal p53 status and apoptosis. Oncogene 9: 3743–3751, 1994.

89.   Darmon AJ, Nicholson DW, Bleackley RC. Activation of the apoptotic protease CPP32 by cytotoxic T-cell-derived granzyme B. Nature 377:446–448, 1995.

C.J. Rosenthal and M. Rotman (Eds.), *Infusion Chemotherapy–Irradiation Interactions*
305

# Potential of antiangiogenic agents in systemic therapy for non-small cell lung cancer

ROY S. HERBST and BEVERLY A. TEICHER

*Dana-Farber Cancer Institute, 44 Binney Street, Boston, MA 02115, USA*

## 1. Introduction

Angiogenesis is the process of growth of the blood vascular system. The blood vascular system provides a distribution network of capillaries through which blood flows and which are the main sites of interchange of gases (oxygen and carbon dioxide) and metabolites (nutrients and metabolic waste) between the tissues and the blood. The basic structure of the vasculature includes an inner lining comprised of a single layer of extremely flattened epithelial cells called endothelial cells supported by a basement membrane and collagenous tissue. Pericytes and fibroblasts are often found associated with capillary endothelial cells. White blood cells pass through the intercellular space between the endothelial cells in some way negotiating the endothelial intercellular junctions.

The vascular patterns of several rodent and human tumors have been studied using vascular casting with a polymer followed by scanning electron microscopy of the casts [1–6]. The vasculature of solid tumors has a number of structural characteristics that typify its abnormality [7–9]. Tumor vessels tend to be devoid of or lacking in smooth muscle, are frequently tortuous and sinusoidal, have increased vascular length and diameter, have an incomplete endothelial cell lining and basement membrane and are prone to spontaneous hemorrhage and/or thrombosis. Since tumor vasculature is most often derived from postcapillary venules, it is tends to be hypotensive [10]. Most normal tissue microvascular beds tend to follow a relatively orderly branching pattern that is usually well described by the diameter and character (arteriolar, capillary, venular) of the vessel [11–13]. Relationships between vessel diameter and other parameters are less well defined in tumor tissues, probably because an orderly branching pattern does not exist uniformly throughout many tumors [14–21].

The trigger for angiogenesis in tumors is still unknown. However, several polypeptides as well as several small molecules secreted by a variety of normal cells and some tumor cells have been shown to be able to induce proliferation of endothelial cells and/or migration of endothelial cells leading to neovascularization [22–31].

The angiogenic proteins identified thus far include: (1) Basic (and acidic) fibroblast growth factors (bFGF, aFGF) which induce the proliferation of a variety of cell types. These factors stimulate endothelial cells to migrate and form tubes and also increase the production of proteases and plasminogen activator [26,32–47]. (2) Vascular endothelial growth factor/vascular permeability factor (VEGF/VPF) induces the proliferation of vascular endothelial cells, increases vascular endothelial cells, increases vascular permeability as well as inducing production of plasminogen activator in endothelial cells [48–65]. (3) Interleukin-8 (IL-8) is a chemoattractant cytokine produced by a variety of tissue and blood cells. Interleuken-8 attracts and activates neutrophils in inflammatory regions, it is also angiogenic in the rat cornea and induces proliferation of endothelial cells [66–71]. (4) Platelet-derived-endothelial cell growth factor (PD-ECGF) stimulates endothelial cell DNA synthesis and chemotaxis and may induce production of FGF by endothelial cells [72]. (5) Angiogenin stimulates endothelial cells to form diacyl-glycerol and to secret prostacyclin by activating phospholipase C and phospholipase $A_2$ [73–75]. Angiogenin also has a ribonucleolytic and proteolytic activities that appear to be necessary for neovascularization [76–79]. (6) Tumor necrosis factor-$\alpha$ (TNF-$\alpha$) induces the production and secretion of bFGF in endothelial cells as well as being a chemoattractant for monocytes and a macrophage activator [80–83]. (7) Angiogenic properties have also been associated with transforming growth factor-$\alpha$ (TGF-$\alpha$) and transforming growth factor-$\beta$ (TGF-$\beta$) [84–87].

Among the small molecules, 1-butyryl glycerol [8], prostaglandins $PGE_1$ and $PGE_2$ [89–92], nicotinamide [93] and related compounds such as adenosine [94,95] are reported to be angiogenic. Adenosine is a vasodilator that accumulates in response to hypoxia. It is not clear how adenosine induces vasoproliferation. Certain degradation products of hyaluronic acid are angiogenic [96]. (12R)-Hydroxyeicosatrienoic acid [97,98] and okadaic acid [99] have been reported to be highly angiogenic.

The signals from the angiogenic factors are transducing through binding to transmembrane receptors primarily on endothelial cells. Many of these receptors are tyrosine kinases [100]. Some, such as the receptors for fibroblast growth factors (FGFR), platelet-derived growth factor-BB (PDGFR$\beta$), transforming growth factor-$\alpha$ (epidermal growth factor receptor, EGFR), and hepatocyte growth factor (Met oncoprotein), are widely expressed in many tissues and cell types, whereas others are strictly endothelial cell specific [101].

## 2. Extracellular matrix

Invasive growth is a hallmark of neoplastic disease. Solid tumors, in order to grow locally, must induce the breakdown of the surrounding extracellular matrix and connective tissue and in order to disseminate must induce the breakdown of host basement membranes [102–106]. The proteolytic enzymes identified in these processes included: (1) metalloproteinases such as collagenases, stromelysins and gelatinases (type IV collagenases) [107–119]; (2) plasminogen activator leading to plasmin [120–130]; (3) cathepsin B [131–135]; (4) elastase [136–141] and (5) glycosidases such as heparanase [142,143]. These enzymes may be secreted by tumor cells or by normal cells such as fibroblasts, macrophages or monocytes [102–106,121,144–150].

Several studies have demonstrated elevated levels of matrix metalloproteinases in human tumor tissue [151–153]. Preclinical studies with an inhibitor of matrix metalloproteinases, TIMP, have shown that this inhibitor can block tumor metastasis to the lungs [154] and can inhibit subcutaneous tumor growth. TIMPs also have been shown to inhibit tumor induced angiogenesis in experimental systems.

## 3. Potential antineoplastic agents directed towards normal cells and normal processes in tumors

The recognition of the critical involvement of stromal cells (endothelial cells, fibroblasts), infiltrating cells (macrophages, monocytes) and extracellular matrix components in neoplastic disease has led to an active search for inhibitors, antagonists and down-regulators of these processes.

The search for antiangiogenic substances has primarily led to the discovery of proteins and small molecules that inhibit various steps in the breakdown of the basement membrane [155,156]. These include naturally occurring proteins such as protamine [157], interferon-$\alpha$ [158,159], interferon-$\gamma$ [160], platelet factor 4 [157,161], tissue inhibitors of metalloproteinases (TIMPs) [162,163], interleukin-12 [164–166], angiostatin [167], peptides derived from cartilages [168,169], vitreous humor [170], smooth muscle [171], and aorta [171], as well as synthetic peptides such as synthetic laminin peptide (CDPG) YIGSR-NH$_2$ [172], somatostatin analogs such as somatoline [173] and antibodies such as MAb LM609 to human integrin $\alpha_v\beta_3$ [174–176]. Antiangiogenic small molecules include naturally occurring heparins [177], a variety of steroids [26,178–180], several retinoids and carotenoids [181–206], warfarin [207], genistein [208–220] and fumagillin [221–240], as well as synthetic agents such as sulfated chitin derivatives [241], sulfated cyclodextrins [177,242,243], linomide [244–253], thalidomide [254] and derivatives of fumagillin [221–240]. Radiation also inhibits blood vessel growth [255–257].

Tumor growth and invasion requires remodeling of surrounding normal tissue and extracellular matrix. The degradation of the extracellular matrix is accomplished by tumor induction of host derived proteinases [156,258,259]. The key enzymes, matrix metalloproteinases, are secreted in latent form by both normal and tumor cells and are activated by cleavage of the amino-terminal of the latent proteinase [162]. Regulation of matrix metalloproteinase activity is very stringent, both at the level of gene expression of the latent enzymes and the secretion of activators of the latent enzymes and of specific inhibitors of the active enzymes. The development of small molecule inhibitors of the matrix metalloproteinases has focused largely on hydroxamic acid-type peptide analogs [260–268]. The most extensively studied of the molecules is batimastat (BB-94, [4-(N-hydroxyamino)-2R-isobutyl-3S-(thiopen-2-ylthiomethyl)-succinyl]-L-phenylalanine-N-methylamide) [262–265, 267,268]. Batimastat has been shown to inhibit the growth of several murine tumors and of human ovarian and colon xenografts as well as to inhibit metastasis in several systems. Batimastat also inhibited angiogenesis in a murine hemangioma [265]. Clinical trials are going forward with marimastat, another non-specific matrix metalloproteinase inhibitor.

It has been recognized for some time that the tetracyclines can inhibit tissue collagenase activity and tetracycline administration has been used in the treatment of periodontal disease [269], gingival collagenolytic activity in diabetes [269,270] and to inhibit joint deterioration in patients with rheumatoid arthritis [271–273]. This inhibitory activity has been associated with both gelatinase (type IV collagenase) and interstitial collagenase [274]. Tamargo et al. [275] first reported that minocycline, a semisynthetic tetracycline with a relatively long circulating half-life, inhibited neovascularization in the rabbit cornea implanted with the VX2 carcinoma. Minocycline has been shown to potentiate the effects of cytotoxic anticancer therapies both alone and in combination with other agents directed towards host "normal" processes involved in tumor growth [233,242,276,277].

In 1987, Sidky and Borden reported that murine interferons inhibited tumor-induced angiogenesis and lymphocyte-induced angiogenesis [278]. The effect of the interferons was species specific suggesting that rather than acting at the endothelial cells, the interferons inhibited the signal inducing angiogenesis at the level of the tumor cells (human or murine). Earlier it was observed that interferon inhibits the locomotion of endothelial cells in vitro [279]. In the clinic, therapy with interferon $\alpha$-2a improved Kaposi's sarcoma, the vascular tumor associated with human immunodeficiency virus (HIV) infection [280–282]. White and colleagues observed remarkable regression of pulmonary hemangiomatosis in a 7-year-old boy after interferon $\alpha$-2a therapy [283]. Orchard et al. reported two cases of hemangioma in infants with thrombocytopenic coagulopathy, one in the pterygopalatine space and the other in the peritoneum. Both tumors regressed after the administration of interferon $\alpha$-2a [284]. Interferon $\alpha$-2a has been used alone and in combination [159,285–289]. Interferon-$\alpha$ and interferon-$\gamma$ have been shown to be potent regulators of both the gelatinase A and B (72 kDa and 92 kDa collagenases) genes in human A2058 melanoma cells, while interferon-$\beta$ and interferon-$\gamma$ suppressed transcription of gelatinase A (72 kDa collagenase) and inhibited invasion of the human renal cell carcinoma cell through reconstituted basement membrane [290].

## 4. A systems approach to cancer therapy for solid tumors

Tumors are dynamic, complex, living tissues undergoing the varied processes of tissue growth under the guidance of aberrant malignant cells. Cytotoxic anticancer therapies have focused solely on the eradication of the malignant cell which is an absolute necessity in cancer therapy; however, even the most heroic therapeutic strategies rarely achieve cure of many tumor types. A broader look at the tumor reminds us that the growth processes of the tumor are normal processes, that the invasion processes of the tumor are normal processes and that it is the inappropriate activation of these processes that comprises the morbidity of malignant disease. The tools are now at hand to make an important step forward in the therapeutic approach to solid tumors to, without losing sight of the importance of eradicating the malignant cell populations, block "normal" processes critical to tumor maintenance and growth (and spread).

The question arises of how to integrate these new therapeutic agents into existing cancer treatment regimens which have been developed through great effort and ingenuity. These additional therapeutic agents are clearly directed towards new targets, that is normal cells and extracellular enzymatic activities. Although these targets are critical to tumor growth it is highly unlikely that agents directed toward these targets will lead to tumor cure. Therefore, the systems approach to therapy of choosing multiple targets to the goal would maintain cytotoxic therapy while incorporating new non-cytotoxic strategies. Several of the agents described above are currently in clinical trial as single agents.

## 5. Lung cancer

Lung cancer is the most prevalent cancer in the United States today. Unfortunately, the majority of lung cancer patients present with inoperable stage III disease or with metastases in distant organs. Indeed, close to 50% of all non-small cell lung cancer patients present with inoperable disease, and relapses in patients initially presenting with early stage disease are quite common. Patients with Stage IV disease cannot be cured with current chemotherapeutic approaches, although a small minority of patients (10–15%) with advanced regional disease may be cured by combined modality therapy.

Among the most widely used agents for the treatment of non-small cell lung cancer, cisplatin has demonstrated a response rate of about 20% in most single agent trials [291]. Numerous investigators have conducted Phase II trials to examine its utility in combination regimens. The first cisplatin containing regimen was CAP, which consisted of cisplatin, cyclophosphamide and adriamycin [292]. Initially, this regimen produced a 39% response rate in 41 previously untreated patients and a 36% response rate in 28 previously treated patients with advanced non-small cell lung cancer. A subsequent study done by the same Mayo Clinic group used cisplatin at a higher dose and showed even better results with a response rate of 48% [293]. These impressive results should, however, be tempered by the fact that the response rates in the earlier trials were defined differently than the response rates determined in later studies, often accepting less than the current standard 50% reduction.

In the 1980s, multiple agents were found to achieve a 15–25% response rate in advanced non-small cell lung cancer, including cisplatin, etoposide and vindesine. Therefore efforts were aimed at developing combination regimens containing these drugs which might increase efficacy while decreasing toxicity. The combination of cisplatin with etoposide in several European studies had produced a response rate of around 40% with a median survival in responders of between 30–60 weeks [294–296]. A similar response rate of 40% was observed by Gralla's group in a trial combining high dose cisplatin with vindesine in patients with good performance status with an observed median survival of 94 weeks in the responding patients [293].

Numerous clinical trials evaluating carboplatin as a single agent or as a component of combination regimens have been performed and the response rates for carboplatin were shown to vary from 9 to 20% in four trials [297,298]. In one of these ECOG trials, carboplatin was associated with a modest but significant survival benefit while severe toxicity was minimal in all of the trials [297]. Meanwhile, a randomized trial was conducted to compare the efficacy of carboplatin and etoposide to cisplatin and etoposide. There were no significant differences observed in response rates or survival duration, but there was a trend for less toxicity with the carboplatin and etoposide regimen [299]. Furthermore, other investigators have evaluated carboplatin and etoposide in three drug combination therapy with vinblastine, or mitoycine in Phase II trials. Response rates ranged from 9 to 17%, suggesting that these combinations were not more effective than carboplatin/etoposide alone [300,301]. Hence, for many years carboplatin plus etoposide was considered the standard regimen for non-small cell lung cancer treatment.

The first of a novel class of antimitotic agents, paclitaxel is derived from the bark of the pacific yew *Taxus brevifolia*. First described in the early 1970s [302], its mechanism of action involves the promotion of microtubule assembly and eventual inhibition of normal disassembly, leading to subsequent paralysis of the mitotic apparatus [303,304]. Clinical trials have demonstrated that paclitaxel has significant activity against ovarian carcinoma, melanoma, breast carcinoma and non-small cell lung cancer [305–309].

Initial phase II studies were performed on chemotherapy-naive patients with advanced non-small cell lung cancer using a 24-h infusion at a relatively high dose of paclitaxel (>200 mg/m$^2$) by the Eastern Cooperative Oncology Group. They studied 24 patients with metastatic disease treated with a 24-h infusion of paclitaxel at 250 mg/m$^2$ given every

3 weeks [308]. Five patients had partial responses (21%) with a median survival time of 24.1 weeks and with a 1-year survival rate of 41.7%.

A Phase II study done by investigators at the Fox Chase Cancer Center involved 53 chemotherapy-naive patients with stage IV or stage IIIB with malignant pleural effusion non-small cell lung cancer treated with paclitaxel and carboplatin [310]. The treatment was repeated at 3-week intervals for a total of 6 cycles with GCSF support being administered. The objective response rate was 62% with 28 partial responses and 5 complete responses; while the median progression-free survival was 28 weeks and the median survival time was 53 weeks. Another phase II study from Vanderbilt involved 51 previously untreated patients with stage IIIB or stage IV non-small cell lung cancer treated with paclitaxel administered by 24 h intravenous infusion on day 1 and 1 h infusion of carboplatin on day 2 [311,312]. This treatment was repeated every 28 days for a total of 6 cycles and hematopoietic growth factors were not routinely used. In this study, there were no complete and 14 partial responses for an overall response rate of 27%. The medium progression-free survival time was 23.8 weeks with a median survival time of 38 weeks while the survival rate at 1 year was 32%. While non-hematologic toxicity was modest, the major toxicity was neutropenia requiring GCSF support in some patients, particularly those treated at the higher paclitaxel dose. There were two treatment-related deaths due to neutropenic sepsis. The relatively lower response rate seen in this study population may reflect patient heterogeneity as well as relative differences in drug dose and dose intensity.

A recent ECOG [313] study randomized patients into three treatment arms: cisplatin plus etoposide at standard dose, taxol at a dose of 225 mg/m$^2$ plus cisplatin with GCSF support and taxol at 135 mg/m$^2$ plus cisplatin, with close to 200 patients enrolled in each arm. The primary endpoints of this study were response rate, median survival and toxicity. Patients with stage IIIB or IV non-small cell lung cancer who demonstrated a performance status of 0 or 1 and who did not have brain metastases were eligible. The response rate for etoposide and cisplatin was 12%, taxol 135/cisplatin was 26% and taxol 250/GCSF/cisplatin was 32% ($P = 0.001$). Improved survival was also observed in patients receiving either taxol combination with median and 1 year survival, respectively, at 7.7 months and 32% for the control, 9.6 and 37% for taxol at 135 mg/m$^2$ and 10.0 and 39% for taxol at 250 mg/m$^2$ ($P = 0.016$). However, there was no statistically significant difference between the two taxol arms. Toxicities included grade 3–4 neutropenia with the highest rate of toxicity found in the group treated with the higher taxol dose.

These results show that there has been progress in the treatment of non-small cell lung cancer through the use of combinations of cytotoxic anticancer drugs and incorporation of newer drugs into the regimens. However, improving our impact on this disease in a major way is likely to require a paradigm shift in treatment strategy. This report describes preclinical studies in the murine Lewis lung carcinoma incorporating the antiangiogenic agents TNP-470 and minocycline into treatment with cytotoxic anticancer therapies.

## 6.  Materials and methods

### 6.1.  Drugs

TNP-470 was obtained as a gift from Dr. K. Kitazawa (Takeda, Osaka, Japan) and subsequently as a gift from Dr. R. Weiss (TAP Pharmaceuticals Inc., Deerfield, IL). Minocycline, cisplatin (*cis*-diamminedichloroplatinum II), cyclophosphamide, carboplatin and paclitaxel (taxol) were purchased from Sigma (St. Louis, MO).

## 6.2.   Tumor growth delay experiments

The Lewis lung tumor [233,236,314] was carried in male C57BL mice (Taconic Farms, Germantown, NY). For the experiments, $2 \times 10^6$ tumor cells prepared from a brei of several stock tumors were implanted subcutaneously into a hind leg of male mice 8–10 weeks of age.

By day 4 after tumor cell implantation, Lewis lung tumors had begun neovascularization. Animals bearing Lewis lung tumors were injected subcutaneously with TNP-470 (30 mg/kg) on alternate days for 8 injections, beginning on day 4 and/or were treated with minocycline (10 mg/kg) intraperitoneally for days 4–18 after tumor implant. When the Lewis lung tumors were approximately 150 mm$^3$ in volume, on day 7 after tumor cell implantation, cytotoxic therapy was initiated. Cisplatin (10 mg/kg) or carboplatin (50 mg/kg) were administered intraperitoneally on day 7. Cyclophosphamide (150 mg/kg) was administered intraperitoneally on days 7, 9 and 11 after tumor implant. Taxol (36 mg/kg) was administered intravenously on days 7–11 after tumor implant.

The progress of each tumor was measured thrice weekly until it reached a volume of 500 mm$^3$. Tumor growth delay was calculated as the days taken by each individual tumor to reach 500 mm$^3$ as compared with the untreated controls. Each treatment group consisted of 6 animals and the experiment was repeated three times. Days of tumor growth delay are the mean ± standard error for the treatment group compared with the control.

## 6.3.   Lung metastases

The external lung metastases from animals treated as described above on day 20 after tumor implant were counted manually and scored as ≥3 mm in diameter. The data shown are the means from 6 pairs of lungs. Untreated control animals died from lung metastases on days 21–25. Parentheses in Table 1 indicate the percentage of total number of metastases that were large [233,242,277].

Table 1

Number of lung metastases on day 20 from subcutaneous Lewis lung tumors after treatment with TNP-470/Minocycline alone or along with cytotoxic anticancer drugs

| Treatment group | Mean number of lung metastases (% large)[a] | | | |
|---|---|---|---|---|
| | Alone | + Mino | + TNP-470 | +TNP-470/ Mino |
| – | 29 (53) | 29 (50) | 30 (52) | 26 (47) |
| Cisplatin (10 mg/kg) day 7 | 13 (58) | 11 (48) | 15 (34) | 14 (50) |
| Cyclophosphamide(150 mg/kg) days 7, 9, 11 | 12 (40) | 6 (33) | 6 (30) | 2 (25) |
| Carboplatin (50 mg/kg) day 7 | 23 (54) | – | – | 18 (44) |
| Taxol (36 mg/kg) days 7–11 | 14 (39) | – | – | 13 (25) |
| Taxol/carboplatin | 14 (50) | – | – | 10 (50) |

[a]Lungs were taken from animals treated as described in Table 1.

*6.4.  Tumor drug levels*

Animals bearing Lewis lung tumors were treated subcutaneously on alternate days with TNP-470 (30 mg/kg) days 4–8 and daily intraperitoneally with minocycline (10 mg/kg) on days 4–8 following tumor implantation. On day 8 these pretreated animals and other tumor-bearing animals that were not pretreated were injected i.p. with $6\,\mu$Ci of [$^{14}$C]cyclophosphamide (300 mg/kg; 52.5 mCi/mmol) or cisplatin (20 mg/kg). Six hours later the animals were killed. Known wet weights of tumor from animals injected with [$^{14}$C]cyclophosphamide were dissolved in tissue solubilizer (Protosol; DuPont NEN Research Products), then counted by liquid scintillation in Aquasol (DuPont NEN Research Products) [315]. Known wet weights of the tumor from the animals injected with cisplatin were dissolved in a tissue solubilizer, then analyzed by flameless atomic absorption spectroscopy. Platinum (Pt) from a $15$-$\mu$l sample of injection volume was atomized from the walls of pyrolytically coated graphite tubes. A Perkin-Elmer Model 2380 atomic absorption spectrophotometer was used in conjunction with a Perkin-Elmer Model 400 graphite furnace (Perkin Elmer Cetus, Norwalk, CT) to measure the absolute mass of Pt in the samples. Each measurement was made in triplicate in three independent experiments [236,315,316].

*6.5.  DNA alkaline elution*

Lewis lung carcinoma-bearing mice were treated subcutaneously with TNP-470 (30 mg/kg) on alternate days 4–8 and minocycline (10 mg/kg) ip daily on days 4–8. Untreated carcinoma-bearing mice were given injections of 0.125 $\mu$Ci/g [*methyl*-$^{14}$C]thymidine (5 mCi/mol; DuPont NEN Research Products) 24 h prior to drug treatment with cyclophosphamide (300 mg/kg) or cisplatin (20 mg/kg) intraperitoneally. At 24 h post-treatment the tumors were excised and a single-cell suspension was prepared as described previously for the tumor excision assay [233,236,317].

Alkaline elution was performed by standard procedures [318,319]. One-half of each group of cells was irradiated on ice with 600 cGy using a Gammacell 40 (Atomic Energy of Canada, Ltd., Ottawa, Ontario, Canada). Approximately $1.5 \times 10^7$ cells per group were placed onto an alkaline elution filter (2.0 $\mu$m pore size) (Millipore, Bedford, MA). As an internal control, $1 \times 10^6$ [$^3$H]thymidine-labeled L1210 cells irradiated with 150 cGy were also placed onto each filter. The cells first were washed with cold PBS, then lysed with 3 ml of 0.2% sodium dodecylsarkosine, 2 M NaCl, 0.04 M EDTA (pH 10), which was allowed to flow through by gravity.

To study DNA–DNA interactions, 0.5 mg/ml proteinase K (Sigma Chemical Company) was added to the lysis solution and incubated on the filters for 60 min at room temperature. Alkaline elution was carried out in the dark using 2% tetrapropylammonium hydroxide (Fisher Scientific Company, Pittsburgh, PA), 0.025 M EDTA at a flow rate of 2.4 ml/h. Fractions were collected at 90-min intervals and were assayed for radioactivity after adding 12 ml of Aquasol. The remaining DNA on the filters was removed by treatment with 0.4 ml 1 M HCl for 60 min at 65°C, and the solution was neutralized with 2.5 ml of 0.4 M NaOH before Aquasol addition. Samples were counted on an LS 7000 Beckman scintillation counter (Beckman Instruments Co., Columbia, MD, USA). Each point was measured in three independent experiments. The DNA cross-linking factor (CLF) was calculated as:

$$CLF = \frac{\log(\text{irradiated control})/\text{control}}{\log(\text{irradiated drug})/\text{control}}$$

## 7.  Results

The Lewis lung carcinoma growing in C57BL mice was chosen for tumor-growth delay studies because this tumor is relatively resistant to many cancer therapies and because it metastasizes avidly to lungs from subcutaneous implants. In order to study tumor growth delay, each of the cytotoxic therapies was administered at full standard dose and schedule. TNP-470, administered subcutaneously on alternate days beginning on day 4 and continuing daily until day 18, was a moderately effective modulator of the cytotoxic therapies. (Table 2). Minocycline and TNP-470 were effective modulators of cisplatin and cyclophosphamide; however, the combination of TNP-470 and minocycline was most effective [235]. With the addition of TNP-470 and minocycline administered on days 4–18 after tumor implant along with cisplatin administered on day 7 there was a 2.4-fold increase in tumor growth delay. In the treatment group treated with TNP-470 and minocycline along with cyclophosphamide on days 7, 9 and 11 after tumor implant there was a 2.3-fold increase in tumor growth delay in animals with growing tumors and in approximately 40% of the animals the primary tumors regressed and these animals were long term survivors (>120 days). The addition of TNP-470 and minocycline administration to treatment with carboplatin resulted in a 2.2-fold increase in tumor growth delay. While the addition of TNP-470 and minocycline to treatment with taxol resulted in a 1.8-fold increase in tumor growth delay. When the taxol and carboplatin treatment regimens were combined, a tumor growth delay of 13 days was achieved which appeared to be a greater-than-additive tumor response. Incorporating TNP-470 and minocycline into that treatment regimen resulted in a 1.5-fold increase in tumor growth delay compared with taxol and carboplatin alone.

Table 2

Growth delay of the Lewis lung carcinoma produced by treatment with TNP-470/minocycline alone or along with cytotoxic anticancer drugs

| Treatment group | Tumor growth delay (days)[a] | | | |
| --- | --- | --- | --- | --- |
| | Alone | +Mino[b] | +TNP-470 | +TNP-470/Mino |
| – | | 1.2 ± 0.4 | 2.1 ± 0.4 | 1.8 ± 0.4 |
| Cisplatin (10 mg/kg) day 7 | 4.5 ± 0.3 | 5.0 ± 0.3 | 6.0 ± 0.5 | 10.9 ± 0.8 |
| Cyclophosphamine (150 mg/kg) days 7, 9, 11 | 19.6 ± 1.6 | 32.4 ± 1.8 | 25.3 ± 2.2 | 44.8 ± 2.8[c] |
| Carboplatin (50 mg/kg) day 7 | 5.2 ± 0.4 | – | – | 11.4 ± 1.5 |
| Taxol (36 mg/kg) days 7–11 | 3.1 ± 0.3 | – | – | 5.6 ± 0.4 |
| Taxol/carboplatin | 13.0 ± 1.3 | – | – | 19.8 ± 1.7 |

[a]Tumor growth delay is the difference in days for treated tumors to reach 500 mm$^3$ compared with untreated control tumors. Untreated control tumors reach 500 mm$^3$ in about 14 days. Mean ± SE of 15 animals.
[b]Minocycline (10 mg/kg) was administered i.p. daily on days 4–18. TNP-470 (30 mg/kg) was administered s.c. on alternate days for 8 injections, beginning on day 4. Cisplatin and carboplatin were administered i.p. on day 7. Cyclophosphamide was administered i.p. on days on days 7, 9 and 11. Taxol was administered i.v. daily on days 7–11.
[c]Long-term survivors 5/12 (>120 days).

The Lewis lung carcinoma metastasizes avidly to the lungs of animals from a subcutaneously implanted tumor. None of the antiangiogenic therapies administered alone altered the
number of lung metastases or the percentage of large (vascularized) lung metastases on day
20 [235]. Each of the cytotoxic anticancer drugs decreased the number of lung metastases
on day 20 compared to the controls. In the case of cyclophosphamide there was a marked
decrease in the number and the percent of large lung metastases when TNP-470 and minocycline were administered along with the drug. Many animals treated with TNP-470 and
minocycline along with cyclophosphamide had zero or very few lung metastases on day 20.
The addition of TNP-470 and minocycline to treatment with the other anticancer drugs resulted in modest or no decrease in lung metastases compared with the anticancer drugs
alone.

Treatment of Lewis lung carcinoma bearing mice with TNP-470 (30 mg/kg) administered subcutaneously on alternate days for three injections beginning on day 4 after tumor
implant and with minocycline (10 mg/kg) administered intraperitoneally for five injections
beginning on day 4 after tumor implant did not alter the growth of the primary tumor compared with untreated controls. To determine whether the TNP-470 and minocycline treatment effected the distribution of cisplatin or cyclophosphamide into the tumors, animals
were injected intraperitoneally with a single dose of cisplatin (20 mg/kg) or with a single
dose of [14C]cyclophosphamide (300 mg/kg) on day 8 and then 6 h later the tumors were
excised and Pt and 14C levels determined (Fig. 1). There was a 5.2-fold greater level of Pt in
the tumors of animals receiving TNP-470 and minocycline along with cisplatin than in those
receiving cisplatin alone. There was a 2.6-fold greater level of 14C in the tumors of animals

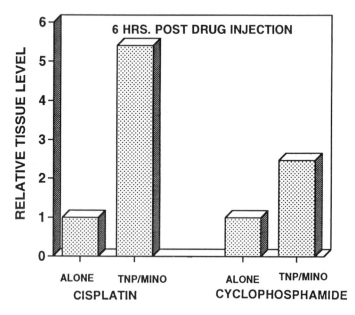

Fig. 1. Relative tumor levels of Pt from cisplatin (20 mg/kg) and 14C from [14C]cyclophosphamide (300 mg/kg)
in C57BL mice bearing Lewis lung tumors subcutaneously in a hind leg 6 h after intraperitoneal administration of
the drug alone or after administration of TNP-470 (30 mg/kg, s.c.) days 4, 6 and 8 and minocycline (10 mg/kg,
i.p.) days 4–8 after tumor implant. Data are expressed as relative to Pt levels or 14C levels in the tumors in animals treated with cisplatin or [14C]cyclophosphamide alone set equal to 1/g tissue.

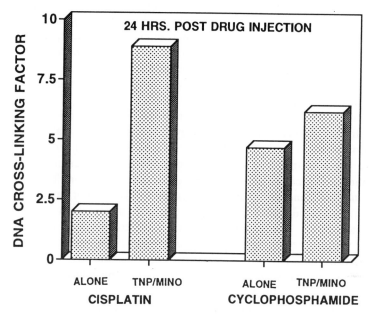

Fig. 2. DNA cross-linking factors from Lewis lung tumors as determined by DNA alkaline elution after treatment of Lewis lung carcinoma bearing animals with TNP-470 (30 mg/kg, s.c.) on days 4, 6 and 8, with minocycline (10 mg/kg, i.p.) daily on days 4–8 and/or with CTX (300 mg/kg, i.p.) or CDDP (20 mg/kg, i.p.) on day 8 after tumor cell implantation. [$^{14}$C]Thymidine was administered i.p. on days 7 and 8. The animals were killed on day 9. A DNA cross-linking factor of 1.0 indicates no cross-links.

receiving TNP-470 and minocycline along with [$^{14}$C]cyclophosphamide compared with [$^{14}$C]cyclophosphamide only.

Both cyclophosphamide and cisplatin are cytotoxic through formation of inter- and intra-strand crosslinks in DNA. To determine whether the increased drug levels observed at 6 h after drug administration resulted in greater drug activity in the tumor, DNA alkaline elution was performed on tumors 24 h after drug administration (Fig. 2) [235]. Animals were treated with TNP-470 and minocycline as described above and then with cisplatin (20 mg/ kg) or cyclophosphamide (300 mg/kg). Treatment with cisplatin (20 mg/kg) alone resulted in a cross-linking factor of 2.0, while treatment with the same dose of cisplatin in animals pretreated with TNP-470/minocycline resulted in a cross-linking factor of 8.9, which extrapolates to equivalency to about 85 mg/kg of cisplatin. Treatment with cyclophosphamide (300 mg/kg) alone resulted in a cross-linking factor of 4.7, while treatment with the same dose of cyclophosphamide in animals pretreated with TNP-470/minocycline resulted in a cross-linking factor of 6.2 which extrapolates to equivalency to about 650 mg/kg of cyclophosphamide.

## 8. Discussion

Despite numerous efforts to produce efficacious treatments, the outcome of patients with advanced non-small cell lung cancer remains poor. More than 15 years after cisplatin was introduced into the treatment of patients with advanced non-small cell lung cancer, drug therapy remains controversial despite multiple randomized trials and meta-analyses to evaluate its efficacy [320–323]. It is only now beginning to be incorporated into standard non-protocol treatments for advanced non-small cell lung cancer. At this time, cisplatin based combinations appear to produce a significant survival advantage compared to the option of best supportive care, although the absolute survival gain is small and may be offset by adverse reactions associated with the treatment [322].

A paradigm shift is needed to markedly improve the impact of systemic therapy on non-small cell lung cancer. There is much evidence to suggest that without the active involvement of the normal cells in the vicinity of a malignant cell "colony" a tumor mass cannot grow. These normal cells are a major component of malignancy [324–332]. They are proliferating and they are actively involved in tumor invasion. The corollary is that both the normal cells and the malignant cells involved in tumor growth as well as the chemical and mechanical signaling pathways that interconnect them are valid targets for therapeutic intervention. The recognized normal tissue compartment targets for therapeutic attack are vascular components, extracellular matrix components, stromal and infiltrating cells [332].

Antiangiogenic agents represent a new class of therapy which act through a novel mechanism. By working to impede growth of the endothelial cells that nourish a tumor, these agents theoretically can shrink tumors with increased specificity and hence decreased toxicity [234,235,237,242,243,277,333]. While several agents are currently in clinical trial (CAI, CM101, $\alpha$-interferon, interleukin-12, marimastat, pentosan sulfate, platelet factor 4, thalidomide and TNP-470) [334] there has to date been only preliminary demonstration of clinical efficacy for these compounds in patients with solid tumors. A large part of this could be due to the inability of the medical community to design clinical trials with suitable endpoints to measure activity of cytostatic agents. However, another equally important problem is that human tumors (especially lung tumors) are often too large and metastatic at presentation. Patients thus are in need of an immediate response to achieve palliation of symptoms and therefore might not have time to tolerate the at best stable disease achieved by antiangiogenic agents alone. Therefore, a fundamental question is to define the use of antiangiogenic agents therapies in combination with cytotoxic drugs as front line therapies.

The Lewis lung carcinoma is a model for non-small cell lung cancer. Although the antiangiogenic therapy TNP-470 and minocycline had no effect on the growth of the primary tumor or on the growth of lung metastases when administered alone, this antiangiogenic therapy potentiated the effects of each of the chemotherapeutic agents with known activity in non-small cell lung cancer [233,234,236,242,277].

Based on these promising preclinical animal studies, we plan a Phase I clinical trial of TNP-470 and taxol. Taxol has emerged as a major new chemotherapeutic agent with activity against a wide variety of tumors. In addition, recent data has also suggested a potent effect of taxol on endothelial cells. Thus, the combination of taxol with TNP-470 offers a potentially promising drug combination to explore in the clinic. The first step in such a trial would be to establish the dosage level and safety of an antiangiogenic/cytotoxic drug therapy in human patients. With success in this initial trial, additional components such as carboplatin and minocycline will sequentially be added to the treatment regimen.

## Summary

*Background.* Non-small cell lung cancer patients often present with inoperable disease. Cisplatin based combination chemotherapy regimens were the first to produce significant response rates in non-small cell lung cancer. More recently treatment of carboplatin in combination with taxol has resulted in increased response rates and improved survival for these patients. However, the benefits are limited and median survival is improved only on the order of 3–6 months. Further improvement in the systemic treatments of non-small cell lung cancer may require a paradigm shift in therapeutic strategy. Antiangiogenic agents represent a new class of drugs with a unique target. *Methods.* Mice bearing the Lewis lung carcinoma were treated with the antiangiogenic agents TNP-470 and minocycline separately or in combination. The response of primary and metastatic disease to cisplatin, carboplatin, cyclophosphamide and taxol alone and along with the antiangiogenic agents was assessed. Tumor levels of [$^{14}$C]cyclophosphamide and platinum from cisplatin as well as DNA cross-linking in the tumors were determined. *Results.* Administration of the antiangiogenic therapy alone to the established tumors did not alter the growth of the primary tumor or significantly decrease the number of lung metastases. Administration of the antiangiogenic therapy along with the cytotoxic chemotherapeutic agents resulted in increased response of both the primary and metastatic disease compared with the cytotoxic agents alone. Examination of drug levels in the tumors of animals treated with the antiangiogenic agents along with cisplatin showed there was a 5-fold increase in the platinum content of the tumors in animals receiving the combination therapy. Similarly, there was a 2.6-fold increase in [$^{14}$C]cyclophosphamide in the tumors of animals receiving the combination therapy. The DNA cross-linking in the tumors from animals receiving the combination therapies was also increased. *Conclusions.* Antiangiogenic agents impede the growth of the endothelial cells that nourish the tumor. Administration of the antiangiogenic combination of TNP-470 and minocycline along with active chemotherapeutic agents markedly improved the response of the Lewis lung carcinoma to systemic therapy. Clinical trial of these agents in non-small cell lung cancer is warranted.

## References

1. Hodde KC, Miodonski A, Bakker C, Veltman WAM. Scanning electron microscopy of microcorrosion casts with special attention on arterio-venous differences and application to the rat's cochlea. Scan Electron Microsc II: 477–484, 1977.
2. Burger PC, Chandler DB, Klintworth GK. Scanning electron microscopy of vascular casts. J Elec Micro Tech 1: 341–348, 1984.
3. Hammersen F, Endrick B, Messmer K. The fine structure of tumor blood vessels. Int J Microcirc Clin Exp 4: 31–43, 1985.
4. Fahrenbach WH, Bacon DR, Morrison JC, Van Buskirk EM. Controlled vascular corrosion casting of the rabbit eye. J Elec Micro Tech 10: 15–26, 1988.
5. Schraufnagel DE, Schmid A. Microvascular casting of the lung. Effects of various fixation protocols. J Elec Micro Tech 8: 185–191, 1988.
6. Falk P. Differences in vascular pattern between the spontaneous and the transplanted C3H mouse mammary carcinoma. Eur J Cancer 18: 155–165, 1982.
7. Warren BA. The vascular morphology of tumors. In: Peterson HI (Ed), Tumor Blood Circulation. Boca Raton, FL: CRC Press, pp. 1–47, 1979.

8.   Falk P. Patterns of vasculature in two pairs of related fibrosarcomas in the rat and their relation to tumour response to single large doses of radiation. Eur J Cancer 14: 237–250, 1978.

9.   Jain RK. Determinants of tumor blood flow: a review. Cancer Res 48: 2641–2658, 1988.

10.  Peters W, Teixeira M, Intaglietta M, Gross JF. Microcirculatory studies in rat mammary carcinoma. I. Transparent chamber method, development of microvasculature and pressures in tumor vessels. J Natl Cancer Inst 65: 631–642, 1980.

11.  Zweifach BW. I. Analysis of pressure distribution in the terminal vascular bed in cat mesentery. Circ Res 34: 843–857, 1974.

12.  House SD, Johnson PC. Diameter and blood flow of skeletal muscle venules during local flow regulation. Am J Physiol 250: H828-H837, 1986.

13.  Schmid-Schoenbein GW, Zweifach BW, Kovalcheck S. The application of stereological principles to morphometry of the microcirculation in different tissues. Microvasc Res 14: 303–317, 1977.

14.  Dewhirst MW, Tso CY, Oliver R, et al. Morphologic and hemodynamic comparison of tumor and healing normal tissue microvasculature. Int J Radiat Oncol Biol Phys 17: 91–99, 1989.

15.  Endrich B, Intaglietta M, Reinhold HS, Gross JF. Hemodynamic characteristics in microcirculatory blood channels during early tumor growth. Cancer Res 39: 17–23, 1979.

16.  Endrich B, Hammersen F, Gotz A, Messmer K. Microcirculatory blood flow, capillary morphology, and local oxygen pressure of the hamster amelanotic melanoma A-Mel-3. J Natl Cancer Inst 68: 475–485, 1982.

17.  Less JR, Skalak TC, Sevick EM, Jain RK. Microvascular architecture in a mammary carcinoma: branching patterns and vessel dimensions. Cancer Res 51: 265–273, 1991.

18.  Skalak TC, Schmid-Schönbein GW. The microvasculature in skeletal muscle. IV. A model of the capillary network. Microvasc Res 32: 333–347, 1986.

19.  Vaupel P. Oxygen supply to malignant tumors. In: Peterson HI (Ed), Tumor Blood Circulation. Boca Raton, FL: CRC Press, pp. 143–168, 1979.

20.  Awwad HK, El Naggar ME, Mocktar N, Barsoum M. Intercapillary distance measurement as an indicator of hypoxia in carcinoma of the cervix uteri. Int J Radiat Oncol Biol Phys 12: 1329–1333, 1986.

21.  Tannock IF, Steel GG. Quantitative techniques for study of the anatomy and function of small blood vessels in tumors. J Natl Cancer Inst 42: 771–782, 1969.

22.  Lauk S, Zietman A, Skates S, et al. Comparative morphometric study of tumor vasculature in human squamous cell carcinomas and their xenotransplants in athymic nude mice. Cancer Res 49: 4557–4561, 1989.

23.  Folkman J. Tumor angiogenesis: therapeutic implications. N Engl J Med 285: 1182–1186, 1971.

24.  Folkman J. Anti-angiogenesis: new concept for therapy of solid tumors. Ann Surg 175: 409–416, 1972.

25.  Voyta JC, Via DP, Butterfield CE, Zetter BR. Identification and isolation of endothelial cells based on their increased uptake of acetylated-low density lipoprotein. J Cell Biol 99: 2034–2040, 1984.

26.  Folkman J, Klagsbrun M. Angiogenic factors. Science 235: 442–447, 1987.

27.  Folkman J. What is the role of angiogenesis in metastasis from cutaneous melanoma? Eur J Cancer Clin Oncol 23: 361–363, 1987.

28.  Folkman J, Watson K, Ingber D, Hanahan D. Induction of angiogenesis during the transition from hyperplasis to neoplasia. Nature 339: 58–61, 1989.

29.  Folkman J. What is the evidence that tumors are angiogenesis dependent? J Natl Cancer Inst 82: 4–6, 1990.

30.  Haimovitz-Friedman A, Vlodavsky I, Chaudhuri A, et al. Autocrine effects of fibroblast growth factor in repair of radiation damage in endothelial cells. Cancer Res 51: 2552–2558, 1991.

31.  Folkman J, Shing Y. Angiogenesis. J Biol Chem 267(16): 10931–10934, 1992.

32.  Shing Y, Folkman J, Haudenschild C, et al. Angiogenesis is stimulated by a tumor-derived endothelial cell growth factor. J Cell Biochem 29: 275–287, 1985.

33.  Thomas KA. Fibroblast growth factors. FASEB J 1: 434–440, 1987.

34.  Rifkin DB, Moscatelli D. Recent developments in the cell biology of basic fibroblast growth factor. J Cell Biol 109(1): 1–6, 1989.

35.  Burgess WH, Maciag T. The heparin-binding (fibroblast) growth factor family of proteins. Ann Rev Biochem 58: 575–606, 1986.

36.  Gospodarowicz D. Fibroblast growth factor and its involvement in developmental processes. Curr Topics Dev Biol 24: 57–93, 1990.

37.  Klagsbrun M, D'Amore PA. Regulators of angiogenesis. Annu Rev Physiol 53: 217–239, 1991.

38.  Montesano R, Vassalli JD, Baird A, et al. Basic fibroblast growth factor induces angiogenesis in vitro. Proc Natl Acad Sci USA 83(19): 7297–7301, 1986.
39.  Thomas KA, Rios-Candelore M, Gimenz-Gallego G, et al. Pure brain-derived acidic fibroblast growth factor is a potent angiogenic vascular endothelial cell mitogen with sequence homology to interleukin 1. Proc Natl Acad Sci USA 82: 6409–6413, 1985.
40.  Lobb RR, Alderman EM, Fett JW. Induction of angiogenesis by bovine brain derived class 1 heparin-binding growth factor. Biochemistry 24(19): 4969–4973, 1985.
41.  Baird A, Ling A. Fibroblast growth factors are present in the extracellular matrix produced by endothelial cells in vitro: implications for a role of heparinase-like enzymes in the neovascular response. Biochem Biophys Res Commun 142: 428–435, 1987.
42.  Shing Y. Heparin-copper biaffinity chromatography of fibroblast growth factors. J Biol Chem 263(18): 9059–9062, 1988.
43.  Moscatelli D, Presta M, Rifkin DB. Purification of a factor from human placenta that stimulates capillary endothelial cell protease production, DNA synthesis, and migration. Proc Natl Acad Sci USA 83(7): 2091–2095, 1986.
44.  Presta M, Moscatelli D, Joseph-Silverstein J, Rifkin DB. Purification from a human hepatoma cell line of a basic fibroblast growth factor-like molecule that stimulates capillary endothelial cell plasminogen activator production, DNA synthesis, and migration. Mol Cell Biol 6(1): 4060–4066, 1986.
45.  Slack JM, Darlington BG, Heath JK, Godsave SF. Mesoderm induction in early Xenopus embryos by heparin-binding growth factors. Nature 326: 197–200, 1987.
46.  Kimmelman D, Kirschner M. Synergistic induction of mesoderm by FGF and TGF-beta and the identification of an mRNA coding for FGF in the early Xenopus embryo. Cell 51(5): 869–877, 1987.
47.  Vlodavsky I, Folkman J, Sullivan R, et al. Endothelial cell-derived basic fibroblast growth factor. synthesis and deposition into subendothelial extracellular matrix. Proc Natl Acad Sci USA 84(8): 2292–2296, 1987.
48.  Ferrara N, Henzel WJ. Pituitary follicular cells secrete a novel heparin-binding growth factor specific for vascular endothelial cells. Biochem Biophys Res Commun 161(2): 851–858, 1989.
49.  Gospodarowicz D, Abraham JA, Schilling J. Isolation and characterization of a vascular endothelial cell mitogen produced by pituitary-derived folliculo stellate cells. Proc Natl Acad Sci USA 86(19): 7311–7315, 1989.
50.  Connolly DT, Heuvelman DM, Nelson R, et al. Tumor vascular permeability factor stimulates endothelial growth and angiogenesis. J Clin Invest 84(5): 1470–1478, 1989.
51.  Pepper MS, Ferrara N, Orci L, Montesano R. Vascular endothelial growth factor (VEGF) induces plasminogen activators and plasminogen activator inhibitor-1 in microvascular endothelial cells. Biochem Biophys Res Commun 181(2): 902–906, 1991.
52.  Leung ZW, Cachianes G, Kuang WJ, et al. Vascular endothelial growth factor is a secreted angiogenic mitogen. Science 246(4935): 1306–1309, 1989.
53.  Plouet J, Schilling J, Gospodarowicz D. Isolation and characterization of a newly identified endothelial cell mitogen produced by AtT-20 cells. EMBO J 8(12): 3801, 1989.
54.  Conn G, Soderman DD, Schaeffer MT, et al. Purification of a glycoprotein vascular endothelial cell mitogen from a rat glioma-derived cell line. Proc Natl Acad Sci USA 87(4): 1323–1327, 1990.
55.  Myoken Y, Kayada Y, Okamoto T, et al. Vascular endothelial cell growth factor (VEGF) produced by A-431 human epidermoid carcinoma cells and identification of VEGF membrane binding sites. Proc Natl Acad Sci USA 88(13): 5819–5823, 1991.
56.  Rosenthal RA, Megyesi J, Henzel WJ, et al. Conditioned medium from mouse sarcoma 180 cells contains vascular endothelial growth factor. Growth Factors 4(1): 53–59, 1990.
57.  Connolly DT, Olander JV, Heuvelman D, et al. Human vascular permeability factor. Isolation from U937 cells. J Biol Chem 264: 20017–20024, 1989.
58.  Keck PJ, Hauser SD, Krivi G, Sanzo K, et al. Vascular permeability factor, an endothelial cell mitogen related to PDGF. Science 246(4935): 1309–1312, 1989.
59.  Conn G, Bayne ML, Soderman DD, et al. Amino acid and cDNA sequences of a vascular endothelial cell mitogen that is homologous to platelet-derived growth factor. Proc Natl Acad Sci USA 87(7): 2628–2632, 1990.
60.  Tischer E, Mitchell R, Hartman T, et al. The human gene for vascular endothelial growth factor. Multiple protein forms are encoded through alternative exon splicing. J Biol Chem 266(18): 11947–11954, 1991.
61.  O'Brien T, Cranston D, Fuggle S, et al. Different angiogenic pathways characterize superficial and invasive bladder cancer. Cancer Res 55: 510–513, 1995.

62. Samoto K, Ikezaki K, Ono M, et al. Expression of vascular endothelial growth factor and its possible relation with neovascularization in human brain tumors. Cancer Res 55: 1189–1193, 1995.

63. Shweiki D, Neeman M, Itin A, Keshet E. Induction of vascular endothelial growth factor expression by hypoxia and by glucose deficiency in multicell spheroids: implication for tumor angiogenesis. Proc Natl Acad Sci USA 92: 768–772, 1995.

64. Plate KH, Breier G, Weich HA, et al. Vascular endothelial growth factor and glioma angiogenesis. coordinate induction of VEGF receptors, distribution of VEGF protein and possible *in vivo* regulatory mechanisms. Int J Cancer 59: 520–529, 1994.

65. Kondo S, Matsumoto T, Yokoyama Y, et al. The shortest isoform of human vascular endothelial growth factor/vascular permeability factor (VEGF/VPF$_{121}$) produced by *Saccharomyces cerevisiae* promotes both angiogenesis and vascular permeability. Biochim Biophys Acta 1243: 195–202, 1995.

66. Luger TA, Schwarz T. Evidence for an epidermal cytokine network. J Invest Dermatol 95: 100S–104S, 1990.

67. Oliveira IC, Sciavolino PJ, Lee TH, Vilcek J. Downregulation of interleukin 8 gene expression in human fibroblasts. unique mechanism of transcriptional inhibition by interferon. Proc Natl Acad Sci USA 89: 9049–9053, 1992.

68. Baggiolini M, Clark-Lewis I. Interleukin-8, a chemotactic and inflammatory cytokine. Fed Eur Biochem Soc 307: 97–101, 1992.

69. Bickel M. The role of interleukin-8 in inflammation and mechanisms of regulation. J Perio Res 64: 456–460, 1993.

70. Koch AE, Polverini PJ, Kunkel SL, et al. Interleukin-8 as a macrophage-derived mediator of angiogenesis. Science 258: 1798–1801, 1992.

71. Aman MJ, Rudolf, G, Goldschmitt J, et al. Type-I interferons are potent inhibitors of interleukin-8 production in hematopoietic and bone marrow stromal cells. Blood 82: 2371–2378, 1993.

72. Ishikawa F, Miyazone K, Hellman U, et al. Identification of angiogenic activity and the cloning and expression of platelet-derived endothelial cell growth factor. Nature 338(6216): 557–562, 1989.

73. Fett JW, Strydom DJ, Lob RR, et al. Isolation and characterization of angiogenin, an angiogenic protein from human carcinoma cells. Biochemistry 24(20): 5480–5486, 1985.

74. Bicknell R, Vallee BL. Angiogenin activates endothelial cell phospholipase. Proc Natl Acad Sci USA 85(16): 5961–5965, 1988.

75. Bicknell R, Vallee BL. Angiogenin stimulates endothelial cell prostacyclin secretion by activation of phospholipase. Proc Natl Acad Sci USA 86(5): 1573–1577, 1989.

76. Shapiro R, Riordan JF, Vallee BL. Characteristic ribonucleolytic activity of human angiogenin. Biochemistry 25(12): 3527–3532, 1986.

77. St. Clair DK, Ryback SM, Riordan JF, Vallee BL. Angiogenin abolishes cell free protein synthesis by specific peptide inactivation of ribosomes. Proc Natl Acad Sci USA 84: 8330–8334, 1987.

78. Hu G-F, Riordan JF, Vallee BL. Angiogenin promotes invasiveness of cultured endothelial cells by stimulation of cell-associated proteolytic activities. Proc Natl Acad Sci USA 91: 12096–12100, 1994.

79. Olson KA, Fett JW, French TC, et al. Angiogenin antagonists prevent tumor growth *in vivo*. Proc Natl Acad Sci USA 92: 442–446, 1995.

80. Leibovich SJ, Polverini PJ, Shepard HM, et al. Macrophage-induced angiogenesis is mediated by tumour necrosis factor-alpha. Nature 329(6140): 630–632, 1987.

81. Frater-Schroder M, Risau W, et al. Tumor necrosis factor type alpha, a potent inhibitor of endothelial cell growth in vitro, is angiogenic in vivo. Proc Natl Acad Sci USA 84(15): 5277–5281, 1987.

82. Okamura K, Sato Y, Matsuda T, et al. Endogenous basic fibroblast growth factor-dependent induction of collagenase and interleukin-6 in tumor necrosis factor-treated human microvascular endothelial cells. J Biol Chem 266(29): 19162–19165, 1991.

83. Beutler B, Cerami A. Cachectin and tumour necrosis factor as two sides of the same biological coin. Nature 320(6063): 584–588, 1986.

84. Schreiber AB, WInkler ME, Derynck R. Transforming growth factor-alpha: a more potent angiogenic mediator than epidermal growth factor. Science 232(4755): 1250–1253, 1986.

85. Derynck R. Transforming growth factor-alpha. Mol Reprod Dev 27(1): 3–9, 1990.

86. Roberts AB, Sporn MB, Assoian RK, et al. Transforming growth factor type beta. rapid induction of fibrosis and angiogenesis in vivo and stimulation of collagen formation in vitro. Proc Natl Acad Sci USA 83(12): 4167–4171, 1986.

87. Sporn MB, Roberts AB. Peptide Growth Factors. Berlin: Springer-Verlag, pp. 419–472, 1990.

88.   Dobson DE, Kambe A, Block E, et al. 1-Butyryl-glycerol. a novel angiogenesis factor secreted by differentiating adipocytes. Cell 61(2): 223–230, 1990.

89.   Form DM, Auerbach R. PGE2 and angiogenesis. Proc Soc Exp Biol Med 172(2): 214–218, 1983.

90.   Ziche M, Jones J, Gullino P. Role of prostaglandin E1 and copper in angiogenesis. J Natl Cancer Inst 69(2): 475–482, 1982.

91.   BenEzra D. Neovasculogenic ability of prostaglandins, growth factors, and synthetic chemoattractants. Am J Opthal 86(4): 455–461, 1978.

92.   Graeber JE, Glaser BM, Setty BNY, et al. 15-Hydroxyeicosatetraenoic acid stimulates migration of human retinal microvessel endothelium in vitro and neovascularization in vivo. Prostaglandin 39(6): 665–673, 1990.

93.   Kull Jr. FC, Brent DA, Parikh I, Cuatrecasas P. Chemical identification of a tumor-derived angiogenic factor. Science 236(4803): 843–845, 1987.

94.   Fraser RA, Ellis M, Stalker AL. Experimental angiogenesis in the chorioallantoic membrane. In: Lewis DH (Ed), Current Advances in Basic and Clinical Microcirculatory Research. Basel: Karger, pp. 25–27, 1979.

95.   Dusseau JW, Hutchins PM, Malbasa DS. Stimulation of angiogenesis by adenosine on the chick chorioallantoic membrane. Circ Res 59(2): 163–170, 1986.

96.   West DC, Hampson IN, Arnold F, Kumar S. Angiogenesis induced by degradation products of hyaluronic acid. Science 228(4705): 1324–1326, 1985.

97.   Masferrer JL, Rimarachin JA, Gerrifsen ME, et al. 12(R)-hydroxyeicosatrienoic acid, a potent chemotactic and angiogenic factor produced by the cornea. Exp Eye Res 52(4): 417–424, 1991.

98.   Laniado-Schwartzman M, Lavrovsky Y, Stoltz RA, et al. Activation of nuclear factor $\kappa$B and oncogene expression by 12(R)-hydroxyeicosatrienoic acid, an angiogenic factor in microvessel endothelial cells. J Biol Chem 269(39): 24321–25327, 1994.

99.   Oikawa T, Suganuma M, Ashino-Fuse H, Shimamura M. Okadaic acid is a potent angiogenesis inducer. Jpn J Cancer Res 83(1): 6–9, 1992.

100.  Mustonen T, Alitalo K. Endothelial receptor tyrosine kinases involved in angiogenesis. J Cell Biol 129(4): 895–898, 1995.

101.  van der Geer P, Hunter T, Lindberg RA. Receptor protein-tyrosine kinases and their signal transduction pathways. Annu Rev Cell Biol 10: 251–337, 1994.

102.  Blood CH, Zetter BR. Tumor interactions with the vasculature: angiogenesis and tumor metastases. Biochim Biophys Acta 1032: 89–118, 1990.

103.  Vlodavsky I, Korner G, Ishai-Michaeli R, et al. Extracellular matrix-resident growth factors and enzymes. possible involvement in tumor metastasis and angiogenesis. Cancer Metastasis Rev 9: 203–226, 1990.

104.  Liotta LA, Steeg PS, Stetler-Stevenson WG. Cancer metastasis and angiogenesis: an imbalance of positive and negative regulation. Cell 64: 327–336, 1991.

105.  Zetter BR. Cell motility in angiogenesis and tumor metastasis. Cancer Invest 8(6): 669–671, 1990.

106.  Dorudi S, Hart IR. Mechanisms underlying invasion and metastasis. Curr Opin Oncol 5: 130–135, 1993.

107.  Liotta LA, Tryggvason K, Garbisa S, et al. Metastatic potential correlates with enzymatic degradation of basement membrane collagen. Nature (London) 284: 67–68, 1980.

108.  Liotta LA, Thorgeirrson UP, Garbisa S. Role of collagenases in tumor cell invasion. Cancer Metastasis Rev 1(4): 277–288, 1982.

109.  Liotta LA, Stetler-Stevenson W. Metalloproteinases and malignant conversion: does correlation imply causality? J Natl Cancer Inst 81(8): 556–557, 1989.

110.  Sanchez-Lopez R, Nicholson R, Gesnel MC, et al. Structure-function relationships in the collagenase family member transin. J Biol Chem 263(24): 11892–11899, 1988.

111.  Muller D, Quantin B, Gesnel MC, et al. The collagenase gene family in humans consists of at least four members. Biochem J 253(1): 187–192, 1988.

112.  Chin JR, Murphy G, Werb Z. Stromelysin, a connective tissue-degrading metalloendopeptidase secreted by stimulated rabbit synovial fibroblasts in parallel with collagenase. Biosynthesis, isolation, characterization, and substrates. J Biol Chem 260(22): 12367–12376, 1985.

113.  Wilhelm SM, Collier IE, Kronberger A, et al. Human skin fibroblast stromelysin. structure, glycosylation, substrate specificity, and differential expression in normal and tumorigenic cells. Proc Natl Acad Sci USA 84(19): 6725–6729, 1987.

114.  Ostrowski LE, Finch J, Krieg P, et al. Expression pattern of a gene for a secreted metalloproteinase during late stages of tumor progression. Mol Carcin 1(1): 13–19, 1988.

115. Paganetti PA, Caroni P, Schwab ME. Glioblastoma infiltration into central nervous system tissue in vitro. involvement of a metalloprotease. J Cell Biol 107(6 Pt 1): 2281–2291, 1988.

116. Chen JM, Chen WT. Fibronectin-degrading proteases from the membranes of transformed cells. Cell 48(2): 193–203, 1987.

117. Werb Z, Tremble PM, Behrendtsen O, et al. Signal transduction through the fibronectin receptor induces collagenase and stromelysin gene expression. J Cell Biol 109: 877–889, 1989.

118. Thorgeirsson UP, Turpeenniemi-Hujanen T, Williams JE, et al. NIH/3T3 cells transfected with human tumor DNA containing activated *ras* oncogenes express the metastatic phenotype in nude mice. Mol Cell Biol 5: 259–262, 1985.

119. Garbisa S, Pozatti R, Mushchel RJ, et al. Secretion of type IV collagenolytic protease and metastatic phenotype: induction by transfection with c-Ha-*ras* but not c-Ha-*ras* plus Ad2-E1a. Cancer Res 47(6): 1523–1528, 1987.

120. Carlsen SA, Ramshaw IA, Warrinton RC. Involvement of plasminogen activator production with tumor metastases in a rat model. Cancer Res 44(7): 1122–1127, 1984.

121. Eisenbach L, Sega S, Feldman M. Proteolytic enzymes in tumor metastasis. II. Collagenase Type IV activity in subcellular fractions of cloned tumor cell populations. J Natl Cancer Inst 74: 87–93, 1985.

122. Sullivan LM, Wuigley JP. An anticatalytic monoclonal antibody to avian plasminogen activator: its effect on behavior of RSV-transformed chick fibroblasts. Cell 45(6): 905–915, 1986.

123. Ramshaw IA, Badenoch-Jones P, Grant A, et al. Enhanced plasminogen activator production by highly metastatic variant cell lines of a rat mammary adenocarcinoma. Invasion Metastasis 6: 133–144, 1986.

124. Ostrowski LE, Ashon A, Suthan BP, et al. Selective inhibition for proteolytic enzymes in an *in vivo* mouse model for experimental metastasis. Cancer Res 46: 4121–4128, 1986.

125. Sappino AP, Busso N, Belin D, Vassali JD. Increase of urokinase-type plasminogen activator gene expression in human lung and breast carcinomas. Cancer Res 47(15): 4043–4046, 1987.

126. Evers JL, Patel J, Madeja JM, et al. Plasminogen activator activity and composition in human breast cancer. Cancer Res 42(1): 219–226, 1982.

127. Ossowoski L, Reich E. Antibodies to plasminogen activator inhibit human tumor metastasis. Cell 35: 611–619, 1983.

128. Ossowski L. Plasminogen activator dependent pathways in the dissemination of human tumor cells in chick embryo. Cell 52(3): 321–328, 1988.

129. Hearing VJ, Law LW, Corti A, et al. Modulation of metastatic potential by cell surface urokinase of murine melanoma cells. Cancer Res 48: 1270–1278, 1988.

130. Axelrod JH, Reich R, Miskin R. Expression activator dependent pathways in the dissemination of human tumor cells in the chick embryo. Mol Cell Biol 9(5): 2133–2141, 1989.

131. Sloane BF, Dunn JR, Honn KV. Lysosomal cathepsin B: correlation with metastatic potential. Science 212(4499): 1151–1152, 1981.

132. Sloane BF, Honn KV, Sadler JG, et al. Cathepsin B activity in B16 melanoma cells: a possible marker for metastatic potential. Cancer Res 42: 980–986, 1982.

133. Koppel P, Baici A, Keist R, et al. Cathepsin B-like enzymes. Subcellular distribution and properties in neoplastic and control cells from human ectocervix. Exp Cell Biol 52(8): 293–299, 1984.

134. Sloane BF, Rozchin J, Johnson K, et al. Association with plasma membrane in metastatic tumors. Proc Natl Acad Sci USA 83: 2483–2487, 1986.

135. Rozhin J, Robinson D, Stevens MA, et al. Mesoderm induction in early Xenopus embryos by heparin-binding growth factors. Cancer Res 40: 550–556, 1987.

136. Kao TR, Stern R. Elastases in human breast carcinoma cell lines. Cancer Res 46(3): 1355–1358, 1986.

137. Nemoto S, Koiso K, Aoyagi K, Takahashi S. Elastase - does this enzyme play any role in bladder cancer invasion? J Urol 134(5): 996–998, 1986.

138. Zeydel M, Nakagawa S, Biempica L, Takahashi S. Collagenase and elastase production by mouse mammary adenocarcinoma primary cultures and cloned cells. Cancer Res 46(12 Pt 1): 6438–6445, 1986.

139. Yusa T, Blood CH, Zetter BR. Tumor cell interactions with elastin. implications for pulmonary metastasis. Am Rev Respir Dis 140(5): 1458–1462, 1989.

140. Kao RT, Wong M, Stern R. Elastin degradation by proteases from cultured human breast cancer cells. Biochem Biophys Res Commun 105(1): 383–389, 1982.

141. Hornebeck W, Brechmeier D, Bollon G, et al. Proteinases and Tumor Invasion. New York: Raven Press, pp. 117–139, 1980.

142. Vlodavsky I, Fuks Z, Bar-Ner M, et al. Lymphoma cell-mediated degradation of sulfated proteoglycans in the subendothelial extracellular matrix: relationship to tumor cell metastasis. Cancer Res 43(6): 2704–2711, 1983.

143. Nakajima M, Irimura T, Di Ferrante D, et al. Heparan sulfate degradation: relation to tumor invasive and metastatic properties of mouse B16 melanoma sublines. Science 220(4597): 611–613, 1983.

144. Corcoran ML, Stetler-Stevenson WG, Brown PD, Wahl LM. Interleukin 4 inhibition of prostaglandin E2 synthesis blocks interstitial collagenase and 92-kDa type IV collagenase/gelatinase production by human monocytes. J Biol Chem 267: 515–519, 1992.

145. Henry N, van Lasmsweerde A-L, Vaes G. Collagen degradation by metastatic variants of Lewis Lung Carcinoma: cooperation between tumor cells and macrophages. Cancer Res 43: 5321–5327, 1983.

146. Templeton NS, Stetler-Stevenson WG. Identification of a basal promoter for the human Mr 72,000 type IV collagenase gene and enhanced expression in a highly metastatic cell line. Cancer Res 51: 6190–6193, 1991.

147. Pyke C, Ralfkiaer E, Huhtala P, et al. Localization of messenger RNA for Mr 72,000 and 92,000 type IV collagenases in human skin cancers by *in situ* hybridization. Cancer Res 52: 1336–1341, 1992.

148. Overall CM, Wrana JL, Sodek J. Transcriptional and post-transcriptional regulation of 72-kDa gelatinase/Type IV collagenase by transforming growth factor-$\beta$1 in human fibroblasts. J Biol Chem 266(21): 14064–14071, 1991.

149. Coucke P, Baramova E, Leprince P, et al. Metalloproteinases and serine proteases activities in mixed spheroids of mouse B16 melanoma cells and fibroblasts. Int J Oncol 5: 1125–1130, 1994.

150. Roskelley CD, Desprez PY, Bissell MJ. Extracellular matrix-dependent tissue-specific gene expression in mammary epithelial cells requires both physical and biochemical signal transduction. Proc Natl Acad Sci USA 91: 12378–12382, 1994.

151. Nakajima M, Welch DR, Wynn DM, et al. Serum and plasma $M_r$ 92,000 progelatinase levels correlate with spontaneous metastasis of rat 13762NF mammary adenocarcinoma. Cancer Res 53: 5802–5807, 1993.

152. Zucker S, Lysik RM, Zarrabi MH, Moll U. $M_r$ 92,000 Type IV collagenase is increased in plasma of patients with colon cancer and breast cancer. Cancer Res 53: 140–146, 1993.

153. Rao JS, Steck PA, Mohanam S, et al. Elevated levels of $M_r$ 92,000 Type IV collagenase in human brain tumors. Cancer Res 53: 2208–2211, 1993.

154. Alvarez OA, Carmichael DF, DeClerck YA. Inhibition of collagenolytic activity and metastasis of tumor cells by a recombinant human tissue inhibitor of metalloproteinases. J Natl Cancer Inst 82: 589–595, 1990.

155. Terranova VP, Hujanen ES, Martin GR. Basement membrane and the invasive activity of metastatic tumor cells. J Natl Cancer Inst 77: 311–316, 1986.

156. Tryggvason K, Hoyhtya M, Salo T. Proteolytic degradation of extracellular matrix in tumor invasion. Biochim Biophys Acta 907: 191–217, 1987.

157. Taylor S, Folkman J. Protamine is an inhibitor of angiogenesis. Nature 297: 307–312, 1982.

158. Groopman JE, Scadden DT. Interferon therapy for Kaposi sarcoma associated with the acquired immunodeficiency syndrome (AIDS). Ann Int Med 110: 335–337, 1989.

159. White CW, Sondheimer HM, Crouch EC, et al. Treatment of pulmonary hemangiomatosis with recombinant interferon alfa-2a. Med Intell 18: 1197–1200, 1989.

160. Strieter RM, Kunkel SL, Arenberg DA, et al. Interferon $\gamma$-inducible protein 10 (IP-10), a member of the C-X-C chemokine family, is an inhibitor of angiogenesis. Biochem Biophys Res Commun 210(1): 51–57, 1995.

161. Kolber DL, Knisely TL, Maione TE. Inhibition of development of murine melanoma lung metastases by systemic administration of recombinant platelet factor 4. J Natl Cancer Inst 87: 304–309, 1995.

162. Stetler-Stevenson WG, Krutzsch HC, Liotta LA. Tissue inhibitor of metalloproteinase (TIMP-2). A new member of the metalloproteinase inhibitor family. J Biol Chem 264: 17374–17378, 1989.

163. Welgus HG, Stricklin GP. Human skin fibroblast collagenase inhibitor. Comparative studies in human connective tissues, serum, and amniotic fluid. J Biol Chem 258: 12259–12264, 1983.

164. Voest EE, Kenyon BM, O'Reilly MS, et al. Inhibition of angiogenesis *in vivo* by interleukin 12. J Natl Cancer Inst 87: 581–586, 1995.

165. Kerbel RS, Hawley RG. Interleukin 12: newest member of the antiangiogenesis club. J Natl Cancer Inst 87(8): 557–558, 1995.

166. Banks RE, Patel PM, Selby PJ. Interleukin 12: a new clinical player in cytokine therapy. Br J Cancer 71: 655–659, 1995.

167. O'Reilly MS, Holmgren L, Shing Y, et al. Angiostatin: a novel angiogenesis inhibitor that mediates the suppression of metastases by a Lewis lung carcinoma. Cell 79: 315–328, 1994.

168. Lee A, Langer R. Shark cartilage contains inhibitors of tumor angiogenesis. Science 221: 1185–1187, 1983.

169. Moses MA, Sudhalter J, Langer R. Identification of an inhibitor of neovascularization from cartilage. Science 248: 1408–1410, 1990.

170. Taylor CM, Weiss JB. Partial purification of a 5.7K glycoprotein from bovine vitreous which inhibits both angiogenesis and collagenase activity. Biochem Biophys Res Commun 133: 911–916, 1985.

171. DeClerck YA. Purification and characterization of a collagenase inhibitor produced by bovine vascular smooth muscle cells. Arch Biochem Biophys 265: 28–37, 1988.

172. Sakamoto N, Iwahana M, Tanaka NG, Osada Y. Inhibition of angiogenesis and tumor growth by a synthetic laminin peptide, CDPGYIGSR-NH$_2$. Cancer Res 51: 903–906, 1991.

173. Bogden AE, Taylor JE, Moreau J-P, et al. Response of human lung tumor xenografts to treatment with a somatostatin analogue (somatuline). Cancer Res 50: 4360–4365, 1990.

174. Brooks PC, Clark RA, Cheresh DA. Requirement of vascular integrin $\alpha_v\beta_3$ for angiogenesis. Science 264: 569–573, 1994.

175. Brooks PC, Montgomery AMP, Rosenfeld M, et al. Integrin $\alpha_v\beta_3$ antagonists promote tumor regression by inducing apoptosis of angiogenic blood vessels. Cell 79: 1157–1164, 1994.

176. Cheresh DA. Human endothelial cells synthesize and express an Arg-Gly-Asp-directed adhesion receptor involved in attachment to fibrinogen and von Willebrand factor. Proc Natl Acad Sci USA 84: 6471–6475, 1987.

177. Folkman J, Weisz PB, Joullie MM, et al. Control of angiogenesis with synthetic heparin substitutes. Science 243: 1490–1493, 1989.

178. Crum R, Szabo S, Folkman J. A new class of steroids inhibits angiogenesis in the presence of heparin or a heparin fragment. Science 230: 1375–1378, 1985.

179. Folkman J, Langer R, Lingardt R, et al. Angiogenesis inhibition and tumour regression caused by heparin or a heparin fragment in the presence of cortisone. Science 221: 719–725, 1983.

180. Lee K-E, Iwamura, M, Cockett ATK. Cortisone inhibition of tumor angiogenesis measured by a quantitative colorimetric assay in mice. Cancer Chemother Pharmacol 26: 461–463, 1990.

181. Ingber D, Folkman J. Inhibition of angiogenesis through modulation of collagen metabolism. Lab Invest 59: 44–51, 1988.

182. Oikawa T, Hirotani K, Nakamura O, et al. A highly potent antiangiogenic activity of retinoids. Cancer Lett 48: 157–162, 1989.

183. Sharpe RJ, Kadin ME, Harmon DC, et al. Complete resolution of Kaposi's sarcoma with systemic etretinate therapy in a patient with mycosis fungoides. J Am Acad Dermatol 20: 1123–1124, 1989.

184. Schwartz JL, Flynn E, Shklar G. The effects of carotenoids on the antitumor immune response in vivo and in vitro with hamster and mouse immune effectors. In: Bendich A, Chandra RK (Eds), Symposium on Micronutrients and Immune Functions. New York: New York Academy of Science, pp. 92–96, 1990.

185. Schwartz JL, Flynn E, Trickler D, Shklar G. Directed lysis of experimental cancer by beta carotene in liposomes. Nutr Cancer 16: 107–112, 1991.

186. Schwartz JL, Shklar G. A cyanobacteria extract and beta carotene stimulates an antitumor immune response against oral cancer cell line. Phytother Res 3: 243–248, 1989.

187. Schwartz JL, Singh R, Teicher B, et al. Induction of a 70-kDa protein associated with the selective cytotoxicity of beta carotene in human epidermal carcinoma. Biochem Biophys 169: 941–946, 1990.

188. Lippman SM, Kavanagh JJ, Paredes-Espinoza M, et al. 13-*cis*-retinoic acid plus interferon-$\alpha$2a in locally advanced squamous cell carcinoma of the cervix. J Natl Cancer Inst 85: 499–500, 1993.

189. Schwartz JL, Suda D, Light G. Beta carotene is associated with the regression of hamster buccal pouch carcinoma and the induction of tumor necrosis factor in macrophages. Biochem Biophys Res Commun 136: 1130–1135, 1986.

190. Shklar G, Schwartz JL. Tumor necrosis factor in experimental cancer regression with vitamin E, B-carotene, canthaxanthin and algae extract. Eur J Cancer 24: 839–850, 1988.

191. Smith MA, Parkinson DR, Cheson BO, Friedman MA. Retinoids in cancer therapy. J Clin Oncol 10: 839–864, 1992.

192. Chiocca E, Davies P, Stein J. The molecular basis of retinoic acid action. J Biol Chem 263: 11584–11589, 1988.

193. Cowan J, Vanhoff D, Dinesman A. Use of a human tumor cloning system to screen retinoids for antineo-plastic activity. Cancer 51: 92–96, 1983.
194. Lotem J, Sachs L. Regulation by *bcl*-2, c-*myc*, and *p53* of susceptibility to induction of apoptosis by heat shock and cancer chemotherapy compounds in differentiation competent and defective myeloid leukemic cells. Cell Growth Differ 4: 41–47, 1993.
195. Schwartz JL. β-carotene induced programmed cell death. J Dent Res 72: 285, 1993.
196. Schwartz JL, Antoniades DZ, Zhao S. Molecular and biochemical reprogramming of oncogenesis through the activity of prooxidant or antioxidants. N Y Acad Sci 686: 262–278, 1993.
197. Alles A, Sulik K. Retinoic acid-induced limb-reduction defects: perturbations of zones of programmed death as a pathogenetic mechanism. Teratology 40: 163–171, 1989.
198. Robertson K, Mueller L, Collins S. Retinoic acid receptors in myeloid leukemia: characterization of re-ceptors in retinoic acid resistant K-562 cells. Blood 77: 340–347, 1991.
199. Tabin C. Retinoids, homeoboxes, and growth factors: toward molecular models for limb development. Cell 66: 199–217, 1991.
200. Schwartz JL, Tanaka J, Khandekar V, et al. β-carotene and/or vitamin E as modulators of alkylating agents in SCC-25 human squamous carcinoma cells. Cancer Chemother Pharmacol 29: 207–213, 1992.
201. Denekamp J. Review article: angiogenesis, neovascular proliferation and vascular pathophysiology as targets for cancer therapy. Br J Radiol 66: 181–196, 1993.
202. Malone TE, Sharpe RJ. Development of angiogenesis inhibitors for clinical applications. Trends Biol Sci 11: 457–461, 1990.
203. Teicher BA, Schwartz JL, Holden SA, et al. *In vivo* modulation of several anticancer agents by β-carotene. Cancer Chemother Pharmacol 34(3): 235–241, 1994.
204. Garewal H, List A, Meyskens F. Phase II trial of fenretinide (N-(4-hydroxyphenyl) retinamide in myelo-dysplasia. Possible retinoid, induced disease acceleration. Leuk Res 13: 339–343, 1989.
205. Hong WK, Lippman SM, Itri LM. Prevention of secondary primary tumors with isotretinoin in squamous cell carcinoma of the head and neck. N Engl J Med 323: 795–801, 1990.
206. Schwartz JL, Antoniades DZ. β-carotene triggers enhanced expression of 70 kD stress protein and tumor suppresser p53 in association with the inhibition of oral carcinogenesis. Cancer Detect Prev, 1995, in press.
207. Majewski S, Szmurlo A, Marczak M, et al. Inhibition of tumor cell-induced angiogenesis by retinoids, 1,25-dihydroxyvitamin D₃ and their combination. Cancer Lett 75: 35–39, 1993.
208. Barnes S, Grubbs C, Setchell KDR, Carlson J. Soybeans inhibit mammary tumor in models of breast can-cer. In: Pariza M, Liss AR (Eds), Mutagens and Carcinogens in the Diet. New York: Wiley-Liss, pp. 239–253, 1990.
209. Akiyama T, Ishida J, Nakawaga S, et al. Genistein, a specific inhibitor of tyrosine-specific protein kinases. J Biol Chem 262(12): 5592–5595, 1987.
210. Okura A, Arakawa H, Oka H, et al. Effect of genistein on toposiomerase activity and on the growth of [Val12] Ha-*ras*-transformed NIH 3Y3 cells. Biochem Biophys Res Commun 157: 183–189, 1988.
211. Zwiller J, Sassone-Corsi P, Kakazu K, Boyton AL. Inhibition of PDGF-induced c-*jun* and c-*fos* expression by a tyrosine protein kinase inhibitor. Oncogene 6: 219–221, 1991.
212. Linassier C, Pierre M, Le Peco J-B, Pierre J. Mechanisms of action in NIH-3T3 cells of genistein, an in-hibitor of EGF receptor tyrosine kinase activity. Biochem Pharmacol 39: 187–193, 1990.
213. Yamashita Y, Kawada S, Nakano H. Induction of mammalian topoisomerase II dependent DNA cleavage by nonintercalative flavonoids, genistein and orobol. Biochem Pharmacol 39: 737–744, 1990.
214. Markovits J, Linassier C, Fosse P, et al. Inhibitory effects of the tyrosine kinase inhibitor genistein on mammalian DNA topoisomerase II. Cancer Res 49(18): 5111–5117, 1989.
215. Peterson G, Barnes S. Genistein inhibition of the growth of human breast cancer cells: independence from estrogen receptors and the multi-drug resistance gene. Biochem Biophys Res Commun 179: 661–667, 1991.
216. McCabe MJ Jr, Orrenius S. Genistein induces apoptosis in immature human thymocytes by inhibiting toposiomerase-II. Biochem Biophys Res Commun 194(2): 944–950, 1993.
217. Kanatani Y, Kasukabe T, Hozumi M, Motoyoshi K. Genistein exhibits preferential cytotoxicity to a leu-kemogenic variant but induces differentiation of a non-leukemogenic variant of the mouse monocytic leu-kemia Mm cell line. Leuk Res 17(10): 847–853, 1993.
218. Fotsis T, Pepper M, Adlercreutz H, et al. Genistein, a dietary-derived inhibitor of *in vitro* angiogenesis. Proc Natl Acad Sci USA 90: 2690–2694, 1993.

219. Sjoberg ER, Chammas R, Ozawa H, et al. Expression of de-*N*-acetyl-gangliosides in human melanoma cells is induced by genistein or nocodazole. J Biol Chem 270(7): 2921–2930, 1995.
220. Uckun FM, Evans WE, Forsyth CJ, et al. Biotherapy of B-cell precursor leukemia by targeting genistein to CD19-associated tyrosine kinases. Science 267: 886–889, 1995.
221. Ingber D, Fujita T, Kishimoto S, et al. Synthetic analogues of fumagillin that inhibit angiogenesis and suppress tumour growth. Nature 348: 555–557, 1990.
222. Kusaka M, Sudo K, Fujita T, et al. Potent anti-angiogenic action of AGM-1470: comparison to the fumagillin parent. Biochem Biophys Res Commun 174: 1070–1076, 1991.
223. Brem H, Ingber D, Blood CH, et al. Suppression of tumor metastasis by angiogenesis inhibition. Surg Forum 42: 439–441, 1991.
224. Brem H, Folkman J. Analysis of experimental antiangiogenic therapy. J Ped Surg 28: 445–451, 1993.
225. Takayamiya Y, Friedlander RM, Brem H, et al. Inhibition of angiogenesis and growth of human nerve sheath tumors by AGM-1470. J Neurosurg 78: 470–476, 1993.
226. Brem H, Gresser I, Grossfeld J, Folkman J. The combination of antiangiogenic agents to inhibit primary tumor growth and metastasis. J Ped Surg 28: 445–451, 1993.
227. Yanase T, Tamura M, Fujita K, et al. Inhibitory effect of angiogenesis inhibitor TNP-470 in rabbits bearing VX-2 carcinoma by arterial administration of microspheres and oil solution. Cancer Res 53: 2566–2570, 1993.
228. Kamei S, Okada H, Inoue Y, et al. Antitumor effects of angiogenesis inhibitor TNP-470 in rabbits bearing VX-2 carcinoma by arterial administration of microspheres and oil solution. J Pharmacol Exp Ther 264(1): 469–474, 1993.
229. Yamaoka M, Yamamoto T, Masaki T, et al. Inhibition of tumor growth and metastasis of rodent tumors by the angiogenesis inhibitor *O*-(Chloroacetyl-carbamoyl)fumagillin (TNP-470; AGM-1470). Cancer Res 53: 4262–4267, 1993.
230. Toi M, Yamamoto Y, Imazawa T, et al. Antitumor effect of the angiogenesis inhibitor AGM-1470 and its combination effect with tamoxifen in DMBA induced mammary tumors in rats. Int J Oncol 3: 525–528, 1993.
231. Yamaoka M, Yamamoto T, Ikeyama S, et al. Angiogenesis inhibitor TNP-470 (AGM-1470) potently inhibits the tumor growth of hormone-independent human breast and prostate carcinoma cell lines. Cancer Res 53: 5233–5236, 1993.
232. Schoof DD, Obando JA, Cusack JC Jr, et al. The influence of angiogenesis inhibitor AGM-1470 on immune system status and tumor growth *in vitro*. Int J Cancer 55: 630–635, 1993.
233. Teicher BA, Holden SA, Ara G, et al. Potentiation of cytotoxic cancer therapies by TNP-470 alone and with other antiangiogenic agents. Int J Cancer 57: 920–925, 1994.
234. Teicher BA, Dupuis N, Kusumoto T, et al. Antiangiogenic agents can increase tumor oxygenation and response to radiation therapy. Radiat Oncol Invest 2: 269–276, 1995.
235. Teicher BA, Holden SA, Dupuis NP, et al. Potentiation of cytotoxic therapies by TNP-470 and minocycline in mice bearing EMT-6 mammary carcinoma. Breast Cancer Res Treatment 36: 227–236, 1995.
236. Teicher BA, Dupuis NP, Robinson M, et al. Antiangiogenic treatment (TNP-470/minocycline) increases tissue levels of anticancer drugs in mice bearing Lewis lung carcinoma. Oncology Res 7(5): 237–243, 1995.
237. Teicher BA, Holden SA, Ara G, et al. Influence of an anti-angiogenic treatment on 9L gliosarcoma. oxygenation and response to cytotoxic therapy. Int J Cancer 61(5): 732–737, 1995.
238. Konno H, Tanaka T, Matsuda I, et al. Comparison of the inhibitory effect of the angiogenesis inhibitor, TNP-470, and mitomycin C on the growth and liver metastasis of human colon cancer. Int J Cancer 61: 268–271, 1995.
239. Hori A, Ikeyama S, Sudo K. Suppression of cyclin D1 mRNA expression by the angiogenesis inhibitor TNP-470 (AGM-1470) in vascular endothelial cells. Biochem Biophys Res Commun 204(3): 1067–1073, 1994.
240. Tanaka T, Konno H, Matsuda I, et al. Prevention of hepatic metastasis of human colon cancer by angiogenesis inhibitor TNP-470. Cancer Res 55: 836–839, 1995.
241. Murata J, Saiki I, Makabe T, et al. Inhibition of tumor-induced angiogenesis by sulfated chitin derivatives. Cancer Res 51: 22–26, 1991.
242. Teicher BA, Alvarez Sotomayor E, Huang ZD, et al. β-Cyclodextrin tetradecasulfate/tetrahydrocortisol ± minocycline as modulators of cancer therapies *in vitro* and *in vivo* against primary and metastatic Lewis lung carcinoma. Cancer Chemother Pharmacol 33: 229–38, 1993.

243. Teicher BA, Holden SA, Ara G, Northey D. Response of the FSaII fibrosarcoma to antiangiogenic modulators plus cytotoxic agents. Anticancer Res 13: 2101–2106, 1993.
244. Larsson EL, Joki A, Stälhandske T. Mechanism of action of the new immunomodulator LS26166 on T-cell responses. Int J Immunopharmacol 9: 425–431, 1987.
245. Harning R, Koo GC, Szalay J. Regulation of the metastasis of murine ocular melanoma by natural killer cells. Invest Ophthalmol Visual Sci 30: 1909–1915, 1989.
246. Kalland T. Effects of the immunomodulator LS-2616 on growth and metastasis of the murine B16-F10 melanoma. Cancer Res 46: 3018–3022, 1986.
247. Harning R, Szalay J. A treatment for metastasis of murine ocular melanoma. Invest Ophthalmol Visual Sci 29: 1505–1510, 1988.
248. Tarkowski A, Gunnarsson K, Nilsson LA, et al. Successful treatment of autoimmunity in MRL/1 mice with LS-2616, a new autoimmunomodulator. Arthritis Rheum 29: 1405–1409, 1986.
249. Ichikawa T, Lamb JC, Christensson PJ, et al. The antitumor effects of the quinoline-3-carboxamide linomide on Dunning R-3327 rat prostatic cancers. Cancer Res 52: 3022–3028, 1992.
250. Vukanovic J, Passaniti A, Hirata T, et al. Antiangiogenic effects of the quinoline-3-carboxamide linomide. Cancer Res 53: 1833–1837, 1993.
251. Karussis DM, Lehmann D, Slavin S, et al. Treatment of chronic-relapsing experimental autoimmune encephalomyelitis with the synthetic immunomodulator linomide (quinoline-3-carboxamide). Proc Natl Acad Sci USA 90: 6400–6404, 1993.
252. Borgström P, Torres Filho IP, Vajkoczy P, et al. The quinoline-3-carboxamide Linomide inhibits angiogenesis *in vivo*. Cancer Chemother Pharmacol 34: 280–286, 1994.
253. Vukanovic J, Isaacs JT. Linomide inhibits angiogenesis, growth, metastasis, and macrophage infiltration within rat prostatic cancers. Cancer Res 55: 1499–1504, 1995.
254. D'Amato RJ, Loughnan MS, Flynn E, Folkman J. Thalidomide is an inhibitor of angiogenesis. Proc Natl Acad Sci USA 91: 4082–4085, 1994.
255. Krishnan EC, Krishnan J, Jewell B, et al. Dose-dependent radiation effect of microvascular and repair. J Natl Cancer Inst 79: 1321–1325, 1987.
256. Krishnan EC, Krishnan L, Jewell WR. Immediate effect of irradiation on microvasculature. Int J Radiat Oncol Biol Phys 15: 147–150, 1988.
257. Prionas SD, Kowalski J, Fajardo LF, et al. Effects of X-irradiation on angiogenesis. Radiat Res 124: 43–49, 1990.
258. Tryggvason K, Höyhtyä M, Pyke C. Type-IV collagenases in invasive tumors. Breast Cancer Res Treatment 24: 209–218, 1993.
259. Cottam DW, Rees RC. Regulation of matrix metalloproteinases: their role in tumor invasion and metastasis (review). Int J Oncol 2: 861–872, 1993.
260. Redwood SM, Liu BC-S, Weiss RE, et al. Abrogation of the invasion of human bladder tumor cells by using protease inhibitor(s). Cancer 69: 1212–1219, 1992.
261. Galardy RE, Grobelny D, Foellmer HG, Fernandex LA. Inhibition of angiogenesis by the matrix metalloproteinase inhibitor N-[2R-2-(Hydroxamidocarbonymethyl)-4-methylpentanoyl)]-L-tryptophan methylamide. Cancer Res 54: 4715–4718, 1994.
262. Davies B, Brown PD, Crimmin MJ, Balkwill FR. A synthetic matrix metalloproteinase inhibitor decreases tumour burden and prolongs survival of mice bearing human ovarian carcinoma xenograft. Cancer Res 53: 2087–2091, 1993.
263. Chirivi RS, Garofalo A, Crimmin MJ, et al. Inhibition of the metastatic spread and growth of B16-BL6 murine melanoma by a synthetic matrix metalloproteinase inhibitor. Int J Cancer 58: 1–5, 1994.
264. Wang X, Fu X, Brown PD, et al. Matrix metalloproteinase inhibitor BB-94 (batimastat) inhibits human colon tumour growth and spread in a patient-like orthotopic model in nude mice. Cancer Res 54: 4726–4728, 1994.
265. Taraboletti G, Garofalo A, Belotti D, et al. Inhibition of angiogenesis and murine hemangioma growth by batimastat, a synthetic inhibitor of matrix metalloproteinases. J Natl Cancer Inst 87: 293–298, 1995.
266. Anderson IC, Shipp MA, Docherty AJP, Teicher BA. Combination therapy including a gelatinase inhibitor and cytotoxic agent reduces local invasion and metastasis of murine Lewis lung carcinoma. Cancer Res., 1996, in press.
267. Watson SA, Morris TM, Robinson G, et al. Inhibition of organ invasion by the matrix metalloproteinase inhibitor batimastat (BB-94) in two human colon carcinoma metastasis models. Cancer Res 55: 3629–3633, 1995.

268. Sledge GW, Qulali M, Goulet R, et al. Effect of matrix metalloproteinase inhibitor batimastat on breast cancer regrowth and metastasis in athymic mice. J Natl Cancer Inst 87: 1546–1550, 1995.

269. Golub LM, Lee HM, Nemiroff LA, et al. Minocycline reduces gingival collagenolytic activity during diabetes. Preliminary observations and a proposed new mechanism of action. J Perio Res 18: 516–526, 1983.

270. Golub LM, McNamara TF, D'Angelo G, et al. A non-antibacterial chemically-modified tetracycline inhibits mammalian collagenase activity. J Dent Res 66: 1310–1314, 1987.

271. Greenwald RA, Golub LM, Lavietes B, et al. Tetracyclines inhibit human synovial collagenase in vivo and in vitro. J Rheumatol 14: 28–32, 1987.

272. Zucker S, Lysik RM, Ramamurthy S, et al. Diversity of melanoma plasma membrane proteinase. inhibition of collagenolytic and cytolytic activities by minocycline. J Natl Cancer Inst 75: 517–525, 1985.

273. Tilley BC, Alarcón GS, Heyse SP, et al. Minocycline in rheumatoid arthritis: a 48-week, double-blind, placebo-controlled trial. Ann Int Med 122: 81–89, 1995.

274. Golub LM, Ramamurthy NS, McNamara TF, et al. Tetracyclines inhibit connective tissue breakdown. new therapeutic implications for an old family of drugs. Crit Rev Oral Biol Med 2: 297–321, 1991.

275. Tamargo RJ, Bok RA, Brem H. Angiogenesis inhibition by minocycline. Cancer Res 51: 672–675, 1991.

276. Alvarez Sotomayor E, Teicher BA, Schwartz GN, et al. Minocycline in combination with chemotherapy or radiation therapy *in vitro* and *in vivo*. Cancer Chemother Pharmacol 30: 377–384, 1992.

277. Teicher BA, Alvarez Sotomayor E, Huang ZD. Antiangiogenic agents potentiate cytotoxic cancer therapies against primary and metastatic disease. Cancer Res 52: 6702–6704, 1992.

278. Sidky YA, Borden EC. Inhibition of angiogenesis by interferons. effects on tumor- and lymphocyte-induced vascular responses. Cancer Res 47: 5155–5161, 1987.

279. Brouty-Boyé D, Zetter BR. Inhibition of cell motility by interferon. Science 208: 516–518, 1980.

280. Real FX, Oettgen HF, Krown SE. Kaposi's sarcoma and the acquired immunodeficiency syndrome. treatment with high and low doses of recombinant leukocyte A interferon. J. Clin Oncol 4: 544–551, 1986.

281. Rios A, Maansell PW, Newell GR, et al. Treatment of acquired immunodeficiency syndrome-related Kaposi's sarcoma with lymphoblastoid interferon. J Clin Oncol 3: 506–512, 1985.

282. Merigan TC. Human interferon as a therapeutic agent: a decade passes. N Engl J Med 318: 1458–1460, 1988.

283. Waddell WR, Ganser GF, Cerise EJ, Loughry RW. Sulindac for polyposis of the colon. Am J Surg 41: 891–894, 1990.

284. Orchard PJ, Smith III CM, Woods WG, et al. Treatment of haemangioendotheliomas with alpha interferon. Lancet 2: 565–567, 1989.

285. Hoffman MA, Wadler S. Mechanisms by which Interferon potentiates chemotherapy. Cancer Invest 11(3): 310–313, 1993.

286. White CW, Wolf SJ, Korones DN, et al. Treatment of childhood angiomatous diseases with recombinant interferon alfa-2a. J Pediatr 118: 59–66, 1991.

287. Ezekowitz RAB, Phil D, Mulliken JB, Folkman J. Interferon alfa-2a therapy for life-threatening hemangiomas of infancy. N Engl J Med 326: 1456–1463, 1992.

288. Toma S, Melioli G, Palumbo R, Rosso R. Recombinant interleukin-2 and $\alpha$-2a-interferon in pre-treated advanced soft tissue sarcomas. Int J Oncol 2: 997–1001, 1993.

289. Iwagaki H, Hizuta A, Yoshino T, et al. Complete regression of advanced liposarcoma of the anterior chest wall with interferon-alpha and tumor necrosis factor-alpha. Anticancer Res 13: 13–16, 1993.

290. Gohji K, Fidler I, Tsan R, et al. Human recombinant interferons-beta and -gamma decrease gelatinase production and invasion by human KG-2 renal-carcinoma cells. Int J Cancer 58: 380–384, 1994.

291. Vokes E, Vijayakumar S, Bitran J. Role of systemic therapy in advanced non-small-cell lung cancer. Proc Am Soc Clin Oncol 13: 331, 1990.

292. Eagen R, Ingle J, Frytak S. Platinum-based polychemotherapy versus dianhydrogalacitol in advanced non-small cell lung cancer. Cancer Treatment Rep 61: 1339–1345, 1977.

293. Gralla R, Casper E, Kelsen D. Cisplatin and vindesine combination chemotherapy for advanced carcinoma of the lung: a randomized trial investigating two dosage schedules. Ann Intern Med 95: 414, 1981.

294. Bunn P. The treatment of non-small-cell lung cancer. current perspectives and controversies, future directions. Semin Oncol 21: 49, 1994.

295. Ruckdeschel J. Etoposide in the management of non-small cell lung cancer. Cancer 67(S): 250–3, 1991.

296. Shepard F. Treatment of non-small cell lung cancer. Semin Oncol 21: 7, 1994.

297. Bonomi P, Finkelstein D, Ruckedschel J. Combination chemotherapy versus single agents followed by a combination chemotherapy in stage IV non-small cell lung cancer. A study of the Eastern Cooperative Oncology Group. J Clin Oncol 7: 1602–13, 1989.

298. Ruckedschel J, Finkelstein D, Ettinger D. A randomized trial of the four most active regimens for metastatic non-small cell lung cancer. J Clin Oncol 4: 14–22, 1986.

299. Klastersky J, Sculier J, Lacroix H. A randomized study comparing cisplatin or carboplatin plus etoposide in patients with advanced non-small cell lung cancer. J Clin Oncol 8: 1556–1562, 1990.

300. Klastersky J, Sculier J, Bureau G. Cisplatin versus cisplatin plus etoposide in the treatment of advanced non-small cell lung cancer. J Clin Oncol 7: 1087–1092, 1989.

301. Klastersky J. Therapy with cisplatin and etoposide for non-small cell lung cancer. Semin Oncol 13(3): 104–114, 1986.

302. Wani M, Taylor H, Wall M. Plant antitumor agents, VI. The isolation and structure of Taxol, a novel antileukemic agent from *Taxus brevifolia*. J Am Chem Soc 93: 2325–2327, 1971.

303. Schiff P, Horowitz S. Taxol stabilizes microtubules in mouse fibroblast cells. Proc Natl Acad Sci USA 77(1561–1565)1980.

304. Schiff P, Fant J, Horowitz S. Promotion of microtubule assembly in vitro by Taxol. Nature 227: 665–667, 1979.

305. McGuire W, Rowinsky E, Rosenshein N. Taxol. A unique antineoplastic agent with significant activity in advanced ovarian epithelial neoplasms. Ann Intern Med 111: 273–279, 1989.

306. Legha S, Ring S, Papadopoulos N. A phase II trial of taxol in metastatic melanoma. Cancer 65: 2478–2481, 1990.

307. Holmes F, Walters R, Theriault R. Phase II trial of taxol, an active drug in the treatment of metastatic breast cancer. J Natl Cancer Inst 83: 1797–1805, 1991.

308. Chang A, Kim K, Glivk J. Phase II study of taxol, merbarone, and piroxantrone in stage IV non-small cell lung cancer. The Eastern Cooperative Oncology Group results. J Natl Cancer Inst 85: 388–393, 1993.

309. Murphy W, Fossella F, Winn R. Phase II study of taxol in patients with untreated advanced non-small cell lung cancer. J Natl Cancer Inst 8: 384–7, 1993.

310. Langer C, Leighton J, Comis R. Paclitaxel and carboplatin in combination in the treatment of advanced non-small cell lung cancer: a phase II toxicity, response and survival analysis. J Clin Oncol 12: 1860, 1995.

311. Johnson D, Paul D, Hande K. Paclitaxel plus carboplatin in advanced non-small cell lung cancer. J Clin Oncol 14: 2054–2060, 1996.

312. Natale R. Preliminary results of a Phase I/II clinical trial of paclitaxel and carboplatin in non-small cell lung cancer. Semin Oncol 23(5 Suppl 12): 2–6, 1996.

313. Bonomi P, Kim K, Chang A. Phase III trial comparing etoposide (E) cisplatin (C) versus taxol (Y) with cisplatin-G-CSF (G) versus taxol-cisplatin in advanced non-small cell lung cancer. An Eastern Cooperative Oncology Group (ECOG) trial. 32nd Meet Am Soc Clin Oncol, Philadelphia, PA, 1996.

314. Steel GG, Nill RP, Peckham MJ. Combined radiotherapy-chemotherapy of Lewis lung carcinoma. Int J Radiat Oncol Biol Phys 4: 49–52, 1978.

315. Teicher BA, Herman TS, Holden SA, et al. Tumor resistance to alkylating agents conferred by mechanisms operative only *in vivo*. Science 247: 1457–1461, 1990.

316. Herman TS, Teicher BA, Cathcart KNS, et al. Effect of hyperthermia on *cis*-diamminedichloro-platinum(II)(Rhodamine 123)2[tetrachloroplatinum(II)] in a human squamous carcinoma cell line and a cis-diamminedichloroplatinum(II)-resistant subline. Cancer Res 48: 5101–5105, 1988.

317. Teicher BA, Holden SA, Jacobs JL. Approaches to defining the mechanism of enhancement by Fluosol-DA 20% with carbogen of melphalan antitumor activity. Cancer Res 47: 513–518, 1987.

318. Kohn KW, Friedman CA, Ewig RAG, Iqbal AM. DNA chain growth during replication of asynchronous L1210 cells. Alkaline elution of large DNA segments from cells lysed on filters. Biochemistry 13: 4134–4139, 1979.

319. Kohn KW, Ewig RAG, Erickson LC, Zwelling LA. Measurement of strand breaks and cross-links in DNA by alkaline elution. In: Friedberg E, Henawalt P (Eds), DNA Repair. A Laboratory Manual of Research Procedures. New York: Marcel Dekker, pp. 379–401, 1981.

320. Rapp E, Pater J, Willan A. Chemotherapy can prolong survival in patients with advanced non-small cell lung cancer-report of a Canadian multicenter randomized trial. J Clin Oncol 6: 633, 1988.

321. Quoix E, Dieterman A, Charbonneau J. Disseminated non-small cell lung cancer: a randomized trial of chemotherapy versus pallative care. Lung Cancer 4: A181, 1988.

322. Stewart L. Chemotherapy in non-small cell lung cancer: a meta-analysis using update data on individual patients from 52 randomized clinical trials. Br Med J 311: 899, 1995.

323. Grilli R, Oxman A, Julian J. Chemotherapy for advanced non-small cell lung cancer: how much benefit is enough? J Clin Oncol 11: 1866, 1993.

324. Mareel MM, Van Roy FM, Bracke ME. How and when do tumor cells metastasize? Crit Rev Oncogen 4(5): 559–594, 1993.

325. Kohn EC. Development and prevention of metastasis. Anticancer Res 13: 2553–2560, 1993.

326. Freitas I, Baronzio GF. Neglected factors in cancer treatment: cellular interactions and dynamic microenvironment in solid tumors. Anticancer Res 14: 1097–1102, 1994.

327. Wellstein A. Growth factor targeted and conventional therapy of breast cancer. Breast Cancer Res Treatment 31: 141–152, 1994.

328. Connolly JL, Ducatman BS, Schnitt SJ, et al. Principles of cancer pathology. In: Holland JF, Frei E III, Bast RC Jr, et al. (Eds), Cancer Medicine. Philadelphia, PA: Lea and Febiger, pp. 432–450, 1993.

329. Cotran RS, Kumar V, Robbins SL. Neoplasia, 4th edn. Philadelphia, PA: WB Saunders, pp. 239–305, 1989.

330. Dvorak HF. Tumors: wounds that do not heal. Similarities between tumor stroma generation and wound healing. N Engl J Med 315: 1650–1659, 1986.

331. Nagy JA, Brown LF, Senger DR, et al. Pathogenesis of tumor stroma generation: a critical role for leaky blood vessels and fibrin deposition. Biochim Biophys Acta 948: 305–326, 1989.

332. Teicher B. A systems approach to cancer therapy (antiangiogenics + standard cytotoxics' mechanism(s) of interaction). Cancer Metastasis Rev 15: 247–72, 1996.

333. Teicher B, Holden S, Ara G, et al. Comparison of several antiangiogenic regimens alone and with cytotoxic therapies in Lewis lung carcinoma. Cancer Chemother Pharmacol 38: 169–177, 1996.

334. Folkman J. Fighting cancer by attacking its blood supply. Sci Am Sept: 150–154, 1996.

C.J. Rosenthal and M. Rotman (Eds.), *Infusion Chemotherapy–Irradiation Interactions*
© 1998 Elsevier Science B.V. All rights reserved

CHAPTER 31

# Gene therapy: its interactions with chemotherapy

RICHARD J. CRISTIANO[1], DAO NGUYEN[1], FRANK SPITZ[2]
and JACK A. ROTH[1]

[1]*Section of Thoracic Molecular Oncology, Department of Thoracic and Cardiovascular Surgery, and*
[2]*Department of Surgical Oncology, University of Texas M.D. Anderson Cancer Center, 1515 Holcombe Blvd.,*
*Houston, TX 77030, USA*

## 1. Introduction

Radiation therapy and chemotherapy have been used for many years to treat cancer. However, these procedures have been relatively ineffective in cancer treatment and may be limited by the ability to adequately affect all tumor cells at sufficient levels to mediate tumor cell death [1]. Gene therapy has now become a possible choice in the methods available for the treatment of human malignancies [2]. This has resulted from the large body of research that has occurred during the past several years, utilizing many types of genes, such as those expressing cytokines or tumor suppressors, to promote tumor cell growth inhibition and apoptosis [3,4]. Unfortunately, gene-mediated therapies for cancer have also been identified to be limited based on the ability to transduce a sufficient number of tumor cells to mediate tumor irradiation. Aspects such as the "bystander effect", which allows non-transduced cells to be affected by transduced cells may contribute to the overall efficacy of gene therapy, however, this may be limited to the use of only certain types of therapeutic genes such as thymidine kinase and the related production of toxic analogues [5].

Our research has focused on the use of tumor suppressors and anti-oncogenes as mediators of tumor cell growth inhibition and apoptosis by gene therapy. The p53 protein has been labeled the "guardian of the cell cycle", since it is a strong tumor suppressor and as we have shown, can generate both growth inhibition as well as apoptosis in tumor cells following high level gene expression [6]. Although it is possible that the expression of p53 may contribute to a bystander effect, the overall therapeutic effect is directly dependent upon the total number of cells that are transduced as well as the overall level of p53 expression in the cell. As a result, both the length and the level of p53 expression is important and can mean the difference between a cell that is transiently growth arrested (by low level p53 expression) or is directed down a pathway towards apoptosis (by high level p53 expression). This has a direct bearing on the success of gene therapy strategies that utilize recombinant adenoviral vectors, since this vector has been shown to mediate high level, but transient gene expression [7,8].

To achieve either a higher therapeutic effect or a higher level of tumor cell transduction, we have investigated alternative methods to enhance tumor suppressor gene therapy. One approach to this problem, would be through the use of improved vectors, however, this aspect has been difficult to achieve and is ongoing [9]. A second and more feasible approach, given current technology, would be to combine present gene delivery systems and therapeutic genes with chemotherapeutics and other common methods for treating cancer. We have focused our research on two potential modes of treatment. The first deals with utilizing the ability of the tumor suppressor p53 to enhance the chemosensitivity of tumor cells to anti-cancer agents such as ionizing irradiation. Many reports in the literature have shown that the tumor suppressor p53 is directly involved in DNA repair as well as having an important function in controlling the cell cycle [10]. This fact as well as the p53 gene being one of the most commonly mutated genes in human malignancies, make it a good choice for use in cancer gene therapy strategies as well as in combination with other anti-cancer agents. The second type of treatment involves the ability of anti-cancer agents to enhance tumor cell transduction. We have identified that DNA-damaging agents such as cisplatin, when given at the correct dose and timing in relation to therapeutic vector administration, can generate higher levels of gene transduction, which in this instance is taken together to represent both the number of cells expressing the transgene as well as the amount of transgene expression. As a result, we have identified that in each of these treatment strategies, a higher level of therapeutic efficacy mediated by the p53 gene can be achieved, allowing for the development of improved methods with which to treat cancer.

## 2. Methods

### 2.1. Cells and culture conditions

The human non-small cell lung carcinoma cell lines H1299 and H460 (gifts from Drs. Adi Gazdar and John Minna) were grown in RPMI-1640 medium supplemented with 5% heat-inactivated fetal calf serum (FCS), 10 mM glutamine, 100 units/ml of penicillin, 100 $\mu$g/ml of streptomycin and 0.25 $\mu$g/ml of amphotericin B. The cell lines H358, H226br (human non-small cell lung carcinoma), SiHa (human cervical cancer cell line), and SW620 (human colorectal cancer cell line) were maintained in complete RPMI-1640 medium similarly supplemented with antibiotics, glutamine, and 10% FCS. The cell line A549 (human, non-small cell lung carcinoma) was grown in Ham's F12 nutrient mixture solution (Gibco BRL, Gaithersburg, MD) similarly supplemented with antibiotics, glutamine and 10% FCS. Primary normal human bronchial epithelial (NHBE) cells (Clonetics Corporation, San Diego, CA), were grown in serum-free optimized growth medium and subcultured under conditions suggested by the manufacturer.

### 2.2. Recombinant adenovirus

The construction and properties of the adenovirus expressing the wild-type p53 gene under the control of the cytomegalovirus (CMV) enhancer and promoter (Adv/p53) have been reported elsewhere [11,12]. The recombinant adenovirus carrying the *Escherichia coli* $\beta$-galactosidase gene under the control of the CMV enhancer/promoter (Adv/$\beta$-gal) was kindly provided by F. Graham, McMaster University, Hamilton, Ontario. The E1A deleted vector dl312 (kindly provided by T. Shenk, Princeton, NJ) was utilized as a control vector. Adenovirus was prepared as previously described [13] and purified by two rounds of cesium chloride ultracentrifugation. Purified virus was mixed with 10% glycerol and dialyzed twice against buffer containing 10 mM Tris–HCl (pH 7.5), 1 mM MgCl$_2$, and 10% glycerol at 4°C. Purified virus was then aliquoted and stored at −80°C until used. Viral titer was determined by UV-spectrophotometric analysis (viral particles/ml) and by plaque assay (pfu/ml) [14]. Final viral concentrations for in vitro and in vivo infections were made by dilution of stock virus in PBS. Adenovirus preparations were free of replication-competent adenovirus as determined by previously described techniques [14].

### 2.3.   In vitro gene delivery and cell proliferation

In vitro gene delivery was performed by incubating cells in six-well plates (Falcon Plastics, Lincoln Park, NJ) for 2 h with Adv/$\beta$-gal in appropriate medium supplemented with 2% FCS. The multiplicity of infection (MOI; number of viral particles per target cell) was based on cell counts of untreated wells. Fresh, complete medium with the appropriate concentration of FCS was then added to the wells at the end of the infection period and cells were then incubated for 20 h at 37°C, with 5% $CO_2$. Histochemical staining for $\beta$-gal expression involved washing the cells with ice-cold PBS, fixing the cells with ice-cold 1.25% glutaraldehyde and then staining with X-gal (5-bromo-4-chloro-3-indolyl-$\beta$-D-galactoside, Gibco BRL) as previously described [15]. The transduction efficiency by Adv/$\beta$-gal was determined by the percentage of positive stained cells (blue) for $\beta$-galactosidase activity (1000 cells counted per well) and the level of transduction enhancement was calculated by dividing the percentage of blue stained cells in the cisplatin treated samples by the percentage of blue stained cells in the non-treated control.

Cell proliferation studies involved the exposure of H1299 cells to cisplatin (0.062 $\mu$g/ml of medium) for 24 h. Cells were then washed twice with PBS, trypsinized and seeded in 6-well plates ($10^5$ cells/well). Forty-eight hours later, cells were infected with Adv/p53 at the MOI of 5 in 1 ml of media containing 2% FCS. The cells were incubated for 2 h at 37°C in a 5% $CO_2$ incubator, after which 2 ml of RPMI-1640 complete medium supplemented with 5% FCS was added. Daily cell counts were performed for 5 days following infection. Controls consisted of untreated cells (PBS only), cells exposed to cisplatin only, cells infected with Adv/p53 only, and cells infected with dl312 (similar MOI) with or without prior cisplatin treatment.

### 2.4.   In vivo tumor models and radiation, cisplatin and Adv/p53 administration

Tumor xenografts involving the cell lines H1299 and SW620 were created by injecting $1 \times 10^7$ and $5 \times 10^6$ cells, respectively, suspended in 100 $\mu$l of PBS into either the dorsal flank subcutaneous space or the hind leg of nude mice that had received 350 rad of total body irradiation prior to injection. Subcutaneous tumor nodules of 200–250 mm³ in size were formed 3–4 weeks later. In vivo radiation experiments were performed on subcutaneous xenograft tumors induced in nude mice of approximately 200 mm³. A uniform injection strategy was utilized for all intratumoral injections. Each injection of purified virus was diluted in a total volume of 200 $\mu$l PBS and was administered in a single pass of a 27-gauge hypodermic needle, using gentle, constant infusion pressure. A total viral dose of $7.5 \times 10^9$ PFU was administered in divided doses on three consecutive days. The treatment of hind leg tumors with irradiation (⁶⁰Co teletherapy unit) consisted of positioning anesthetized animals in the irradiation field such that only the hind leg bearing the tumor was in the field and the rest of the body was shielded by a lead block. For cisplatin studies, different combinations of cisplatin and Adv/p53 were studied for their tumoricidal efficacy: (a) intraperitoneal (i.p.) cisplatin (5 $\mu$g/g body weight) given on day 0, followed by intratumoral Adv/p53 injections of 3 equally divided doses of $5 \times 10^9$ viral particles/100 $\mu$l PBS on days 2, 4, and 6; (b) simultaneous cisplatin (i.p.) and Adv/p53 administration (3 equally divided doses) and (c) i.p. cisplatin given 3 days after completion of intratumoral Adv/p53 injections. The divided dose regime was designed to address issues that may limit the use of high virus titer such as toxicity and volume of injectate to accommodate low titer viral stocks. The controls consisted of tumors injected with either PBS, Adv/p53 without prior systemic cisplatin, dl312 with or without prior i.p. cisplatin or tumor-bearing animals receiving i.p. cisplatin only. Tumor sizes were measured every 2 days for 32 days and tumor volumes were estimated by assuming a spherical shape with the average tumor diameter calculated as the square root of the product of the orthogonal diameters. All mice were euthanized when tumors grew to 4000 mm$^3$.

## 2.5. Statistical analysis

Results were presented as mean ± standard deviation. Analysis of variance (ANOVA) and two-tailed Student's $t$-test were used for statistical analysis of multiple groups and pair-wise comparison respectively, $P < 0.05$ is considered significant.

## 3. Results

### 3.1. Enhancement of tumor cell sensitivity to irradiation

The high prevalence of mutations in the p53 gene in many tumor types as well as the fact that p53 expression in normal cells in non-toxic, makes it a good choice for use in gene therapy. In lung cancer, mutations can occur in 40–60% of tumors, while in colon cancer, this can reach as high as 80% [16]. Both lung and colon tumors are also relatively insensitive to treatments such as ionizing irradiation [17,18]. As a result, the cell lines SW620 (colon, mutant p53 expression) and H1299 (lung, deleted for p53 expression) were utilized to determine if expression of p53 could enhance the sensitivity of the cell lines to irradiation. Previously we have shown that when a clonogenic assay is performed, cell lines that are infected with an adenovirus carrying the gene for the tumor suppressor p53 (Adv/p53) and then irradiated with a dose of 5 Grey(Gy), showed the lowest number of surviving colonies, while those cells treated with either 5 Gy alone or in combination with a control adenovirus demonstrated significantly higher numbers of colonies that were capable of growth (data not shown) [19]. This observation is true for both the cell line SW620 as well as the cell line H1299.

To confirm that p53 can enhance the sensitivity of these cell lines to irradiation in an in vivo model, subcutaneous tumors generated with the cell line H1299 (250 mm$^3$) were injected with Adv/p53 and then localized irradiation of the tumor with a dose of 5 Gy was done 2 days later. Measurement of tumor growth over a 36 day period identified that tumors treated with the combined treatment were much smaller than tumors treated with Adv/p53 only, 5 Gy irradiation only, or similar treatments involving the control virus dl312 (Fig. 1). This result is similar to that achieved when experiments were done using the colon cancer cell line SW620 [19]. Further analysis of animals in the experiments involving the treatment of SW620 tumors has identified that after 100 days, 40% of the animals are either tumor free or have very slow growing tumors (Fig. 2). In comparison, animals that were treated

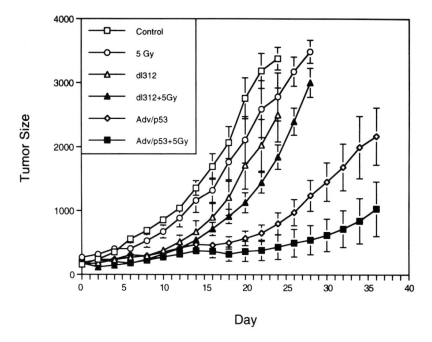

Fig. 1. The effect of Adv/p53 administration and 5 Gy irradiation on H1299 subcutaneous tumor growth in nude mice. Tumor size equals volume in mm$^3$ and was measured every 2 days. $n = 5$ animals/group.

with Adv/p53 only, 5 Gy only, or combinations involving the control virus dl312, had to be euthanized after approximately 30–40 days, as the tumors had reached the maximum allowable size of 1.5–2 cm (Fig. 2). Overall, this shows that exogenous p53 expression in cell lines bearing mutations in the p53 gene can result in enhanced sensitivity of those cell lines to irradiation and an overall increase in the survival of treated animals.

## 3.2. Enhancement of tumor cell transduction by cisplatin

As an alternative to using p53 expression to enhance the sensitivity of tumors to DNA-damaging agents, we have also analyzed agents that can be used to increase the transduction and potentially the overall level of therapeutic gene expression in tumor cells. The goal again is to increase both the number of cells that are expressing the transgene as well as the amount of transgene expression, generating a better overall effect on tumor growth. The DNA-damaging agent cisplatin was investigated to determine if it could be used as an agent to enhance the gene transduction of cancer cells.

In our initial analysis, two non-small cell lung adenocarcinoma cell lines (H1299 and H460) were incubated with cisplatin at several different concentrations for 24 h prior to infection with Adv/β-gal at 24, 48, 72 and 96 h after drug treatment. A brief 24-h exposure of H1299 and H460 cells to cisplatin (0.062 μg/ml), followed by infection with Adv/β-gal 48 h after drug removal resulted in a 2–3-fold increase of gene transduction in target cells infected by Adv/β-gal as quantitated by X-gal staining and ONPG analysis (data not shown) [20]. To determine whether enhancement could be achieved using cell lines of different origins, several malignant cell lines were treated with the optimal conditions for maximal

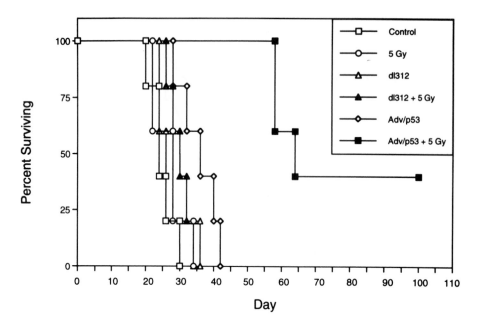

Fig. 2. Survival curve of nude mice bearing SW620 subcutaneous tumors that were injected with Adv/p53 and irradiated with 5 Gy. Animals were euthanized when tumor size reach the maximum volume of 4000 mm$^3$.

enhancement of gene expression (cisplatin concentration of 0.062 $\mu$g/ml and gene transfer at 48 h after drug treatment). The magnitude of maximal enhancement was dependent on the cell line tested (ranging from 1.6 (A549) to 2.7 (H1299) fold), but it consistently occurred when gene transfer was performed 48 h after exposure to 0.062 $\mu$g/ml of cisplatin (Fig. 3). Similar exposure of stationary primary human bronchial epithelial cells that were 90% confluent in culture, to a low concentration (0.062 $\mu$g/ml) of cisplatin, failed to enhance gene expression in these normal cells after Adv/$\beta$-gal infection (Fig. 3). However, at higher drug concentrations (1 and 4 $\mu$g/ml), a dose-dependent elevation of the percentage of $\beta$-gal-positive cells that was 1.5–2.5 fold higher than that observed in unexposed NHBE cells occurred (data not shown). In all cell lines tested, the window for the enhancement of transduction was short-lived as the percentage of positively stained, treated cells, infected on day 4 or 5 after cisplatin exposure was similar to that of the control (data not shown).

### 3.3. The effect of cisplatin treatment on Adv/p53-mediated gene delivery

To determine if the combination of cisplatin and Adv/p53-mediated gene transfer would result in an enhancement of tumor cell growth inhibition by p53, H1299 cells were treated with a combination of sequential cisplatin and Adv/p53 infection and then analyzed by a cell proliferation assay (Table 1). Treating H1299 cells with cisplatin (0.0625 $\mu$g/ml) for 24 h had no effect on cell growth in vitro, nor did infection with dl312 with or without prior cisplatin treatment. However, exposure of H1299 cells to cisplatin 48 h prior to infection with Adv/p53 resulted in a 61% and a 55% increase in inhibition of tumor proliferation on day 3 and 5 after p53 transfer when compared to control H1299 cells similarly infected with Adv/p53 (Table 1).

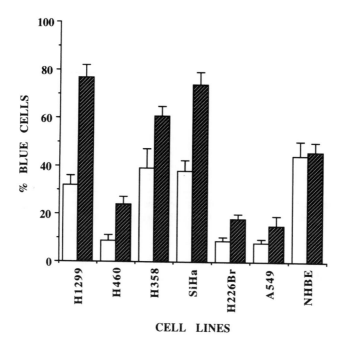

**CELL LINES**

Fig. 3. The effect of cisplatin treatment on the transduction of various cell types. Different malignant and normal cells were infected with Adv/$\beta$-gal 48 h following exposure to cisplatin (hatched bar) or PBS (open bar). MOI = 1 (H1299, SiHa), 5 (H460, NHBE), 10 (H358, H226br, A549); mean ± SD ($n = 6$; results of 2 experiments, with triplicate samples). Cells were stained for $\beta$-gal expression, 24 h after infection.

To confirm this observation in vivo, tumor bearing animals were given a single intraperitoneal injection of cisplatin followed by injections of Adv/p53 (3 doses of $5 \times 10^9$ viral particles, total dose of $1.5 \times 10^{10}$ viral particles) and then tumor size was measured over a 32-day period (Table 2). Tumors grew rapidly in groups of control animals receiving only i.p. cisplatin or intratumoral PBS with tumor sizes reaching the maximal allowable volume

Table 1

In vitro H1299 tumor cell proliferation

| Sample | Day | | |
|---|---|---|---|
| | 1 | 3 | 5 |
| PBS | $6.8 \times 10^5 \pm 1.1 \times 10^5$ | $3.21 \times 10^6 \pm 4.2 \times 10^5$ | $6.6 \times 10^6 \pm 5.0 \times 10^5$ |
| CDDP | $6.3 \times 10^5 \pm 1.0 \times 10^5$ | $3.05 \times 10^6 \pm 3.6 \times 10^5$ | $6.92 \times 10^6 \pm 7.0 \times 10^5$ |
| PBS/d1312 | $6.2 \times 10^5 \pm 1.3 \times 10^5$ | $2.95 \times 10^6 \pm 5.6 \times 10^5$ | $6.2 \times 10^6 \pm 7.5 \times 10^5$ |
| CDDP/d1312 | $6.4 \times 10^5 \pm 2.5 \times 10^5$ | $2.75 \times 10^6 \pm 6.0 \times 10^5$ | $5.9 \times 10^6 \pm 7.0 \times 10^5$ |
| PBS/Advp53 | $4.3 \times 10^5 \pm 7.0 \times 10^4$ | $5.4 \times 10^5 \pm 4.0 \times 10^4$ | $1.34 \times 10^6 \pm 1.7 \times 10^5$ |
| CDDP/Advp53 | $4.7 \times 10^5 \pm 8.0 \times 10^4$ | $2.1 \times 10^5 \pm 5.0 \times 10^4$ | $6.5 \times 10^5 \pm 2.0 \times 10^5$ |

Values represent the total number of cells counted at each time point. Each time point represents the average of at least 2 experiments that were performed with the counting of duplicate wells.

Table 2

In vivo H1299 tumor cell growth

| Sample | Day | | |
|---|---|---|---|
| | 2 | 16 | 32 |
| PBS | 333 ± 55 | 2432 ± 242 | N.D. |
| CDDP | 253 ± 97 | 2262 ± 193 | N.D. |
| PBS/dl312 | 305 ± 38 | 2014 ± 219 | N.D. |
| CDDP/dl312 | 255 ± 33 | 1828 ± 222 | N.D. |
| PBS/Advp53 | 271 ± 51 | 644 ± 112 | 3357 ± 391 |
| CDDP/Advp53 | 241 ± 30 | 243 ± 66 | 1597 ± 221 |
| CDDP+Advp53 | 284 ± 33 | 615 ± 100 | 2300 ± 275 |
| Advp53/CDDP | 274 ± 28 | 563 ± 100 | 2820 ± 457 |

Values represent volume in $mm^3$ of tumors measured at each time point. A minimum of 5 tumors were analyzed for each group. N.D., not determined (animals were euthanized prior to this time point as tumor size was $\geq 4000$ $mm^3$).

of 4000 $mm^3$ 22–26 days after treatment. Tumors injected with dl312, with or without prior i.p. cisplatin, showed some degree of growth retardation secondary to vector toxicity. Injections of Adv/p53 resulted in inhibition of tumor growth during and immediately after the treatment. These tumors reached a mean tumor volume of 3357 ± 391 $mm^3$, 32 days after the onset of therapy. Intraperitoneal cisplatin administration given 2 days prior to the beginning of the gene therapy schedule resulted in a more pronounced inhibition of tumor development. There was a regression of tumor mass that lasted for 14–16 days before the tumor growth resumed, which occurred at a much slower rate than Adv/p53 injected tumors. At the end of the observation period, the average tumor size was 1597 ± 221 $mm^3$ ($P < 0.001$ versus Adv/p53 without prior cisplatin). Systemic cisplatin administration prior to p53 gene replacement therapy, therefore, resulted in a synergistic effect of tumor growth inhibition that was responsible for at least 52% further reduction in tumor size. This increased level of tumor growth inhibition is due to an increase in the number of cells that are transduced in the tumor. This was identified by performing a similar treatment strategy, but replacing the injection of Adv/p53 with an injection of Adv/$\beta$-gal. Histochemical analysis of sections through the Adv/$\beta$-gal injected tumors have identified that at least a two-fold increase in gene transduction occurs (data not shown). To illustrate the importance of the timing of cisplatin administration in relation to p53 gene transfer, cisplatin (5 $\mu$g/ml) was given either at the same time as the injections of Adv/p53 ($1.5 \times 10^{10}$ total viral particles) (cisplatin + Advp53) or 3 days after adenovirus-mediated p53 gene transfer (Advp53/cisplatin). The combination of sequential cisplatin and Adv/p53 showed the most significant tumor growth inhibition, with the mean tumor volume of 1597 ± 221 $mm^3$ as compared to a mean tumor volume of 2300 ± 275 $mm^3$ when cisplatin was given concurrently with Adv injections and 2820 ± 457 $mm^3$ when cisplatin was given after adenovirus-mediated p53 gene transfer ($P < 0.001$ by ANOVA and Student's $t$-test) (Table 2). The combination of sequential cisplatin and Adv/p53 significantly prolonged the survival of treated animals after the onset of therapy as compared to either tumor-bearing mice injected with control virus with or without cisplatin as well as PBS and cisplatin injected controls. The prolonging of survival was also longer than in Adv/p53 injected animals, since these animals were close to the cut-off for tumor size of 4000 $mm^3$ by the 32nd day of the experiment.

## 4. Discussion

The ability to transduce target cells both specifically and efficiently, continues to be one of the limiting aspects for the use of gene therapy in the treatment of cancer. Present vectors such as recombinant adenovirus and retrovirus have provided the means with which initial clinical studies have been started, however, the limitations of these vectors has confined the use and effectiveness of many gene therapy strategies [21]. The problems associated with transducing cells can certainly be overcome through the use of improved gene delivery vectors. Vectors such as molecular conjugates, which provide for the ability to target certain cell types through the use of a specific ligand, have been pursued as "synthetic viruses" [22]. When the molecular conjugates are combined with DNA, the resulting protein–DNA complex has the capability of cell specific targeting combined with components that mediate gene delivery, however, without the presence of side effects associated with viral vectors [23]. As an alternative approach, we have chosen to combine present gene delivery systems and therapeutic genes with commonly used cancer treatment agents in an attempt to enhance the efficiency of these systems.

Our results show that tumor suppressor p53 expression in malignant cells bearing p53 mutations can enhance the sensitivity of those cells to DNA-damaging agents such as irradiation. This observation is clearly due to p53 expression, since similar studies involving the use of a control virus had a limited effect. Further analysis of SW620 tumors treated with Adv/p53 and 5 Gy irradiation has also shown that the enhanced effect is due to higher levels of apoptosis, mediated by p53 [19]. These results are similar to the studies of Fujiwara et. al. in which p53 was used to enhance the chemosensitivity of lung cancer cells to cisplatin [11]. More recent studies have also shown that human ovarian carcinoma cells treated with p53 have an enhanced sensitivity to ionizing radiation [24]. Again, in each of these studies, enhancement is due to p53 expression and its role in interacting with damaged DNA in the cell. However, recent work has now shown that there are many other proteins that interact with p53 to mediate programmed cell death such as Bcl2 and Bax [25,26]. It is quite possible that these proteins are also playing a role in this model, aiding in the degree of apoptosis generated. However, this is all dependent upon the level of expression of these proteins in the cell lines used and is now currently being investigated. Although in our analysis, tumor growth does start to reoccur, strategies such as repeated administration of both Adv/p53 and irradiation could be done, however, the immune response that is generated against adenoviral vectors in humans may limit this strategy [27]. It is also possible that other therapeutic genes either administered alone or together with p53, may mediate even higher levels of chemosensitivity.

As an alternative approach, we have used cisplatin to increase gene expression specifically in tumor cells. We have shown that low-level doses of cisplatin can mediate a 2–3 fold increase in gene expression in cancer cells from many different origins, as well as mediating a higher level of p53 expression in both in vitro and in vivo models. Further analysis of cells treated by this strategy in both of these models have shown that the higher level of efficacy is due to both a higher level of p53 as well as a higher level of apoptosis (data not shown).

The mechanism associated with the enhancement of tumor cell transduction by cisplatin treatment prior to vector administration has not been identified. While p53 gene expression may be contributing to the enhanced effect through increased chemosensitivity in combination with cisplatin, it is clear from the transduction studies using $\beta$-gal, that a different mechanism is involved. We are currently attempting to identify what this mechanism is and if identified, this mechanism could be manipulated to generate even higher levels of transduction. Similar studies using DNA-damaging agents have been done by Son et al. in which treatment of cisplatin insensitive ovarian carcinoma cells with a different dosing protocol, resulted in as much as a 30-fold increase in gene expression [28]. This study involved the use of lipid–DNA complexes, while other studies have shown that normal cells treated with high doses of cisplatin can be infected at much higher levels with recombinant adeno-associated vectors [29]. Our studies have also identified that the enhancement with cisplatin as shown here in combination with recombinant adenoviral vectors can also occur with a modified adenovirus–DNA complex and with lipid–DNA complexes as well [20]. As a result, the mechanism is clearly not associated with the type of vector, nor the type of cell line that is used. The studies to identify the mechanism must be designed to cover all aspects of DNA, RNA, and protein production and maintenance in the cells. One major conclusion that can be made is that this treatment strategy is resulting in previously non-transduced cells becoming transduced as well as generating higher levels of p53 expression to force growth arrested cells into programmed cell death or apoptosis. Overall, these treatment strategies as presented here, provide for improved methods with which to treat cancer in the clinical setting, combining current methodologies with new strategies such as gene therapy.

## Summary

*Background*: The ability to treat cancer by tumor suppressor gene replacement therapy has recently been shown in human trials. The overall efficiency of any cancer gene therapy strategy is dependent upon the level of tumor cell transduction, which may be limiting. To enhance the transduction of tumor cells or the efficacy of this type of therapy, we have attempted to combine the use of chemotherapeutics with tumor suppressor gene therapy. *Methods*: Cultured tumor cells and subcutaneous tumor models in nude mice were infected with recombinant adenoviral vectors expressing either $\beta$-gal or the tumor suppressor p53 and were combined with either irradiation or treatment with cisplatin in varying combinations and with varying doses. Levels of transduction were measured by histochemical staining for $\beta$-gal and by analyzing cell proliferation and tumor growth for p53. *Results*: The expression of p53 in tumor cells prior to irradiation resulted in a higher level of tumor growth inhibition and prolonged survival, while treatment of tumor cells with cisplatin prior to gene transfer resulted in a higher level of gene expression which also resulted in increased tumor growth inhibition. *Conclusions*: The combination of chemotherapeutics with gene therapy provides improved methods with which cancer can be treated in the clinical setting.

## Acknowledgements

This study was partially supported by grants from the National Cancer Institutes and the National Institute of Health (R01 CA45187) (J.A.R.); Specialized Program of Research Excellence (SPORE) in Lung Cancer (P50-CA70907); by gifts to the Division of Surgery and Anesthesiology from Tenneco and Exxon for the Core Laboratory Facility; by the UT M.D. Anderson Cancer Center Support Core Grant (CA16672); and by a grant from the Mathers Foundation.

# References

1.  Vaughn DJ, Haller DG. Nonsurgical management of recurrent colorectal cancer (review). Cancer 71: 4278–4292, 1993.
2.  Roth JA, Cristiano RJ. Gene therapy for cancer: what have we done and where are we going? J Natl Cancer Inst 89: 21–39, 1997.
3.  Zier KS, Gansbacher B. IL-2 gene therapy of solid tumors: an approach for the prevention of signal transduction defects in T cells. J Mol Med 74: 127–134, 1996.
4.  Zhang W, Fang X, Mazur W, et al. High-efficiency gene transfer and high-level expression of wild-type p53 in human lung cancer cells mediated by recombinant adenovirus. Cancer Gene Ther 1: 5–13, 1994.
5.  Gagandeep S, Brew R, Green B, et al. Prodrug-activated gene therapy: involvement of an immunological component in the "bystander effect". Cancer Gene Ther 3: 83–88, 1996.
6.  Spitz FR, Nguyen D, Skibber JM, et al. In vivo adenovirus-mediated p53 tumor suppressor gene therapy for colorectal cancer. Anticancer Res 16: 3415–3422, 1996.
7.  Li Q, Kay MA, Woo SLC. Assessment of recombinant adenoviral vectors for hepatic gene therapy. Hum Gene Ther 4: 403–409, 1993.
8.  Cusack JC, Spitz FR, Nguyen DM, et al. High levels of gene transduction in human lung tumors following intralesional injection of recombinant adenovirus. Cancer Gene Ther 3: 245–249, 1996.
9.  Fisher KJ, Choi H, Burda J, et al. Recombinant adenovirus deleted of all viral genes for gene therapy of cystic fibrosis. Virology 217: 11–22, 1996.
10. Marx J. How p53 suppresses cell growth. Science 262: 1644–1645, 1995.
11. Fujiwara T, Grimm EA, Mukhopadhyay T, et al. Induction of chemosensitivity in human lung cancer cells in vivo by adenoviral-mediated transfer of the wild-type p53 gene. Cancer Res 54: 2287–2291, 1994.
12. Zhang WW, Fang X, Branch CD, et al. Generation and identification of recombinant adenovirus by liposome-mediated transfection and PCR analysis. Biotechniques 15: 868–872, 1993.
13. Graham F, Previc L. Manipulation of adenovirus vectors. In: Murray EJ (Ed), Methods in Molecular Biology: Gene Transfer and Expression Protocols, Vol. 7. Clifton, NJ: Humana Press, pp. 205–225, 1991.
14. Zhang W, Alemany R, Wang J, et al. Safety evaluation of Ad5CMV-p53 in vitro and in vivo. Hum Gene Ther 6: 155–164, 1995.
15. MacGregor GR, Mogg AE, Burke JF, Caskey CT. Histochemical staining of clonal mammalian cell lines expressing *E. Coli* B Galactosidase indicates heterogeneous expression of the bacterial gene. Somat Cell Mol Genet 13: 253–265, 1987.
16. Takahashi T, Nau MM, Chiba I, et al. p53: a frequent target for genetic abnormalities in lung cancer. Science 246: 491–494, 1989.
17. Green MR. Multimodality therapy in unresected stage III non-small cell lung cancer: the American cooperative groups' experience (review). Lung Cancer 1: 87–94, 1995.
18. DeCosse JJ, Cennerazzo W. Treatment options for the patient with colorectal cancer (review). Cancer 70: 1342–1345, 1992.
19. Spitz FR, Nguyen DM, Skibber JM, et al. Adenoviral-mediated wild-type p53 gene expression sensitizes colorectal cancer cells to ionizing radiation. Clin Cancer Res 2: 1665–1671, 1996.
20. Nguyen D, Kataoka M, Wiehle S, et al. The enhancement of tumor cell transduction by treatment with DNA-damaging agents, (in preparation).
21. Mulligan RC. The basic science of gene therapy. Science 260: 926–932, 1993.
22. Cristiano RJ, Roth JA. Molecular conjugates: a targeted gene delivery vector for molecular medicine. J Mol Med 73: 479–486, 1995.
23. Cristiano RJ, Roth J. Epidermal growth factor mediated DNA delivery into lung cancer cells via the epidermal growth factor receptor. Cancer Gene Ther 3: 4–10, 1996.
24. Gallardo D, Drazan KE, McBride WH. Adenovirus-based transfer of wild-type p53 gene increases ovarian tumor radiosensitivity. Cancer Res 56: 4891–4893, 1996.
25. Leake R. The cell cycle and regulation of cancer cell growth (review). Ann N Y Acad Sci 784: 252–262, 1996.
26. Sakakura C, Sweeney EA, Shirahama T, et al. Overexpression of bax sensitizes human breast cancer MCF-7 cells to radiation-induced apoptosis. Int J Cancer 67: 101–105, 1996.
27. Amalfitano A, Begy CR, Chamberlain JS. Improved adenovirus packaging cell lines to support the growth of replication-defective gene-delivery vectors. Proc Natl Acad Sci USA 93: 3352–3356, 1996.

28. Son K, Huang L. Exposure of human ovarian carcinoma to cisplatin transiently sensitizes the tumor cells for liposome-mediated gene transfer. Proc Natl Acad Sci USA 91: 12669–12672, 1994.
29. Alexander IE, Russell DW, Miller AD. DNA-damaging agents greatly increase the transduction of nondividing cells by adeno-associated virus vectors. J Virol 68: 8282–8287, 1994.

C.J. Rosenthal and M. Rotman (Eds.), *Infusion Chemotherapy–Irradiation Interactions*
© 1998 Elsevier Science B.V. All rights reserved

343

# CHAPTER 32

# Cellular targets in SV40-mediated transformation

## JAMES A. DECAPRIO

*Assistant Professor of Medicine, Dana-Farber Cancer Institute, Harvard Medical School,
44 Binney Street, Boston, MA 02115, USA*

## 1. Cellular transformation by small DNA tumor viruses

The small DNA tumor viruses, including simian virus 40 (SV40), adenovirus (Ad), and human papilloma virus (HPV) have proven themselves to be excellent subjects for studying oncogenic mechanisms. Investigations centered on these virus's ability to transform cells has led to the identification of several important cellular growth regulatory processes. While these viruses are not related to each other, they have independently evolved to inactivate the retinoblastoma (pRB) and p53 tumor suppressors. It has been proposed that viral transformation is mediated, at least in part, by the functional inactivation of these and perhaps additional cellular tumor suppressors. This review focuses on the potential role of the pRB-related proteins, p130 and p107, as two additional targets in viral-mediated transformation.

The transforming proteins SV40 large T Ag, Ad E1a, and HPV E7 each can bind to the retinoblastoma tumor suppressor (pRB) via their conserved Leu-X-Cys-X-Glu residues (Fig. 1) [1–4]. Mutations within the LXCXE domain of the viral proteins inactivates their ability to bind to pRB and reduces their ability to transform cells. These results suggest that viral

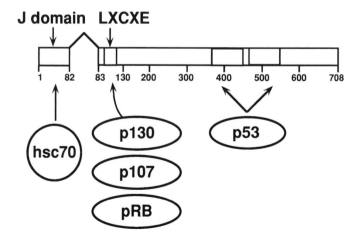

Fig. 1. LXCXE domain where X is any amino acid.

protein binding to pRB leads to the inactivation of the growth suppressive properties of pRB. Inactivation of pRB function leads to continued cellular proliferation despite less than ideal growth conditions. Inactivation of pRB function may also lead to an inability for a cell to complete its differentiation program.

These three viruses also target the p53 tumor suppresser. While SV40 large T Ag also binds to both pRB and p53, the Ad E1a or HPV E7 does not bind to p53. Instead, the adenovirus and papilloma virus express additional proteins that bind p53. The 55 kDa protein of Ad E1B and the E6 HPV protein binds to p53. Remarkable, each of these three viruses inactivate p53 in a unique fashion. SV40 T Ag has a bipartite p53-binding domain extending from residues 350 to 550. When SV40 T Ag binds to p53, it alters the DNA binding specificity of p53 and decreases its ability to transactivate genes that lead to growth arrest such as p21 and Bax. While the Ad E1b 55 kDa protein binds to a different region of p53 that T Ag binds, it also alters its DNA binding specificity. In contrast, the HPV E6 protein targets p53 for rapid degradation by the ubiquitin-proteasome pathway [5–7]. Inactivation of p53 function is also thought to promote cellular growth as well as to inhibit apoptosis.

## 2.  The pRB family of tumor suppressors

It was noted earlier that the viral transforming proteins can bind to pRB, p107 and p130. The frequent association of *Rb-1* mutations in human tumors has confirmed its role as an important tumor suppressor. The retinoblastoma tumor suppressor gene (*Rb-1*) is mutated in nearly all retinoblastomas and in many other malignancies. In contrast, it is uncertain whether the pRB-related proteins, p107 or p130, are tumor suppressors. Although p130 and p107 are highly homologous to pRB by primary sequence analysis, there have been no reports of a spontaneous mutations in the p107 or p130 gene found in any human tumor sample examined to date [8].

There is strong laboratory research that supports the notion that pRB can suppress tumor formation. For example, re-introduction of wild-type pRB into SaOS-2 cells, a human osteosarcoma cell line deleted for *Rb-1* (RB −/−), by transfection with an RB cDNA expression plasmid or microinjection of purified pRB protein results in a growth arrest [9–11]. Expression of pRB blocked exit from the G1 phase and entry into the cell cycle and inhibited the ability of these cells to proliferate. This assay defined several domains within RB that are required for growth suppression. For example, many of the naturally occurring, tumor-specific, mutations that affect residues 373–579 and 637–772 of pRB, known as the pocket domain, were not capable of inducing a growth arrest in SaOS-2 cells [9,12,13]. In a manner similar to pRB, transient expression of p107 or p130 in SaOS-2 cells leads to a growth arrest in G1, despite the presence of wild type p107 and p130 in these cells [14–17].

The growth inhibitory functions of pRB are regulated by cell cycle dependent phosphorylation. During G0 and early G1, when pRB exerts its growth suppressive functions, pRB appears hypophosphorylated. Upon entry into the cell cycle, during the G1/S transition, pRB becomes phosphorylated and remains hyperphosphorylated throughout S and G2 phases [18,19]. Notably, SV40 T Ag binds specifically to the G1, underphosphorylated, form of pRB [20,21]. In a transformed cell, T Ag dissociates from phosphorylated pRB during S and G2 phases and re-associates with pRB when it undergoes dephosphorylation in mitosis. These observations led to the hypothesis that the growth suppressing function of underphosphorylated pRB can be relieved by phosphorylation in normal cells or by binding to T Ag in transformed cells. It has also been demonstrated that p107 and p130 undergo cell cycle dependent phosphorylation and this effect is correlated with relief of their growth suppressing properties [14,16,22].

Several lines of evidence suggest that pRB is an important substrate for the cyclin dependent kinase, cyclin D/cdk4. Cyclin D/cdk4 or cyclin D/cdk6 activity peaks in the mid-G1 phase of the cell cycle, near the time that pRB becomes phosphorylated [23,24]. In addition, microinjection of antibodies against cyclin D blocked cell cycle progression in pRB +/+ cells but not in RB −/− cells [25]. Furthermore, the cdk 4 kinase inhibitor, p16$^{INK4a/MTS1}$, is frequently deleted in tumor cells that contain normal pRB leading to the hyperphosphorylation and inactivation of pRB [26,27]. Cyclin D/cdk 4 activity may also regulate p107 and p130 activity [14,16,28]. The p16$^{MTS/INK4a}$ is an inhibitor of cyclin D/cdk4 and loss of the p16 tumor suppressor leads to increase activity of cyclin D/cdk4 and hyperphosphorylation of pRB as well as p130 and p107. Therefore, it is possible that the loss of p16 activity could lead to inactivation of all three members of the pRB family.

Many hematologic malignancies are accompanied by the specific genetic loss of p16$^{MTS/INK4a}$. In a large fraction of acute T-cell leukemia, in lymphoid blast crisis of adult chronic myelogenous leukemia and in a fraction of B-cell non-Hodgkin's lymphoma, several groups have reported deletions or mutations in both alleles of the p16 gene [29–31]. Since the loss of p16$^{MTS/INK4a}$ may lead to inactivation of all members of the pRB family, it is important to decipher the specific contribution of each to tumor suppression.

## 3.  SV40 T Ag inactivates the pRB-related proteins, p107 and p130

It has been demonstrated that SV40 T Ag, AD E1a, and HPV E7 proteins each can bind to all three members of the pRB family. Furthermore, each of these viral proteins bind to pRB family members through the LXCXE motif. Mutations within the LXCXE motif render the viral protein transformation defective. Presumably, at least part of the transforming activity of the LXCXE domain is due to inactivation of the pRB tumor suppresser. However, since the LXCXE domain also participates in binding to p107 and p130, it is been difficult to determine whether the specific interaction with each of the pRB-related proteins contributes to transformation.

In an attempt to address this question, we asked whether SV40 T Ag could transform fibroblasts derived from mouse embryos homozygously deleted for *Rb-1* (RB−/−). For example, if the *Rb-1* tumor suppressor gene was already inactivated by targeted mutagenesis, was there a requirement for an intact LXCXE domain in transformation by T Ag? If so, then it would suggest that the LXCXE domain targeted other cellular proteins in addition to pRB during transformation. We prepared RB−/− fibroblasts from embryos derived from the mating of a male and female mice that were each heterozygote for a mutant *Rb-1* allele [32]. We transfected these fibroblasts with plasmids that expressed either wild type T Ag or a T Ag that contained a mutation in the LXCXE domain but was otherwise intact (i.e., a mutant T Ag that remained capable of binding to and inactivating p53). Clones of cells that expressed each of the T Ag constructs were generated.

The growth characteristics of each T Ag established clone was tested in several transformation assays. In high (10%) or low (1%) serum-containing media, lines expressing wild type T Ag had a readily detectable growth advantage compared to lines expressing any of the LXCXE mutations. In every case, wild type T Ag expressing cells grew faster and to a higher cell density than cells expressing a T Ag with a defective LXCXE domain. This growth advantage of wild type T Ag was evident in both RB +/+ and RB −/− lines. In addition, wild type T Ag-expressing lines were able to overgrow a monolayer and form colonies in soft agar with high efficiency. Conversely, every LXCXE mutant T Ag line, whether in an RB +/+ or RB −/− background, had high serum requirement for growth and was unable to form colonies in soft agar.

These observations suggested that an intact LXCXE domain was required for transformation of both RB +/+ and −/− MEFs. The defect in transformation by the LXCXE mutation of T Ag could be rescued by expression of wild type HPV 16 E7 in both RB +/+ or RB −/− MEF. Conversely, an HPV 16 E7 containing a deletion in the LXCXE domain was unable to induce transformation when expressed in a mutant T Ag line. These results suggested that other cellular proteins, in addition to pRB, were targeted by the LXCXE domain in T Ag-mediated transformation. Since the LXCXE domain could also bind to p107 and p130, we considered that they could be the relevant targets. Although we and others been reported that T Ag can bind to the pRB-related proteins, p130 and p107 [33–37], it did not prove that disruption of p107 or p130 function was an essential component of T Ag-mediated transformation.

## 4. SV40 T Ag perturbs the phosphorylation state of p130 and p107

We pursued the possibility that SV40 T Ag could inactivate the potential growth suppressive functions of p130 and p107. Normally, p130 and p107 undergo cell cycle-dependent phosphorylation. At the transition between the G1 and S phase of the cell cycle, both p130 and p107 undergo an increase in the amount of serine and threonine phosphorylation. This phosphorylation may be due to cyclin D and cdk kinase activity. We compared the state of p130 and p107 in the lines transformed by wild type T Ag and by the LXCXE mutations. We were greatly surprised when the phosphorylation state of p130 and p107 in MEFs established by wild type T Ag was examined. These cells appeared to contain only hypophosphorylated p130 and p107. Conversely, in cells expressing an LXCXE mutation, p130 and p107 appeared to be normally phosphorylated, similar to what we had observed in naive NIH 3T3 cells [38]. Since the MEFs expressing LXCXE mutations of T Ag appeared to contain normally phosphorylated p130, we suspected that the disappearance of phosphorylated p130 depended upon binding to the LXCXE domain of T Ag. We were able to confirm this in a transient expression assay by co-transfecting plasmids that expressed an epitope-tagged version of wild type p130 and either wild type T Ag or various LXCXE mutations. Similar to the lines that stably expressed T Ag, only hypophosphorylated p130 was present when transiently expressed with wild type T Ag [38]. In contrast, expression of any one of several LXCXE mutations of T Ag that were unable to p130 in a co-precipitation assay had no detectable effect on the overall p130 phosphorylation status.

To determine if other residues within T Ag were also necessary, we tested the ability of deletion mutations of T Ag with an intact LXCXE domain to affect p130 phosphorylation. We found that expression of the first 147 residues of T Ag reduced the levels of phosphorylated p130 at least as well as full-length T Ag. In contrast, T Ag constructs that deleted or substituted residues within the N-terminus of T Ag, were unable to affect p130 phosphorylation. For example, expression of $T_{83-708}$, a deletion of the first exon with addition of an initiating methionine at residue 83, did not affect the p130 phosphorylation despite retaining the ability to bind p130. Significantly, $T_{83-708}$ has been reported to be transformation defective [39,40] and this correlation suggests that the specific effect of T Ag on the phosphorylation status of p130 and p107 may be a part of T Ag's transformation activity.

## 5.   The N-terminus of SV40 T Ag has homology to the J domain of DnaJ

It has been appreciated that the N-terminus of T Ag shares significant homology with the DnaJ family of heat shock (hsp40) or molecular chaperone, proteins [41]. DnaJ homologues have been found in most, if not all, prokaryotic and eukaryotic species. DnaJ homologues can interact with various members of the hsp70 family. All members of the DnaJ family share an N-terminal region of approximately 70 residues known as the J domain [42]. The J domain contains several highly conserved residues, including the HPDK motif with the HPD residues absolutely conserved in all known DnaJ homologues as well as all papova viral T Ags, including SV40 large T Ag. In addition, the N-terminus of T Ag binds to hsc70, a constitutively expressed member of the hsp70 family [43,44]. However, it is no known whether the association with this highly expressed cellular protein is required for transformation.

We considered the possibility that the N-terminus of T Ag behaved as a DnaJ molecular chaperone. We tested the ability of T Ag with substitutions in the conserved HPDK domain to reduce p130 phosphorylation. For example, substitution of a glutamine residue for histidine (H33Q) in the *Escherichia coli* DnaJ homologue disrupted the ability to support l-replication. The homologous T Ag mutation, H42Q, was constructed and found to be defective in reducing the levels of p130 phosphorylation [49].

Does the N-terminus of T Ag behave as a J domain? To test this possibility, we performed a J swap experiment, substituting the first 82 residues of T Ag with the J domain from two different human DnaJ homologues, DNAJ2 and HSJ1. Each of the constructions expressed similar levels of T Ag, were stable proteins, and were able to co-precipitate p130. Notably, both DnaJ-T Ag chimeras reduced the level of phosphorylated p130. To test that each chimera contributed a specific J domain activity, the corresponding histidine to glutamine substitution in the HPDK domain was generated by site-directed mutagenesis. In contrast to the wild type chimeras, neither the DNAJ2- T HQ or the HSJ1-T HQ mutation could reduce the levels of phosphorylated p130, similar to the defect of the H42Q mutation in wild type T Ag. This result implies that T Ag's ability to reduce the level of p130 phosphorylation can be mediated by a J domain. Furthermore, it suggests that the N-terminus of T Ag contains a J domain activity.

How does wild type T Ag reduce the levels of phosphorylated p130? Several mechanisms could be proposed to explain this effect. T Ag could specifically inhibit a p130 kinase or activate a phosphatase. Alternatively, T Ag could reduce the half-life of phosphorylated p130. To address this question, we performed a pulse chase experiment to determine the half-life of p130 in the presence or absence of T Ag. U2OS cells were transfected with plasmids expressing HA-tagged p130 and wild type T Ag, an LXCXE mutation, or a point mutation in the N-terminus (H42Q). One day after transfection, replica plates were pulse-labeled with [$^{35}$S]methionine for 20 min and chased with excess cold methionine for intervals up to 10 h. The half-life of p130 alone or in the presence of an LXCXE mutation of T Ag was approximately 5 h. In contrast, p130 had a half-life of less than 1 h in the presence of wild type T Ag. The half-life of p130 increased to approximately 10 h in the presence of the H42Q mutation of T Ag. Therefore, the N-terminus of T Ag, in conjunction with the LXCXE domain, not only contributed to the reduction of phosphorylated p130, but it also reduced the overall half-life. These results suggest that T Ag targets p130 for rapid degradation.

The effect of T Ag on p107 and p130 phosphorylation and p130 stability could not be separated genetically in our assays, and we believe they are both manifestations of the same T Ag activity. Based on the requirement for a J-domain, we can speculate that the mechanism of these effects may involve an associated hsp70. An association has been demonstrated between the N-terminal region of T Ag and hsc70, a constitutively expressed form of mammalian hsp70, and recent work has demonstrated that the HPD motif is critical to this interaction . The J-domain of DnaJ proteins has been shown to activate the intrinsic ATPase activity of associated hsp70 ATP hydrolysis may contribute to the ability of certain DnaJ homologues to modulate the folding of multimeric protein complexes. In the case of T Ag, activation of the associated hsc70 ATPase could alter the folding of the associated p107 and p130 and interfere with cyclins and their associated cyclin dependent kinases. Furthermore, the J-domain-hsc70 complex could, directly or indirectly, target p130 for proteasome-mediated degradation.

## 6. Role of the small DNA tumor viruses in human cancer

Of all human cancers, cervical cancer is the most closely linked with a viral cause. In a recent international survey of invasive cervical cancers, 95% contained human papilloma virus (HPV) DNA [45]. In addition, 95% of these specimens contained HPV from a high risk serotype, including the HPV16 and HPV 18 groups [45,46]. It has been demonstrated the development of invasive cervical cancer is dependent on expression of at least two viral proteins, E7 and E6 [46]. The molecular biology of the specific inactivation of pRB and p53 by these viral proteins supports the epidemiologic evidence that HPV contributes to carcinogenesis.

The role of SV40 in human cancers has been of some concern. More than 1 million people were vaccinated in the late 1950s and early 1960s with polio vaccine prepared in monkey cells that potentially contained the SV40 virus. Several epidemiological studies have failed to find evidence that having received a potentially contaminated vaccine led to an increased risk for developing cancer. Nevertheless, several investigators have found evidence for SV40 viral DNA in a variety of human cancers including ependymoma and mesotheliomas [47,48]. Whether SV40 contributed to the development of these tumors and whether T Ag was expressed in any of those tumors has not yet been determined.

SV40 T Ag and HPV E7 specifically target the three known-members of the pRB family of tumor suppressors. We have demonstrated that the LXCXE domain of T Ag and E7 is necessary for transformation, even in the setting of the specific targeted loss of pRB. These results imply that the pRB-related proteins, p107 and p130, may be additional targets of the viral oncoproteins. In addition, our preliminary data suggests that SV40 T Ag targets p130 for rapid degradation. The experiments highlighted in this review strengthen the hypothesis that p130 and p107, in addition to pRB, are targeted by T Ag and HPV E7 during transformation. Perhaps T Ag targets p130 for degradation in manner similar to the mechanism used by HPV E6 to reduce levels of the p53 tumor suppressor. If T Ag and E6 utilize similar pathways, then comparison of the two systems may yield important new insights into viral-mediated oncogenesis, and ultimately to improved methods for detection, prevention, and treatment of human cancer.

## Summary

The retinoblastoma (pRB) family of tumor suppressors includes the two closely related proteins, p130 and p107. While pRB has been found to be mutated in a wide variety of human tumors, p107 and p130 are rarely, if ever, affected. Therefore, given the lack of genetic evidence, it was uncertain whether p107 and p130 were capable of behaving as tumor suppressors. The viral proteins, SV40 T antigen and the human papilloma virus E7, have provided clues that suggests that p107 and p130 contribute to tumor suppression. T antigen can bind to all three members of the pRB family. Our investigations have focused on whether the inactivation of the growth suppressive properties of p107 and p130 is required for transformation by T antigen. We have recently reported (J Virol 70: 2781–2788, 1996) that the expression of SV40 T Ag reduces the cellular levels of phosphory-lated p130 and p107. We have found that this effect requires two domains of T Ag; the LXCXE domain, required for binding to p130, and the N-terminal domain. Both of these domains are required for transformation by T antigen. The N-terminus of T Ag shows significant homology with DnaJ, a class of heat shock proteins (Hsp40) present in most, if not all, organisms from bacteria to mammals. The J domain of DnaJ binds to and activates Hsp70 and participates in protein folding. We demonstrate that T antigen is a DnaJ homologue by substitution of the N-terminus of T Ag with the J domain from two different human DnaJ homologues, HSJ1 and DNAJ2. These chimeric proteins were capable of reducing the levels of phosphorylated p130 and p107 in a manner similar to wild type T antigen. Furthermore, we have evidence that T antigen decreases the half-life of p130. This reduction in the half-life of p130 is dependent on the DnaJ homology region. We have tested the ability of T antigen to transform fibroblasts derived from mice with the genes knocked-out for pRB, p107 or p130. Using a combination of various T antigen mutants and knockout cells, we have found that the J domain of T antigen was required to specifically inactivate both p107 and p130. Therefore, the loss of p107 and p130 function, either by genetic loss or by viral-mediated degradation is required for transformation by T antigen. These results demonstrate that the SV40 virus has evolved to borrow a component of the heat shock family to specifically inactivate the functions of the p130 and p107 tumor suppressors. These observations may lead to novel approaches to the treatment of viral infections and viral-induced cancer.

## Acknowledgements

This work was supported by Public Health Service grant (CA 63113) from the National Cancer Institute and funding from the Women's Cancer Program of the Dana-Farber Cancer Institute.

## References

1.  DeCaprio JA, Ludlow JW, Figge J, et al. SV40 large T antigen forms a specific complex with the product of the retinoblastoma susceptibility gene. Cell 54: 275–283, 1988.
2.  Dyson N, Howley PM, Munger K, Harlow E. The human papilloma virus-16 E7 oncoprotein is able to bind to the retinoblastoma gene product. Science 243: 934–937, 1989.
3.  Whyte P, Buchkovich KJ, Horowitz JM, et al. Association between an oncogene and an antioncogene: the adenovirus E1A proteins bind to the retinoblastoma gene product. Nature 334: 124–129, 1988.
4.  Whyte P, Williamson NM, Harlow E. Cellular targets for transformation by the adenovirus E1A proteins. Cell 56: 67–75, 1989.
5.  Scheffner M, Werness BA, Huibregtse JM, et al. The E6 oncoprotein encoded by human papillomavirus types 16 and 18 promotes the degradation of p53. Cell 63: 1129–1136, 1990.
6.  Scheffner M, Huibregtse JM, Vierstra RD, Howley PM. The HPV-16 E6 and E6-AP complex functions as a ubiquitin-protein ligase in the ubiquitination of p53. Cell 75: 495–505, 1993.
7.  Scheffner M, Nuber U, Huibregtse JM. Protein ubiquitination involving an E1-E2-E3 ubiquitin thioester cascade. Nature 373: 81–83, 1995.
8.  Claudio PP, Howard CM, Baldi A, et al. p130/pRb2 has growth suppressive properties similar to yet distinctive from those of retinoblastoma family members pRb and p107. Cancer Res 54: 5556–5560, 1994.
9.  Qin X-Q, Chittenden T, Livingston DM, Kaelin WGJ. Identification of a growth suppression domain within the retinoblastoma gene product. Genes Dev 6: 953–964, 1992.
10. Hinds PW, Mittnacht S, Dulic V, et al. Regulation of retinoblastoma protein functions by ectopic expression of human cyclins. Cell 70: 993–1006, 1992.
11. Goodrich DW, Wang NP, Qian Y-W, et al. The retinoblastoma gene product regulates progression through the G1 phase of the cell cycle. Cell 67: 293–302, 1991.
12. Hu Q, Dyson N, Harlow E. The regions of the retinoblastoma protein needed for binding to adenovirus E1A or SV40 large T antigen are common sites for mutations. EMBO J 9: 1147–1155, 1990.
13. Kaelin WG Jr, Ewen ME, Livingston DM. Definition of the minimal simian virus 40 large T antigen- and adenovirus E1A-binding domain in the retinoblastoma gene product. Mol Cell Biol 10: 3761–3769, 1990.
14. Beijersbergen RL, Carlée L, Kerhoven RM, Bernards R. Regulation of the retinoblastoma protein-related p107 by G1 cyclin complexes. Genes Dev 9: 1340–1353, 1995.
15. Hijmans EM, Voorhoeve PM, Beijersbergen RL, et al. E2F-5, a new E2F family member that interacts with p130 in vivo. Mol Cell Biol 15: 3082–3089, 1995.
16. Xiao Z-X, Ginsberg D, Ewen M, Livingston DM. Regulation of the retinoblastoma protein-related protein p107 by G1 cyclin-associated kinases. Proc Natl Acad Sci USA 93: 4633–4637, 1996.
17. Zhu L, Enders G, Lees JA, et al. The pRB-related protein p107 contains two growth suppression domains: independent interactions with E2F and cyclin/cdk complexes. EMBO J 14: 1904–1913, 1995.
18. DeCaprio JA, Ludlow JW, Lynch D, et al. The product of the retinoblastoma susceptibility gene has properties of a cell cycle regulatory element. Cell 58: 1085–1095, 1989.
19. Buchkovich K, Duffy LA, Harlow E. The retinoblastoma protein is phosphorylated during specific phases of the cell cycle. Cell 58: 1097–1105, 1989.
20. Ludlow JW, DeCaprio JA, Huang C-M, et al. SV40 Large T antigen binds preferentially to an underphosphorylated member of the retinoblastoma susceptibility gene product family. Cell 56: 57–65, 1989.
21. Ludlow JW, Shon J, Pipas JM, et al. The retinoblastoma susceptibility gene product undergoes cell cycle-dependent dephosphorylation and binding to and release from SV40 large T. Cell 60: 387–396, 1990.
22. Mayol X, Garriga J, Graña X. Cell cycle-dependent phosphorylation of the retinoblastoma-related protein p130. Oncogene 11: 801–808, 1995.
23. Matsushime H, Quelle DE, Shurtleff SA, et al. D-type cyclin-dependent kinase in mammalian cells. Mol Cell Biol 14: 2066–2076, 1994.
24. Meyerson M, Harlow E. Identification of G1 kinase activity for cdk6, a novel cyclin D partner. Mol Cell Biol 14: 2077–2086, 1994.
25. Lukus J, Bartkova J, Rohde M, et al. Cyclin D1 is dispensable for G1 control in retinoblastoma gene-deficient cells independently of cdk4 activity. Mol Cell Biol 15: 2600–2611, 1995.
26. Serrano M, Hannon GJ, Beach D. A new regulatory motif in cell-cycle control causing specific inhibition of cyclin D/CDK4. Nature 366: 704–707, 1993.
27. Parry D, Bates S, Mann DJ, Peters G. Lack of cyclin D-Cdk complexes in Rb-negative cells correlates with high levels of p16$^{INK4/MTS1}$ tumor suppressor gene product. EMBO J 14: 503–511, 1995.

28.   Claudio PP, De Luca A, Howard CM, et al. Functional analysis of pRb2/p130 interaction with cyclins. Cancer Res; 56: 2003–2008, 1996.

29.   Ogawa S, Hangaishi A, Miyawaki S, et al. Loss of the cyclin-dependent kinase 4-inhibitor (p16; MTS1) gene is frequent in and highly specific to lymphoid tumors in primary human hematopoietic malignancies. Blood 86: 1548–1556, 1995.

30.   Uchida T, Watanabe T, Kinoshita T, et al. Mutational analysis of the CDKN2 (MTS/p16ink4A) gene in primary B-cell lymphomas. Blood 86: 2724–2731, 1995.

31.   Sill H, Goldman JM, Cross NC. Homozygous deletions of the p16 tumor-suppressor gene are associated with lymphoid transformation of chronic myeloid leukemia. Blood 85: 2013–2016, 1995.

32.   Jacks T, Fazelli A, Schmitt EM, et al. Effects of an *Rb* mutation in the mouse. Nature 359: 295–300, 1992.

33.   Dyson N, Buchkovich K, Whyte P, Harlow E. The cellular 107K protein that binds to adenovirus E1A also associates with the large T antigens of SV40 and JC virus. Cell 58: 249–255, 1989.

34.   Ewen ME, Ludlow JW, Marsilio E, et al. An N-terminal transformation-governing sequence of SV40 large T antigen contributes to the binding of both p110RB and a second cellular protein, p120. Cell 58: 257–267, 1989.

35.   Ewen ME, Xing Y, Lawrence JB, Livingston DM. Molecular cloning, chromosomal mapping, and expression of the cDNA for p107, a retinoblastoma gene product-related protein. Cell 66: 1155–1164, 1991.

36.   Hannon GJ, Demetrick D, Beach D. Isolation of the Rb-related p130 through its interaction with CDK2 and cyclins. Genes Dev 7: 2378–2391, 1993.

37.   Zalvide J, DeCaprio JA. Role of pRb-related proteins in simian virus 40 large-T-antigen-mediated transformation. Mol Cell Biol 15: 5800–5810, 1995.

38.   Stubdal H, Zalvide J, DeCaprio JA. Simian virus 40 large T antigen alters the phosphorylation state of the RB-related proteins p130 and p107. J Virol 70: 2781–2788, 1996.

39.   Montano X, Millikan R, Milhaven JM, et al. Simian virus 40 small tumor antigen and an amino-terminal domain of large tumor antigen share a common transforming function. Proc Natl Acad Sci USA 87: 7448–7452, 1990.

40.   Marsilio E, Cheng SH, Schaffhausen B, et al. The T/t common region of simian virus 40 large T antigen contains a distinct transformation-governing sequence. J Virol 65: 5647–5652, 1991.

41.   Kelley W, Landry SJ. Chaperone power in a virus? Trends Biol Sci 19: 277–278, 1994.

42.   Silver PA, Way JC. Eukaryotic DnaJ homologs and the specificity of Hsp70 activity. Cell 74: 5–6, 1993.

43.   Michalovitz D, Fisher-Fantuzzi L, Vesco C, et al. Activated Ha-*ras* can cooperate with defective simian virus 40 in the transformation of nonestablished rat embryo fibroblasts. J Virol 61: 2648–2654, 1987.

44.   Sawai ET, Butel J. Association of a cellular heat shock protein with simian virus 40 large T antigen in transformed cells. J Virol 63: 3961–3973, 1989.

45.   Bosch FX, Manos MM, Muñoz N, et al. Prevalence of human papillomavirus in cervical cancer: a worldwide perspective. J Natl Cancer Inst 87: 796–802, 1995.

46.   Lowy DR, Kirnbauer R, Schiller JT. Genital human papillomavirus. Proc Natl Acad Sci USA 91: 2436–2440, 1994.

47.   Bergsagel DJ, Finegold MJ, Butel JS, et al. DNA sequences similar to those of simian virus 40 in ependymomas and choroid plexus tumors of childhood. N Engl J Med 326: 988–993, 1992.

48.   Carbone M, Pass HI, Rizzo P, et al. Simian virus 40-like sequences in human pleural mesothelioma. Oncogene 9: 1781–1790, 1994.

49.   Stubdal H, Zalvide J, Campbell KS, et al. Inactivation of pRB-related proteins p130 and p107 mediated by the J domain of simian virus 40 large T antigen. Mol Cell Biol 17: 4979–4990, 1997.

# SECTION IV

# CHEMO–RADIATION INDUCED CARCINOGENESIS

*"Science commits suicide when it adopts a creed."*
Thomas Henry Huxley

C.J. Rosenthal and M. Rotman (Eds.), *Infusion Chemotherapy–Irradiation Interactions*
© 1998 Elsevier Science B.V. All rights reserved

# Mechanisms of mammalian cell mutagenesis by ionizing radiation and chemical agents

BARRY S. ROSENSTEIN

*Department of Radiation Oncology, Mount Sinai School of Medicine of the City University of New York, New York, NY 10029, USA*

As increasing numbers of cancer patients, particularly young people, are cured through the use of chemotherapeutic agents and radiotherapy, there is increasing concern that these treatments may cause the induction of new tumors. In fact, radiation and many drugs used in cancer therapy have been shown to be carcinogenic in both rodent model systems as well as humans [1–4].

The goal of radiotherapy or chemotherapy is to sterilize the primary tumor of all clonogenic cells as well as the elimination of any metastases which may be present when treatment is initiated. Although great efforts may be made to specifically target the radiation or drug to the tumor cells, it is always true that non-malignant cells comprising normal tissues will also be affected. If large numbers of these cells are inactivated, then the particular tissue or organ system may malfunction and result in a debilitating complication associated with therapy. However, many of the cells which sustain some level of DNA damage will also survive, particularly those which may have received only a portion of the full therapeutic dose of the agent. If a DNA lesion is produced within an oncogene or tumor suppressor gene in a particular cell, then this cell may advance on the pathway to the formation of a new tumor due to the inappropriate expression of the oncogene or inactivation of the tumor suppressor gene [5,6].

The initial events associated with the interaction of cells and X-rays used in radiotherapy may be ionization of DNA components resulting in alterations within this molecule. This is referred to as the direct action of radiation and accounts for approximately one-third of the damage detected in the DNA of irradiated cells. The remaining two-thirds of the DNA alterations arise due to the indirect effect of radiation which involves radiolysis of water molecules within the vicinity of DNA resulting in the formation of free radicals, such as hydroxyl radicals, which then go on to react with DNA [7,8]. In addition, the presence of oxygen increases the types and numbers of damages formed in DNA [9,10].

One class of damage induced through these processes is base damage which often is produced from attack of hydroxyl radicals upon the C-5, C-6 double bond in thymine [10,11] This results in various ring saturated derivatives and fragmentation products. In addition, damage to the deoxyribose sugar also occurs, which may be of particular importance as this can result in the breakage of the phosphodiester chain [7]. These DNA strand breaks, particularly double strand breaks, may be an important mutagenic event as this can cause the breakage and possible rearrangement of chromosomes. If breaks occur in the vicinity of an oncogene, this can potentially lead to activation of the oncogene by disassociating this gene from its normal control mechanism. Alternatively, it can result in placement of the oncogene under the control of a strong promoter so that it is inappropriately expressed. In addition, breakage of a chromosome within the region of a tumor suppressor gene may cause loss of activity of this gene.

Many drugs used in cancer treatment also produce their cytotoxic effects through the creation of lesions in DNA. For example, alkylating drugs are electrophilic agents which react with nucleophilic sites in DNA resulting in the addition of an alkyl group to a DNA base [12–14]. These agents may be monofunctional and react with only one site in DNA. Alternatively, alkylating agents can be bifunctional in which case each drug molecule may react with two DNA sites resulting in either intrastrand or interstrand crosslinks. Another example of a crosslinking agent used in chemotherapy is *cis*-platinum. In this instance, it becomes an electrophilic agent through loss of chloride from the compound and then reacts with DNA to form either monoadducts or crosslinks [15,16].

However, cells are not passive in the face of DNA damage and possess an impressive array of enzymatic systems whose function it is to remove the DNA lesions or allow the cell to survive through tolerance of the damage. Briefly, there are three general mechanisms through which cells repair DNA damage. The first type of repair process involves the direct reversal of the DNA damage. Probably the most detailed example of this is repair of the alkylation damage $O^6$-methylguanine that is produced following exposure to alkylating agents. In this system, $O^6$-methylguanine DNA methyltransferase, a suicide enzyme that is consumed in the process, transfers the methyl group from guanine to a cysteine residue in the enzyme thereby restoring the guanine back to its original state [17–19].

In fact direct reversal is able to address only a small number of possible DNA damages and the vast majority of repair takes place through excision repair for which there are two principal mechanisms, base excision repair and nucleotide excision repair [20]. The first step in base excision repair involves recognition of the damaged base by a DNA glycosylase which causes hydrolysis of the N-glycosylic bond between the altered base and the deoxyribose sugar leaving an apurinic or apyrimidinic (AP) site [21,22]. Attack at such sites then takes place by a 5′ AP endonuclease [23] resulting in a break in the DNA strand with a 5′ terminal deoxyribose-phosphate which is then excised by a DNA deoxyribophosphodiesterase [24]. This leaves a single nucleotide gap which is resynthesized by a DNA polymerase [25] using the complementary strand to determine the correct base and the remaining nick sealed through the action of a DNA ligase [26]. Base excision repair is responsible for the correction of a limited spectrum of DNA lesions as each DNA glycosylase recognizes a specific type of DNA alteration. Therefore, the number of damages addressed by base excision repair is relatively small as a different enzyme must be synthesized to remove each type of damage.

In contrast, nucleotide excision repair is far more general in its scope and is responsible for repair of a large variety of DNA lesions. In this system [27], a complex of enzymes first recognizes that the DNA has been damaged and then an endonucleolytic activity produces breaks separated by approximately 30 nucleotides both 3′ and 5′ to the damage [28,29], so that a piece of DNA corresponding to this length is removed. The final steps are similar to base excision repair in that the gap produced is eliminated through repair synthesis and the nick sealed by DNA ligase.

The repair processes outlined above, which are relatively error free and do not generally result in the formation of mutations, will eliminate much of the DNA damage induced by chemicals and radiation. Nevertheless, it is likely that many DNA alterations will still be present when a cell attempts to replicate its DNA in S phase of the cell cycle and it therefore may be necessary for DNA synthesis to take place using a damaged genetic template. This is the period in which most errors occur resulting in mutations as the DNA polymerase may not place the correct base in the growing DNA chain as the strand being replicated may contain non-coding or incorrect base sequence information [30,31].

One way in which an incorrect base may be inserted within the nascent DNA strand is due to mispairing of the damaged base with the incorrect complementary base. For example, the $O^6$-methylguanine produced by treatment of cells with alkylating agents may incorrectly pair with thymine rather than cytosine as two hydrogen bonds can now form between this altered form of guanine and thymine [32], although evidence has been obtained that the explanation for this incorrect base pairing may be more complex [33].

A more general mechanism resulting in mutation formation is translesion DNA synthesis which appears to involve a relaxation in the fidelity of the DNA polymerase permitting the synthesis of DNA past a damaged and non-coding region in DNA [34–36]. This allows the cell to replicate its DNA and divide to form two new cells, possibly resulting in the insertion of an incorrect base at the site of the damaged base. Therefore, although the cell may survive, the individual may pay a high price for this act of survival as the mutation may occur in an oncogene or tumor suppressor gene and represent an important step in the formation of a new tumor.

Typically errors in DNA synthesis can result in point mutations which fall into two classes, transition and transversion mutations [20]. Transition mutations are those in which one purine is substituted for another or one pyrimidine for another. In contrast, transversion mutations involve the substitution of a purine for a pyrimidine or pyrimidine for a purine. If a point mutation occurs in a coding region of a gene, this may cause a missense mutation in which a codon for a particular amino acid is changed so that a different amino acid is now encoded. Another possibility is for a nonsense mutation in which the codon for an amino acid is changed to a stop codon which results in premature termination of synthesis of the nascent polypeptide chain. In addition, a frameshift mutation may occur in which the translational reading frame has been altered through the addition or deletion of $3n \pm 1$ base pairs so that an incorrect series of amino acids is encoded along with a likely stop codon resulting in termination of protein synthesis.

This paper represents a brief review of the mechanisms involved in mammalian cell mutagenesis which operate in cells exposed to radiation or chemicals. The interested reader is encouraged to consult the references listed below to explore in greater depth any of the topics presented.

## Summary

Radiation and many of the chemical agents used in the treatment of malignancies have been shown to be carcinogenic. It is likely that an early step in this process of neoplastic transformation is the creation of DNA damages within oncogenes or tumor suppressor genes resulting in the inappropriate expression of oncogenes or the inactivation of tumor suppressor genes. Although cells possess mechanisms to remove these damages, DNA replication may take place prior to the removal of all DNA alterations. Hence, either non-coding or improperly coding regions may be present at the time of DNA replication causing the insertion of an incorrect base in the nascent DNA strand and result in a mutation. The purpose of this paper is to briefly review the mechanisms involved in the creation of mutations in mammalian cells exposed to radiation and chemicals.

## References

1.  Ludlum DB. Therapeutic agents as potential carcinogens. In: Cooper CS, Grover PL (Eds), Chemical Carcinogenesis and Mutagenesis I. Berlin: Springer, pp. 153–175, 1990.
2.  Casciato DA, Scott JL. Acute leukemia following prolonged cytotoxic agent therapy. Medicine 58: 32–47, 1979.
3.  Marselos M, Vainio H. Carcinogenic properties of pharmaceutical agents evaluated in the IARC monographs programme. Carcinogenesis 12: 1751–1766, 1991.
4.  International Agency for Research on Cancer. Monographs on the evaluation of carcinogenic risks to humans: overall evaluations of carcinogenicity. An Updating of IARC Monographs, Vols. 1–42. Lyons: International Agency for Research on Cancer, 1987.
5.  Bishop JM. Cellular oncogenes and retroviruses. Annu Rev Biochem 52: 301–354, 1983.
6.  Marshall CJ. Tumor suppressor genes. Cell 64: 313–3266, 1991.
7.  Ward JF. DNA damage produced by ionizing radiation in mammalian cells: identities, mechanisms of formation and reparability. Prog Nucleic Acid Res Mol Biol 35: 95–125, 1988.
8.  Goodhead DT. The initial damage produced by ionizing radiations. Int J Radiat Biol 56: 623–634, 1989.
9.  Frankenberg-Schwager M, Frankenberg D, Blocher D, Adamczyk C. The influence of oxygen on the survival and yield of DNA double-strand breaks in irradiated yeast cells. Int J Radiat Biol 36: 261–270, 1979.
10. von Sonntag C. The Chemical Basis of Radiation Biology. London: Taylor & Francis, 1987.
11. Teoule R. Radiation-induced DNA damage and its repair. Int J Radiat Biol 51: 573–589, 1987.
12. Lawley PD. Mutagens as carcinogens: development of current concepts. Mutat Res 213: 3–25, 1989.
13. Singer B. The chemical effects of nucleic acid alkylation and their relation to mutagenesis and carcinogenesis. Prog Nucleic Acid Res Mol Biol 15: 219–284, 1975.
14. Singer B, Kusmierek JT. Chemical mutagenesis. Annu Rev Biochem 51: 655–693, 1982.
15. Chu G. Cellular responses to cisplatin. J Biol Chem 269: 787–790, 1994.
16. Eastman A. The formation, isolation and characterization of DNA adducts produced by anticancer platinum complexes. Pharmacol Ther 34: 155–166, 1987.
17. Boulden AM, Foote RS, Fleming GS, Mitra S. Purification and some properties of human DNA-$O^6$-methylguanine methyltransferase. J Biosci 11: 215–224, 1987.
18. Harris AL, Karran P, Lindahl T. $O^6$-methyl-guanine-DNA methyltransferase of human lymphoid cells: structural and kinetic properties and absence in repair-deficient cells. Cancer Res 43: 3247–3252, 1983.
19. Pegg AE. Mammalian $O^6$-alkylguanine-DNA alkyltransferase: regulation and importance in response to alkylating carcinogenic and therapeutic agents. Cancer Res 50: 6119–6129, 1990.
20. Friedberg EC, Walker GC, Siede W. DNA Repair and Mutagenesis. American Society for Microbiology, 1995.
21. Duncan BK. DNA glycosylases. In: Boyer PD (Ed), The Enzymes, 3rd edn. New York: Academic Press, pp. 565–586, 1981.
22. Lindahl T. DNA glycosylases, endonuclease for apurinic/apyrimidinic sites and base excision-repair. Prog Nucleic Acid Res Mol Biol 22: 135–192, 1979.
23. Doetsch PW, Cunningham RP. The enzymology of apurinic/apyrimidinic endonucleases. Mutat Res 236: 173–201, 1990.
24. Franklin WA, Lindahl T. DNA deoxyribophosphodiesterase. EMBO J 7: 3617–3522, 1988.
25. Kornberg A, Baker T. DNA Replication. New York: WH Freeman, 1991.
26. Lindahl T, Barnes DE. Mammalian DNA ligases. Annu Rev Biochem 61: 251–281, 1992.
27. Hoeijmakers JHJ. Nucleotide excision repair II: from yeast to mammals. Trends Genet 9: 211–217, 1993.
28. Symkowski DE, Hajibagheri MAN, Wood RD. Electron microscopy of DNA excision repair patches produced by human cell extracts. J Mol Biol 231: 251–260, 1993.

29.   Huang J-C, Svoboda DL, Reardon JT, Sancar A. Human nucleotide excision nuclease removes thymine dimers from DNA by incising the 22nd phosphodiester bond 5′ and the 6th phosphodiester bond 3′ to the photodimer. Proc Natl Acad Sci USA 89: 3664–3668, 1992.

30.   Kaufmann WK. Pathways of human cell post-replication repair. Carcinogenesis 10: 1–11, 1989.

31.   Rossman TG, Klein CB. From DNA damage to mutation in mammalian cells: a review. Environ Mol Mutagen 11: 119–133, 1988.

32.   Loveless A. Possible relevance of O-6-alkylation of deoxyguanosine to the mutagenicity and carcinogenicity of nitrosamines and nitrosamides. Nature 223: 206–207, 1969.

33.   Swann PF. Why do $O^6$-alkylguanine and $O^4$-alkylthymine miscode? The relationship between the structure of DNA containing $O^6$-alkylguanine and $O^4$-alkylthymine and the mutagenic properties of these bases. Mutat Res 233: 81–94, 1990.

34.   Spivak G, Hanawalt PC. Translesion DNA synthesis in the dihydrofolate reductase domain of UV-irradiated CHO cells. Biochemistry 31: 6794–6800, 1992.

35.   Carty MP, Hauser J, Levine AS, Dixon K. Replication and mutagenesis of UV-damaged DNA templates in human and monkey cell extracts. Mol Cell Biol 13: 533–542, 1993.

36.   Thomas DC, Nguyen DC, Piegorsch WW, Kunkel TA. Relative probabilities of mutagenic translesion synthesis on the leading and lagging strands during replication of UV-irradiated DNA in a human cell extract. Biochemistry 32: 11476–11482, 1993.

C.J. Rosenthal and M. Rotman (Eds.), *Infusion Chemotherapy–Irradiation Interactions*

# CHAPTER 34

# Chemo-radiation induced carcinogenesis: the bone marrow transplant model

BRENDA SHANK

*Radiation Oncology Department, Box 1236, Mount Sinai Medical Center, One Gustave L. Levy Place, New York, NY 10029-6574, USA*

## 1. Introduction

Many studies have called attention to the increased risk of developing a secondary malignancy after bone marrow transplantation [1–16]. In these studies it has often been difficult to ascertain whether the increased risk is due to the immunosuppression of the transplant regimen alone or whether it is due to one or more of the agents used for cytoreduction prior to transplantation. The genetic predisposition to a secondary malignancy in someone with a first malignancy or a genetic disorder is also difficult to assess. Types of secondary malignancies range from lymphomas and leukemias to skin cancers and other solid tumors. In this study, a review of the literature has been done of not only secondary malignancies which develop after marrow transplantation but also those which occur after other organ transplantations or other treatments for similar malignancies with the hope of shedding some light on the mechanism of the development of these malignancies after bone marrow transplantation.

## 2. Methods

A review of the literature was done regarding the development of secondary malignancies after marrow transplantation, other organ transplantation, or chemotherapy and radiation treatment of the same diseases treated for marrow transplantation. Issues which were examined included the distribution of types of secondary malignancies, the agents that were used for treatment or transplantation, the delay of development of secondary malignancies under these various conditions, the incidence of the various types of secondary malignancies and risk factors for their development such as age, immunosuppressive agents, types of chemotherapy, use of radiation, use of splenectomy, the patient's platelet count, family history and initial diagnosis. Based on all of these studies, an attempt at reaching some general conclusions about the etiology of the secondary malignancies was made.

## 3. Results

### 3.1. Distribution of secondary malignancies after marrow transplantation

Several studies have shown that lymphomas and skin tumors are the most common forms of

Table 1

Distribution of secondary malignancies (SM) after BMT

| Study | No. BMT | No. SM | Types (%) | | | | |
|---|---|---|---|---|---|---|---|
| | | | Lymphomas | Leukemias | Skin | Brain | Other |
| IBMTR [9] | 14783 | 166 | 44 | 9 | 18 | – | 29 |
| Princess Margaret Hospital [10] | 557 | 10[a] | 10 | 10 | 30 | – | 50 |
| EBMT [16] | 1211 | 47 | 6 | – | 28 | 9 | 62 |
| Seattle [7] | 2246 | 35 | 46 | 17 | 11 | 9 | 17 |
| U. Minn. [14] | 2150 | 52 | 48[b] | 21 | – | – | 33 |

[a]In 9 patients.

[b]Most (22/25) were EBV-related B-cell type.

secondary malignancies seen after marrow transplantation (Table 1) [7,9,10,14,16]. However, there is also a high incidence of leukemias, brain tumors, and other solid tumors. In a study by Kolb et al. in 1992 [5] it was found that of 116 patients who developed second malignancies after marrow transplantation, 73 were leukemias and lymphomas. This proportion was similar to that found with organ transplantation in which only immunosuppression is used. This suggests that immunosuppression is a major factor in the etiology of these tumors. In the study from the University of Minnesota [14] most of the lymphomas were Epstein-Barr-virus (EBV)-related B-cell type (22/25) also suggesting a predominant role of immunosuppression per se in the development of these malignancies.

Both of the two studies which assess the incidence of brain tumors had an incidence of 9% in marrow transplant patients [7,16]. In a study of childhood acute lymphoblastic leukemia (ALL) treated on a variety of multimodality protocols of the Children's Cancer Study Group, the majority of tumors were central nervous system (CNS) tumors [17]. These patients had been treated with a variety of regimens and it was found that the ratio of observed to expected CNS tumors in these patients was 21.7 compared with only 3.9 for leukemias and lymphomas. It is important that, in these CNS secondary neoplasms, 39 of the patients had received prior CNS radiation either at the time of diagnosis of their ALL or at the time of relapse. Also, it would appear that there is a role of host susceptibility in the secondary CNS tumors after treatment of leukemia. It was found that there was a 2.8-fold excess risk of hematopoietic neoplasms in siblings of children with CNS tumors and an 8-fold excess risk of such neoplasms in siblings of children with medulloblastoma.

## 3.2. Incidence

The incidence of second malignancies reported in different studies varies by the length of followup. Crude incidences reported in several studies have ranged between 1.1% and 3.9% (Table 1), but this does not consider the true patients at risk, i.e., those who have not died of their primary disease, or been lost to followup. When most of the patients were transplanted for malignancies rather than for the anemias, the actuarial incidence rate is in the range of 10–12% at 11–13 years [10,14].

It is clear also that the primary diagnosis of the patient who received marrow transplantation is an important consideration in the incidence rate of secondary malignancies. One paper which caused much concern in the transplantation community was that of Socie et al.

who reported in a small group of patients with either aplastic anemia (107 patients) or Fanconi's anemia (40 patients) a cumulative incidence rate of 22% at 8 years. The preparative regimen used was cyclophosphamide and thoraco-abdominal irradiation (TAI) to a dose of 6 Gy. Due to the small number of events the standard error was quite large, ±11% [1].

Shortly thereafter, the group from Seattle analyzed their data for aplastic anemia and Fanconi's anemia patients and published it in a letter [2]. They had 318 patients with severe aplastic anemia and 12 with Fanconi's anemia. The cumulative incidence rate at 5 years for a secondary cancer was only 0.4% and at 10 years 1.4%. Their cases had a long followup; thus they were able to report a 15-year incidence of second malignancies, 4.2%. They pointed out that in their regimen they used cyclophosphamide alone as a conditioning agent. In their study they had considerably fewer Fanconi's anemia patients who were found to develop tumors even without treatment. They suggested that the difference in their study compared with the French study was the use of irradiation and recommended that radiation be avoided in marrow transplantation for non-malignant diseases. In a recent publication from Seattle, it was felt that the highest risk of developing a solid tumor was associated with diagnosis of Fanconi's anemia [13].

In response to the original Seattle letter [2], Socie et al. pointed out that their incidence rate increased to 25% at 8 years with the development of another cancer in a male. In a followup article, the French group analyzed the radiation doses and fields in relationship to the development of secondary tumors [15]. They found that all five of their tumors had occurred within the radiation field penumbra and the estimates of doses received varied from 2.5 Gy for four of the tumors to 6 Gy for one tumor within the field. It was suggested that tumors may arise in the penumbra zone. Since the tumors were either epidermoid carcinomas (4 cases) or in one case a mucoepidermoid carcinoma, it was suggested that irradiation may promote the development of epidermoid carcinoma. However, such tumors are common in immunosuppression alone, as discussed below.

Since there is a high incidence of secondary lymphomas and leukemias in patients who have undergone marrow transplantation, it has been felt that this is more suggestive of an immunosuppressive effect rather than a direct effect of the chemotherapy and/or radiation {5,16}. In the Seattle study all of the secondary cancers were squamous cell carcinomas as well, three in the head and neck region, one in an extremity and one in the vulva.

## 3.3. Immunosuppression

As was mentioned above, the high incidence of leukemias and lymphomas after transplantation is similar to that after immunosuppression for treatment of other diseases. In addition, it is found that skin tumors after organ transplantation, i.e., heart or kidney, are the most common tumors after immunosuppression and these are also commonly seen after marrow transplantation with the use of immunosuppressive agents to prevent rejection (Table 1) [18,19].

In organ transplantation, it is felt that the skin tumors and lymphomas that are seen might well be a result of the immunosuppressive agents allowing oncogenic viruses such as EB to transform cells [19]. In one study of the development of malignant neoplasms after marrow transplantation, it was found that, of 51 patients who developed secondary malignancies, 22 cases were B-cell lymphoproliferative disorders [14]. In these, the histologic appearance was similar to EBV-induced polymorphic B-cell proliferation which is seen after solid organ transplantation or which occurs in normal primary immunodeficiency. In a multivariate analysis there were several statistically significant risk factors which were independently associated with an increased risk of developing these B-cell lymphoproliferative disorders, namely in vitro T-cell depletion of the marrow prior to transplant, HLA mismatched transplants, the use of ATG either for GVHD prophylaxis or as part of the preparative regimen. There was a trend also for marrow deficiency as a primary diagnosis leading to a higher incidence of these neoplasms ($P = 0.06$).

One very interesting study of patients registered in the European Bone Marrow Transplantation-Severe Aplastic Anemia Working Party was able to have sufficient patients available for a credible analysis of risk factors. They had 860 patients who were treated by immunosuppression only and 748 patients who had received bone marrow transplantation for the treatment of severe aplastic anemia [6]. In these patients, 42 malignant conditions were reported in the 860 patients who received immunosuppressive therapy and 9 were reported in the 748 patients who received bone marrow transplants. In the bone marrow transplant group, 7 of the 9 cases were solid tumors and there were only 2 cases of acute leukemia. In the immunosuppression group, 19 of the 42 cases were myelodysplastic syndrome (MDS); 15, acute leukemia; 1, non-Hodgkin's lymphoma; and 7, solid tumors. The incidence of solid tumors was essentially the same in both groups whereas the incidence of the leukemias and lymphomas were far greater in the immunosuppression group. When only cases of leukemia were considered, the relative risk in the immunosuppression group was 7.57 compared with the transplantation group. No statistically significant difference between groups was observed for the number of solid tumors.

### 3.4. Delay to development of secondary malignancies (latency)

After transplantation for malignant disease (lymphomas or leukemias) it is found that the development of myelodysplastic syndrome, acute myelogenous leukemia or acute lymphocytic leukemia tend to occur very early after transplantation with some tumors appearing in the first year and others occurring as late as 8 years. The median in three studies was 3–4 years [8,11,14]. In patients who are transplanted for aplastic anemia including some Fanconi's anemias, lymphoid malignancies tend to occur within the first 2 years after transplantation [6,13]. In one of the studies after immunosuppression only, it was found that MDS and acute leukemia occurred any time from the first year to 10 years following the initiation of the therapy with the median being about 4 years [6]. This was quite different from marrow transplantation alone, after which only two acute leukemias developed, both within the first 3 years.

For comparison, one can look at the SEER data for all patients with a variety of malignancies grouped together treated with chemotherapy and/or radiation therapy (Table 2) [20] It is found that generally there appears to be a deficit of leukemias in the first year following treatment, but risk increases by the second year and continues out to at least 7 years, being somewhat higher in the third to seventh years. The risks are similar whether radiation is given or chemotherapy is given and are greater than that for patients who received neither of these agents. This is discussed further later. The principal tumor in these patients was acute non-lymphocytic leukemia (ANLL) which accounted for all of the leukemic excess in the radiation therapy group and in the chemotherapy alone group.

When one looks at the development of solid tumors, a very different pattern of delay emerges. Although solid tumors may occur in the first year after transplantation, there tends to be a sharp increase after 8 years and they may continue to develop as far out as 13 years

Table 2
Relative risk of second primary leukemias as a function of initial treatment and latency (time from primary[a] diagnosis)

| Latency (year) | Radiation alone | Chemotherapy alone | Radiation + chemotherapy | None |
|---|---|---|---|---|
| 1 | 0.6 | 0.8 | 0.7 | 0.9 |
| 2 | 1.4 | 2.0 | 2.2 | 0.8 |
| 3–7 | 2.2 | 5.2 | 10.9 | 1.2 |

[a]All first primary sites combined. SEER data [20].

in studies which have long followup [14]. The median time to solid tumor development was 4 years compared with a median of 3 years for the MDS and acute leukemias, which plateau at 4 years. In patients transplanted for aplastic anemia, the development of solid tumors also occurs late, any time from the first year out to 8 or 9 years after transplantation. The median interval in two studies was 52 months and 99 months [6,13].

### 3.5. Influence of chemotherapy and radiation

#### 3.5.1. Chemotherapy

There is a considerable body of evidence to indicate that chemotherapy contributes to the development of MDS or leukemias. Many of the agents used in marrow transplantation are known carcinogenic drugs, such as busulfan, cyclophosphamide, procarbazine, thiotepa and adriamycin. Some of these agents are used prior to marrow transplantation during induction or consolidation; others are used in the cytoreductive schema for transplantation. On a chromosomal level, epipodophyllotoxins are known to cause 11q23 rearrangements, and alkylating agents are known to cause chromosome 5 and 7 aberrations [11].

In the non-Hodgkin's lymphoma transplant setting, we see an increase in risk of MDS with increased duration of exposure to chemotherapeutic agents pre-transplant and with increased duration of exposure to alkylating agents [12].

When one looks at the treatment of Hodgkin's disease patients excluding transplantation, there is an increase in leukemias, in particular ANLL, with chemotherapy. Kaldor et al. has shown that the risk of developing leukemia was nine times the risk with radiation therapy alone, and was found to be 13 times the risk with radiation therapy if more than six cycles of chemotherapy were given (which included procarbazine and mechlorethamine) [21]. Tura et al. showed that the incidence of ANLL after treatment of Hodgkin's disease increased with the number of MOPP courses [22]. SEER data for the development of leukemias after any kind of cancer treatment demonstrated that ANLL significantly increased after chemotherapy for breast cancer, ovarian cancer and multiple myeloma [20]. The increase of MDS and leukemias in the transplant setting is not surprising, therefore, considering the amount of prior chemotherapy, as well as cytoreductive chemotherapy, in these patients.

#### 3.5.2. Radiation therapy

In contrast to chemotherapy, radiation appears to be a risk factor for the development of solid tumors in nearly all of the studies where it was examined. Several studies have now shown a strong trend or a statistically significant increased risk of development of solid tumors after the use of large field irradiation in preparative regimens for transplantation, regardless of the initial diagnosis [3,6,10,13,14]. One example is from the European transplant group which showed that when TBI, TAI, or total lymphoid irradiation (TLI) were used in aplastic anemia patients, there was a higher risk by multivariate analysis of the development of solid tumors, with $P = 0.05$ [6]. Another study, which was predominantly with leukemias, lymphomas and some aplastic anemia patients, showed a trend towards an increased risk for solid tumors with the use of TBI [14].

The increase in solid tumors with radiation-containing transplant regimens is also not a surprising finding considering that there have been other results in the literature which suggest that radiation is a risk factor for the development of solid tumors. In children with ALL treated with a variety of regimens including chemotherapy or cranial prophylaxis (and transplant in a few cases), there was an increased risk for solid tumor development with the use of irradiation especially for CNS tumors which occurred only in children who had had prophylactic cranial irradiation [17]. SEER data shows that there appears to be an increase in leukemias especially ANLL with the use of irradiation. This was particularly evident in patients with endometrial cancer who would have had a larger amount of bone marrow in their pelvis treated [20]. In marrow transplantation in patients with NHL, one study showed that the use of radiation therapy, in particular pelvic irradiation, prior to transplantation increased the risk of MDS [12]. Similarly, in another study, there was an increase in MDS and AML with the use of TBI for transplantation in NHL and Hodgkin's disease patients [8]. Eight percent of the patients who had TBI developed either MDS/AML versus none who did not have TBI. This was only found for patients who were 40 years old and older.

One interesting study in dogs showed a significant increase in cancer deaths secondary to TBI ($P < 0.0001$), with higher doses, larger fraction sizes, and shorter treatment schedules enhancing earlier tumor development [5]. Chemotherapy also increased cancer deaths ($P = 0.06$).

## 3.6.  Other risk factors

### 3.6.1.  Age
Quite a few studies have shown that older age in itself is a risk factor for the development of secondary malignancies. In the transplant setting, regardless of primary diagnosis, it has been shown that older age is significant for the development of MDS and/or AML, with studies using cutoffs of ages ranging from 35 to 40 years [8,12,14]. Also some analyses have been done for the development of solid tumors which shows that increasing age is a risk factor for the development of these [6,13]. In children with ALL therapy of any type, it is found that age less than or equal to 5 years old is a risk factor for development of second malignancies which is all the more reason to be concerned about transplantation in such young children [17].

### 3.6.2.  Splenectomy
In a study of aplastic anemia patients who were transplanted it was found that the incidence of MDS increased with splenectomy and was the most significant factor [6]. Outside of the transplant setting, it has been found that there is an increase in ANLL in splenectomized Hodgkin's disease patients who were treated with combined modality therapy [22]. It has also been reported that there have been increasing cases of leukemia post traumatic splenectomy; this was reported in a letter to the editor by Demeter and Lehoczky [23].

### 3.6.3.   GVHD and its therapy

In one study, it has been shown that patients have an increased incidence of secondary cancers after the development of acute graft-versus-host-disease (GVHD) greater than or equal to grade II. Most of these malignancies were epithelial in origin [10]. Treatment for graft-versus-host-disease may play a role, such as the use of azathioprine, ATG or CD3 monoclonal antibody [3,13]. The addition of androgens to ATG and methylprednisolone for the treatment of GVHD increased the incidence of MDS and acute leukemia and it was found that two or more courses of immunosuppression was also a factor [6].

### 3.6.4.   Miscellaneous factors

Other factors which are difficult to explain and may play a role in enhancing the development of secondary malignancies include male sex for solid tumors in aplastic anemia patients [6], and platelets less than 152 000 at the time of autologous transplant in non-Hodgkin's lymphoma patients [12].

## 4.   Conclusions

Secondary malignancies after transplantation are a serious consequence of aggressive therapy. Identifying the factors involved may help one change cytoreductive regimens with the hope of lessening this risk. Although secondary MDS and ANLL may be treated successfully with bone marrow transplantation [24], it would be wise to try to avoid this complication at the outset if possible. From analysis of the characteristics of these second malignancies, including the distribution of malignant types, incidence, latency, and risk factors involved, several important factors emerge. For the development of MDS and leukemias, it is quite clear that chemotherapy plays a major role not only in transplantation but in the primary treatment of cancer. Radiation therapy also appears to be a contributing factor in the development of these tumors especially when combined with chemotherapy.

For the development of solid tumors, radiation is a major risk factor, and these tumors are often not seen until many years after transplantation. This risk appears to increase with age, but it is not clear that replacing radiation with chemotherapy in the older age group would improve upon this. Immunosuppression per se also plays a role since patients who undergo transplantation with any kind of cytoreduction are immunosuppressed for a time. Many are given immunosuppressive agents following transplantation to prevent or treat GVHD. It is hoped that with analyses such as these, one will be able to eventually arrive at regimens which will be less leukemogenic and carcinogenic.

## Summary

*Background*: Many publications have cited the increased number of second malignancies (SM) that develop after bone marrow transplantation (BMT) for leukemias, lymphomas, and benign diseases such as aplastic anemia. Similar increases in SMs occur after chemotherapy, and/or irradiation, or immunosuppression alone. *Methods*: A review of the literature has been done regarding the development of SMs after BMT, other organ transplantations, or chemotherapy and radiation treatment of the same diseases for which marrow transplantation is used. Risk factors were examined and results summarized. *Results*: Genetic factors play a large role in the development of SMs in Fanconi's anemia patients who are transplanted. Immunosuppression is a consequence of marrow transplantation regimens per se as well as of prophylaxis against graft-versus-host-disease (GVHD) and contributes to the development of lymphoid and myeloid malignancies. Chemotherapy and large field irradiation play a significant role in the development of leukemias/myelodysplasia and solid tumors respectively. Other factors include age and the use of splenectomy. *Conclusions*: Although no one factor emerges as the primary cause of secondary malignancies after BMT, it is likely that chemotherapy, both prior to transplant and as a part of the cytoreductive regimen, contribute largely to the development of myelodysplasia and acute non-lymphocytic leukemias, with large field irradiation adding to this risk in older patients ($\geq$40 years old). Irradiation as part of the cytoreductive regimen is most likely the major contributor to the development of solid tumors which occur later. Immunosuppression also contributes, especially in patients who develop GVHD.

## References

1. Socie G, Henry-Amar M, Cosset JM, et al. Increased incidence of solid malignant tumors after bone marrow transplantation for severe aplastic anemia. Blood 78: 277, 1991.
2. Witherspoon RP, Storb R, Pepe M, et al. Cumulative incidence of secondary solid malignant tumors in aplastic anemia. Blood 79: 289, 1992.
3. Sullivan KM, Mori M, Sanders J, et al. Late complications of allogeneic and autologous marrow transplantation. Bone Marrow Transplant 10: 127, 1992.
4. Socie G, Henry-Amar M, Bacigalupo A, et al. Malignancies occurring after the treatment for aplastic anemia: a survey on 1680 patients conducted by the European Group for Bone Marrow Transplantation (EBMT) - Severe Aplastic Anemia Working Party (abstr.) Blood 80: 169a, 1992.
5. Kolb HJ, Guenther W, Duell T, et al. Cancer after bone marrow transplantation. Bone Marrow Transplant 10: 135, 1992.
6. Socie G, Henry-Amar M, Bacigalupo A, et al. Malignant tumors occurring after treatment of aplastic anemia. N Engl J Med 329: 1152, 1993.
7. Witherspoon RP, Fisher LD, Schoch G, et al. Secondary cancers after bone marrow transplantation for leukemia or aplastic anemia. N Engl J Med 321: 784, 1989.
8. Darrington DL, Vose JM, Anderson JR, et al. Incidence and characterization of secondary myelodysplastic syndrome and acute myelogenous leukemia following high-dose chemoradiotherapy and autologous stem-cell transplantation for lymphoid malignancies. J Clin Oncol 12: 2527, 1994.
9. Dicke KA. Late effects after allogeneic bone marrow transplantation. Bone Marrow Transplant 14(Suppl 4): S11, 1994.
10. Lowsky R, Lipton J, Fyles G, et al. Secondary malignancies after bone marrow transplantation in adults. J Clin Oncol 12: 2187, 1994.
11. Miller JS, Arthur DC, Litz CE, et al. Myelodysplastic syndrome after autologous bone marrow transplantation: an additional late complication of curative cancer therapy. Blood 83: 3780, 1994.
12. Stone RM, Neuberg D, Soiffer R, et al. Myelodysplastic syndrome as a late complication following autologous bone marrow transplantation for non-Hodgkin's lymphoma. J Clin Oncol 12: 2535, 1994.
13. Deeg HJ, Socie G, Schoch G, et al. Malignancies after marrow transplantation for aplastic anemia and Fanconi anemia: a joint Seattle and Paris analysis of results in 700 patients. Blood 87: 386, 1996.
14. Bhatia S, Ramsay NKC, Steinbuch M, et al. Malignant neoplasms following bone marrow transplantation. Blood 87: 3633, 1996.
15. Pierga J-Y, Socie G, Gluckman E, et al. Secondary solid malignant tumors occurring after bone marrow transplantation for severe aplastic anemia given thoraco-abdominal irradiation. Radiother Oncol 30: 55, 1994.
16. Kolb HJ, Duell T, Socie G, et al. New malignancies in patients surviving more than 5 years after marrow transplantation (abstr.) Blood 86: 460a, 1996.

17. Neglia JP, Meadows AT, Robison LL, et al. Second neoplasms after acute lymphoblastic leukemia in childhood. N Engl J Med 325: 1330, 1991.
18. Penn I. Cancers of the anogenital region in renal transplant patients. Cancer 58: 611, 1986.
19. Couetil J-P, McGoldrick JP, Wallwork J, English TAH. Malignant tumors after heart transplantation. J Heart Transplant 9: 622, 1990.
20. Curtis RE, Hankey BF, Myers MH, Young JL Jr. Risk of leukemia associated with the first course of cancer treatment: an analysis of the surveillance, epidemiology, and end results program experience. J Natl Cancer Inst 72: 531, 1984.
21. Kaldor JM, Day NE, Clarke EA, et al. Leukemia following Hodgkin's disease. N Engl J Med 322: 7, 1990.
22. Tura S, Fiacchini M, Zinzani PL, et al. Splenectomy and the increasing risk of secondary acute leukemia in Hodgkin's disease. J Clin Oncol 11: 925, 1993.
23. Demeter J, Lehoczky D. Splenectomy and the risk of developing leukemia (letter). J Clin Oncol 11: 375, 1993.
24. Longmore G, Guinan EC, Weinstein HJ, et al. Bone marrow transplantation for myelodysplasia and secondary acute nonlymphoblastic leukemia. J Clin Oncol 8: 1707, 1990.

# SECTION V

# ADVANCES IN CANCER CHEMO-PREVENTION

*"Four steps to achievement: plan purposefully, prepare prayerfully, proceed positively, pursue persistently."*
William A. Ward

C.J. Rosenthal and M. Rotman (Eds.), *Infusion Chemotherapy–Irradiation Interactions*

# CHAPTER 35

# Chemoprevention of lung cancer

BONNIE S. GLISSON, FADLO R. KHURI, JONATHAN M. KURIE,
SCOTT M. LIPPMAN and WAUN K. HONG

*Department of Thoracic/Head and Neck Medical Oncology, The University of Texas, M. D. Anderson Cancer
Center, 1515 Holcombe Blvd., Box 80, Houston, TX 77030, USA*

## 1. Introduction

Cancer occurring in the respiratory tract is a major public health problem throughout the
world, with more than 165 000 estimated attributable deaths from lung cancer in the United
States alone in 1997 [1]. Despite massive efforts to the contrary, 5-year survival rates and
presumed cure for patients with these cancers is currently 13%, a rate which has not improved significantly in more than three decades [2]. Further, successful control of early
stage disease with surgery is all too frequently only preamble to a second primary tumor
(SPT) arising in the carcinogen-damaged mucosa. Given the poor outcome of treatment for
advanced stage disease and the frequent incidence of SPTs in patients successfully treated
for early stage disease, much effort in the past 10–15 years has been targeted at prevention
of these highly morbid and mortal cancers. Chemoprevention, the use of chemical agents to
prevent cancer, has been the focus of much research originating in both the clinical and basic environments. These efforts have been facilitated by collaboration between investigators
in both arenas reflecting translational research at its best. Advances in knowledge of lung
cancer biology and of upper aerodigestive tract chemoprevention have supplied the foundation of current research.

## 2. Epidemiology

Studies conducted over the last four decades have convincingly demonstrated a causative
link between cigarette smoking and lung carcinoma [3]. Approximately 87% of lung carcinomas are attributable to tobacco exposure, and the relative risk for lung carcinoma in current smokers is as much as 20-fold greater than for those who have never smoked [3]. Lung
carcinoma risk in all cohorts of former smokers, although lower than for current smokers,
remains greater than for never smokers, even for those former smokers who quit in their
thirties [3].

The close correlation between smoking and lung cancer has led the National Cancer Institute's Division of Cancer Prevention and Control to make prevention of smoking and
smoking cessation the primary strategies in the control of lung cancer. Public education regarding the hazards of cigarette smoking has resulted in a substantial reduction in the percentage of adults who smoke in the United States [4]. Since 1965, when the first National

Health Interview Survey (NHIS) was initiated, there has been a 77% decrease in the number of people who smoke. The most recent data available (from 1991) revealed that 43.5 million adults in the United States are former smokers and that, among those in the current US population who ever smoked, 48.5% are now former smokers.

It is notable that former smokers remain at significantly enhanced risk for developing lung cancer, and they account for a rising percentage of lung cancer cases in the United States. Analysis of data from both M.D. Anderson Cancer Center and Harvard University-affiliated hospitals demonstrated that more than 50% of lung cancer cases occur in former smokers [5]. Thus, the risk of lung cancer among former smokers poses an increasing public health problem in the United States, one that is likely to persist for many years to come.

Although an association between cigarette smoke and lung cancer has been observed since the late 1940s [6], it was not until 1950 that a causal relationship was determined by two well designed epidemiological studies, one from the United States [7] and one from Great Britain [8]. These population-based findings were buttressed by the work of Auerbach et al. whose pathologic evaluation of the tracheobronchial trees of chronic smokers who died of lung cancer represents the seminal work in the biology of lung cancer [9,10]. This research, while identifying diffuse epithelial damage, was most important for the finding of carcinoma in situ in 15% of the tissue sections from patients dying from lung cancer. Further, this lesion was strongly associated with smoking for which a dose-response effect was documented.

## 3. Tobacco-related carcinogenesis and field effect

The findings of Auerbach et al. are clearly analogous to the work by Slaughter who had previously defined the theory of "field cancerization" based on his study of patients with oral cavity squamous cell cancer [11]. More recently, the tools of molecular biology have been applied and provide even more support for the concept of field carcinogenesis related to tobacco exposure. A spectrum of genetic abnormalities commonly found in lung cancer specimens, such as allelic deletion of 3p, 9p, and 17p and mutations of the tumor suppressor gene *p53* have now also been identified in premalignant lesions of the tracheobronchial epithelium in patients with lung cancer [12–15]. Perhaps, more significantly, many of these genetic abnormalities can be found in the bronchial epithelium of smokers and former smokers who have no evidence of lung cancer [16]. It is of note that particular changes, such as loss of heterozygosity at 9p and 17p, appear to persist despite smoking cessation, perhaps reflecting permanent tobacco-related genetic damage. These findings underscore the potential impact of an effective chemopreventive intervention in former smokers.

The most direct evidence implicating tobacco in respiratory carcinogenesis comes from the work of Denissenko et al. who demonstrated that treatment of HeLa cells and bronchial epithelial cells with benzo[*a*]pyrene diol epoxide, a carcinogen found in tobacco, resulted in DNA adducts which were non-randomly distributed on the exons of the *p53* gene at major mutational hot spots in lung cancer (codons 157, 248, and 273) [17]. This targeted adduct formation with a tobacco carcinogen strongly supports an etiologic role for smoking and the development of lung cancer.

## 4. Retinoid biology and pharmacology

Epidemiological studies have demonstrated that vitamin A deficiency is associated with an increased incidence of lung cancer in humans [18]. Vitamin A deficiency also induces squamous metaplasia in the mucosa of the upper aerodigestive tract [19] that is similar to the premalignant changes in this mucosa that are found in heavy smokers [20]. Dietary vitamin A supplementation reversed squamous metaplasia in the trachea of vitamin A deficient animals in vivo [21], and various retinoids exhibited a similar activity in vitro [22].

Vitamin A derivatives, or retinoids, are a family of compounds that have complex biologic effects, including the modulation of differentiation, proliferation, and apoptosis within both normal and neoplastic tissues. The complexity of their function affects not only the diversity of the retinoid ligands but also the diversity of the nuclear retinoid receptors that mediate their activity. Retinoids bind and activate retinoid receptors to function as transcription factors. These receptors are expressed at varying levels in different cell types and thus this differential expression ultimately affects downstream gene expression.

There are two classes of nuclear retinoid receptors: the retinoic acid receptors (RARs) and the retinoid x receptors (RXRs). There are three subclasses: $\alpha$, $\beta$, and $\gamma$, with each divided further into a large number of isoforms produced through differential promoter usage and alternative splicing of receptor transcripts [23,24]. Specific isoforms of RARs and RXRs appear to have different functions, activating different downstream target genes. RXRs form homodimers and heterodimers with RARs or a host of other receptors such as those for vitamin D and thyroid hormones and a variety of orphan receptors [23]. Because RXR is a ligand binding partner in combination with orphan receptors, RXR ligands appear to be more versatile than RAR ligands in the activation of retinoid and other pathways.

Natural retinoids, including all-*trans*, 13-*cis*, and 9-*cis* retinoic acid, exist as stereoisomers, spontaneously interconverting in the intracellular space. For that reason, treatment with these retinoids non-selectively activates RARs and RXRs. In contrast, synthetic retinoids are being developed that are capable of binding specifically to individual nuclear retinoid receptors, thus allowing a degree of selectivity in the enhancement of the desired effects of certain retinoids and the reduction of the undesired effects. For example, a retinoid specific only for RAR-$\beta$ may avoid inducing dermatologic side effects that have been caused by activation of RAR-$\gamma$. The goal is to enhance the potential therapeutic effects of specific retinoids while limiting the toxicity caused by the widely used natural retinoids [25].

It is thought that retinoid receptors affect gene transcription either directly or indirectly. This phenomenon is illustrated by the receptor interaction with activator protein-1 (AP-1), an important regulator of cellular proliferation and inflammation. The mechanism of this interaction was recently elucidated by Kamei et al. [26], who demonstrated that retinoid-mediated inhibition of AP-1 activity appears to be the result of competition between nuclear retinoid receptors and AP-1 for binding to a transcriptional co-activator. This co-activator is found in limited quantities in the cell and is thus the rate limiting step for both the retinoid receptors and AP-1. Synthetic retinoids have been developed that selectively inhibit AP-1 without activating nuclear receptors. These AP-1 selective synthetic retinoids have been found to be potent antiproliferative agents in a number of tumor-derived cell lines [27–29] and are capable of reversing the squamous differentiation of bronchial epithelial cells [30]. Their toxicity profile may be favorable as retinoid toxicity has been linked to retinoid receptor activation.

Further work in the area of retinoid biology and pharmacology has focused on the study of retinoid resistance. Clinical de novo retinoid resistance occurs in 40% of oral premalignant lesions and appears to develop over time in many lesions that had previously responded to retinoid treatment [25]. The mechanisms that underlie retinoid resistance are not yet well defined. However, the frequency with which clinical resistance is encountered has resulted in evaluation of novel retinoids such as 4-*N*-(hydroxyphenyl) retinamide (4-HPR) which does not appear to bind any of the retinoid receptors but is a potent in vitro inducer of apoptosis [25,31]. Retinoids also appear to have potent effects when combined with other cytotoxic or cytostatic agents. Shalinsky et al. [32] demonstrated that 9-cRA combined with cisplatin in human oral squamous carcinoma xenografts in nude mice shows enhanced anti-tumor efficacy bordering on synergism.

Thus, retinoids alone or in combination with other cytotoxic [32] or biologic [33,34] agents have the intriguing potential to reverse preneoplastic lesions. The preclinical demonstration of efficacy as well as the extensive epidemiologic data previously cited has led to integration of retinoids into clinical chemoprevention trials in upper aerodigestive tract cancers as well as lung cancer.

## 5.  Chemoprevention trials

The ability of vitamin A derivatives to reverse premalignant lesions of the upper aerodigestive tract and to prevent SPTs in patients with an index squamous cancer of the head and neck forms much of the basis for investigation of these same approaches in patients at risk for and/or diagnosed previously with lung cancer.

### 5.1.  Reversal of premalignancy

One of the major difficulties in studies attempting to reverse premalignancy has been the absence of consensus regarding the definition of premalignancy in the bronchial epithelium. Investigators have used both cytologic changes in sputum and histologic changes in bronchial biopsies, from metaplasia to dysplasia, as markers of risk. Reversal of these changes to normal has been regarded as a potential intermediate endpoint for prevention of cancer.

In general, studies focused on sputum analysis from chronic smokers have shown wide spontaneous variation in the degree of atypia over time and no consistent effect from retinoids [35–37]. In an effort to develop a more dependable, semi-quantitative assay, Mathe et al. described the metaplasia index (MI) to quanititate the degree of squamous metaplasia in bronchial biopsies from six specific anatomic sites [38]. The MI was defined as the number of samples with metaplasia divided by the total number of samples analyzed, multiplied by 100. MIs were documented pre- and post-treatment in a single arm trial of smokers receiving etretinate 25 mg/day for 6 months [38]. This trial did demonstrate a decrease in the MI following etretinate therapy. These findings, however, are overshadowed by those of Lee et al. [39]. In this trial 93 smokers with metaplasia or dysplasia, quantitated at baseline using the MI, were randomized to 13-*cis* retinoic acid (13cRA) or placebo for 6 months. Post-treatment biopsies demonstrated a similar rate of decrease in the MI in both arms, most strongly associated with smoking cessation, calling the findings of Mathe et al. into question. Clearly, future trials of this sort should be placebo-controlled to correct for variables such as smoking cessation, sampling differences and spontaneous regression.

## 5.2.   Primary prevention

Based on epidemiologic data which indicated an inverse correlation between cancer risk and dietary $\beta$-carotene and serum retinol levels, $\beta$-carotene has been the major agent studied in primary prevention of lung cancer [40]. Three large primary prevention trials using $\beta$-carotene with or without $\alpha$-tocopherol or retinol have been completed and two of the three trials have documented an increased incidence of lung cancer in the treatment arms with $\beta$-carotene.

The Finnish ATBC trial randomized 29 133 male smokers aged 50–69 years old to one of four regimens, using a $2 \times 2$ factorial design. The regimens were $\alpha$-tocopherol (50 mg/day) alone, $\beta$-carotene (20 mg/day) alone, both agents, or placebo [41]. The participants in the ATBC trial continued this intervention for 5–8 years. Over the course of the study, 876 new cases of lung cancer were diagnosed. Patients receiving $\beta$-carotene had an 18% increased incidence of lung cancer and an 8% increased mortality rate. $\alpha$-Tocopherol administration failed to significantly alter either lung cancer incidence or overall mortality. Subsequent analysis of these data demonstrated a trend to increased risk for $\beta$-carotene treatment in heavy smokers ($\geq 1$ pack/day) and in those who had high ethanol intake ($>11$ g/day) [42].

Accrual to a second primary prevention trial performed in the US was stopped early due to similar findings. The CARET study randomized a total of 18 314 smokers, former smokers, and people with a history of asbestos exposure to a combination of $\beta$-carotene (30 mg/day) and retinol (25 000 IU/day) in the form of retinyl palmitate or placebo in a double-blind trial [43]. After a mean followup of 4 years accrual was suspended due to a relative risk of lung cancer and death from lung cancer in the treatment arm of 1.28 and 1.46, respectively. Similar to the ATBC trial, there was association of excess lung cancer incidence with current smoking and the highest quartile of ethanol intake [43].

A third trial of US male physicians, of whom only 11% were current smokers, randomized 22 071 participants to $\beta$-carotene (50 mg qod) or placebo [44]. Neither benefit nor harm was demonstrated from the intervention in terms of the incidence of malignant neoplasms, cardiovascular disease, or death from all causes.

The mechanism of enhancement of lung carcinogenesis by supplemental $\beta$-carotene (alone or in combination with retinol) in smokers has yet to be defined. The most plausible theory at this time implicates a potential pro-oxidant effect of $\beta$-carotene in the damaged lungs of individuals who continue to smoke heavily [45]. In light of the data from the CARET and ATBC trials, current smokers should not use $\beta$-carotene supplements. These results also emphasize that randomized clinical trials of high-risk patients should be the only setting for high-dose supplementation with compounds of unproven clinical efficacy.

## 5.3.   Prevention of second primary tumors

Three randomized trials designed to reduce the incidence of SPTs in patients with an index cancer of the head and neck or lung have now been completed. Two of these three trial have demonstrated an impact on tobacco-related cancer with retinoid treatment.

In a seminal study by Hong et al., 103 patients with a prior diagnosis of squamous cell cancer of the head and neck were randomized patients to receive either high dose 13cRA (50–100 mg/m$^2$ per day) or placebo for 1 year [46]. Although originally conceived as an adjuvant trial, this study did not demonstrate any impact of treatment on the locoregional recurrence or metastatic disease. However, with a median followup period of 32 months, second primary tumors developed in only 2 (4%) of the treated patients as opposed to 12 (24%) of patients receiving placebo. Of particular note, 93% (13 of 14) of the second primary tumors observed were in the carcinogen-exposed field of the upper aerodigestive tract, lungs, and esophagus. Recent reanalysis of this trial at a median followup of 4.5 years indicated most striking results for the impact of 13cRA treatment on tumors in the "condemned mucosa" with 3 versus 13 SPTs in the retinoid and placebo arms, respectively [47]. This effect of 13cRA persisted for approximately 3 years, after which time the incidence of SPT equalized in both arms. These promising results are offset somewhat by the significant mucocutaneous toxicity associated with 13cRA such that one-third of patients required significant dose reduction during 1 year of therapy.

A second trial by Bolla et al. randomized 316 patients with a prior squamous cell cancer of the oral cavity or oropharynx to etretinate (50 mg/day for 1 month, followed by 25 mg/day for 2 years) or placebo [48]. After a median followup of 41 months, no treatment effect was observed either in incidence of SPTs or recurrent disease. The results of this trial were notable for the high rate of SPTs (24% of patients), 79% of which were clearly tobacco-related.

In the only completed study of patients with an index diagnosis of lung cancer, Pastorino et al. randomized 307 patients who had been surgically cured of stage I non-small cell lung cancer to receive either retinyl palmitate (300 000 IU/day for 1 year) or placebo [49]. The retinyl palmitate treatment was associated with an overall reduction in second primary tumors, 18 versus 29 SPTs in the retinyl palmitate and placebo arms, respectively. Considering only tobacco-related tumors, rates were 13 versus 25 SPTs/arm. In contrast to 13cRA, the retinyl palmitate was well-tolerated with compliance during 1 year of treatment exceeding 80%.

Building on the results of these two positive trials, current trials include an NCI- (US) sponsored phase III trial of low dose 13cRA (30 mg/day for 3 years) versus placebo in patients who have undergone curative resection for stage I non-small cell lung cancer. Patients will be followed for 4 years following treatment to assess reduction in SPT incidence. Similarly, the Euroscan study is evaluating the efficacy of retinyl palmitate (300 000 IU/day) and the antioxidant $N$-acetylcysteine (600 mg/day), in the prevention of second primary tumors following the definitive therapy of early stage squamous cell carcinoma of the head and neck or fully resected stage I, II, or IIIA (T3N0 only) non-small lung cancer. This study has a $2 \times 2$ factorial design in which study participants receive either retinyl palmitate or $N$-acetylcysteine alone, both drugs, or placebo for 2 years and then have 4 years of followup.

## 6. Future directions

While the data from these ongoing phase III trials is anxiously awaited, it is clear that clinical chemoprevention research would be significantly advanced by the development of intermediate endpoints as surrogates for cancer incidence. Time, cost, and lives lost to cancer could conceivably all be reduced if studies such as these could be interpreted more quickly. However, discovery and validation of an intermediate marker will require a more precise molecular model of lung carcinogenesis than currently exists. Studies in progress evaluating markers of retinoid-responsiveness, such as RAR-$\beta$, genetic markers such as deletions of 3p, 9p, and 17p, and mutations of tumor suppressor genes such as $Rb$ and $p53$ will hopefully shed light on the complex multistep process that precedes frank lung cancer. These data can then be applied in clinical trials of promising chemopreventive agents to quicken the pace of progress and reduce death from the tobacco pandemic.

## Summary

A growing body of molecular biologic and epidemiologic evidence now complements the previous population-based information linking tobacco smoke causally with the development of lung cancer. Although current smokers clearly have the highest risk, former smokers, who represent a growing segment of the population, remain at increased risk for lung cancer, many for their lifetime. Further epidemiologic data suggests that retinoids and carotenoids are effective dietary inhibitors of carcinogenesis. Clinical trials of retinoids as chemopreventive agents in the aerodigestive tract for the reversal of premalignancy and prevention of second primary tumors have yielded promising results. However, clinical trials of high dose $\beta$-carotene in the primary prevention of cancer in active smokers have introduced a cautionary note for the direct application of diet-based epidemiologic data in clinical trials with pharmacologic doses of single nutrients. Further studies of retinoid biology and aerodigestive tract carcinogenesis are necessary to increase the selectivity and effectiveness of chemopreventive interventions.

## References

1. Parker SL, Tong T, Bolden S, et al. Cancer statistics, 1996. CA: Cancer J Clin 46: 5, 1996.
2. Ginsberg RJ, Kris MG, Armstrong JG. Cancer of the lung. In: DeVita VT, Hellman S, Rosenberg SA (Eds), Cancer: Principals and Practice of Oncology, 4th edn. Philadelphia, PA: Lippincott, p. 673, 1994.
3. Shopland DR, Eyre HJ, Pechacek TF. Smoking attributable cancer mortality in 1991: is lung cancer now the leading cause of death among smokers in the United States? J Natl Cancer Inst 83: 1142, 1991.
4. Office of Smoking and Health, U.S. Centers for Disease Control. Morbid Mortal Weekly Rep 43: 50, 1994.
5. Kurie JM, Spitz MR, Hong WK. Lung cancer chemoprevention: targeting former rather than current smokers. Cancer Prev Int 2: 55, 1995.
6. Ochsner A, DeBakey M. Carcinoma of the lung. Arch Surg 42: 209, 1941.
7. Wynder EL, Graham EA. Tobacco smoking as a possible etiologic factor in bronchogenic carcinoma: a study of six hundred and eighty four proved cases. J Am Med Assoc 143: 329, 1950.
8. Doll R, Hill AB. Smoking and carcinoma of the lung: preliminary report. Br Med J 2: 739, 1950.
9. Auerbach O, Gere JB, Forman JB, et al. Changes in bronchial epithelium in relation to smoking and cancer of the lungs a report of progress. N Engl J Med 256: 97, 1957.
10. Auerbach O, Stout AP, Hammond EC, et al. Changes in bronchial epithelium in relation to cigarette smoking and in relation to lung cancer. N Engl J Med 265: 253, 1961.
11. Slaughter DP, Southwick HW, Smejkal W. "Field cancerization" in oral stratified squamous epithelium: clinical implications of multicentric origin. Cancer 6: 963, 1953.
12. Hung J, Kishimoto Y, Sugio K, et al. Allele-specific chromosome 3p deletions occur at an early stage in the pathogenesis of lung cancer. J Am Med Assoc 273: 558, 1995.
13. Kishimoto Y, Sugio K, Hung JY, et al. Allele-specific loss in chromosome 9p loci in preneoplastic lesions accompanying non-small cell lung cancers. J Natl Cancer Inst 87: 1224, 1995.
14. Sozzi G, Miozzo M, Donghi R, et al. Deletions of 17p and p53 mutations in preneoplastic lesions of the lung. Cancer Res 52: 6079, 1992.
15. Mao L, Hruban RH, Boyle JO, et al. Detection of oncogene mutations in sputum precedes diagnosis of lung cancer. Cancer Res 54: 1634, 1994.

16.    Mao L, Lee JS, Kurie JM, et al. Clonal genetic alterations in the lungs of current and former smokers. J Natl Cancer Inst 89: 857, 1997.

17.    Denissenko MF, Pao A, Tung M, et al. Preferential formation of benzo [a] pyrene adducts at lung cancer mutational hotspots in p53. Science 274: 430, 1996.

18.    Hong WK, Itri LM. Retinoids and human cancers. In: Sporn MB, Roberts AB, Goodman DS (Eds), The Retinoids, New York: Raven Press, p. 597, 1994.

19.    Wolbach SB, Howe PR. Tissue changes following deprivation of fat-soluble A vitamin. J Exp Med 62: 753, 1925.

20.    Auerbach O, Hammond EC, Garfinkel L. Changes in bronchial epithelium in relation to cigarette smoking, 1955–1960 vs 1970–1977. N Engl J Med 300: 381, 1979.

21.    Wolbach SB. Effects of vitamin A deficiency and hypervitaminosis in animals. In: Sebrell, WH, Harris RS (Eds), The Vitamins, Vol. 1. New York: Academic Press, p. 106, 1956.

22.    Sporn MB, Newton DL. Chemoprevention of cancers with retinoids. Fed Proc 38: 2528, 1979.

23.    Mangelsdorf DJ, Umesono K, Evans RM. The retinoid receptors. In: Sporn MB, Roberts AB, Goodman DS (Eds), The Retinoids. New York: Raven Press, p. 319, 1994.

24.    Chambon P. The retinoid signaling pathway: molecular and genetic analyses. Semin Cell Biol 5: 115, 1994.

25.    Mayne ST, Lippman SM. Retinoids and carotenoids. In: DeVita VT, Hellman S, Rosenberg SA (Eds), Cancer: Principles and Practice of Oncology, 5th edn. Philadelphia, PA: Lippincott, 1997, in press.

26.    Fanjul A, Dawson MI, Hobbs PD, et al. A new class of retinoids with selective inhibition of AP-1 inhibits proliferation. Nature 372: 107–111, 1994.

27.    Li JJ, Dong Z, Dawson MI, Colbum NIL. Inhibition of tumor promoter-induced transformation by retinoids that transrepress AP-1 without transactivating retinoic acid response element. Cancer Res 56: 483–489, 1996.

28.    Angel P, Karin M. The role of Jun, Fos and the AP-1 complex in cell-proliferation and transformation. Biochim Biophys Acta 1072: 129–157, 1991.

29.    Kamei Y, Xu I, Heinzel T, et al. A CBP integrator complex mediates transcriptional activation and AP-1 inhibition by nuclear receptors. Cell 85: 403–414, 1996.

30.    Lee HY, Dawson MI, Walsh GL, et al. Retinoic acid receptor- and retinoid x receptor-selective retinoids activate signaling pathways that converge on AP-1 and inhibit squamous differentiation in human bronchial epithelial cells. Cell Growth Dev 7: 997–1004, 1996.

31.    Oridale N, Lotan D, Xu XC, et al. Differential induction of apoptosis by all-*trans*-retinoic acid and *N*-(4-hydroxyphenyl) retinamide in human head and neck squamous cell carcinoma cell lines. Clin Cancer Res 2: 855–863, 1996.

32.    Shalinsky DR, Bischoff ED, Gregory ML, et al. Enhanced antitumor efficacy of cisplatin in combination with ALRT 1057 (9-*cis* retinoic acid) in human oral squamous carcinoma xenografts in nude mice. Clin Cancer Res 2: 511–520, 1996.

33.    Lippman SM, Parkinson DR, Itri LM, et al. 13-cis-retinoic acid and interferon alpha-2a: effective combination therapy for advanced squamous cell carcinoma of the skin. J Natl Cancer Inst 84: 235–241, 1992.

34.    Lippman SM, Kavanagh JJ, Paredes-Espinoza M, et al. 13-cis-retinoic acid plus interferon alpha-2a: highly active systemic therapy for squamous cell carcinoma of the cervix. J Natl Cancer Inst 84: 241–245, 1992.

35.    Saccomanno G, Moran PG, Schmidt RD, et al. Effect of 13-cis-retinoic acid on premalignant and malignant cells of lung origin. Acta Cytol 26: 78–85, 1982.

36.    Heimburger DC, Alexander CB, Burch R, et al. Improvement in bronchial squamous metaplasia in smokers treated with folate and vitamin B12. Report of a preliminary randomized, double-blind intervention trial. J Am Med Assoc 259: 1525, 1988.

37.    Heimburger DC, Krumdieck CL, Alexander CB, et al. Localized folic acid deficiency and bronchial metaplasia in smokers: hypothesis and preliminary report. Nutr Int 2: 54, 1987.

38.    Mathe G, Gouveia J, Hercend TM, et al. Correlation between precancerous bronchial metaplasia and cigarette consumption, and preliminary results of retinoid treatment. Cancer Detect Prev 5: 461–466, 1982.

39.    Lee JS, Lippman SM, Benner SE, et al. Randomized placebo controlled trial of isotretinoin in chemoprevention of bronchial squamous metaplasia. J Clin Oncol 12: 937, 1994.

40.    Peto R, Doll R, Buckley JD, Sporn MB. Can dietary $\beta$-carotene materially reduce human cancer rates? Nature 290: 201–208, 1981.

41.  The effect of vitamin E and beta carotene on the incidence of lung cancer and other cancers in male smok-
     ers. The Alpha-Tocopherol, Beta Carotene Cancer Prevention Study Group. [See comment citation in
     Medline]. N Engl J Med 330: 1029, 1994.
42.  Albanes D, Heinonem OP, Taylor PR, et al. Alpha-tocopherol, beta carotene cancer prevention study:
     effects of baseline characteristics and study compliance. J Natl Cancer Inst 88: 1560, 1996.
43.  Omenn GS, Goodman GE, Thornquist MD, et al. Risk factors for lung cancer and for intervention effects in
     CARET, the Beta-Carotene and Retinol Efficacy Trial. J Natl Cancer Inst 88: 1500–1509, 1996.
44.  Hennekans CH, Buring JE, Manson JE, et al. Lack of long-term supplementation with Beta-Carotene on
     the incidence of malignant neoplasms and cardiovascular disease. New Engl J Med 334: 1145, 1996.
45.  Mayne ST, Handleman GJ, Beecher G. $\beta$-Carotene and lung cancer promotion in heavy smokers a plausi-
     ble relationship. J Natl Cancer Inst 88: 1513, 1996.
46.  Hong WK, Lippman SM, Itri LM, et al. Prevention of second primary tumors with isotretinoin in
     squamous-cell carcinoma of the head and neck. N Engl J Med 323: 795–801, 1990.
47.  Benner SR, Pajak TF, Lippman SM, et al. Prevention of second primary tumors with isotretinoin in patients
     with squamous cell carcinoma of the head and neck: long-term followup. J Natl Cancer Inst 86: 140–141,
     1994.
48.  Bolla M, Lofur R, Ton Van K, et al. Prevention of second primary tumors with etretinate in squamous cell
     carcinoma of the oral cavity and oropharynx. Results of a multicentric double-blinded randomised study.
     Eur J Cancer 30A: 767–772, 1994.
49.  Pastorino U, Infante M, Maioli M, et al. Adjuvant treatment of stage I lung cancer with high-dose vitamin
     A. J Clin Oncol 11: 1216–1222, 1993.

C.J. Rosenthal and M. Rotman (Eds.), *Infusion Chemotherapy–Irradiation Interactions*
© 1998 Elsevier Science B.V. All rights reserved

# CHAPTER 36

# Testing the worth of antiestrogens to prevent breast cancer

MONICA MORROW and V. CRAIG JORDAN

*Department of Surgery and the Robert H. Lurie Cancer Center,*
*Northwestern University Medical School, Chicago, IL 60611, USA*

## 1. Introduction

Twenty years ago tamoxifen was shown to prevent the induction [1,2] and promotion [3] of carcinogen-induced mammary cancer in rats. Similarly tamoxifen prevents the development of mammary cancer induced by ionizing radiation in rats [4]. These laboratory observation, coupled with the emerging preliminary clinical observation that adjuvant tamoxifen would prevent contralateral breast cancer in women [5], provided a rationale for Dr. Trevor Powles at the Royal Marsden Hospital in England to establish a vangard study to test whether tamoxifen could prevent breast cancer in high risk women [6]. It is now clear from the Overview Analysis that tamoxifen reduces contralateral breast cancer by 38% [7] in women who have had unilateral breast carcinoma. This chapter explores the progress that has been achieved in the last decade to answer the question "Does tamoxifen have worth in the prevention of breast cancer in selected high risk women?" This question can only be answered by carefully organized double-blind placebo-controlled clinical trials. The design and preliminary results of the three international trials that are currently being conducted – the Royal Marsden Study, the NSABP/NCI study, and an Italian study – are described.

## 2. Royal Marsden Study

Powles and co-workers have completed recruitment to a pilot randomized placebo controlled trial using tamoxifen 20 mg daily for up to 8 years in healthy women at increased risk of developing breast cancer. The trial was undertaken to evaluate the problems of accrual, acute symptomatic toxicity, compliance, and safety as a basis for subsequent large national multicenter trials designed to test whether tamoxifen can prevent breast cancer.

From October 1986 until June 1993, 2012 healthy women with an increased risk of developing breast cancer were recruited [8]. Healthy women aged 30–70 years were eligible provided they had a family history of breast cancer on their maternal side with at least one first degree relative (sister, mother, daughter) who had developed breast cancer under the age of 45 years, or had developed bilateral breast cancer, or with a first degree relative, as well as at least one other maternal relative. Women with two affected first degree relatives of any age were also eligible, as were women with a first degree relative and a history of previous biopsy for benign breast disease. Women with a past history of venous thrombosis, any previous malignancy, or a estimated life expectancy of less than 10 years were excluded.

Acute symptomatic toxicity was low for participants on tamoxifen or placebo, and compliance remained correspondingly high: 77% of women on tamoxifen and 82% of women on placebo remained on medication at 5 years, as predicted. Patients on tamoxifen had a significant increase in hot flashes (34 versus 20%), primarily in premenopausal women ($P < 0.005$), vaginal discharge (16 versus 4%, $P < 0.005$), and menstrual irregularities (14 versus 9%, $P < 0.005$), compared to those on placebo. Until their report in 1994 [13], the Marsden group had no thromboembolic episodes; a detailed analysis of other coagulation parameters in a sequential subset of women also found no significant changes in Protein S, Protein C, or cross-linked fibrinogen degradation products.

A number of other effects were observed in women on tamoxifen. A significant fall in total plasma cholesterol occurred within 3 months of beginning therapy and was sustained over 5 years of treatment [9–11] in postmenopausal women. The decrease affects low density lipoprotein, with no change in apolipoproteins A and B or high density lipoprotein cholesterol. In addition, tamoxifen produced variable effects on bone density, depending on menopausal status. In premenopausal women early results demonstrate a small but significant ($P < 0.05$) loss of bone in both the lumbar spine and hip at 3 years [11]. It will be most important to evaluate the results at 5 and 8 years of therapy, as the current indications suggest bone stabilization rather than continued loss. In contrast, postmenopausal women have increased bone mineral density in the spine ($P < 0.005$) and hip ($P < 0.001$) compared to non-treated women.

Finally, the Marsden group has made an extensive study of gynecological complications associated with tamoxifen treatment in healthy women. Since ovarian and uterine assessment by transvaginal ultrasound became available some time after the start of the trial, many subjects did not have a baseline evaluation. Ovarian screening demonstrated a significantly increased risk ($P < 0.005$) of benign ovarian cysts in premenopausal women who had received tamoxifen for more than 3 months compared to controls. There were no changes in ovarian appearance in postmenopausal women [8].

A careful examination of the uterus with transvaginal ultrasonography using color Doppler imaging in women taking tamoxifen showed that the organ was usually larger and the endometrium was significantly thicker [12]. Of particular interest in this regard is the recent observation that tamoxifen, 20 mg daily, exerts a time-dependent proliferation of the endometrium in premenopausal and early postmenopausal women. This effect appears to be mediated by the stromal component, since no cases of cancer or even epithelial hyperplasia were observed among the tamoxifen treated group in a recent Italian study with 33 women [13].

Although the vangard study is providing invaluable information about the biological effects of tamoxifen in healthy women, the trial was not designed to answer the question of whether tamoxifen will prevent breast cancer. Larger national trials will provide this information. In the United Kingdom, an expanded study has started to enroll 20 000 women nationwide.

## 3. NSABP/NCI Study

This study opened in the US and Canada in May 1992, with an accrual goal of 16 000 women to be recruited throughout North America at 100 sites. The study design is illustrated in Fig. 1. Those eligible for entry include any woman over the age of 60, or women between the ages of 35 and 59 whose 5-year risk of developing breast cancer, as predicted

## Potential Participants

>60 years old - with/without risk factors
35-59 years old - with risk factors

• LCIS

• 1o relative with breast cancer

• Breast biopsies

• atypical hyperplasia

• Over 25 years old before
  birth of first child

• no children

• menarche before age 12

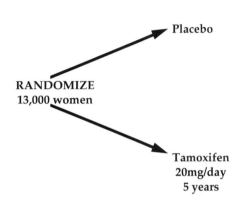

Fig. 1. The entry requirements and study design of the NSABP trial to test the worth of tamoxifen as a preventive for breast cancer. The study will only recruit 13 000 volunteers as the RR is calculated to be higher than originally anticipated.

by the Gail model [14] equals that of a 60-year-old women. Additionally, any woman over age 35 with a diagnosis of lobular carcinoma in situ (LCIS) treated by biopsy alone is eligible for entry to the study. In the absence of LCIS, the risk factors necessary to enter the study vary with age, such that a 35-year-old woman must have a relative risk (RR) of 5.07, whereas at 45 the RR must be 1.79. Although recruitment to the study has been slow, more than 10 000 women have already been processed and randomized to the study. Health care evaluations are extremely rigorous and, most importantly, all women will have routine endometrial biopsies to evaluate the role of tamoxifen in the detection of pre-existing endometrial conditions.

The breast cancer risk of the women already enrolled in the study is extremely high, with no age group, including those over 60, with a relative risk of less than 4. Recruitment is also balanced, with about one-third of the participants younger than 50 years of age, one third between 50 and 60 years old, and one-third older than 60 years of age. A full evaluation of lipid and cholesterol profiles is being made, as well as bone density determinations in select groups. Most importantly, the study will provide the first information about the role of genetic markers in the etiology of breast cancer and will determine whether tamoxifen can have a role to play in the treatment of women who are found to carry somatic mutations in the BRCA1 gene. The initial results from this study should be available by the turn of the century.

### 4. Italian Study

This study is recruiting 20 000 normal women over the age of 45 to be randomized to 20 mg tamoxifen daily or a placebo for 5 years. Only hysterectomized women are admitted to the trial to avoid issues of pregnancy and endometrial pathologies. To date, more than 4000 women have been randomized in Italy, and the trial is being opened to other Europe nations.

## 5. Toxicological concerns

### 5.1. Liver

Tamoxifen at high doses given for prolonged periods, has been shown to produce liver tumors in rats. Such tumors have not been noted in other species and there is no evidence that tamoxifen can cause liver tumors in women. Although millions of women have been exposed to tamoxifen treatment for long periods, only a few (approximately three) liver tumors have been noted worldwide. Since hepatocellular carcinoma is a rare tumor in the Western world (5 per 100 000), any new potentially causative agent like tamoxifen would be quickly implicated by an increase in national statistics. This has not occurred; nevertheless, the issue of the relevance of rat studies for the risks of human liver carcinogenesis has been extensively reviewed [15,16]. It is now clear that the effects of tamoxifen in the liver are unique to the rat. It is also clear that if today's concerns about tamoxifen and carcinogenesis had been expressed 20 years ago, tens of thousands of women would have died prematurely from breast cancer because tamoxifen specifically, and antiestrogens in general, would never have been developed [15]. Fortunately, this is not the case, and the successful re-evaluation of tamoxifen safety should reassure both breast cancer patients and healthy participants in new clinical prevention trials.

### 5.2. Endometrium

In the past decade there have been a number of reports regarding the interaction of tamoxifen with the female reproductive tract. While endometrial cancer has been the main focus, tamoxifen has also been associated with minor changes in gonadotrophin levels, amenorrhea and oligomenorrhea, ovarian hyperstimulation in premenopausal women occasionally leading to ovarian cysts, exacerbation or regression of endometriosis, promotion of the growth of uterine leiomyomas and endometrial polyps, and there are even isolated case reports of women who developed ovarian or fallopian tube tumors and had a history of tamoxifen intake [17]. In general, the gynecologic concerns are mainly anecdotal. Estrogenic effects of tamoxifen have been demonstrated in the vaginal epithelium and increased endometrial proliferation has been observed in about one third of treated postmenopausal women [17]. The major clinical problem, however, has been the inability to predict which women will respond to tamoxifen as an estrogen-like substance and which will not.

Since 1985, a number of reports linking tamoxifen to endometrial cancer have appeared in the world literature. Many of these are non-controlled case reports which were collected retrospectively. In addition, a number of double-blind randomized trials have documented an increased frequency of endometrial cancer in tamoxifen-treated patients. These trials, however, were not designed to specifically answer the question of an association between tamoxifen and endometrial cancer. A number of biases may thus confound the results of these studies [18]. In none of these trials did the patients have a baseline endometrial screening for any existing lesions before they started taking tamoxifen, nor were they ran-

Table 1

Detection and distribution of uterine malignancies in patients exposed to tamoxifen [18]

| | |
|---|---|
| Endometrial carcinomas | 349 |
| Mixed Müllerian tumors | 18 |
| Sarcomas | 9 |
| Patients | |
|   Postmenopausal | 200 |
|   Premenopausal | 2 |
| Duration of tamoxifen therapy | |
|   ≤2 years | 91 |
|   ≥2 years | 108 |

domized with respect to major risk factors for the development of endometrial cancer. The possibility cannot be excluded that a significant number of these women had an undetected endometrial malignancy prior to beginning tamoxifen therapy. In support of this notion are the findings of a large autopsy study that showed that the incidence of occult endometrial cancer was five times higher than the reported rate for the same geographical area during the same period of time [19].

We have previously reviewed the literature and found a total of only 349 endometrial carcinomas reported in tamoxifen-treated patients (Table 1) [17,18]. A number of sarcomas and mixed Mullerian tumors (MMT) have also been reported in association with tamoxifen treatment and are listed separately. Contrary to recent concerns expressed with regard to the potentially detrimental endometrial effects of tamoxifen in premenopausal women [20], the vast majority of the reported endometrial cancers have occurred in postmenopausal women. Although the duration of tamoxifen therapy is not reported for all cases, it appears that both short-term (≤2 years) and long term (>2 years) treatment is implicated in the higher frequency of endometrial tumors. The daily dose of tamoxifen administered to these patients varies among the different reports, with 20 mg as the prevailing dosage. Some investigators have suggested that doses higher than the current standard (20 mg/day) may lead to an increase in the detection of endometrial cancer, however, our database provides no clear-cut evidence of such a relationship.

Concern has been raised that tamoxifen may promote the development of a more aggressive form of endometrial cancer, primarily due to a case-control study from Yale that was published in the *Journal of Clinical Oncology* [21] in 1993. The authors conducted a retrospective search of the Yale/New Haven tumor registry for the decade 1980–1990. After screening 3457 records, they identified 53 breast cancer patients who later developed a uterine tumor. Fifteen of these patients had a history of 40 mg/day of tamoxifen intake for an average of 4.2 years. Ten of these tumors (67%) were of aggressive histologic type (high-grade endometrioid carcinoma, MMT, clear cell carcinoma, papillary serous carcinoma) and one-third of the patients died of endometrial cancer. The authors concluded that "…women receiving tamoxifen are at risk for high-grade endometrial cancers that have a poor prognosis…"

This report created a lot of concern among clinicians as it challenged the long-standing belief that endometrial tumors arising in tamoxifen-treated patients have a favorable outcome, as do endometrial tumors in patients with a history of estrogen replacement therapy (ERT).

Table 2

Distribution of the stage of endometrial cancer in the Yale study [21], a review of the international literature [18] and the SEER database [22]

|  | Yale (%) | Review (%) | Seer % |
|---|---|---|---|
| Stage 1 | 7/9 (78) | 184/234 (79) | 74 |
| Stage 2 | 2/9 (22) | 50/234 (21) | 26 |

To address this issue, we have gathered all the available published data on stage and grade of endometrial carcinomas occurring in tamoxifen-treated patients [18]. Stage is reported for 234 of these patients and grade is reported for 225 of them. In Table 2 we have compared the stage of endometrial tumors as reported in the Yale study [21] with the data from our literature review [18] as well as the SEER data [22]. There is general agreement that endometrial cancer detected in tamoxifen-treated women is typically confined to the uterus. Comparing the same three data sources, we have depicted the data on grade in Fig. 2. As the figure shows, there is significant discrepancy among the three data sources. Contrary to the Yale data, which showed a predominance of high-grade tumors, our review shows that, similar to the SEER data, endometrial cancer developing in patients treated with tamoxifen is of low (grade 1) or intermediate (grade 2) grade. Indeed, no other clinical study supports the Yale study.

The first large-scale prospective clinical trial that offered evidence of a possible association between tamoxifen and endometrial cancer was the Stockholm trial [23]. A total of 1846 patients were randomized to receive either 40 mg of tamoxifen or placebo for 2 years. Patients who were initially randomized to take tamoxifen for 2 years were offered the option to be re-randomized to receive tamoxifen for another 3 years, for a total of 5 years. Although tamoxifen proved beneficial in controlling second primary breast cancer, there was an increase in the incidence of endometrial cancer. Four years later, the same group published an update of their findings, containing the individual characteristics of all the patients

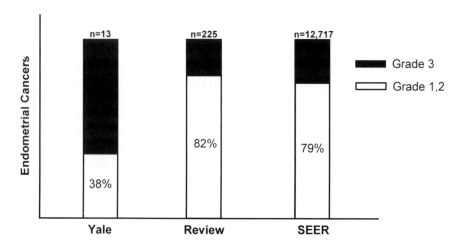

Fig. 2. A comparison of the grade of the patients in the Yale study compared with the distribution of grades found in the review conducted by Assikis et al. [18] and the national SEER data.

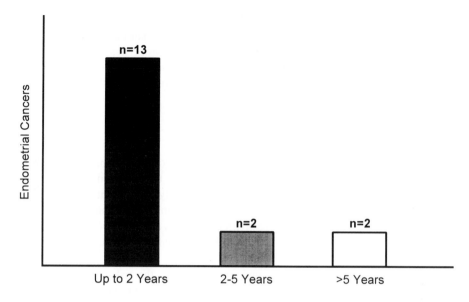

Fig. 3. A re-evaluation conducted by Jordan and Morrow [25] of the detection of endometrial cancer in the Stockholm trial [23,24].

afflicted with endometrial cancer [24]. Seventeen endometrial cancers were diagnosed in the tamoxifen-treated group and five in the control group. This increase was reported to be higher for the long-term tamoxifen therapy (>2 years) group than the short-term ($\leq$2 years) group and lead the authors to conclude that "...the cumulative frequency of endometrial cancer was significantly greater in patients who continued on tamoxifen than in those who stopped at 2 years". Interestingly, plotting the actual data (Fig. 3) leads to a conclusion different than the one reported by the Stockholm group. It is apparent from Fig. 3 that the majority of endometrial cancer cases (13/17) occurred in patients who had actually been treated with tamoxifen for 2 years or less [25].

The results of the NSABP B-14 trial [26] showed that although an increased incidence of endometrial carcinoma was observed, most tumors were of low grade and stage and the rate of detection of endometrial cancer was constant over time on the drug. Interestingly, there are clinical trials, concerning both short-term (Christie Hospital trial) and long-term therapy (Scottish trial), that have failed to detect an increase in the frequency of endometrial cancer in association with tamoxifen treatment [17]. With thousands of women having taken or currently receiving tamoxifen, there would have been an "epidemic" of endometrial malignancies by now should the effect of tamoxifen be as detrimental to the endometrium as some investigators have suggested [27]. Clearly, this is not the case. Based on the findings of the world's literature and those of randomized clinical trials, we believe that tamoxifen treatment confers a two- to three-fold increase in the detection of endometrial cancer [17,18, 25].

In the past decade a great number of investigators have looked into the association of tamoxifen with endometrial growth. Although the exact mechanisms by which tamoxifen exerts its growth-promoting effects in some patients and growth-inhibiting effects in others are yet to be identified, there is evidence of an association between tamoxifen therapy and an increase in the detection of endometrial malignancies. The existing findings point more towards a stimulation of an already initiated uncontrolled endometrial growth rather than a carcinogenic insult. In support of this notion is the fact that human uterine samples contain no [28] or barely detectable [29] DNA adducts. Estrogenic properties of the drug are believed to account for this growth-promoting effect on the uterus, but current evidence suggests that tamoxifen's effect on the uterine tissues is more complicated than those typically seen with ERT.

*5.3.  Conclusions about tamoxifen safety*

We have reviewed the world's literature and found that endometrial cancer detected in tamoxifen-treated women is not an aggressive malignancy but usually produces symptoms at early stages and can, therefore, be dealt with quite effectively. Taking into account the frequency of endometrial cancer reported in prospective trials, in conjunction with the findings of case-control studies, we conclude that tamoxifen produces a 2/1000 woman-years annual risk for endometrial cancer. The concern is mainly confined to post-menopausal women, and the dose of the drug does not seem to play a role.

Aggressive screening of tamoxifen-treated women carries the risk of identifying large numbers of patients with benign endometrial changes which do not require therapy and cannot be justified on the basis of cost-effectiveness. It is of utmost importance that physicians taking care of tamoxifen-treated women are well aware of these effects and do not consider stopping tamoxifen prematurely out of fear of an overestimated risk of secondary malignancies. The benefits of tamoxifen in the treatment of breast cancer far outweigh any adverse gynecological effects. It is imperative that patients with breast cancer are not denied the benefits of tamoxifen. The risk of dying from endometrial cancer is far less than the risk of dying from recurrence of breast cancer.

The World Health Organization, which lists tamoxifen as an essential medicine for the treatment of breast cancer, has recently evaluated the evidence for the carcinogenic potential of tamoxifen. They concluded that there is insufficient evidence to identify carcinogenic risks other than an elevation in the risk of detecting endometrial cancer. They also stated, however, that no woman should be denied tamoxifen treatment based on this risk because the clinical benefits with respect to treatment of breast cancer far outweigh any toxicological risks.

*6.  A new approach to prevention*

By the late 1980s, the information we had acquired about the potential beneficial effects of tamoxifen on bones and coronary heart disease could have heralded a new era for the prevention of pathologies associated with the menopause [30]. However, concerns about the increased risk of endometrial cancer have limited the enthusiasm for the widespread use of tamoxifen in healthy women. Hormone replacement therapy can dramatically reduce the risk of coronary heart disease and the development of osteoporosis, but the risks of developing breast cancer are unaltered, or, in some studies, very slightly increased.

We have proposed the development of the ideal antiestrogen that would be targeted to produce specific actions at different sites around a woman's body. The properties of the ideal agent are summarized in Fig. 4. Such an agent would have all the benefits of estrogen for the postmenopausal woman but with the added advantage of preventing breast and endometrial cancer [31].

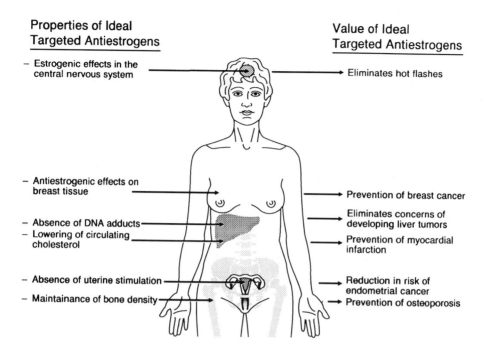

Properties of Ideal
Targeted Antiestrogens

– Estrogenic effects in the
  central nervous system

– Antiestrogenic effects on
  breast tissue

– Absence of DNA adducts
– Lowering of circulating
  cholesterol

– Absence of uterine stimulation
– Maintainance of bone density

Value of Ideal
Targeted Antiestrogens

Eliminates hot flashes

Prevention of breast cancer

Eliminates concerns of
developing liver tumors

Prevention of myocardial
infarction

Reduction in risk of
endometrial cancer
Prevention of osteoporosis

Fig. 4. The design of an ideal hormone replacement using the concept of a targeted antiestrogen. The primary goal is to prevent osteoporosis and coronary heart disease, but the inhibition of breast and endometrial cancer will be beneficial side effects.

At present, two compounds that might fit our criteria, raloxifene and droloxifene, are being tested clinically for the prevention of osteoporosis in older women. It is clear that future drug development in this area will result in appropriate new hormone replacement therapies that might also protect women from breast cancer. A single maintenance medicine for postmenopausal women to prevent osteoporosis and coronary heart disease might conceivably prevent breast and endometrial cancer as a beneficial side effect. There is no doubt that the development of tamoxifen over the past quarter of a century has revolutionized this strategy and the overall prospects for women's health care.

## Acknowledgements

This work was supported in part by Breast Cancer Program Development Grant R 21 CA 65734 and the Lynn Sage Breast Cancer Foundation of Northwestern Memorial Hospital, Chicago.

## References

1.  Jordan VC. Antitumour activity of the antioestrogen ICI 46,474 (tamoxifen) in the dimethylbenzanthracene (DMBA) induced rat mammary carcinoma model. J Steroid Biochem 5: 354, 1974.

2.  Jordan VC. Effect of tamoxifen (ICI 46,474) on initiation and growth of DMBA-induced rat mammary carcinomata. Eur J Cancer 12: 419–425, 1976.
3.  Jordan VC, Allen KE, Dix CJ. Pharmacology of tamoxifen in laboratory animals. Cancer Treatment Rep 64: 745–759, 1980.
4.  Welsch CW, Goodrich-Smith M, Brown CK, et al. Effect of an estrogen antagonist (tamoxifen) on the initiation and progression of gamma radiation - induced mammary tumors in female Sprague-Dawley rats. Eur J Cancer 17: 1255–1258, 1981.
5.  Cuzick J, Baum M. Tamoxifen and contralateral breast cancer. Lancet ii: 282, 1985.
6.  Powles TJ, Hardy JR, Ashley SE, et al. A pilot trial to evaluate the acute toxicity and feasibility of tamoxifen for prevention of breast cancer. Br J Cancer 60: 126–133, 1989.
7.  Early Breast Cancer Trialists' Collaborative Group. Systematic treatment of early breast cancer by hormonal, cytotoxic, or immune therapy: 133 randomized trials involving 31000 recurrences and 24000 deaths in 75000 women. Lancet 33: 1–15, 71–85, 1992.
8.  Powles TJ, Jones AL, Ashley SE, et al. The Royal Marsden Hospital pilot tamoxifen chemoprevention trial. Breast Cancer Res Treatment 31: 73–82, 1994.
9.  Jones AL, Powles TJ, Treleaven J, et al. Haemostatic changes and thromboembolic risk during tamoxifen therapy in normal women. Br J Cancer 66: 744–747, 1992.
10. Powles TJ, Tillyer CP, Jones AL, et al. Prevention of breast cancer with tamoxifen - an update on the Royal Marsden pilot program. Eur J Cancer 26: 680–684, 1990.
11. Powles TJ, Hickish T, Kanis JA, et al. Effect of tamoxifen on bone mineral density measured by dual-energy X ray absorptiometry in healthy premenopausal and postmenopausal women. J Clin Oncol 14: 78–84, 1996.
12. Kedar, RP, Bourne, TH, Powle TJ, et al. Effects of tamoxifen on uterus and ovaries of postmenopausal women in a randomized breast cancer prevention trial. Lancet 343: 1318–1321, 1994.
13. Decensi A, Fontant V, Bruno S, et al. Effect of tamoxifen on endometrial proliferation. J Clin Oncol 14: 434–440, 1996.
14. Gail MH, Binton LA, Byar DP, et al. Projecting individualized probabilities of developing breast cancer for white females who are being examined annually. J Natl Cancer Inst 81: 1879–1886, 1989.
15. Jordan VC. What if tamoxifen (ICI 46,474) had been found to produce liver tumors in rats in 1973? Ann Oncol 6: 29–34, 1995.
16. Jordan VC. Tamoxifen and tumorigenicity: a predictable concern. J Natl Cancer Inst 87: 623–626, 1995.
17. Assikis VJ, Jordan VC. Gynecologic effects of tamoxifen and the association with endometrial carcinoma. Int J Gynecol Obstet 49: 241–257, 1995.
18. Assikis VJ, Neven P, Jordan VC, et al. A realistic clinical perspective of tamoxifen and endometrial carcinogenesis. Eur J Cancer 32A: 1464–1476, 1996.
19. Horwitz, RI, Fienstein AR, Horwitz SM, et al. Necropsy diagnosis of endometrial cancer and detection-bias in case/control studies. Lancet 2: 66–68, 1981.
20. Sasco AJ. Tamoxifen and menopausal status: risks and benefits. Lancet 347: 761, 1996.
21. Magriples U, Naftolin F, Schwartz PE, et al. High-grade endometrial carcinoma in tamoxifen-treated breast cancer patients. J Clin Oncol 11: 485–490, 1993.
22. National Cancer Institute. SEER Cancer Statistics Review 1973–1990, Document 932789. Bethesda, NM: National Cancer Institute, 1993.
23. Fornander T, Rutqvist LE, Cedermark B, et al. Adjuvant tamoxifen in early breast cancer: occurrence of new primary cancers. Lancet 1: 117–120, 1989.
24. Fornander T. Helistrom AC, Moberger B. Descriptive clinicopathologic study of 17 patients with endometrial cancer during or after adjuvant tamoxifen in early breast cancer: J Natl Cancer Inst 85: 1850–1855, 1993.
25. Jordan VC, Morrow M. Should clinicians be concerned about the carcinogenic potential of tamoxifen? Eur J Cancer 30A: 1714–1721, 1994.
26. Fisher B, Costantino JP, Redmond CK, et al. Endometrial cancer in tamoxifen-treated breast cancer patients: findings from the National Surgical Adjuvant Breast and Bowel Project (NSABP) B-14. J Natl Cancer Inst 186: 527–537, 1994.
27. DeGregorio MW, Maenpaa JU, Wiebe VJ. Tamoxifen for the prevention of breast cancer: no. In: DeVita VT, Hellman S, Rosenberg SA (Eds), Important Advances In Oncology. Philadelphia, PA: JP Lippincott, 1995.

28.   Carmichael PL, Ugwumada AHN, Neven P, et al. Lack of gentoxicity of tamoxifen in human en-
      dometrium. Cancer Res 56: 1475–1479, 1996.
29.   Hemminki K, Rajaniemi H, Lindahl B, et al. Tamoxifen induced DNA adducts in endometrial samples for
      breast cancer patients. Cancer Res 56: 4374–4377, 1996.
30.   Lerner LJ, Jordan VC. Development of antiestrogens and their use in breast cancer: Eighth Cain Memorial
      Award Lecture. Cancer Res 50: 4177–4189, 1990.
31.   Tonetti DA, Jordan VC. Targeted antiestrogens to treat and prevent diseases in women. Mol Med Today 2:
      218–223, 1996.

28.

29.

30.

31.

C.J. Rosenthal and M. Rotman (Eds.), *Infusion Chemotherapy–Irradiation Interactions*

# CHAPTER 37

# Activity of retinoids, interferons and tamoxifen and their association in human breast cancer

SALVATORE TOMA[1,2], GIOVANNI BERNARDO[3], GIUSEPPE CANAVESE[1],
GIUSEPPE DASTOLI[4], LAURA ISNARDI[5], GUIDO NICOLÒ[1],
RAFFAELLA PALUMBO[1], PATRIZIA RAFFO[5],
MARIO REGAZZI-BONORA[6] and CARLO VECCHIO[1]

[1]*National Institute for Cancer Research, Genova, Italy,* [2]*Department of Experimental and Clinical Oncology, University of Genova, Genova, Italy,* [3]*Department of Medical Oncology, University of Pavia, Pavia, Italy,* [4]*Roche S.p.A., Milano, Italy,* [5]*Pre-Clinical Oncology Laboratory, Advanced Biotechnology Center (ABC), Genoa, Italy and* [6]*Department of Pharmacology, S. Matteo Hospital, Pavia, Italy*

The incidence of mammary carcinoma is increasing everywhere; in spite of large scale screening programs, locally advanced breast cancer, representing about 20–30% of total cases, remains an important public health problem. At present, it is currently accepted that breast carcinoma is microscopically spread at diagnosis in a considerable percentage of cases, mostly when metastases in regional nodes are present. Therefore, besides surgery and radiotherapy, chemotherapy and hormone therapy and, more recently, the use of new compounds with a different mechanism of action with respect to traditional cytostatic/cytotoxic drugs are becoming increasingly important. In the two past decades, a potential therapeutic activity has emerged for the class of biological response modifiers and, among these, a promising role for retinoids, natural and synthetic derivatives of vitamin A, such as various types of interferons (IFNs) has been suggested.

While many studies have been reported on effects of tamoxifen (TAM) in both pre-clinical [1] and clinical breast cancer models [2,3] only a small amount of evidence is available in the literature concerning the activity of retinoids (RAs) or IFNs. The antiproliferative effects of different RAs, in particular of all-*trans*-retinoic acid (tRA), have been showed by in vitro studies on human breast cancer cell lines [4–6], while in vivo experiences have demonstrated the ability of these agents to induce a regression of chemically induced mammary epithelium displasia in different animal models [7–11]. An antiproliferative activity of IFNs on breast cancer cell lines has also been showed by several experimental studies [12–15].

From a clinical point of view, only a few trials have tested 13-*cis*-retinoic acid (13cRA), fenretinide or retinyl-acetate as single agents in patients with advanced and/or metastatic breast cancer, failing to show a significant activity [16–18], while preliminary clinical data on IFNs are contrasting [19–21]. A synergic antiproliferative activity between RAs and TAM has been suggested in several breast cancer preclinical models [22–24], while a synergy of action between RAs and IFNs has been recently supported by in vitro and in vivo

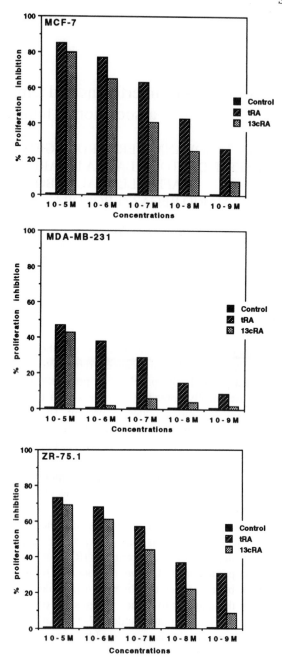

Fig. 1. Antiproliferative effect of tRA and 13cRA treatment in ER⁺ (MCF-7 and ZR-75.1) and ER⁻ (MDA-MB-231) cell lines. Data refer to cells cultured for 8 days with RAs.

studies on different hematological and solid tumors, including breast carcinoma [25,26]. On the other hand, an increased estrogen receptor (ER) expression in various breast cancer cell lines after IFN administration has been showed by in vitro experiences [15,27,28], such as a

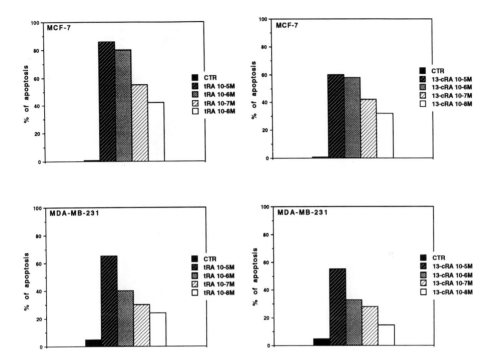

Fig. 2. Dose-dependent induction of apoptosis in ER$^+$ MCF-7 and ER$^-$ MDA-MB-231 cells. Data refer to cells cultured for 6 days with tRA and 13cRA, at different concentrations. Apoptosis was determined by flow-cytometric analysis of propidium iodide stained cells. Percentages indicate cells with hypodiploid DNA content, consistent with apoptosis, and are the mean of three independent experiments.

more than additive effect of IFNs when combined with TAM in inhibiting tumor cell growth in ER$^+$ mammary carcinoma cell lines [28,29].

In the clinical setting, different combinations of such agents have been tested in a small number of trials on advanced and/or metastatic breast cancer patients; encouraging, even if isolated results have been reported with TAM plus RAs [30,31] and IFNs plus TAM association [32–35].

To further confirm the above results, our group has performed two in vitro studies to evaluate the potentiating and/or synergistic antitumor effects among RAs, TAM and $\alpha$-interferon 2a ($\alpha$-IFN 2a) on human breast cancer cell lines.

In the first study [36], we have investigated the effect of different RAs (essentially 13cRA and tRA) on various breast cancer cell lines, both ER$^+$ (MCF-7 and ZR 75.1) and ER$^-$ (MDA.MB.231) (Fig. 1); our results showed that both RAs were able to inhibit mammary cancer cell proliferation, being more effective on ER$^+$ lines. The antiproliferative effect was clearly dose-dependent, and tRA was significantly more potent than 13cRA, thus suggesting a priority of use of the first retinoid in further in vitro–in vivo studies. Concerning the mechanism of cell proliferation inhibition, we showed that both RAs were able to induce apoptosis in MCF-7 (with concomitant reduction of bcl-2 levels) and MDA.MB.231 cells (Fig. 2), while in ZR 75.1 the same compounds produced cellular differentiation (demonstrated by ER level reduction), without apoptosis induction. These results seem to

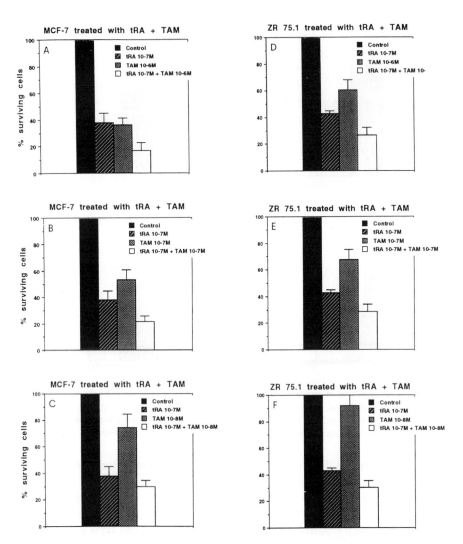

Fig. 3. Breast carcinoma cell lines: MCF-7 (a–c) and ZR-75.1 (d–f) treated with tRA (at a concentration of $10^{-7}$ M), TAM (at concentrations ranging from $10^{-6}$ to $10^{-8}$ M), and their combination, for 8 days. Histograms show the percentage of surviving cells with respect to untreated cells. Mean ± standard deviation of three separate experiments are shown.

indicate that breast carcinoma is a complex cellular model, in which RAs may act in different and alternative ways, either inducing apoptosis or producing cellular differentiation. Further studies are now in progress to better understand the biological mechanisms implicated in the effects of RAs on mammary carcinoma cell lines.

Regarding the effects of combining RAs with other therapeutic agents, in a second study [37] our group has evaluated the in vitro effect on the same breast cancer cell lines of a combined treatment with RAs and TAM and/or $\alpha$-IFN 2a. Our results showed different results among the different cells tested; in ER+ cell lines (MCF-7 and ZR 75.1) all the agents mentioned were effective when used in monotherapy ($\alpha$-IFN 2a was less effective in ZR

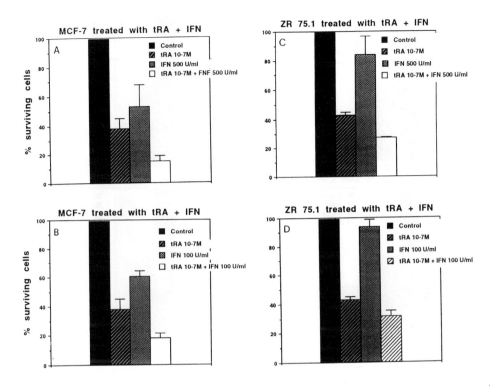

Fig. 4. Breast carcinoma cell lines: MCF-7 (a,b) and ZR-75.1 (c,d) treated with tRA (at a concentration of $10^{-7}$ M), $\alpha$-IFN (at a concentration of 500 and 100 IU/ml), and their combination, for 8 days. Histograms show the percentage of surviving cells with respect to untreated cells. Mean ± standard deviation of three separate experiments are shown.

75.1), while in the ER⁻ cell line only $\alpha$-IFN 2a showed a potent antiproliferative effect. As far as a combined treatment is concerned, in ER⁺ cells the association of TAM and RAs displayed an additive activity (Fig. 3), that of RAs and $\alpha$-IFN 2a a synergistic effect (Fig. 4), and that of TAM and $\alpha$-IFN 2a additivity or synergism depending on the tested cell line (ZR 75.1 or MCF-7) (Fig. 5). A combination of all three agents produced a further increase of antiproliferative activity (Fig. 6). In ER⁻ cells, no association seemed able to potentiate the effect of $\alpha$-IFN 2a used alone. These positive drug interactions may be explained by several biological mechanisms, essentially the modulation of ER by RAs and IFNs and that of retinoic acid receptors (RARs) by IFNs; we are now further investigating the complex biological interactions among these drugs at a molecular level.

The hypothesis of a synergism among RAs, TAM and IFNs prompted us to undertake two pilot studies testing the safety and activity of both 13cRA + TAM and 13cRA + TAM + $\alpha$-IFN 2a combination in advanced breast cancer patients. In both trials we demonstrated a good treatment compliance, with low and quickly reversible toxicity. A surprisingly high objective response (OR) rate of 78% was observed with the 13cRA + TAM association, significantly superior than that reported in previous studies [30,31]. However, the different drugs and administration schedules used make these trials incomparable. In our second study, a promising clinical activity of the 13cRA + TAM + $\alpha$-IFN 2a combination was also

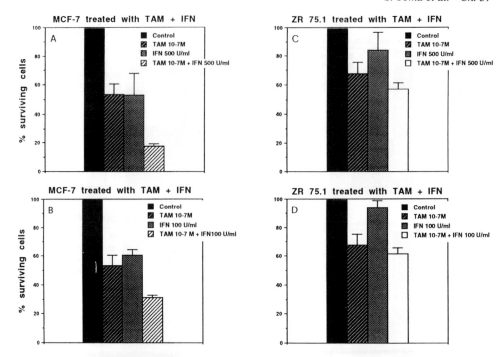

Fig. 5. Breast carcinoma cell lines: MCF-7 (a,b) and ZR-75.1 (c,d) treated with TAM (at a concentration of $10^{-7}$ M), $\alpha$-IFN (at a concentration of 500 and 100 IU/ml), and their combination, for 8 days. Histograms show the percentage of surviving cells with respect to untreated cells. Mean ± standard deviation of three separate experiments are shown.

achieved, consisting of 54% OR rate, maintained over a median period of 10 months [37]. Our results are in agreement with those of a previous phase II study, in which an OR rate of 55% was achieved with the combination of TAM, retinyl-palmitate and $\beta$-IFN on a series of 49 stage IV breast cancer patients [38].

Although several Groups are testing the in vitro and in vivo activity on breast cancer of RAs, when given alone or in combination with IFNs or TAM, no controlled study has been performed to evaluate the in vivo biological modulations among such agents and the potential mechanisms of actions supporting the mutual interactions. Therefore, we started a clinical phase IB study to verify the biological activity and safety of a combined treatment with tRA ± TAM ± $\alpha$-IFN 2a in patients with locally advanced operable breast cancer. The following biological parameters are evaluated on bioptical specimens at the study entry and on surgical pieces of tumor exeresis, after 3 weeks of treatment: ER and PgR status, histologic grade, Ki67, $G_0$–$G_1$ phase, TGF-$\beta$ type 1 and 2, RARs expression. Pharmacokinetic analysis is carried out at day 1, 7 and 21 of the treatment. Preliminary data are available on the first completed 15 cases. A biological activity of tRA is already detectable at the lower tested doses of 15 mg/m²; a down-grading, from G3 to G2, was observed in 2 of the 5 patients treated at the first tRA dose level; an increased ER and/or PgR expression was found in 5 patients, while TGF-$\beta$ levels were increased in 4 patients. From a clinical point of view, treatment toxicity was low, quickly reversible and not dose-related, consisting of WHO grade I–II hypercholesterolemia in 7 patients and mild headache in 3 patients. Preliminary pharmacokinetic data show that the intermittent schedule of tRA administration (days 1, 3,

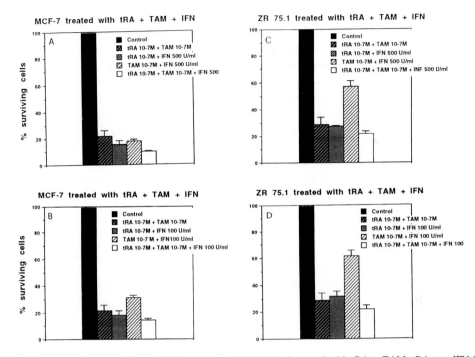

Fig. 6. Breast carcinoma cell lines: MCF-7 (a,b) and ZR-75.1 (c,d) treated with tRA + TAM, tRA + α-IFN 2a, TAM + α-IFN 2a, and tRA + TAM + α-IFN 2a, for 8 days. Histograms show the percentage of surviving cells with respect to untreated cells. Mean ± standard deviation of three separate experiments are shown.

5, 7 per week, over 3 consecutive weeks) adopted maintains adequate plasma drug concentrations. The analysis of the completed cases at the higher tRA dose levels (45 and 75 mg/m²) and that of the following treatment group (tRA combined with a flat dose of TAM) is presently ongoing.

In conclusion, the in vitro–in vivo evidence reported here suggests that triple combination of RAs with IFNs and TAM is adequate for testing in both breast cancer preclinical models and clinical trials. In our own experience, in vitro antitumor activity of the combinations tested was detectable, in terms of antiproliferative effects. The mutual biological modulations of these drug associations need to be further investigated, also in view of a better selection of patients as potential candidate for such treatment.

## Summary

*Background.* While a large amount of data is available on tamoxifen effects in postmenopausal breast cancer patients, little evidence exists concerning the activity of interferons and retinoids in such a tumor type. On the other hand, recent in vitro data support a more than additive and/or synergistic effect of these agents when used in combination. *Methods.* The literature available on in vitro and in vivo data on retinoids, tamoxifen and interferons in human breast cancer, used alone and in association, are reviewed. Our own experiences, concerning preclinical and clinical studies with all-*trans*-retinoic acid, tamoxifen, α-interferon 2a, and their associations, are also presented. *Results.* Laboratory and clinical studies reported suggest that the triple combination of retinoids, tamoxifen and interferons is adequate for testing in both preclinical breast cancer models and clinical trials. Specifically, our personal data showed an evident antitumor activity of such a combination in vitro, while a good treatment compliance with low toxicity has been demonstrated in our two pilot trials on advanced, pretreated breast cancer patients. *Conclusions.* The mutual biological modulations among the agents tested need to be further investigated, to identify the in vivo activity of retinoids, tamoxifen and interferons combination in human breast cancer, also in view of a better selection of patients who might potentially benefit from these treatments. Preliminary pharmacokinetic results of our ongoing phase IB study on patients with advanced, operable breast cancer suggest that the intermittent schedule of all-*trans*-retinoic acid administration allows adequate drug plasma concentrations to be achieved.

## References

1.  Jordan VC, Lababidi MK, Lanyan-Fahey S. The suppression of mouse mammary tumorigenesis by long-term tamoxifen therapy. J Natl Cancer Inst 83: 492–496, 1991.
2.  Jordan VC. Chemosuppression of breast cancer with long-term tamoxifen therapy. Prev Med 20: 3–14, 1991.
3.  Mouridsen HT. Endocrine therapy of advanced breast cancer. In: Cavalli F (Ed), Endocrine Therapy of Breast Cancer. Berlin: Springer, pp. 79–90, 1986.
4.  Ueda H, Takenawa T, Millan JC, et al. The effects of retinoids on proliferative capacities and macromolecular synthesis in human breast cancer MCF-7 cells. Cancer 46: 2203–2209, 1980.
5.  Fontana JA, Miksis G, Miranda DM, et al. Inhibition of human mammary carcinoma cell proliferation by retinoids and cAMP elevating compounds. J Natl Cancer Inst 78: 1107–1112, 1987.
6.  Fontana JA, Hobs PD, Dawison MI. Inhibition of mammary carcinoma growth by retinoic acid derivatives. Exp Cell Biol 56: 254–263, 1988.
7.  Moon RC, Grubbs CJ, Sporn MB. Inhibition of 7,12-dimethyl-benz(a)anthracene-induced mammary carcinogenesis by retinyl acetate. Cancer Res 36: 2626–2630, 1976.
8.  Grubbs DJ, Moon RC, Sporn MB, et al. Inhibition of mammary cancer by retinyl methyl esters. Cancer Res 37: 599–602, 1987.
9.  Moon RC, Thompson HJ, Becci PJ, et al. *N*-(4-Hydroxyphenyl)retinamide, a new retinoid for prevention of breast cancer in the rat. Cancer Res 39: 1339–1346, 1979.
10. McCormick DL, Moon RC. Influence of delayed administration of retinyl acetate on mammary carcinogenesis. Cancer Res 42: 2639–2643, 1982.
11. Lacroix A, Daskes C, Bhat P. Inhibition of growth of established N-methyl nitrosourea-induced mammary cancer in rats by retinoic acid and ovariectomy. Cancer Res 50: 5731–5734, 1990.
12. Marth C, Mayer I, Bock G, et al. Effects of human interferon alpha-2a and gamma on proliferation, estrogen receptor content and sensitivity of antiestrogens of cultured breast cancer cells. In: Dianzani F, Rossi GB (Eds), Interferon Systems, Vol. 24. New York: Raven Press, pp. 367–371, 1981.
13. Dimitrov N, Meyer CJ, Strander H, et al. Interferon as a modifier of estrogen receptors. Ann Clin Lab Sci 14: 32–39, 1984.
14. Iacobelli S, Natoli C, Arno E, et al. An antiestrogenic action of interferons in human breast cancer cells. Anticancer Res 6: 1392–1394, 1986.
15. Sica G, Natoli V, Stella C, Del Bianco S. Effects of natural beta-interferon on cell proliferation and steroid receptor level in human breast cancer cells. Cancer 60: 2419–2423, 1987.
16. Cassidy J, Lippman M, Lacroix A, Peck G. Phase II trial of 13-cis-retinoic acid in metastatic breast cancer. Eur J Cancer Clin Oncol 18: 925–928, 1982.
17. Modiano M, Dalton W, Lippmann SM, et al. Phase II study of fenretinide (n-{4-hydroxyphenyl}-retinamide) in advanced breast cancer and melanoma. Invest New Drugs 8: 317–319, 1990.
18. Resasco M, Canobbio L, Trave F, et al. Plasma retinol levels and side effects following high-dose retinyl acetate in breast cancer patients. Anticancer Res 8: 1319–1324, 1988.

19.  Pouillart P, Palangie T, Jouve M, et al. Administration of fibroblast interferon to patients with advanced breast cancer: possible effects on skin metastases and on hormone receptors. Eur J Cancer 18: 929–935, 1982.

20.  Laszlo J, Hood L, Goodwin B. A randomized trial of low doses of alpha interferon in patients with breast cancer. J Biol Respir Mod 5: 206–210, 1986.

21.  Fentiman IS, Balkwill FR, Cuzick J, et al. A trial of human alpha interferon as an adjuvant agent in breast cancer after loco-regional recurrence. Eur J Surg Oncol 13: 425–428, 1987.

22.  Whetherall NT, Taylor CM. The effects of retinoid treatment and antioestrogens on the growth of T47D human breast cancer cells. Eur J Cancer Clin Oncol 22: 53–59, 1986.

23.  Ratko TA, Detrisac CJ, Dinger NM, et al. Chemopreventive efficacy of combined retinoid and tamoxifen treatment following surgical excision of primary mammary cancer in female rats. Cancer Res 49: 4472–4476, 1989.

24.  Fontana JA, Burrows Mezu A, Cooper BN, Miranda D. Retinoid modulation of estradiol-stimulated growth and of protein synthesis and secretion in human breast carcinoma cells. Cancer Res 50: 1997–2002, 1990.

25.  Toma S, Monteghirfo S, Tasso P, et al. Antiproliferative and synergistic effect of alpha-interferon 2a, retinoids and their association in established human cancer cell lines. Cancer Lett 82: 209–216, 1994.

26.  Moore DM, Kalvakolanu DV, Lippman SM, et al. Retinoic acids and interferon in human cancer: mechanistic and clinical studies. Semin Hematol 31: 31–37, 1994.

27.  Van den Berg HW, Leahey WJ, Lynch M, et al. Recombinant human interferon alpha increases oestrogen receptor expression in human breast cancer cells (ZR 75.1) and sensitizes them to the antiproliferative effects of tamoxifen . Br J Cancer 55: 255–257, 1987.

28.  Goldstein D, Brushmeyer SM, Witt PL, et al. Effects of type I and II interferons on cultured human breast cells: interaction with estrogen receptors and with tamoxifen. Cancer Res 49: 2698–2702, 1989.

29.  Bezwoda WR, Meyer K. Effect of interferon, $17\beta$-estradiol, and tamoxifen on estrogen receptor concentration and cell cycle kinetics of MCF-7 cells. Cancer Res 50: 5387–5391, 1990.

30.  Boccardo F, Canobbio L, Resasco M, et al. Phase II study of tamoxifen and high-dose retinyl-acetate in patients with advanced breast cancer. I Cancer Res Clin Oncol 116: 503–506, 1990.

31.  Cobleigh MA, Dawlatshahi K, Deutsch AT, et al. Phase I/II trial of tamoxifen with or without fenretinide, an analog of vitamin A, in women with metastatic breast cancer. J Clin Oncol 11: 474–477, 1993.

32.  Porzsolt F, Otto AM, Trauschel B, et al. Rationale for combining tamoxifen and interferon in the treatment of advanced breast cancer. J Cancer Res Clin Oncol 115: 465–469, 1989.

33.  Macheledt JE, Buzdar AU, Hortobagy GN, et al. Phase II evaluation of interferon added to tamoxifen in the treatment of metastatic breast cancer. Breast Cancer Res Treatment 18: 165–170, 1991.

34.  Buzzi F, Brugia M, Rossi G, et al. Combination of beta-interferon and tamoxifen as a new way to overcome clinical resistance to tamoxifen in advanced breast cancer. Anticancer Res 12: 869–872, 1992.

35.  Seymour L, Bezwoda WR. Interferon plus tamoxifen treatment for advanced breast cancer: *in vivo* biologic effects of two growth modulators. Br J Cancer 68: 352–356, 1993.

36.  Toma S, Isnardi L, Raffo P, et al. Effects of all-*trans*-retinoic acid and 13-*cis*-retinoic acid on breast cancer cell lines: growth inhibition and apoptosis induction. Int J Cancer 70: 619–627, 1997.

37.  Toma S, Raffo P, Isnardi L, et al. Associations of retinoids, tamoxifen and $\alpha$-interferon 2a in human breast cancer: in vitro and in vivo studies. Int J Oncol 10: 597–607, 1997.

38.  Recchia F, Sica G, De Filippis S, et al. Interferon-beta, retinoids, and tamoxifen in the treatment of metastatic breast cancer: a phase II study. J Interferon Cytokine Res 15: 605–610, 1995.

C.J. Rosenthal and M. Rotman (Eds.), *Infusion Chemotherapy–Irradiation Interactions*

# CHAPTER 38

# Aspirin and other prostaglandin inhibitors for the prevention of colon cancer

## KOYAMANGALATH KRISHNAN[1], MACK T. RUFFIN IV[2] and DEAN E. BRENNER[3]

[1]*Division of Hematology-Oncology, Department of Internal Medicine, James H. Quillen College of Medicine and Veterans Affairs Medical Centre, East Tennessee State University, Johnson City, TN, USA,* [2]*Department of Family Practice and* [3]*Division of Hematology-Oncology, Department of Internal Medicine, University of Michigan Medical School and Veterans Affairs Medical Center, Ann Arbor, MI, USA*

## 1. Introduction

Cancer chemoprevention, a term coined by Sporn et al., is a new, developing science based on the pharmacological ability of certain agents to prevent, inhibit or reverse carcinogenesis [1]. In the past few years, several new agents of chemopreventive interest have been identified and characterized and some of their potential mechanisms of action as it pertains to carcinogenesis and its prevention have also been elucidated [2–9]. The field of cancer chemoprevention involves close multidisciplinary collaboration between several different allied fields and offers unique challenges which are not seen in standard chemotherapy trials with cytotoxic drugs. Several recent reviews on cancer chemoprevention provide convincing evidence that this approach can realistically reduce the incidence of various types of cancer [2–11]. Current systemic cytotoxic treatments for many common solid tumors remain largely ineffective. Hence a strong rationale exists for diverting research time, preclinical and clinical resources, and multidisciplinary expertise to the prevention of cancer.

Recent case-controlled epidemiological studies, in vitro animal and preclinical studies provided initial evidence of the potential for non-steroidal anti-inflammatory drugs (NSAIDs) like aspirin to significantly reduce the incidence of sporadic colorectal cancer in the general population. Anti-carcinogenic effects of NSAIDs were also demonstrated in elegant animal chemical models of colon cancer in the early 1980s. These initial observations from epidemiological and experimental studies were the driving force for pursuing the effects of NSAIDs in the prevention and reduction of colorectal cancer. Although recent molecular studies have provided us further insights into the different mechanisms of NSAID effects on normal and abnormal cells, we still do not know the precise mechanism of NSAID-mediated chemoprevention. The characterization of molecular abnormalities in several human neoplasia continues to occur at a rapid pace. Interaction of hereditary predisposition and environmental influences like diet are being better understood. It is feasible to identify cohorts of susceptible patients at high risk for a particular type of cancer (e.g., the BRCA-1 and BRCA-2 mutations for ovarian and breast cancer, APC mutations for familial adenomatous polyposis, etc.) although several practical, ethical and psychological issues have yet to be resolved.

In this chapter, we summarize the general aspects of chemoprevention and the epidemiological, experimental and recent molecular evidence in support of NSAIDs (aspirin, sulindac, sulindac sulfone, ibuprofen, piroxicam, curcumin) as colorectal cancer chemopreventive agents.

## 2.  Unique aspects of cancer chemoprevention [12]

Cancer chemoprevention is directed at the inhibition, retardation or reversal of carcinogenesis in apparently healthy, asymptomatic individuals identified to be at risk of developing neoplasia at some time in the future. Criteria for the identification of high risk individuals at risk for developing a particular type of neoplasm include the presence of premalignant lesions, previous history of cancer in the individual, strong family history of malignancy or mutations of tumor suppressor genes or presence of tumor promoting genes on genetic susceptibility testing. Cancer chemotherapy is directed at the treatment of previously existing malignant lesions in symptomatic patients with the intention of eradicating the tumor or palliating symptoms in advanced disease.

Cancer chemopreventive agents are carefully tested in preclinical and early clinical trials for its safety. Ideally, these agents should have minimal or no side effects. This is an essential attribute to ensure adherence, since the drugs would have to be administered over an extended period of time to healthy people. In addition even minor side-effects could have profound impact on the health of the population given the large number of people potentially involved. Cytotoxic chemotherapy treats people with established disease and significant side-effects are accepted as trade-offs for a potential cure of a fatal disease. Since most cytotoxic chemotherapy drugs are administered intravenously, adherence is ensured. Adherence is a major issue in cancer chemoprevention trials since drugs are being administered to an asymptomatic cohort in the general population selected to be at increased risk.

Clinical efficacy of cytotoxic drugs is monitored by surrogates like reduction in the palpable physical findings or radiological abnormalities. Toxicity is used as a surrogate of drug effect. There are no readily measurable physical or radiological surrogates to evaluate chemopreventive efficacy.

## 3.  Advances in molecular biology and colorectal cancer chemoprevention

Rapid advances in molecular biology have made significant contributions to our understanding of cancer chemoprevention and the interactions of genetic predisposition and dietary influences in colorectal carcinogenesis [13]. Epidemiological and experimental observations have molecular explanations now for some of their observed effects. Advances in molecular biology will continue to provide new insights on several aspects of importance in colorectal cancer chemoprevention including: (a) pathways of carcinogenesis, (b) genetic abnormalities in colon cancer, (c) mechanisms of drug action, (d) interaction of genetics and environmental influences, (e) potential new target sites for chemopreventive agents, and (f) influence the development of a new generation of chemopreventive agents with increased selectivity and decreased toxicity.

## 3.1.   Impact of molecular genetics on colorectal cancer chemoprevention

The Vogelstein laboratory proposed a multistep process of colorectal carcinogenesis in which histological progression from a normal epithelium through the stages of hyperproliferative epithelium and adenomatous change to frank cancer was shown to occur through the acquisition of multiple genetic abnormalities [14]. Fifteen percent of colorectal cancers have a known genetic basis; familial adenomatous polyposis (FAP) and hereditary non-polyposis colorectal cancer (HNPCC) are the best defined genetic syndromes. Insights gained from these two syndromes have provided information on the genetic mechanisms involved in carcinogenesis.

Genes of the replication-signaling pathway (K-ras, APC, and DCC) and genes involved in maintenance of DNA fidelity (*mutHLS* genes namely *h*MSH2, *h*MLH*1*, *h*PMS*1*, hPMS2, and p53) have now been identified to be involved in colorectal carcinogenesis [15–19]. The genetic defect in FAP involves the APC gene and leads to the production of a truncated protein; mutation of the APC gene affects its gatekeeper function and influences tumor initiation. The *mutHLS* genes are involved in genetic "proof-reading" and prevent the accumulation of mismatched base-pairs; the defect in HNPCC affects tumor progression. A large proportion of patients with hereditary non-polyposis colorectal cancer (HNPCC) and approximately 15% of patients with sporadic colorectal cancer have abnormalities in the *mutHLS* genes. Vogelstein et al demonstrated that loss of heterozygosity (LOH) or allelic loss is common in colorectal cancer. He showed that allelic losses of 5q (APC), 18q (DCC) and 17p (p53) were common. The mechanism of allelic loss in sporadic colorectal cancer is not clear.

The inheritance of a susceptibility gene for colon cancer alone does not suffice to develop cancer. All patients with germ-line mutations of the APC gene do not develop malignancy. Hence additional modifying factors, environmental or additional genetic changes, are essential. In the *Min* mouse model of FAP, it has been shown that a modifying gene called *MOM1* determines the number of polyps that the mice develop [20]. The *MOM1* locus codes for secreted phospholipase A2 (sPLA2) [21]. The discovery of MOM1 offers a link between lipids in diet, and heredity in colorectal cancer and a stronger support for the prostaglandin pathway in colon carcinogenesis. This is a good example of how genetic studies have provided information on interaction of genetics and environment.

Molecular studies in non-human systems like eukaryotes continue to unravel the functions of these genes. The wild-type APC gene appears to function as a "gatekeeper" gene and its inactivation may lead to uncontrolled growth of colonic epithelial cells [13]. APC may control apoptotic processes; introduction of wild-type APC into a cell line with mutant APC restores apoptosis [22]. APC also interacts with $\beta$-catenin, a protein essential in cadherin-mediated cell adhesion. APC may therefore influence cell adhesion through its effects on $\beta$-catenin [23,24].

Although the molecular changes underlying neoplastic transformation of the normal colonic epithelium can occur in any order, K-*ras* mutations and deletions of DCC gene and p53 are probably late events. Genetic screening for APC mutation in familial adenomatous polyposis (FAP) and *mutHLS* genes in hereditary non-polyposis colorectal cancer (HNPCC) kindreds is now possible although the practical problems have yet to be resolved [25,26]. Currently, there are no genetic screening methods available for the more common sporadic human colorectal cancer. Genetic screening in the selection of high risk subjects for colorectal cancer chemoprevention trials can only be one aspect of selection of high risk subjects. The problem of genetic mutations associated with early onset of colorectal cancer presents a therapeutic dilemma. Should early colectomy be performed on all these subjects? Should these subjects be enrolled in long term chemoprevention trials? The interested reader is referred to an excellent review on hereditary colorectal cancer by Vogelstein et al. [13].

## 3.2. Emerging role of cyclooxygenase-2 (COX-2) isoform in colorectal tumorigenesis

Several important studies have been recently published that establishes a pivotal role for COX-2 in colonic tumorigenesis (reviewed in detail by DuBois et al.) [27]. This information will have a significant bearing on our understanding of the role of prostaglandin inhibitors in colorectal cancer chemoprevention. There are two isoforms of cyclooxygenase, COX-1 and COX-2; COX-1 is a 'house-keeping' gene and is normally present in all cells at a low level of activity. COX-2 on the other hand is an inducible gene and its expression is increased by inflammatory and mitogenic stimuli. Although these two enzymes are closely related they may serve different functions.

COX-2 has been shown to have the following characteristics: (i) COX-2 mRNA is not detectable in normal colonic epithelium in both mice and humans but COX-2 mRNA is overexpressed in colorectal cancer and adenomas [28,29], (ii) COX-2 is localized at a different site at the subcellular level when compared to COX-1 [30], (iii) gene 'knockout' mice models of COX-1 and COX-2 genes result in different phenotype manifestations. The COX-2 null mice (homozygous COX-2 mutant mice) have variety of defects in ovaries, heart and kidneys including absence of corpora lutea, cardiac fibrosis, renal dysplasia, female infertility and increased susceptibility to peritonitis. COX-1 knock out models showed less gastric pathology, less incidence of indomethacin-induced gastric toxicity, decreased platelet aggregation and decreased inflammatory response to arachidonic acid [31–33] and (iv) when COX-2 was overexpressed in rat intestinal epithelial cells (RIE), it was shown to confer phenotypic changes in these cells including alterations in cell adhesion and resistance to apoptosis.

Sulindac corrects these phenotypic changes and decreases COX-2 expression [34], (vi) in APC knockout mice, COX-2 begins to be overexpressed at a very early stage of polyp development while COX-1 is not [35]. Mice carrying an APC mutation were bred with mice carrying a disrupted COX-2 gene. All mice were Apc+/−. The mice with wildtype COX-2 gene developed the maximum number of polyps while the COX-2 deficient mice developed fewer polyps. Treatment of the mice with a selective COX-2 inhibitor reduced the polyp number [36]. These data lend strong support to an important role of COX-2 in colorectal tumorigenesis. Can a mutation of wild-type APC gene influence COX-2 expression? It has been suggested though not proven that a mutated APC gene may cause COX-2 overexpression through LEF-1, a transcription factor [37].

From the available evidence, COX-2 appears to be a suitable "biomarker" in colorectal cancer chemoprevention and deserves further study. There is also sufficient evidence to support the vigorous search for a selective COX-2 inhibitor in colorectal cancer chemoprevention.

## 3.3. Regulation of cell cycle and chemoprevention

As our understanding of cell cycle regulation increases, potential new sites for pharmacological intervention will be available. For example, the overexpression of COX-2 in colorectal carcinoma [28,29] may cause resistance to apoptosis. D-type cyclins are crucial for G1 progression in the mammalian cell cycle. Recently, DuBois et al. have shown a delay in G1 progression and a decrease in cyclin D1 protein in rat intestinal epithelial cells (RIE) transfected to overexpress COX-2 protein [28]. Hence, inhibition of COX-2 expression by NSAIDs may promote G1 progression and programmed cell death (apoptosis). Better understanding of the genetic and molecular mechanisms of cell cycle regulation, cell proliferation and chemopreventive drug action, will lead to a more rational and scientific utilization of chemopreventive methods.

## 4. Important attributes of current chemoprevention trials

The Chemoprevention Branch of the National Cancer Institute (NCI) has identified three key factors of importance in the development of drugs for chemoprevention trials which include the following [12,38].

### 4.1. Chemopreventive agents

A suitable candidate chemopreventive should have the following characteristics before being tested in large clinical trials:
–   demonstration of chemopreventive efficacy at the target site in preclinical models of carcinogenesis,
–   demonstration of a low toxicity profile; hence adequate preclinical efficacy data, toxicity, pharmacokinetic and pharmacodynamic data and or long established clinical use is required,
–   early clinical dosing studies are required to establish the minimum and optimal dosage required,
–   a putative mechanism of action of the candidate chemopreventive should be known; this is useful in targeting the drug and also to identify markers of drug effect. For example, NSAIDs are known to suppress prostaglandin metabolism through its effects on cyclooxygenase enzyme and knowledge of this mechanism offers potential biochemical parameters that can be monitored to follow drug effect.

### 4.2. Intermediate "biomarkers" in chemoprevention

Validated reliable surrogate "biomarkers" have to be established for each type of cancer; modulation of these biomarkers should have a good correlation with cancer incidence. The development of clinically recognizable cancer takes decades. Therefore, it is not practical to use the occurrence of cancer as an end-point in the evaluation of the chemopreventive efficacy of a putative agent in a clinical trial and alternate "surrogate" markers are required.
–   The term "biomarker" or "intermediate end-point" refers to a biological or chemical property which can be measured and is known to be correlated with cancer incidence and progression [39–42].
–   Examples of potential "biomarkers" include genetic and molecular markers (micronuclei formation, genetic mutations), proliferation/differentiation markers, apoptotic and cell cycle markers, histological markers (colon polyps, aberrant crypt foci) and biochemical markers (prostaglandin levels, COX-2mRNA expression etc.).

–   Several potential "biomarkers" have been identified but none have been validated in clinical trials as being reliable. Hence there is a critical need to characterize and standardize useful "biomarkers" in colorectal cancer chemoprevention research.

### 4.3. Cohorts

Cohorts of patients at risk for a particular type of neoplasm need to be identified for testing of putative chemopreventive drugs in clinical efficacy studies. For example in colorectal cancer chemoprevention clinical trials, these patients would be those with an increased risk of colon cancer and would include:

–   patients with previous history of colon cancer treated by surgery or adjuvant therapy and are disease free,
–   history of previously resected colorectal adenomas greater than 2 cm diameter,
–   family history of colon cancer in first-degree relatives,
–   familial basis for colorectal cancer, e.g. FAP and HNPCC syndromes.

As our understanding of the genetic basis of colon cancer and our ability to test for genetic cancer susceptibility improves, we would be able to improve our ability to identify such high risk cohorts.

## 5.  Epidemiological evidence for NSAIDs in colorectal cancer chemoprevention

Substantial epidemiological evidence derived from case-controlled studies exist to support the significant effects of NSAIDs in the prevention of colon cancer [43]. Most of the studies published so far show reduction in either colorectal polyp formation or colorectal cancer in subjects who use aspirin [44–53]. Two studies show an increased risk [54–55]. Figure 1 depicts the published studies and relative risk reduction in each study.

The North American Study of the American Cancer Society (Cancer Prevention Study II, CPS II) was a large, landmark. prospective cohort mortality study of 662 424 adults [45]. Information on frequency and duration of aspirin use and death rates from colon cancer were measured from 1982 to 1988. Death rates from colon cancer decreased with increased aspirin use in both men and women. The relative risk among individuals who used aspirin 16 or more times a month for at least 1 year was 0.60 in men (95% confidence interval, 0.40–0.89) and 0.58 in women (95% confidence interval, 0.37–0.90). This would indicate approximately halving the death rate from colon cancer in this population even among individuals taking aspirin every other day.

The study was commendable for its prospective design, large size of the sample population (over 650 000 adult Americans), its precise evaluation of risk reduction and an almost complete followup. Its drawbacks included the following: (i) it assessed the mortality of colon cancer and not the incidence; the lower rate of mortality from colon cancer could have been due to increased survival and not decreased incidence; (ii) the mortality from rectal cancer was not measured; a decrease in the mortality due to rectal cancer would have added further support to the data since it shares several common features with colon cancer; (iii) the possibility of selection bias in the study could not be completely excluded since a significant proportion of the subjects did not answer questions on aspirin use and the information on diet and exercise were not complete; (iv) the study could not exclude completely the issue of whether pain or bleeding from colon cancer may have made patients avoid aspirin

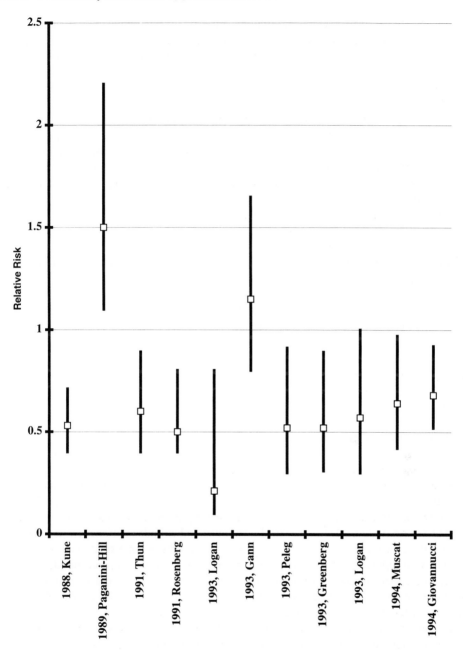

Fig. 1. Epidemiological studies of NSAID use and risk of colorectal cancer.

or that aspirin-induced bleeding may have made patients seek earlier intervention; (v) the mechanisms of aspirin's action and the least effective dose were also uncertain from this study. Nevertheless, this was an important epidemiological study in colorectal cancer prevention.

Published epidemiological studies highlight the following issues of importance in planning future interventional trials in colorectal cancer chemoprevention:

–   epidemiological studies show chemopreventive benefit only with aspirin and not the other NSAIDs,
–   chemopreventive intervention with a NSAID like aspirin probably has to be initiated at an early step in colon carcinogenesis for it to be effective,
–   regular use of aspirin is essential for it to be effective but the studies do not identify the optimal dose and frequency of aspirin,
–   prolonged use of aspirin for at least 10 years may be required for risk reduction,
–   data from controlled epidemiological studies although informative may not be fully applicable to the heterogeneous general population. Prospective data from a randomised study on the efficacy of NSAIDs like aspirin in prevention of sporadic colorectal cancer in the general population is essential.

## 6.  Experimental evidence for NSAIDs in colorectal cancer chemoprevention

The evidence for the chemopreventive effects of NSAIDs from studies on animal models of chemically-induced colon cancer indicate that several of the NSAIDs (aspirin, ibuprofen, piroxicam, sulindac, sulindac sulfone, curcumin) have anti-carcinogenic properties. Sulindac sulfone, a metabolite of sulindac without the COX-suppressive properties, also has anti-carcinogenic effects. This suggests that multiple chemopreventive mechanisms that affect cellular proliferative and apoptotic events may be involved in NSAID-mediated chemoprevention. A single best NSAID cannot be identified from the available experimental data.

### 6.1.  Aspirin, indomethacin and piroxicam

#### 6.1.1.  Evidence in animal carcinogenesis models
The earliest experiments with aspirin and other NSAIDs and its potential to inhibit chemical carcinogenesis in animal models were conducted in the mid-1970s. Colonic tumorigenesis induced by numerous chemical carcinogens can be suppressed by several different NSAIDs including aspirin, indomethacin, piroxicam, sulindac and sulindac sulfone. Dimethylhydrazine, dimethylnitrosamine, and methylazoxymethanol-induced intestinal tumors in male F344 rats were suppressed by treatment with indomethacin, piroxicam, and sulindac. Piroxicam suppressed azoxymethane-induced colon tumors; Reddy et al. have demonstrated linear relationships between piroxicam dose and tumor suppression. Synergy was also shown between piroxicam and difluoro-methylornithine (DFMO) [56–62].

Treatment of rats with indomethacin or ASA at doses that suppress colonic PG production increases the uptake of tritiated thymidine into mucosal DNA in colon, gastric fundus, small intestine and duodenum [63]. When male F344 rats with azoxymethane-induced colon tumors were fed ASA in their diet significant suppression of colonic mucosal $PGE_2$ levels occurred which was associated with inhibition in the incidence and number of these tumors [64]. Chemopreventive agents have been shown to have a regional effect on AOM-induced rat colon tumors; piroxicam suppressed proximal tumors more than distal tumors (82% versus 57%) while agents like DFMO and oltipraz suppressed distal tumors more than proximal colon tumors [65].

Piroxicam inhibits AOM-induced aberrant crypt foci and colon cancer in rats. Periera et al. [66] have also shown recently that aberrant crypt foci formation was inhibited in AOM-treated male Fischer 344 rats (30 mg/kg body weight) fed piroxicam at a dose of 0.125 g/kg in their diet. Piroxicam not only inhibits the formation of colon tumors but also caused regression of aberrant crypt foci (the putative precursor lesion of colon cancer) in this model.

### 6.1.2.   Evidence from in vitro experimental studies

The cyclooxygenases (COX-1 and COX-2) catalyze both oxidative and reductive reactions in the prostaglandin synthesis pathway. ASA completely inhibits bis-oxygenation of arachidonate by COX-1. In contrast, ASA-treated COX-2 metabolizes AA to 15-HETE (a leukotriene with anti-inflammatory and anti-mitogenic properties) instead of PGH2 [67]. Indomethacin, sulindac sulfide, and piroxicam preferentially inhibited COX-1. Ibuprofen, flurbiprofen and meclofenamate inhibit both enzymes with equal efficacy. COX-1 and not COX-2, is expressed at a low level in quiescent 3T3 fibroblasts [67].

In cultured HT-29 colon cancer cells, aspirin, indomethacin and piroxicam were shown to alter cell cycle phase distribution of these cells in a time- and concentration-dependent manner; they reduced the proliferation and altered the morphology of these cells [68]. ASA and piroxicam can slow the cell cycle by reduction in levels of two cyclin-dependent kinases which are essential for normal cell cycle progression (p34cdc2 and p33cdk2) [68]. All the NSAIDs studied, except aspirin, were also shown to induce apoptosis in HT-29 cells. These data, further discussed in the next section, offer alternate pathways of anti-carcinogenic effects of these compounds. Why aspirin did not induce apoptosis is an important question to answer.

## 6.2.   Sulindac and sulindac sulfone

Sulindac, a non-steroidal anti-inflammatory indene derivative, undergoes reversible reduction to a sulfide metabolite and irreversible oxidation to a sulfone (SN) metabolite. The drug undergoes enterohepatic circulation with the excretion of oxidized forms in the bile. The bacterial flora in the gut convert sulindac to sulindac sulfone and sulindac sulfide. As an anti-inflammatory, the sulfide metabolite is active biologically and inhibits prostaglandin production [69,70] but the sulfone metabolite is inactive and does not affect prostaglandin synthesis [71]. New data indicate that sulindac sulfone through its effects on apoptotic pathways may possess prostaglandin pathway-independent chemopreventive properties as discussed below [68,72,73].

### 6.2.1.   Evidence from animal carcinogenesis models

This is described earlier in Section 6.1.

### 6.2.2.   Evidence based on in vitro experimental data and molecular studies

The anti-carcinogenic properties of sulindac have been shown in experiments in cultured colon cancer cell lines, transfection studies, the *Min* model of colon cancer and genetic "knockout" studies.

Sulindac sulfide and sulfone inhibit the growth of tumor cells in culture with reduction in cell number in confluent and preconfluent HT-29 cell cultures [68]. Cell proliferation was not affected under growth inhibitory conditions. Both the metabolites induce apoptosis but not cell differentiation.

Reduction in proportion of cells in the S phase, and increase in cells in the $G_0/G_1$ phase has been seen in HT-29 colon adenocarcinoma cells. Sulindac and sulindac sulfone cause alterations in levels of *bcl-2* and *bax*, induction of apoptosis and inhibition of cell cycle progression in HT-29 colon cancer cell lines [74]. In a group of 22 patients randomized to either 150 mg of sulindac or placebo, sulindac caused an increased in the subdiploid apoptotic fraction after 3 months with no change in cell proliferation (studied by immunohistochemistry for PCNA) [75]. DuBois et al in transfection experiments overexpressed COX-2 in rat intestinal epithelial (RIE) cells and demonstrated increased adhesion of RIE cells to extracellular matrix proteins and inhibition of apoptosis; this was reversed by sulindac sulfide [34].

These data suggest that the mechanism of action of sulindac may be solely through apoptotic induction. It is conceivable that the effects of sulindac on apoptosis are mediated through cyclooxygenase or prostaglandins. The observation that sulindac sulfone, a metabolite without prostaglandin suppressive properties, also had anti-proliferative effects on HT-29 colon cancer cells would suggest that these alternate pathways may be important in NSAID chemoprevention. But the sulfone is almost 10 times less potent than the sulfide in its effects. Interestingly, aspirin, a compound known to have chemopreventive properties based on animal experiments and epidemiological data did not induce apoptosis. This further suggests that apoptosis is perhaps not the only pathway of chemoprevention and other mechanisms are also involved. Whether an effective chemopreventive compound for this site should have antiproliferative, pro-apoptotic activity or both remains the subject of intense investigation and speculation at this time.

### 6.2.3. Evidence from "knockout" and animal models of colon cancer

Overexpression of COX-2 has been associated with an increased incidence of colon cancer. COX-2 is overexpressed in 90% of cancers and 40% of premalignant colorectal adenomas and not expressed in normal colon tissues [76]. Boolbol et al. [35] studied C57BL/6J-*Min*/+(Min) mice (a strain with a fully penetrant dominant *Apc* gene mutation). This strain develops intestinal polyps by 110 days of age. The mice were fed sulindac and sacrificed at 110 days of age. The sulindac-fed mice had significantly less tumors when compared to controls ($0.1 \pm 0.1$ tumors per mouse versus $11.9 \pm 7.8$ tumors per mouse). The sulindac-fed mice demonstrated decreased amounts of $PGE_2$ and COX-2 and restoration of normal apoptosis. Oshima et al. [36] demonstrated suppression of intestinal polyposis in $Apc^{\Delta716}$ knockout mice by a selective COX-2 inhibitor (MF tricyclic, a furanone derivative) and sulindac. It was also shown in this experiment that suppression of polyp formation with the selective COX-2 inhibitor was better than with sulindac. When a null mutation of the COX-2 gene (*Ptgs2*) was introduced into this model, there was a reduction in the number and size of polyps [36].

### 6.3. Curcumin

Curcumin, a commonly used spice in Asia, is the major yellow pigment extracted from turmeric, the rhizome of the herb, *Curcuma longa*. It is used as a cooking spice for many dishes. In India and Southeast Asia, curcumin has long been used as treatment (as turmeric) for inflammation, skin wounds and tumors [77].

### 6.3.1. Evidence from animal experiments

Curcumin has potent anti-inflammatory activity in an acute model inflammation test

[78,79]. It inhibits lipid peroxidation induced by carcinogens in liver homogenates of ede-matous mice [80]. Curcumin has broad spectrum chemopreventive activity in preclinical models. Curcumin inhibited tumor formation in rat models of skin cancer, oral cancer, and papillomas [81–86].

Huang et al. [83,87] have demonstrated that a dose of 0.5–4.0% commercial grade (98%) curcumin inhibited azoxymethane-induced colonic tumors by 51–62% in CF-1 mice. Reddy et al. have found a reduction in invasive tumor multiplicity and adenomas in azoxymethane-treated rats at a dose of 2000 ppm without toxicity [88] with reduction in ornithine decar-boxylase activity, tyrosine protein kinase activity, cyclooxygenase and 5-lipoxygenase ac-tivity.

## 7.   How do NSAIDs prevent colorectal carcinogenesis?

The exact mechanisms by which aspirin and other NSAIDs suppress carcinogenesis is not known. The dose of the NSAID, type of NSAID and frequency of administration may be important. Several new possible cell regulatory targets of NSAID action have been identi-fied recently. It is apparent that NSAIDs have profound effects on cell regulation and tran-scription that may be the result of acetylation of the cyclooxygenase enzyme at its Ser530 position or may be cyclooxygenase-independent or both.

### 7.1.   Restoration of COX-2 mediated abnormalities of epithelial cell function

As discussed earlier, COX-2 has an important role in colon tumorigenesis with increased expression in colon adenomas and carcinomas [28,29]. COX-2 overexpression leads to fail-ure of apoptosis and changes in cell phenotype [34,68]. NSAIDs directly suppress the ex-pression of COX-2 mRNA and correct these abnormalities [34].

### 7.2.   Suppression of prostaglandin products involved in cell growth

Prostaglandins may influence immune responsiveness and promote tumor growth. High levels of prostaglandins especially of the E series are present in both experimental and hu-man tumors probably due to increased activity of COX-2 [89]. Suppression of prostaglandin production may therefore retard tumor growth although recent evidence suggests that it is probably not the main mechanism and that effects at the transcriptional level are probably more important mechanistically.

### 7.3.   Reduction of intracellular oxygen stress induced by cyclooxygenase activity

Oxidation of arachidonic acid and other fatty acids via the COX or lipoxygenase pathways produces reactive moieties like superoxide in the colonic mucosa. Generation of malondial-dehyde, a potent mutagen and carcinogen, occurs through the metabolism of the COX pathway. Malondialdehyde produces frame shifts and base pair substitutions, principally $G \rightarrow T$ transversions and $C \rightarrow T$ and $A \rightarrow G$ transitions. $C \rightarrow T$ transitions are frequently associated with p53 mutations in the human colon. Other carcinogens also appear to be acti-vated through COX activity [90]. The characterization of the gene that encodes secreted phospholipase (sPLA2), *MOM1*, in the Min mouse as a modifying gene influencing polyp number, offers a link between dietary products, arachidonic metabolism and heredity [20,21]. NSAIDs may therefore neutralize dietary mutagens activated through this pathway.

## 7.4. Generation of 15-HETE by aspirin

Lipoxygenase products may be pro-inflammatory or anti-inflammatory. Lipoxygenase products are mitogenic in bovine aortic endothelial cells and Friend erythroleukemia cell lines [91–93]. They directly oxygenate phospholipids including lipids in biological membranes to their corresponding hydroperoxides which could activate carcinogens. Mammalian lipoxygenases which are able to produce unsaturated fatty-acid derived peroxy radicals may activate aflatoxin $B_1$ to a DNA-binding metabolite. Generation of 15-HETE, a leukotriene with anti-inflammatory and anti-mitogenic properties, by aspirin could be anti-carcinogenic. Such an effect is aspirin specific as other NSAIDs do not induce the production of 15-HETE.

## 7.5. Suppression of NF-kB activation by aspirin and salicylic acid

NF-kB, inducible eukaryotic transcription factor of the *rel* family exists in an inactive form in the cytoplasm, bound to an inhibitory protein, I-kB. In response to many stimulants, it dissociates from I-kB and translocates from the cytoplasm to the nucleus and binds to DNA [94]. It regulates the transcription of key immune and inflammatory response genes (e.g., IL-1, 6, 8, interferon-$\beta$, tumor necrosis factor $\alpha$, cell adhesion molecules). Activation of NF-kB is inhibited by high ($\geq 2$ mM) intracellular aspirin and salicylic acid concentrations [95]. Reduction of cellular production of mediators of inflammation on a chronic basis may reduce cellular oxygen stress. The high intracellular drug and metabolite concentrations required for this effect support NF-kB's role in aspirin's antiinflammatory effects; however, the low doses and infrequent dosing schedules of aspirin (most of those surveyed were taking low doses of aspirin as a cardiovascular disease preventive) that have been associated with reduction of colorectal cancer incidence in recently published epidemiologic studies reduces support to the idea that NF-kB plays a pivotal role in colorectal carcinogenesis.

## 7.6. Induction of apoptosis and inhibition of cell proliferation

NSAIDs influence programmed cell death (apoptosis) in the human gastrointestinal tract. Reduction in proportion of cells in the S phase, and increase in cells in the $G_0/G_1$ phase has been seen in HT-29 colon adenocarcinoma cells [68]. ASA and piroxicam can slow the cell cycle by reduction in levels of two cyclin dependent kinases which are essential for normal cell cycle progression (p34cdc2 and p33cdk2). Sulindac and sulindac sulfone cause alterations in levels of *bcl-2* and *bax*, induction of apoptosis and inhibition of cell cycle progression in HT-29 colon cancer cell lines [74].

## 7.7. Abrogation of cytokine expression by salicylates

Salicylates are capable of abrogating the expression of certain cytokines (IL-11, IFN-$\alpha$, TNF-$\alpha$, IL-1$\beta$ and GM-CSF) in the colonic epithelium in HT-29 and HCT-116 cell lines [96]. This suggests that cytokines may mediate NSAID action in the colonic epithelium. Moreover, the presence of increased amounts of COX-2 in the interstitial cells rather than intestinal epithelial cells of polyps [36] suggests that COX-2 may promote colon tumorigenesis through a paracrine loop involving perhaps cytokines.

## 8.   Current colorectal cancer chemoprevention trials

National Cancer Institute (NCI) sponsored clinical trials with an emphasis on biochemical, molecular and pathologic surrogates for cancer risk reduction are in progress evaluating the effects of NSAIDs (sulindac and aspirin) in patients with previous history of polyps and those with a previous history of colon cancer. Current surrogates of interest are adenoma number and size, proliferation indices (PCNA), tissue prostaglandin concentrations and differentiation surrogates. Results from these early trials should provide validation data on the predictive power of these surrogates while testing the potential efficacy of chemopreventive agents. At this time, no agents have reduced colorectal cancer risk.

### 8.1.   Aspirin [97]

The authors' group at the University of Michigan have completed phase I trials in normal human subjects to identify the lowest dose of aspirin that is necessary to modulate rectal prostaglandin levels (unpublished data). The phase I study shows that a single daily aspirin dose of 81 mg suppresses rectal prostaglandins and its effects are prolonged.

A phase III low dose aspirin study from the United States Physicians Health Study closed early because of the significant effects of aspirin in reducing the incidence of myocardial infarction. Aspirin's ability to reduce the incidence of colorectal cancer remains undetermined in this study. Investigators in Boston are evaluating a combination of 50 mg of $\beta$-carotene, 600 IU vitamin E or 100 mg of aspirin for 4 years on the incidence of epithelial cancers and vascular events. A Phase II chemoprevention trial in Dallas is evaluating the effects of a proliferation biomarker ([3H]thymidine labeling) in colon adenomas. There is no strong evidence in human trials to identify any of the NSAIDs as being the most efficacious colorectal cancer chemopreventive. Aspirin is a strong choice based on its popularity, easy availability, demonstrated efficacy as a cardiovascular protective, low cost and minimal toxicity.

### 8.2.   Sulindac [98]

Sulindac is effective in the induction of polyp regression in familial adenomatous polyposis (FAP) [98–102]. Sulindac promotes regression and inhibition of adenoma recurrence in FAP with a dramatic reduction in size and number of the polyps. But polyps recur if the drug is discontinued. Similar effects occur with rectal administration [103]. Proliferation indices are not affected by sulindac administration [104]. A decrease in the number of adenomatous polyps was reported in a crossover controlled study of five patients with FAP and previous ileorectal anastomosis [105]. Polyp number increased in the placebo arm. Proliferation indices were not changed. Sulindac (300 mg/day) or placebo was given in this study in two 4-month periods with a 1-month wash out period. In another controlled trial of 24 patients, sulindac was given to 24 patients with subtotal colectomy and ileorectal anastomosis. Polyps were visualized by video assessment and proliferation by bromodeoxyuridine labelling. A significant fall in proliferation indices and polyp count was observed [106]. A study in patients with sporadic colonic adenomas showed no benefit [107].

The issues to be addressed in sulindac and sulindac sulfone chemoprevention include characterization of the role of sulindac in the apoptosis pathway, the effects of sulindac sulfone on cell proliferation and the effects of these compounds in sporadic human colorectal cancer and not just polyp reduction.

### 8.3. Curcumin

Clinical chemoprevention trials with curcumin are not available. Phase 1 studies in normal human subjects on curcumin pharmacokinetics and "biomarker" modulation are in progress at the University of Michigan (Dr. Brenner).

## 9. Summary and future directions

The science of chemoprevention has made tremendous progress over the last two decades. NSAIDs represent a class of chemopreventive agents with realistic potential to reduce the incidence of colorectal carcinoma. The information obtained from epidemiological studies and early animal experiments support NSAID anti-carcinogenic effects. The mechanisms by which NSAIDs exert their anticarcinogenic effects are unclear, but rapidly accumulating data support the concept that cyclooxygenases, particularly cyclooxygenase-2, play an important role in cellular proliferation and apoptotic control. These drugs may directly inhibit genetic transduction as well as alter epigenetic events of cellular growth regulation and apoptosis.

The data to date are insufficient to support the regular use of aspirin or other NSAIDs as colorectal cancer chemopreventives. Risk reduction in humans is unproven. The optimal NSAID dose to recommend is unclear. If COX-2 plays a significant role in colorectal tumorigenesis, would a selective inhibitor of COX-2 be a more effective and safer chemopreventive than the current NSAIDs? Would a combination of chemopreventives with different sites of action in the carcinogenesis pathway be more efficacious than single agent therapy? When should chemopreventive agents be administered, how much and for how long? How do we follow the subjects and monitor the response in asymptomatic people? When do we know that a particular agent is effective? When do we know that a particular agent is ineffective? Answers to these questions and several others are being actively sought in several research centers and will hopefully give us further insights into colorectal cancer chemoprevention.

### Acknowledgements

This study received grant support from the Department of Veterans Affairs, VA Merit Review, American Cancer Society Grant EDT-55, National Cancer Institute CN-25429 and the University of Michigan Cancer Center Munn Fund.

### References

1.   Sporn M. Approaches to prevention of epithelial cancer during the preneoplastic period. Cancer Res 36: 2699–2702, 1976.

2. Greenwald P, Nixon D, Malone W, et al. Concepts in cancer chemoprevention research. Cancer 65: 1483–1490, 1990.

3. Greenwald P, Kelloff G, Burch-Whitman C, Kramer B. Chemoprevention. CA Cancer J Clin 45: 31–49, 1995.

4. Kelloff G, Johnson J, Crowell J, et al. Approaches to the development and marketing approval of drugs that prevent cancer. Cancer Epidemiol, Biomarkers Prev 4: 1–10, 1995.

5. Lippman S, Benner S, Hong W. Cancer chemoprevention. J Clin Oncol 12: 851–873, 1994.

6. Lippman S, Hittelman W, Lotan R, et al. Recent advances in cancer chemoprevention. Cancer Cells 3: 59–65, 1991.

7. Szarka C, Grana G, Engstrom P. Chemoprevention of cancer. Curr Prob Cancer 18: 6–78, 1994.

8. Wattenberg L. Chemoprevention of cancer. Cancer Res 45: 1–8, 1985.

9. Weinstein IB. Cancer prevention: recent progress and future opportunities. Cancer Res. 51: 5080–5085, 1991.

10. Krishnan K, Brenner DE. Chemoprevention of colorectal cancer. Gastroenterol Clin North Am 25: 821–858, 1996.

11. Boone CW, Kelloff GJ, Malone WE. Identification of candidate chemopreventive agents and their evaluation in animal models and human clinical trials. Cancer Res 50: 2–9, 1990.

12. Kelloff GJ, Hawk ET, Crowell JA, et al. Strategies for identification and clinical evaluation of promising chemopreventive agents. Oncology 10: 1471–1480, 1996.

13. Kinzler KW, Vogelstein B. Lessons from hereditary colorectal cancer. Cell 87: 159–170, 1996.

14. Fearon ER, Vogelstein B. A genetic model for colorectal tumorigenesis. Cell 61: 759–767, 1990.

15. Nishisho I, Nakamura Y, Miyoshi Y, et al. Mutations of chromosome 5q21 genes in FAP and colorectal cancer patients. Science 253: 665–669, 1991.

16. Groden J, Thliveris A, Samowitz W, et al. Identification and characterization of the familial adenomatous polyposis coli gene. Cell 66: 589–560, 1991.

17. Spirio L, Olshwang S, Groden J, et al. Alleles of the APC gene: an attenuated form of familial polyposis. Cell 75: 951–957, 1993.

18. Leach FS, Nicolaides NC, Papadopoulos N, et al. Mutations of a mutS homolog in hereditary nonpolyposis colorectal cancer. Cell 75: 1215–1225, 1993.

19. Parsons R, Li G, Longley M, et al. Hypermutability and mismatch repair deficiency in RER+ tumor cells. Cell 75: 1227–1236, 1993.

20. Dietrich WF, Lander ES, Smith JS, et al. Genetic identification of *Mom-1*, a major modifier locus affecting Min-induced intestinal neoplasia in the mouse. Cell 75: 631–639, 1993.

21. MacPhee M, Chepenik K, Liddell R, et al. The secretory phospholipase A2 gene is a candidate for the *Mom1* locus, a major modifier of ApcMin-induced intestinal neoplasia. Cell 81: 957–966, 1995.

22. Morin PJ, Vogelstein B, Kinzler KW. Apoptosis and APC in colorectal tumorigenesis. Proc Natl Acad Sci USA 93: 7950–7954, 1996.

23. Rubinfeld B, Souza B, Albert I, et al. Association of the APC gene product with beta-catenin. Science 262: 1731–1734, 1993.

24. Su LK, Vogelstein B, Kinzler KW. Association of the APC tumor suppressor protein with catenins. Science 262: 1734–1737, 1993.

25. Powell S, Peterson G, Krush A, et al. Molecular diagnosis of familial adenomatous polyposis. N Engl J Med 329: 1982–1987, 1993.

26. Liu B, Parsons R, Papadopoulos N, et al. Analysis of mismatch repair genes in hereditary non-polyposis colon cancer. Nat Med 2: 169–174, 1996.

27. Williams CS, DuBois RN. Prostaglandin endoperoxide synthase: why two isoforms? Am J Physiol 270: G393–400, 1996.

28. Eberhart CE, Coffey RJ, Radhika A, et al. Up-regulation of cyclooxygenase 2 gene expression in human colorectal adenomas and adenocarcinomas. Gastroenterology 107: 1183–1188, 1994.

29. Kargman S, O'Neill G, Vickers P, et al. Expression of prostaglandin G/H synthase-1 and -2 protein in human colon cancer. Cancer Res 55: 2556–2559, 1995.

30. Morita I, Schindler M, Regier MK, et al. Different intracellular locations for prostaglandin endoperoxide H synthase-1 and -2. J Biol Chem 270: 10902–10908, 1995.

31. Dinchuk JE, Car BD, Focht RJ, et al. Renal abnormalities and an altered inflammatory response in mice lacking cyclooxygenase II. Nature (London) 378: 406–409, 1995.

32. Langenbach RS, Morham SG, Tiano HF, et al. Prostaglandin synthase-1 gene disruption in mice reduces arachidonic acid induced inflammation and indomethacin induced gastric ulceration. Cell 83: 483–492, 1995.
33. Morham SG, Langenbach R, Loftin CD, et al. Prostaglandin synthase-2 gene disruption causes severe renal pathology in the mouse. Cell 83: 473–482, 1995.
34. Tsujii M, DuBois R. Alterations in cellular adhesion and apoptosis in epithelial cells overexpressing Cox-2. Cell 83: 493–450, 1995.
35. Boolbol SK, Dannenberg AJ, Chadburn A, et al. Cyclooxygenase-2 overexpression and tumor formation are blocked by sulindac in a murine model of familial adenomatous polyposis. Cancer Res 56: 2556–2560, 1996.
36. Oshima M, Dinchuk JE, Kargman SL, et al. Suppression of intestinal polyposis in Apc$^{\Delta716}$ knockout mice by inhibition of cyclooxygenase 2 (COX-2). Cell 87: 803–809, 1996.
37. Prescott SM, White RL. Self-promotion? Intimate connections between APC and prostaglandin H synthase-2. Cell 87: 783–786, 1996.
38. Kelloff GJ, Boone CW, Crowell JA, et al. Surrogate endpoint biomarkers for phase II cancer chemoprevention trials. J Cell Biochem 19: 1–9, 1994.
39. Boone C, Kelloff G. Intraepithelial neoplasia, surrogate endpoint biomarkers, and cancer chemoprevention. J Cell Biochem 17: 37–48, 1993.
40. Lipkin M, Levin B, Kim Y, Kelloff G. Intermediate biomarkers of precancer and their application in chemoprevention. J Cell Biochem Suppl: 1–196, 1992.
41. Lipkin M. Current trends in chemoprevention research. Eur J Cancer Prev 3: 368–371, 1994.
42. Lippman S, Lec J, Lotan R, et al. Biomarkers as intermediate endpoints in chemoprevention trials. J Natl Cancer Inst 82: 555–560, 1990.
43. Thun MJ. NSAID use and decreased risk of gastroenteric cancers. Gastroenterol Clin North Am 25: 333–348, 1996.
44. Kune G, Kune S, Watson L. Colorectal cancer risk, chronic illnesses, operations and medications: case control results from the Melborne Colorectal Cancer Study. Cancer Res 48: 4399–4404, 1988.
45. Thun MJ, Namboodiri MM, Heath CW Jr. Aspirin use and reduced risk of fatal colon cancer. N Engl J Med 328: 1593–1596, 1991.
46. Rosenberg L, Palmer JR, Zauber AG, et al. A hypothesis: nonsteroidal anti-inflammatory drugs reduce the incidence of large-bowel cancer. J Natl Cancer Inst 83: 355–358, 1991.
47. Greeneberg ER, Baron JA, Freeman D Jr, et al. Reduced risk of large-bowel adenomas among aspirin users. The Polyp Prevention Study Group. J Natl Cancer Inst 85: 912–916, 1993.
48. Giovannucci E, Rimm EB, Stampfer MJ, et al. Aspirin use and the risk for colorectal cancer and adenoma in male health professionals. Ann Int Med 121: 241–246, 1994.
49. Muscat JE, Stellman SD, Wynder EL. Nonsteroidal antiinflammatory drugs and colorectal cancer. Cancer 74: 1847–1854, 1994.
50. Greenberg E, Baron J, Freeman D, et al. Reduced risk of large-bowel adenomas among aspirin users. J Natl Cancer Inst 85: 912–916, 1993.
51. Logan RFA, Little J, Hawtin PG, Hardcastle JD. Effect of aspirin and non-steroidal anti-inflammatory drugs on colorectal adenomas: case-control study of subjects participating in the Nottingham faecal occult blood screening programme. Br Med J 307: 285–289, 1993.
52. Peleg I, Maibach H, Brown S, Wicox C. Aspirin and nonsteroidal anti-inflammatory drug use and risk of subsequent colorectal cancer. Arch Intern Med 154: 394–399, 1994.
53. Martnez M, McPherson R, Levin B, Annegers J. Aspirin and other non-steroidal anti-inflammatory drugs and risk of colorectal adenomatous polyps among endoscoped individuals. Cancer Epidemiol, Biomark Prev 4: 703–707, 1995.
54. Paganini-Hill A, Chao A, Ross R, Henderson B. Aspirin use and chronic diseases a cohort study of the elderly. Br Med J 299: 1247–1250, 1989.
55. Gann PH, Manson JE, Glynn RJ, et al. Low-dose aspirin and incidence of colorectal tumors in a randomized trial. J Natl Cancer Inst 85: 1220–1224, 1993.
56. Craven PA, DeRubertis FR. Effects of aspirin on 1,2-dimethylhydrazine-induced colonic carcinogenesis. Carcinogenesis 13: 541–546, 1992.
57. Moorghen M, Ince P, Finney KJ, et al. The effect of sulindac on colonic tumour formation in dimethylhydrazine-treated mice. Acta Histochem Suppl 34: 195–199, 1990.

58. Pollard M, Luckert PH. Treatment of chemically-induced intestinal cancer with indomethacin. Proc Soc Exp Biol Med 167: 161–164, 1981.

59. Pollard M, Luckert PH. Effect of indomethacin on intestinal tumor induced in rats by the acetate derivative of dimethylnitrosamine. Science 214: 558–559, 1981.

60. Pollard M, Luckert PH, Schmidt MA. The suppressive effect of piroxicam on autochronous intestinal tumors in the rat. Cancer Lett 21: 57–61, 1983.

61. Reddy BS, Rao CV, Rivenson A, Kelloff G. Inhibitory effect of aspirin on azoxymethane-induced colon carcinogenesis in F344 rats. Carcinogenesis 14: 1493–1497, 1993.

62. Lynch NR, Castes M, Astoin M, Salomon JC. Mechanism of inhibition of tumour growth by aspirin and indomethacin. Br J Cancer 38: 503–512, 1978.

63. Craven PA, Thornburg K, DeRubertis FR. Sustained increase in the proliferation of rat colonic mucosa during chronic treatment with aspirin. Gastroenterology 94: 567–575, 1988.

64. DeRubertis FR, Craven PA. Early alterations in rat colonic mucosal cyclic nucleotide metabolism and protein kinase activity induced by 1,2-dimethylhydrazine. Cancer Res 40: 4589–4598, 1980.

65. Liu T, Mokuolo AO, Rao CV, et al. Regional chemoprevention of carcinogen-induced tumors in rat colon. Gastroenterology 109: 1167–1174, 1995.

66. Pereira MA, Barnes LH, Steele VE, et al. Piroxicam induced regression of azoxymethane-induced aberrant crypt foci and prevention of colon cancer in rats. Carcinogenesis 17: 373–376, 1996.

67. Meade EA, Smith WL, DeWitt DL. Differential inhibition of prostaglandin endoperoxide synthase (cyclooxygenase) isozymes by aspirin and other non-steroidal anti-inflammatory drugs. J Biol Chem 268: 6610–6614, 1993.

68. Schiff SJ, Koutsos MI, Qiao L, Rigas B. Nonsteroidal antiinflammatory drugs inhibit the proliferation of colon adenocarcinoma cells: effects on cell cycle and apoptosis. Exp Cell Res 222: 179–188, 1996.

69. Marnett LJ. Aspirin and the potential role of prostaglandins in colon cancer. Cancer Res 52: 5575–5589, 1992.

70. Duggan SE, Hooke KF, Risley EA, et al. Identification of the biologically active form of sulindac. J Pharmacol Exp Ther 201: 8–13, 1977.

71. Thompson HJ, Briggs S, Paranka NS, et al. Inhibition of mammary carcinogenesis in rats by sulfone metabolite of sulindac. J Natl Cancer Inst 16: 1259–1260, 1995.

71. Shiff S, Qiao L, Tsai L, Rigas B. Sulindac sulfide, an aspirin-like compound, inhibits proliferation, causes cell cycle quiescence, and induces apoptosis in HT-29 colon adenocarcinoma cells. J Clin Invest 96: 491–503, 1995.

73. Piazza G, Rahm A, Krutzsch M, et al. Antineoplastic drugs sulindac sulfide and sulfone inhibit cell growth by inducing apoptosis. Cancer Res 55: 3110–3116, 1995.

74. Goldberg Y, Pittas K, Reed JC, et al. Sulindac and sulindac sulfide alter the levels of *bcl-2* and *bax* proteins in HT-29 colon cancer cells. Gastroenterology 108: A475, 1995.

75. Pasricha P, Bedi A, O'Connor K, et al. The effects of sulindac on colorectal proliferation and apoptosis in familial adenomatous polyposis. Gastroenterology 109: 994–998, 1995.

76. Sano H, Kawahito Y, Wilder RL, et al. Expression of cyclooxygenase-1 and -2 in human colorectal cancer. Cancer Res 55: 3785–3789, 1995.

77. Ammon HPT, Wahl MA. Pharmacology of curcumin. Planta Med 57: 1–7, 1991.

78. Donatus IA, Sardjoko, Vermeulen NPE. Cytotoxic and cytoprotective activities of curcumin. Biochem Pharmacol 39: 1869–1875, 1990.

79. Srimal RC, Dharvan BN. Pharmacology of curcumin. A non-steroidal and anti-inflammatory agent. J Pharm Pharmacol 25: 447–452, 1973.

80. Sharma SC, Muhktar H, Skarun SK, Murti CRCK. Lipid peroxide formation in experimental inflammation. Biochem Pharmacol 21: 1210–1214, 1972.

81. Huang M-T, Lysz T, Ferraro T, et al. Inhibitory effects of curcumin on in vitro lipoxygenase and cyclooxygenase activities in mouse epidermis. Cancer Res 51: 813–819, 1991.

82. Rao CV, Simi B, Reddy BS. Inhibition of dietary curcumin of azoxymethane induced ornithine decarboxylase, tyrosine, protein kinase, arachidonic acid metabolism and aberrant crypt foci formation in the rat colon. Carcinogenesis 14: 2219–2225, 1993.

83. Huang M-T, Wang ZY, Georgiadis CA, et al. Inhibitory effects of curcumin on tumor initiation by benzo-[a]pyrene and 7,12-dimethylbenz[a]anthracene. Carcinogenesis 13: 2183–2186, 1992.

84. Huang M-T, Lou Y-R, Ma W, et al. Inhibitory effects of dietary curcumin in forestomach, duodenal, and colon carcinogenesis in mice. Cancer Res 54: 5841–5847, 1994.

85. Lu YP, Change RL, Huange M-T, Conney AH. Inhibitory effect of curcumin on 12-O-tetradecanoyl-phorbol-13-acetate induced increase in ornithine decarboxylase mRNA in mouse epidermis. Carcinogenesis 14: 293–297, 1993.

86. Nagabhushan M, Bhide SB. Curcumin as an inhibitor of cancer. J Am Coll Nutr 11: 192–198, 1992.

87. Huang M-T, Wang ZY, Georgiadis CA, et al. Inhibitory effect of curcumin chlorogenic acid caffeic acid and ferulic acid on tumor promotion in mouse skin by 12-O-tetradecanoylphorbol-13-acetate. Cancer Res 48: 5941–5946, 1988.

88. Rao CV, Rivenson A, Simi B, Raddy BS. Chemoprevention of colon carcinogenesis by dietary curcumin, a naturally, occurring plant phenolic compound. Cancer Res 55: 259–266, 1995.

89. Tutton PJM, Barkla DH. Influence of prostaglandin analogues on epithelial cell proliferation and xenograft growth. Br J Cancer 41: 47–45, 1980.

90. Marnett LJ. Aspirin and the role of prostaglandins in colon cancer. Cancer Res 52: 5575–5589, 1992.

91. Yamamoto S. Mammalian lipooxygenases: molecular structures and functions. Biochem Biophys Acta 1128: 117–131, 1992.

92. Haliday EM, Ramesha CS, Ringold G. TNF induces c-fos via a novel pathway requiring conversion of arachidonic acid to a lipoxygenase metabolite. EMBO J 10: 109–115, 1991.

93. Setty BNY, Graever JE, Stuart MJ. The mitogenic effect of 15- and 12-hydroxyeicosatetraeinoic acid on endothelial cells may be mediated via diacylglycerol kinase inhibition. J Biol Chem 262: 1613–1622, 1987.

94. Grilli M, Chiu JJ-S, Lenardo MJ, et al. NF-kappa B and Rel: participants in a multiform transcriptional system. Int Rev Cytol 143: 1–62, 1993.

95. Kopp E, Ghosh S. Inhibition of NF-kB by sodium salicylate and aspirin. Science 265: 956–958, 1994.

96. Finley G, Melhem M, Dagnet AL, Meisler A. Cytokine expression in colorectal adenocarcinoma and mucosa. Proc Am Assoc Cancer Res 37: A1090, 1996.

97. Kelloff GJ, Crowell JA, Boone CW, et al. Clinical development plan: aspirin. J Cell Biochem Suppl 20: 74–85, 1994.

98. Kelloff GJ, Crowell JA, Boone CW, et al. Clinical development plan: sulindac. J Cell Biochem Suppl 20: 240–251, 1994.

99. Wadell WR, Ganser GF, Cerise EJ, Loughry RW. Sulindac for polyposis of the colon. Am J Surg 157: 175–178, 1989.

100. Friend W. Sulindac suppression of colorectal polyps in Gardner's syndrome. Am Fam Phys 41: 891–894, 1990.

101. Giardiello FM, Hamilton SR, Krush AJ, et al. Treatment of colonic and rectal adenomas with sulindac in familial adenomatous polyposis. N Engl J Med 328: 1313–1316, 1993.

102. Giardiello FM. NSAID-induced polyp regression in familial adenomatous polyposis patients. Gastroenterol Clin North Am 25: 349–362, 1996.

103. Winde G, Gumbinger H, Osswald H, et al. The NSAID sulindac reverses rectal adenomas in colectomized patients with familial adenomatous polyposis: clinical results of a dose-finding study on rectal sulindac administration. Int J Colon Dis 8: 13–17, 1993.

104. Spagnesi M, Tonelli F, Dolara P, et al. Rectal proliferation and polyp recurrence in patients with familial adenomatous polyposis after sulindac treatment. Gastroenterology 106: 362–366, 1994.

105. Labayle D, Fischer D, Vielh P, et al. Sulindac causes regression of rectal polyps in familial adenomatous polyposis. Gastroenterology 101: 635–639, 1991.

106. Nugent K, Farmer K, Spigelman A, et al. Randomized controlled clinical trial of sulindac on intestinal polyposis in FAP. Br J Surg 80: 1618–1619, 1994.

107. Hixson L, Earnest D, Fennerty M, Sampliner R. NSAID effect on sporadic colon polyps. Am J Gastroenterol 88: 1652–1656, 1993.

C.J. Rosenthal and M. Rotman (Eds.), *Infusion Chemotherapy–Irradiation Interactions*

423

# Omeprazole and clarithromycin for *Helicobacter pylori* eradication for the prevention of gastric carcinoma

CLARENCE B. VAUGHN[1], M. BRIAN FENNERTY[2], MANUAL R. MADIANO[3] and GRANT N. STEMMERMAN[4]

[1]*Southfield Oncology Institute, 27211 Lahser Road, Southfield, MI 48034, USA,* [2]*Oregon Health Science University, OR, USA,* [3]*Department of haematology and Oncology, University of Arizona, Tucson, AZ, USA and* [4]*University of Cincinnati, Cincinnati, OH, USA*

## *1. Helicobacter pylori gastric cancer*

Although a marked decline in the incidence of gastric carcinoma is observed in many industrialized nations, cancer of the stomach remains the second most common cause of cancer-related death in the world. The incidence of gastric cancer was the highest in Asia, South America and Europe with about 2:1 male predominance (Fig. 1). The decline in the death rate from gastric cancer has been more marked in Japan who for decades had the highest in the world. Recent statistics show that the highest death rate from this disease is in Costa Rica followed by Andeans and Europeans (Fig. 2) [2].

The minorities, Native American and African American, and immigrants from Northern Europe, Asia and Latin American display a higher risk for gastric cancer in the United States and this is depicted in Table 1 for several key cities in the United States [3]. The death rate from gastric cancer has been increasing in this country and the American Cancer

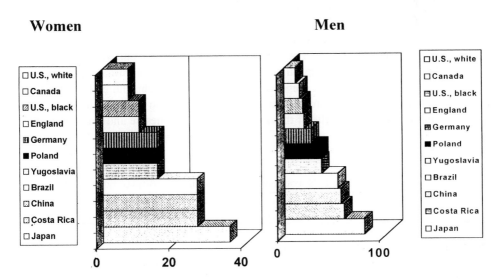

Fig. 1. Annual incidence of gastric cancer (cases per 100 000 population).

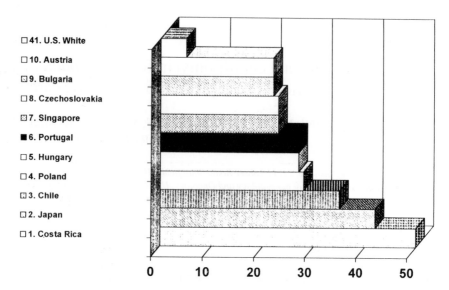

| □ 41. U.S. White |
| □ 10. Austria |
| ☑ 9. Bulgaria |
| □ 8. Czechoslovakia |
| ☒ 7. Singapore |
| ■ 6. Portugal |
| □ 5. Hungary |
| □ 4. Poland |
| ☑ 3. Chile |
| □ 2. Japan |
| □ 1. Costa Rica |

Fig. 2. Gastric cancer rates males, 1984–1985 (rate per 100 000 population).

Society estimates that in 1996 22 800 Americans will be diagnosed with gastric carcinoma and 14 000 will die from the disease [4].

Gastric cancer in an endemic area is located primarily in the distal stomach [5]. Cancer in the distal stomach showed a reduction in incidence from 1930 to 1976 which resulted in a decrease in gastric carcinoma. In the United States there has been a steady rise in cancer of the proximal stomach and gastro-esophageal junction. Gastric cancer with its origin in the proximal portion is associated with Barrett's esophagus and is frequently encountered in white men [5]. The rise in incidence of proximal gastric cancer in the white male, an increase incidence of gastric cancer in minorities and the increase immigrants from the endemic areas of the world for distal gastric have caused an increase in gastric cancer and a major health problem in the United States.

There are two types of adenocarcinoma with stomach, intestinal and diffuse [6]. The diffuse type has a similar incidence throughout the world while the intestinal type is prevalent in the areas of high incidence of adenocarcinoma of the stomach. The cells of the diffuse type lack cohesiveness and produce an infiltrative lesion which starts in the cardia of the stomach. On the other hand, cells of the intestinal type are cohesive and produce bulky ul-

Table 1

Gastric cancer incidence rates, males, 1978–1982, per 100 000 population

|  | White | Black | Other |  |
| --- | --- | --- | --- | --- |
| Atlanta | 6 | 16 |  |  |
| New Orleans | 7 | 17 |  |  |
| New Mexico | 6 |  | 16 (Hispanic) | 19 (Indian) |
| Los Angeles | 9 | 16 | 15 (Hispanic) | 25 (Japanese) |
| Hawaii | 12 |  | 31 (Hawaiian) | 28 (Japanese) |

Table 2

Gastric adenocarcinoma types

|  | Diffuse | Intestinal |
|---|---|---|
| World distribution | Universal | High risk regions |
| Age | Young | Elderly |
| Morphology | Infiltrative | Gland formation |
| Cells | Lack cohesion | Cohesive |
| Gastric lesion | Thick wall | Ulcerative |
| Location | Entire stomach (cardia) | Antrum |

cerative lesions in the antrum of the stomach (Table 2). The intestinal type of gastric cancer is often preceded by a long precancerous phase.

Correa [7] has proposed a model for carcinogenesis of gastric cancer which was widely accepted. In this model, cancer develops from atrophic gastritis produced by nitrites and salt in food and decrease the ascorbic acid and carotenoids in the diet. The atrophy of the gastric mucosa evolves into the intestinal metaplasia which is a precursor lesion for the intestinal type of cancer of the stomach (Fig. 3). The reports of several investigators [8–10] have shown that *Helicobacter pylori* infections produce a superficial gastritis which is associated with atrophic gastritis and an increase incidence of gastric cancer in the distal stomach. *H. pylori* infection stimulates the infiltration lymphocytes, plasma cells and neutrophils in the upper lamina propria which persist for years. This step is followed by a reduction in the size

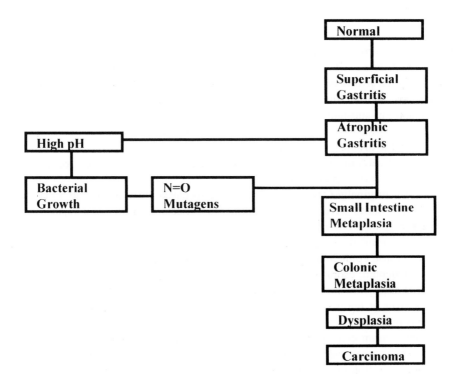

Fig. 3.

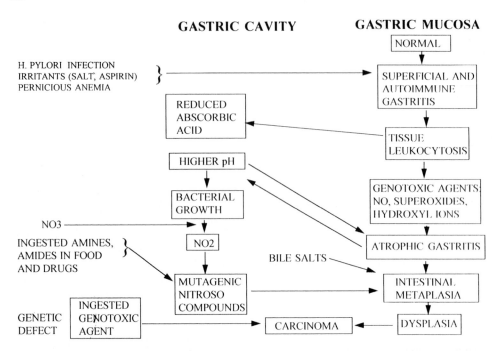

Fig. 4. The inclusion of the role of leukocyte and genotoxic substances in the carcinogenesis of distal gastric cancer.

and number of the pyloric glands and atrophic gastritis. The stem cells of the glands are replaced and become surface cells which resemble cells of the small intestines, intestinal metaplasia. The *H. pylori* infection is a chronic infection and is associated with low socio-economic status. Stemmermann [11] propose that the *H. pylori* elaborates a mutagen which causes a genotoxic substance to be elaborated by the infiltrating leukocytes. This factor works in concert with nitrates and the deficiency of the antioxidants which lead to cancer development in the distal stomach (Fig. 4).

This modified carcinogenic pathway of distal gastric cancer is the basis for the present strategy for gastric cancer prevention.

*H. pylori* was originally *Campylobacter pyloridis* because it was an enteric bacterium. *C. pyloridis* characteristics were different from the other bacteria in this genus and it was assigned to a new genus, *Helicobacter*.

*H. pylori* is a spiraled-shaped flagellated gram-negative bacterium found only in the mucous layer of gastric epithelium. The organism can also produce infection in ectopic gastric mucosa, in duodenum, esophagus rectum and Meckel's diverticulum. *H. pylori* has unique properties that allow it to survive the acid medium of the stomach and penetrate the protective mucous layer of the gastric mucosa to produce an infection in the epithelial cell. The bacterium has high concentrations of urease on the cell surface. Urease is an enzyme which degrades urea to ammonia and bicarbonate. These two chemical substances produce an alkaline microenvironment around the organism and protect it from the acid medium. The flagella, spiral morphology and ammonia production are properties of *H. pylori* which increase it motility in the mucous layer of the gastric mucosa.

Table 3

Diagnostic tests for *H. pylori* infection

| | Invasive |
|---|---|
| Breath test | |
|   Carbon-13 ($^{13}$C) | – |
|   Carbon-14 ($^{14}$C) | – |
| Biopsy urease | + |
| Histology | + |
| Culture | + |
| Serologic | + |

The diagnosis of *H. pylori* infection can be established by several non-invasive and invasive tests (Table 3) which utilize the unique properties of the organism. These tests can be used to document the presence of infection and confirm the response of the infection to therapy.

*H. pylori* infection can be eradicated in 92% of the patients with disease with omeprazole and clarithromycin [12]. This combination is well tolerated and will be used in this proposal to treat the *H. pylori* infection.

## 2.  Proposal

*Title*: A pilot study of omeprazole and clarithromycin followed by supplements of ascorbic acid, beta-carotene and alpha-tocopherol versus observation for the prevention of gastric cancer resulting from *Helicobacter pylori*.

*Objective*: To assess the effectiveness of the above program in reducing metaplasia and cancer of the stomach.

*Study design*: The proposal will be accomplished by the following of ethnic groups: American Indian, Oriental, African-American and Hispanic who are undergoing routine endoscopy for clinical reasons and have a positive rapid urease test. Members of the above mentioned ethnic population undergoing endoscopy would have mappings of their stomach done in a systematic fashion (biopsies of the antrum along the lesser and greater curvatures, and biopsies of the body along the lesser or greater curvature) (Fig. 5). These patients would have serum drawn for pepsinogen assays (an indicator of atrophic gastritis). The subjects will also have their serum analyzed for the antibody for *Helicobacter pylori* (a more sensitive means of detecting the infection) and/or histological evidence of infection. Additionally, 24 h urine sodium could be obtained for studying salt intake in this population. The subjects would receive 2 weeks of therapy with omeprazole, 20 mg twice a day and clarithromycin 500 mg t.i.d. Repeat antibody (IgA/IgG) in 12 months for evidence of eradication of *H. pylori*. Additionally, patients would then have their diet supplemented with

Table 4

Treatment

| 1. Omeprazole | 20 mg b.i.d. | >14 days |
|---|---|---|
| 2. Clarithromycin | 500 mg t.i.d. | >14 days |
| 3. Ascorbic acid | 500 mg q.d. | 2 years |
| 4. $\beta$-Carotene | 30 mg q.d. | 2 years |
| 5. $\alpha$-Tocopherol | 300 mg q.d. | 2 years |

Recommended sites for gastric biopsies:

① Greater curve, antrum, 3cm
    proximal to pyloric ring*
② Incisura**
③ Antro-corpus junction, anterior wall
④ Antro-corpus junction, posterior wall
⑤ Lesser curve, proximal corpus***
⑥ Greater curve, proximal corpus
⑦ Samples from specific lesions
    (eg. ulcer margins, tumor, polyps)

   * Site most likely to show incomplete
    metaplasia and an indication of
    extensive IM

   ** First area (with 3 and 4) to become
    metaplastic and most likely to be of
    the complete type
   *** Positive when antral metaplasia is very
    extensive
   **** Greater curve must show atrophy and
    IM at this site to justify a diagnosis of
    pernicious anemia

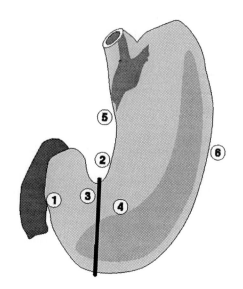

Fig. 5. Recommended biopsy sites, gastric endoscopy.

ascorbic acid (500 mg once a day), $\beta$-carotene (30 mg once a day) and $\alpha$-tocopherol (300 mg once a day) for 2 years (Table 4). At the end of this treatment period, the subjects would undergo repeat endoscopy with rapid urease testing and biopsy, following the identical protocol that was used as baseline (study entry) (Fig. 6).

## Subjects:

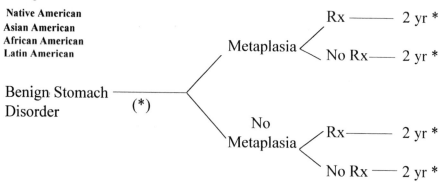

Native American
Asian American
African American
Latin American

Benign Stomach Disorder (*)

Metaplasia
   Rx ——— 2 yr *
   No Rx—— 2 yr *

No Metaplasia
   Rx——— 2 yr *
   No Rx —— 2 yr *

1. Biopsy
2. Serum pepsinogen assay
3. Serum antibody, H. Pylori
4. 24 hour urine Na

* Endoscopy + Biopsy

Fig. 6.

This research study will answer a very important question whether intestinal metaplasia can be reversed by eradicating the *H. pylori* infection and using antioxidants. The completion of the study will add to the understanding of carcinogenesis of the lesions in the antrum of the stomach.

## References

1.  Whelan SL, Parkin DM, Masuyer E (Eds). Trends in Cancer Incidence and Mortality. Lyons, France: IARC Scientific Publications, 1993.
2.  Kurihara M, Aoki K, Hisamichi S. Cancer mortality statistics in the world 1950–1985. Nagoya, Japan: The University of Nagoya Press, 1989.
3.  Muir C, Waterhouse J, Mack T, et al. Cancer Incidence in Five Continents, Vol. 5. Scientific Publications No. 88. Lyons, France: International Agency for Research on Cancer, 1987.
4.  American Cancer Society. Facts and Figures 1996. Atlanta, GA: American Cancer Society, 1996.
5.  Fuchs CS, Mayer RJ. Gastric carcinoma. N Engl J Med 333: 32–41, 1995.
6.  Lauren P The two histological main types of gastric carcinoma: diffuse and so-called intestinal type of carcinoma. Acta Pathol Microbiol Scand 64: 31–49, 1963.
7.  Correa P. Human gastric carcinogenesis: a multistep and multifunctional process - First American Cancer Society Award Lecture on Cancer Epidemiology and Prevention. Cancer Res 52: 6735–6740, 1992.
8.  Nomura A, Stemmerman GN, Chyou P-H, et al. Helicobacter pylori infection and gastric carcinoma among Japanese Americans in Hawaii. N Engl J Med 325: 1132–1136, 1991.
9.  Parsonnet J, Friedman GD, Vandersteen DP, et al. Helicobacter pylori infection and the risk of gastric carcinoma. N Engl J Med 325: 1127–1131, 1991.
10. Forman D, Newell DG, Fullerton F, et al. Association between infection with Helicobacter pylori and risk of gastric cancer: evidence from a prospective investigation. Br Med J 302: 1302–1305, 1991.
11. Stemmermann GN. The role of Helicobacter pylori in the etiology of gastric cancer. Cancer Prevention, October 1991. Philadelphia, PA: JB Lippincott, pp. 1–7, 1991.
12. Logan RPH, Gummett PA, Hegarty BT, et al. Clarithromycin and Omeprazole for Helicobacter pylori. Lancet 340: 239, 1992.

# SECTION VI

# COMPUTER TECHNOLOGY IN RESEARCH
# AND CLINICAL PRACTICE

*"To know what has to be done, then to do it comprises the
whole philosophy of practical life."*

Sir William Osler

C.J. Rosenthal and M. Rotman (Eds.), *Infusion Chemotherapy–Irradiation Interactions*

# CHAPTER 40

# The use of computer technology in oncologic research and practice

EDWARD P. AMBINDER

*Department of Medicine, Mount Sinai School of Medicine, 1 Gustave Levy Place, New York, NY 10029, USA*

## 1. Introduction

We are on the threshold of having a molecular definition of cancer. This will translate into a diverse array of more capable clinical tools to detect and combat cancer. It will require us to assimilate these findings into our daily clinical practice and research activities which are already under enormous pressure to become more cost effective, while we continue to improve its quality for a much more sophisticated consumer and payer. Today, the medical, radiation, and surgical oncologist must be a clinician, researcher, educator, businessperson, statistician, healthcare administrator, and an "informatition" who must interact with the whole patient as both a cancer specialist and primary caregiver. For over 200 different cancer types oncologists must be expert in the prevention, natural history, diagnosis, staging, and treatment of cancer with chemotherapy, surgery, radiation therapy, immunotherapy, and biologic response modifiers.

In 1997, all oncologists will experience unprecedented challenges to their research, therapeutic and practice management skills as summarized in Table 1. There are two over-riding general themes that will have a marked impact on our professional life. First is the necessity to manage the geometric increase in medical information. With over 17 000 medical textbooks and 22 000 active medical journals publishing over 420 000 articles this year and medical knowledge doubling every 12 years, it is impossible for the medical oncologist to keep current. Figure 1 illustrates the dramatic increase in medical citations listed in MEDLINE over the past 30 years. Second is the striking changes in the clinical practice of oncology brought on by managed competition and the public perception that medical care is expensive and inefficient. It will imperil our ability to perform clinical and basic science research, provide medical care and educate the future physician. Our academic institutions are under siege merging with one another, designing integrated healthcare systems and reorienting their training programs from emphasizing medical subspecialization to general medicine. All this with their continuing needs to modernize their primitive information systems.

New practice models are being introduced throughout the country. For example, there is a relatively new phenomenon, the "corporatization" of medicine. It seeks to acquire clinical practices, invest in upgrading where necessary, consolidate duplicative facilities, increase administrative efficiencies, take advantage of economies of scale, integrate vertically and horizontally, and develop powerful local referral networks. As pointed out by Berwick, the lack of emphasis on the needs of the individual physician and the patient in this ongoing financial and structural reorganization of medicine require five guiding principles: (1) focus-

Table 1

Challenges facing medical, radiation and surgical oncologists in 1997

*Therapeutic challenges*
- Utilize new genetic risk and prevention data based on the explosion in the identification of cancer genes
- Apply molecular knowledge to an aging population with rising cancer incidence rates
- Use combined surgical, radiotherapeutic, chemotherapeutic and biologic agents to maximize organ salvage and cancer cell kill
- Integrate the novel uses of maturational agents, gene replacement therapy, anti-angiogenic agents, antisense oligonucleotides, and cell cycle regulators into our clinical armamentarium

*Research challenges*
- Find ways to prevent second malignancies caused by our therapies and the cancer patient's propensity to develop other cancers
- Combat the reduction of support for basic science and clinical research

*Clinical practice challenges*
- Develop and implement critical pathways and practice guidelines in the practice of oncology
- Comprehend and effectively use the economic components of medical practice and clinical research in a managed competition environment
- Practice cost-effective medicine with admittedly expensive and some marginally effective therapies
- Work together in larger groups and accept less autonomy
- Shift from a patient-based to a population-based medical paradigm
- Reconcile the at times differing needs of the individual patient and her health care organization in this cost-containment environment
- Remain effective in the lives of individual cancer patients in an era of increasing patient advocacy
- Increase public awareness about provider outcomes and procedure-specific guidelines
- Increase patient accrual on clinical trials (<3% newly diagnosed patients with metastatic disease enter trials)

ing on integrating experiences, not just structures; (2) learning to measure improvement, not just measuring judgment; (3) developing better ways to learn from one another, not just discovering "best practices"; (4) reducing total costs, not just local costs; and (5) competing against disease, not against each other [1].

Our success in extending the life expectancy of our cancer patients, along with modern medicine's achievements with many other chronic diseases, has provided us with an aging

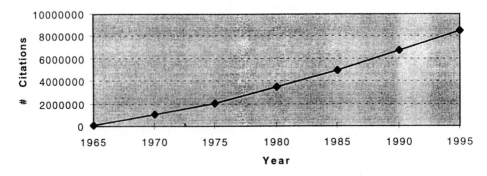

Fig 1. Medical information growth 1967–1996.

population fraught with an increasing number of complex diseases. Treatment requires greater access to, and tracking of, detailed medical data. Disease management clinical guidelines for cancer patients are being introduced which require the micromanagement of patients and the need for oncologists to appreciate the true costs of providing medical care [2]. Managed competition as well as clinical trials research demand more intense recording of patient medical information, while our reimbursements and time available for each patient is diminished. Our clinical trials must show not only progression-free and overall survival benefits but also cost-effectiveness and patient satisfaction [3,4]. We must be able to show that a treatment is both effective (when performed under usual circumstances) and efficacious (when performed under ideal circumstances). Clinical treatment outcomes become multidimensional by measuring not only mortality and toxicity, but also the functional, physiologic, mental, physical, social and satisfactional state of the patient. All of this taking place in a legal and regulatory climate mandating a rationale to support decision-making with zero tolerance for error.

Information technology has transformed every discipline with medicine being one of the last to be affected. Computers are no longer bookkeeping and writing tools. Together they offer the means to radically transform patient care and the education, research and economics of medicine. All of society's major institutions are experiencing monumental changes in the economics of information. The personal computer, the ability to network or connect computers, the digitalization of information and the rapid electronic interchanging of information on a worldwide basis are recognized as the hallmark of a new order in society. For oncologists to master these profound changes, it is necessary to understand and use effectively the tools of the Information Age. These tools include the computer which acts as the gateway and integrator, the electronic medical record which is the translator and repository of our clinical information gathering and the Internet's World Wide Web which coordinates interactive information resources and personal communication.

## 2.  The central role of the computer

Oncologists require a tool to efficiently and easily capture, process, manipulate, output and communicate data. Data when organized produces information, which can be defined as something that makes a difference. When information is meaningful it produces knowledge that, when linked to other knowledge is called intelligence. Intelligence when combined with experience is known as wisdom. The computer is a tool that integrates digital data, communication technologies and the experience of the user to give rise to wisdom. The computer takes a repetitive, time consuming and exhaustive task performing it over and over again, accessing information in any form irrespective of time, place or person without becoming tired or bored, freeing the oncologist to think and reason about the patient. As exemplified by the mainframe computer, computers were originally designed as a "one to many" paradigm where the unitary mainframe communicated with many computer terminals. As microcomputers developed in the 1980s, the paradigm shifted to a "one to one and a one to many" model. Recently with the explosive growth of the Internet and information providers, the paradigm has shifted again to the "many to many" or distributed model.

Today, the computer is our most efficient device for obtaining timely information and has become our most effective decision-making tool. It has become an integrated information device that has merged video, audio, telephone, printers, scanners, faxes, copiers, and filing cabinets. Interested readers are referred to *Medical Informatics: Computer Applications in Health Care* [5] for a comprehensive review of the general medical informatics field and to *Oncology and the Information Revolution* [6] for oncologic-specific informatics. Two excellent resources for medical hardware and software are the *Medical Hardware & Software Buyers' Guide* [7] and the *Directory of Medical Hardware and Software Companies* [8].

## 3. Laws of the Information Age

It is necessary to understand the three basic laws that have governed the Information Age since its inception in the early 1950s in order to understand why computers have become so indispensable in the 1990s. These laws help explain how the declining cost and increasing efficiency of processing, storing and transmitting information has changed more rapidly then any prior human endeavor. Gordon Moore's Law states that the performance of semiconductor technology, as exemplified by microprocessor chips, where data are stored and manipulated, will double every 18 months. Since 1950, this increase has continued unabated. As demonstrated by the Internet, Bob Metcalfe's Law states that the power of a network rises by the square of the number of terminals attached to it. Finally the Law of the Telecosm, as formulated by George Gilder, combines Metcalfe's Law with Moore's law of the Microcosm [9]. It ordains that the cost-effectiveness of computer terminals will rise by the square of the number of additional transistors integrated on a single chip. Amplified by the Law of the Microcosm, the Law of the Telecosm signifies the rise in the cost-effectiveness of a network in proportion to the resources deployed on it and the number of potential nodes and routers (connectors) available to it. In the 50 years since the development of ENIAC, the first electronic computer, the efficiency of information technology has increased 100 octillion times (100 000 000 000 000 000 000 000 000 000 000). Figures 2–5 illustrate the unprecedented growth in information technology and its cost efficiency as illustrated by the microprocessor chip and telecommunication speeds between 1972 and 1997.

Medicine has always been conservative in adopting change as noted by Martensen [10] who comments today in a *Journal of the American Medical Association* editorial on "The slowness with which important medical discoveries are generally put to practical use" pub-

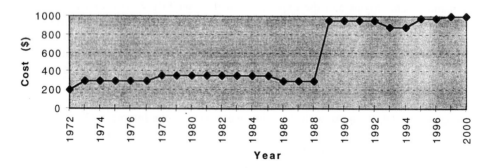

Fig. 2. Microprocessor cost in dollars from 1972–2000 (est.).

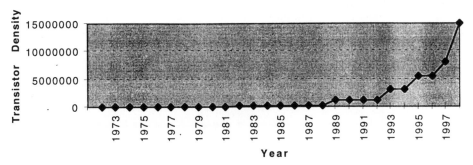

Fig. 3. Transistor density per microprocessor chip 1972–1997.

lished in 1896 [11]. Medicine has been slow to grasp the reality of the Laws of the Information Age but, with the changes induced by managed competition, a revolution in the practice management of oncology is underway. We must take advantage of the information technology explosion propelled by the computer and its connection to the Internet. We must use the computer to communicate with patients and healthcare providers possibly utilizing a Community Health Information Network (CHIN). We must continue to utilize our training in clinical trials that gives our specialty a unique advantage to apply the principles of care plans, practice guidelines, biostatistics and data management to managed competition.

## 4. Electronic medical records

The placement of patient charts on the computer is not only inevitable, but also the best way for the oncologist to contend with this new order. To capture medical data at the point of care, then access it where and whenever needed is essential to making accurate, well-informed decisions and providing quality care. We must wholeheartedly accept the concept of computerized patient medical records that are integrated with our practice management

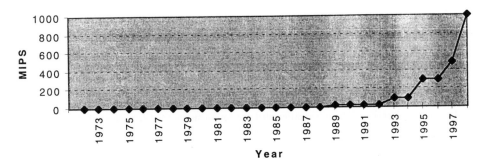

Fig. 4. Speed that microprocessors handle instructions in millions of instructions per second (MIPS) from 1972 to 1997.

## Telecommunication Speed (bauds per seconds)

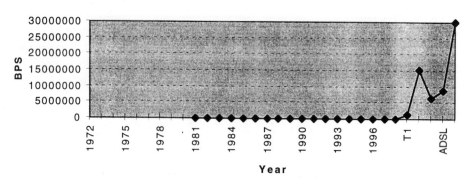

Fig. 5. Network telecommunication speed in bauds per second for transferring information from 1972–1997.

software. This will allow us to practice more cost-effective and efficient medicine, thus permitting us to increase the number of patients on clinical trials and survive in a managed competition atmosphere by simplifying the torments of data management requirements. For the first time, oncologists will be able to comprehend the economics of medical practice management permitting us to effectively compete for the healthcare dollar with large managed care and healthcare networks. Table 2 summarizes the advantages of electronic medical records.

Implementing electronic medical records requires changing our habits, adjusting to new work processes and producing significant initial hardware and software expenditures, which will be quickly recouped. As modern medicine becomes more of a team approach, the patient record must be accessible to multiple users at multiple locations. In the past we were accustomed to having parts of the individual patient's paper records for review but with computerization, records can be viewed integrating information from several medical sources for a single patient or a group of patients selected by appropriate searching and sorting qualifications. Instead of viewing a patient's history one episode at a time, computers can review patient problems and clinical information across episodes. Direct cost savings become apparent when one compares the time lost trying to obtain information from paper

Table 2

The advantages of electronic medical records

- Patient information accessible anytime, anywhere and by anyone with appropriate security clearance
- Coordinate communication between caregivers
- Enforce documentation, standardization and security to improve accuracy of data collection and limit malpractice exposure and audit liabilities
- Produce a personalized view of the same data for each caregiver either in text, data base, or flow sheet format
- Make available diagnostic tools such as differential diagnosis assistance and decision support that can provide reminders, screening alerts, drug formulary information, drug–drug interactions, and allergy checking
- Analyze practice expense and revenue
- Perform cost-effective analyses
- Facilitate clinical outcome and quality of life determinations
- Monitor quality assurance, patient preferences and referral tracking

records and the elimination of dictation costs when using the electronic medical record along with improved reimbursement for thorough documentation in traditional fee-for-service practice.

Several medical centers have determined that with paper records, the unavailability of information occurs 35% of the time. How often do we practice medicine blindly with no knowledge of the patient's history, recent test results, or drug allergies? These cost savings, along with the capability of recently developed user-friendly medical record software that takes no longer to document a patient encounter than the paper-based or dictated methods, will make it easier for oncologists to computerize. If we do not then managed competition, which require more documentation than paper records can give, integrated delivery systems that requires vast amount of information to be moved among its sites and community networks will drag us along.

Since 1973, Neugut et al. using data taken from the Connecticut Tumor Registry, reported that the incidence of second cancers has more than doubled [12]. They report that second and higher order cancers made up more than 14% of all cancer cases in the United States. The age adjusted death rate held constant during this period, suggesting that the increased incidence was due to environmental and genetic influences on treated cancer patients who have longer survival due to our earlier detection and improving therapies. Thus using electronic medical records and cancer registries should facilitate the monitoring of cancer patients for second malignancies.

## 5.   The Internet

No recent phenomenon has captured the world's attention more swiftly than the Internet, the "Information Superhighway" and its World Wide Web with its linked matrix of information resources and its ability to network different computer networks, all using the same interconnection technology [13,14]. Currently there are over 40 000 networks (1/2 commercial, 1/3 educational and 1/5 research), 5 million host computers, 40 million users and 230 000 World Wide Web sites [13]. The Web displays data as pages of multimedia objects. These objects include text, graphics, animation, audio and video linked together with hypertext pointers so that data stored on computers in vastly different locations can be pulled in over the network and be viewed on the requesting computer. It is a universal multiplatform that runs on most existing operating systems using a standard communication protocol (TCP/IP). The Web has built-in security using digital signatures, passwords and encryption technology.

Using the Hypertext Mark-up Language (HTML) format for presenting information, words and pictures in a document, one can be linked to other words and pictures on other computers irrespective of time, place or person. The Web uses a client-server model where the client program, the browser, processes the location of servers, receives the Web page, interprets the HTML code to build a page, communicates with a Web server that stores Web pages and manages user access. In the near future browsers will become part of all computer operating systems. Table 3 lists a summary of the more popular topics found on the Internet.

The Web has begun to cause a paradigm shift in the distribution of information and its cost structure. For over 500 years, one took information, put it on a substrate such as a book, newspaper or CD-ROM and shipped it around. Today it is not necessary to put information

Table 3

General information categories available on the Internet

| | |
|---|---|
| Adult education | Magazines |
| Airlines | Mail/address and zip directories: national and world |
| Arts: directories, artists, galleries, auction houses | Maps and locators |
| Automobiles: information and purchase | Media |
| Books: locate and purchase | Money |
| Business/Finance: finance information, investment | Movies |
|   tools, corporations, stock quotes | Museums |
| Classifieds: jobs, real estate | Music |
| Computers: hardware and software | News |
| Corporations | Newsgroups: find a newsgroup on any topic with |
| Cruises |   guides to ongoing on-line discussions. |
| Destinations | People |
| Directory services | Pets |
| Disease | Phone directories: national and world |
| Drugs | Photography |
| Education: high schools, colleges, professional | Politics |
|   schools, institutions | Radio stations |
| Elections | Real estate: locate and purchase |
| Engineering | Recreation |
| Entertainment | Reference |
| Environment | Regional |
| Fashion | Religion |
| Fitness | Science |
| Food and drink | Shopping malls |
| Games | Society |
| Global search: these tools will conduct a | Space |
|   Web-wide search for a single word | Sports |
| Governmental publications and databases | Search services |
| Health/medicine | Taxes |
| Hobbies | Teaching |
| Home improvement | Travel |
| Insurance | TV stations |
| Internet | Weather |
| Intranet | White pages: on-line white pages to help locate people |
| Law |   on the Internet |
| Life and style | Wine |
| Live chats | Women's health |
| Live web events | Yellow pages: searchable listings for businesses and |
| Lodging |   services in the US |

on a substrate. It is only necessary to put information in any form on the Internet and it can be accessed immediately by anyone connected to the Internet. Time and place does not matter.

In addition to the World Wide Web, there are five other tools available on the Internet. The most commonly used resource is E-mail which is the asynchronous (time independent) electronic equivalent of postal mail. List Servers or Mail Servers include discussion groups to share ideas and knowledge on a subject that is available by request. USENETs are newsgroups that access thousands of topic-based discussion groups that are available without permission. File Transfer or "ftp" permits the placing and retrieving of files on the Internet.

Table 4

Medical resources available on the Internet

| | |
|---|---|
| AIDS resources | Medical decision support |
| Atlases: Geographic maps of diseases or procedures | Medical schools |
| CANCERLIT | MEDLINE |
| Clinical Trials Cooperative Groups | Molecular Biology databases |
| Community Health Information Networks | News: Current and archived |
| Corporations | Newsletters |
| Differential Diagnosis software | Organizations |
| Disease-specific sites | Patient groups: Information and support |
| Drug formulary information | PDQ |
| Economics | Physician credentialing |
| Electronic medical records | Physician locator |
| Government references and databases | Practice Guidelines |
| Grants | Practice Management: Vendors, Payers |
| Hospital information systems | and Government Organizations |
| | Preventative Medicine |
| Human Genome Study | SEER database |
| Informatics | Telemedicine |
| Medical journals | Textbooks: Reference and Purchase |
| Managed Care | Travel |
| Manuals and training guides | |

Finally, Telenet or remote log-in provides a connection onto another computer permitting remote control of that computer.

General medical [15–19] and oncology specific [20] uses of the Internet are limited only by one's imagination. Table 4 lists some useful medical resources found on the Internet. Using the Internet with work group software, elaborate coordination of investigators, irrespective of their world-wide location, can facilitate common studies and publication development. This ability to bring together on a world-wide basis disparate proprietary data systems, linking them in real-time and allowing the transfer of information is what makes the Internet so enticing.

To simplify the Internet and to make it more resemble television, which is a broadcast medium, Web sites are using "content-push" or "webcasting" software to automatically broadcast at user-defined selected intervals individually chosen topics to any computer desktop. Currently, these topics include national and international news, politics, business with stock ticker, stock charts and specific company information, worldwide and local weather, sports news and ticker, specific industries including computer, electronics, entertainment, healthcare and hospitals, household and consumer, Internet and on-line sources, and medical and computer software.

Over the past year, the tools of the Internet have become available inside institutions or among networks of providers. When this private Internet network is set up behind a firewall, or security barrier, for the use of authorized individuals it is called an Intranet. Providers can use the Intranet for connecting to the Internet for local e-mail, messaging, conferences, bulletin boards, video and audio conferences, consult requests and reports, and electronic medical records.

Telecommunication speed today is limited by bandwidth which is the amount of information that can be transferred between computers in a medium, i.e., copper wire, glass fiber or the atmosphere. Text can be sent instantaneously but pictures may take many seconds and X-

rays and medical imaging videos may take many minutes to hours to be received. As Fig. 2
illustrates, within the next 2 years a dramatic increase in bandwidth will provide us from our

Table 5

World Wide Web resources for the oncologist

| Internet resources | Addresses (URL) |
| --- | --- |
| *Oncologic resources* | |
| AECC Cancer Newsletter 1995 | http://www.ca.aecom.yu.edu/newsletter-fall.html |
| ATSDR Cancer Policy Framework | http://atsdr1.atsdr.cdc.gov:8080/cancer.html |
| Breast Cancer Information | http://nysernet.org/breast/Default.html |
| Cancer (Medical Specialties) | http://galaxy.einet.net/galaxy/Medicine/ |
| Medical-Specialties/Cancer.html | |
| Cancer Center Newsletter - Fall 1994 | http://www.ca.aecom.yu.edu/newsletter-fall.html |
| CancerGuide: Steve Dunn's Cancer Information Page | http://bcn.boulder.co.us/health/cancer/canguide. html |
| CancerNet | http://biomed.nus.sg/Cancer/welcome.html |
| Detecting Breast Cancer | http://nysernet.org/bcic/detecting/detecting.html |
| Fred Hutchinson Cancer Research Center | http://www.fhcrc.org/ |
| H. Lee Moffitt Cancer Center | http://daisy.moffitt.usf.edu/ |
| IARC | http://www.iarc.fr/ |
| M.D. Anderson | http://rpisun1.mda.uth.tmc.edu |
| National Cancer Institute home page | http://www.nci.nih.gov/ |
| NCCS guide to cancer resources: cansearch | http://www.access.digex.net/~mkragen/cansearch. html |
| OncoLink, The University of Pennsylvania Cancer Resource | http://cancer.med.upenn.edu:80/ |
| Oncology Online | http://www.mecklerweb.com/onco/home.html |
| Quick Information about Cancer for Patients and Families | http://asa.ugl.lib.umich.edu/chdocs/cancer/ |
| CANCERGUIDE.HTML | |
| Regional Breast Cancer Support Groups | http://nysernet.org:80/breast/nabco/resource-list/support-groups.html |
| Telematics Services in Cancer | http://telescan.nki.nl/ |
| *Medical resources* | |
| American Medical Association | http://www.ama-assn.org/home/amahome.htm |
| Atlas of Hematology | http://pathy.fujita-hu.ac.jp/~ichihasi/Pictures/ atoras.html |
| BioMedNet | http://www.cursci.co.uk/BioMedNet/biomed.html |
| Center for Disease Control | http://www.cdc.gov/ |
| Diagnostic Test Information Server | http://dgim-www.ucsf.edu/TestSearch.html |
| Duke University Medical Center | http://www.mc.duke.edu/ftp/standards/html |
| DXplain differential diagnosis | http://camis.stanford.edu/people/bdetmer/ dxplain.html |
| Emerging Infectious Diseases | http://www.cdc.gov/ncidod/EID/eid.htm |
| Federally-Funded Research in the U.S. | http://medoc.gdb.org/best/fed-fund.html |
| Grants (Reference and Interdisciplinary Information) | http://www.einet.net/galaxy/Reference-and- |
| Interdisciplinary-Information/Grants.html | |
| Health network | http://www.sarnoff.com/sarnoff/spin-off/healthnet.shtml |
| Health Services/Technology Assessment Text (HSTAT) | http://text.nlm.nih.gov/index.html |
| Hospital.Net | http://hospital.net/ |
| HospitalWeb | http://dem0nmac.mgh.harvard.edu/ hospitalweb.html |
| HyperDOC: The National Library of Medicine (NLM) | http://www.nlm.nih.gov/ |
| Johns Hopkins | gopher://welchlink.welch.jhu.edu/ |

Jonathan Tward's Multimedia Medical Reference Library
http://www.tiac.net/users/jtward/index.html

Mayo Clinic
http://www.mayo.edu/

MCW International Travelers Clinic
http://www.intmed.mcw.edu/travel.html

Medical Center
http://www-sci.lib.uci.edu/~martindale/Medical.html

Medical Matrix- Guide to Internet Medical Resources
http://kuhttp.cc.ukans.edu/cwis/units/medcntr/Lee/homepage.html

Medicine – TheYellowPages
http://theyellowpages.com/medicine.htm

MEDLINE
http://ncbi.nlm.nih.gov/cgi-bin/medline

Medscape
http://www.medscape.com/

MedSearch America's Physician Finder Online
http://msa2.medsearch.com/pfo/

Morbidity and Mortality Weekly Report
http://www.crawford.com/cdc/mmwr/mmwr.html

National Science Foundation
http://www.nsf.gov/

National Institutes of Health
http://www.nih.gov/

National Library of Medicine HyperDOC
http://www.nlm.nih.gov/

Pharmaceutical Information Network
http://pharminfo.com/

PharmWeb - Pharmacy Information Resources
http://sunsite.unc.edu/pwmirror/

Physician's Online
http://www.po.com/Welcome.html

PosterNet(tm)
http://pharminfo.com/poster/

The British Medical Journal
http://www.bmj.com/bmj/

The Mount Sinai School of Medicine
http://www.mssm.edu/

The National Center for Biotechnology Information
http://www.ncbi.nlm.nih.gov/

The Virtual Hospital
http://vh.radiology.uiowa.edu/

The Whole Brain Atlas
http://www.med.harvard.edu:80/AANLIB/home.html

The World-Wide Web Virtual Library: Biosciences
http://golgi.harvard.edu/biopages/all.html

*Biomedical resources*

Biologists's Control Panel
http://kiwi.imgen.bcm.tmc.edu:8088/bio/bio_home.html

BMEnet Biomedical Engineering Resource
http://fairway.ecn.purdue.edu/bme/

EMBnet: European Molecular Biology Network
http://beta.embnet.unibas.ch/embnet/info.html

Primer on Molecular Genetics (Department of Energy)
http://www.gdb.org/Dan/DOE/intro.html

The Mouse Genome Informatics Project
http://www.informatics.jax.org/

The National Center for Biotechnology Information
http://www.ncbi.nlm.nih.gov/

*Directories, Indices and Searching Tools*

Access ET
http://www.telegraph.co.uk/login.html

Argus/University of Michigan Clearinghouse
http://www.lib.umich.edu/chhome.html

AT&T Internet Toll Free 800 Directory
http://www.tollfree.att.net/dir800/

Awesome Lists (makulow@trainer.com)
http://www.clark.net/pub/journalism/awesome.html

Colorado Area Research Library
http://www.carl.org/

Directory
https://www6.internet.net/cgi-bin/getNode?node = 1and
session = −144

E-mail Discussion Groups
http://www.nova.edu/Inter-Links/listserv.html

FileList
http://l0pht.com/~spacerog/filelist.html#ustCoolStuff

Four11 White Page Directory (SLED)
http://www.four11.com/

Home Page - TheYellowPages.com(tm)
http://theyellowpages.com/

InfoSeek Home Page
http://www.infoseek.com/Home

Internet Guide by Franklin
http://ug.cs.dal.ca:3400/newbie.html

Internet Search
http://home.netscape.com/home/internet-search.html

Lycos Server- Carnegie-Melon
http://lycos.cs.cmu.edu/

| | |
|---|---|
| NYNEX Interactive Yellow Pages | http://www.vtcom.fr/nynex/ |
| Phonebooks | gopher://merlot.gdb.org/11/phonebooks |
| Search E-mail addresses | http://www.four11.com/ |
| Search the World Wide Yellow Pages(tm) | http://www.yellow.com/cgi-bin/SearchWWYP |
| Stanford Netnews Filtering Service | http://woodstock.stanford.edu:2000/ |
| THE LIST | http://thelist.com/ |
| The World Factbook 1994 | http://www.ic.gov/94fact/fb94toc/fb94toc.html |
| WebCrawler Searching | http://webcrawler.com/ |
| Work Media: Work Software Yellow Pages | http://planetcom.com/workmedia/wsyp.html |
| World Factbook (CIA) | http://www.ic.gov/94fact/fb94toc/fb94toc.html |
| Yahoo:Health:Medicine:Cancer | http://www.yahoo.com/Health/Medicine/Cancer/ |
| Yahoo:Health:Medicine | http://akebono.stanford.edu/yahoo/Health/ Medicine |

homes and offices the capability to increase the speed of transporting information by 1000-fold! True multimedia medical documents will be transmitted over networks in seconds. Readers interested in further information on the Internet are referred to Table 5 which lists useful sites and their Universal Resource Locator (URL) or address for oncologic, medical, and biomedical resources in addition to general Internet directories, indices, and search tools.

If we are to promote the exchange of novel ideas, facilitate the development of cooperative experimental and clinical projects and promote the interaction between scientists and clinicians we must not lose sight of our mission to heal, do research, to educate and to be our patient's advocate in our individual quests for economic survival. If we as clinical investigators and medical practitioners are to promote and facilitate future ideas, projects and collaborations among ourselves in a rapidly changing medical universe, we must understand the Laws of the Information Age and invest the time and energy to harness the vast untapped powers of computers, electronic medical records, and the Internet.

## Summary

All oncologists are faced with the need to manage a geometrically increasing amount of medical and basic science research and practice management information while the traditional methods of education, research, teaching, and clinical practice are being radically transformed by the forces of managed competition and business. In order for oncologists to continue their clinical and basic science research studies to elucidate the mechanism of interactions between chemotherapy and radiation, to reduce treatment toxicities by organ salvage and to monitor for and prevent second primary neoplasms, the medical tools of the Information Age, which include the vast untapped powers of computers, electronic medical records, and the Internet, must be understood and used effectively and efficiently. Only then, can oncologists, as clinical investigators and medical practitioners, promote and facilitate their future ideas, projects and collaborations among themselves in a rapidly changing medical universe.

# *References*

1.  Berwick DM. Quality comes home. Ann Intern Med 125: 839–843, 1996.
2.  Winn RJ. National Comprehensive cancer network oncology practice guidelines. Oncology (Suppl): 1–317, 1996.
3.  Gotay CC. Trial-related quality of life: using quality-of-life assessment to distinguish among cancer therapies. Monogr Natl Cancer Inst 20: 1–6, 1996.
4.  Weeks J. Taking quality of life into account in health economic analyses. Monogr Natl Cancer Inst 20: 23–27, 1996.
5.  Shortliffe EH, Perreault LE. Medical Informatics: Computer Applications in Health Care. Reading, MA: Addison-Wesley, 1990.
6.  Ambinder EP. Oncology and the information revolution. In: Holland JF, Frei T, Bast RC, et al. (Eds), Cancer Medicine. Baltimore, MD: Williams and Wilkins, pp. 3371–3386, 1996.
7.  The 13th Annual Medical Hardware and Software Buyers Guide. MD Computing: 485–576, 1996.
8.  The 13th Annual Directory of Medical Hardware and Software Companies. MD Computing: 227–270, 1996.
9.  Gilder G. The coming software shift. Forbes ASAP August 28: 147–162, 1995.
10. Martensen RL. The effect of medical conservatism on the acceptance of important medical discoveries. J Am Med Assoc 1996: 276, 1933.
11. Editorial. J Am Med Assoc 1896: 27: 1210–1211.
12. Neugut AI, Ahsan, H, Robinson E. Increased incidence of second malignancies: a sign of success? Proc Am Soc Clin Oncol 15: 194, 1996.
13. Martin JA. Speeding up the world wide wait. Macworld January: 169–171, 1997.
14. Grove AS. Is the Internet overhyped? Forbes September 23: 108–117, 1996.
15. Lowe HJ, Lomax EC, Polonkey SE. The World Wide Web: a review of an emerging Internet-based technology for the distribution of biomedical information. J Am Med Informatic
s Assoc 3: 1–14, 1996.
16. Hersh WR, Brown KE, Donohoe LC, et al. Cliniweb: managing clinical information on the World Wide Web. J Am Med Informatics Assoc 3: 273–280, 1996.
17. Glowniak JV. Medical resources on the Internet. Ann Int Med 123: 123–131,1995.
18. Sondak NE. An Internet strategy for physicians. Phys Comput June: 30–37, 1996.
19. Glowniak JV, Bushway MK. Computer networks as a medical resource. J Am Med Assoc 271: 1934–1956, 1994.
20. Glode LM. Challenges and opportunities of the Internet for medical oncology. J Clin Oncol 14: 2181–2186, 1996.

# Subject index